Bruno Reichart,
Roland Fasol, John Odell, Ulrich von Oppell
Hermann Reichenspurner, Peter Zilla

Department of Cardiothoracic Surgery
Groote Schuur Hospital

RECENT ADVANCES IN CARDIOVASCULAR SURGERY

Groote Schuur Hospital
20 Years of Heart Transplantation

RECENT ADVANCES
IN
CARDIOVASCULAR SURGERY

Editors:
Bruno Reichart,
Roland Fasol,
John Odell,
Ulrich von Oppell,
Hermann Reichenspurner,
Peter Zilla

R. S. SCHULZ

Figure on cover:
"Orthotopic heart transplantation"
Illustration by Prof. Leopold Metzenbauer, Vienna
from the book
"Herz- und Herz-Lungen-Transplantation"
by Prof. Dr. Bruno Reichart
Verlag R. S. Schulz

Figures on backside cover:
first row: Heart- and Lung-transplantation (left), Laser therapy (right)
second row: Ventricular assist devices (left), Endothelial cell lining (right)

The dosages of the various drugs mentioned in this book
were carefully checked and reflect mainly the experiences
of the authors.
The reader of this book is, however, courteously asked to check
the package insert before use.

Copyright © 1989 by Verlag R. S. Schulz
Publisher: Dr. jur. h. c. Rolf S. Schulz
8136 Percha am Starnberger See, Berger Straße 8 bis 10
8136 Kempfenhausen am Starnberger See, Seehang 4
Telephone (08151) 149-0, Telex 526427 buch
Federal Republic of Germany

ISBN 3-7962-0502-X

Reader:
Floyd Daniel
Rudolf Stieglmeier

Design und Desktop Publishing:
Brigitte Groh
Matthias Stieglmeier

All rights reserved; this includes multiplying and translation.
No parts of the book may be reproduced without permission of the publisher.

Printed by Kastner & Callwey, Munich.

You also can reach us by

Table of Contents

		Page
	List of Authors	9
	Twenty Years of Human Heart Transplantation - A Foreword B Reichart, H Reichenspurner, J Odell, U von Oppell, P Human, R Fasol, P Zilla, DH Boehm	19
1.	**Transplantation**	25
1.1.	**Clinical Advances**	27
1.1.1.	**Allogeneic and Xenogeneic Heart Transplantation in Infants** LL Bailey, S Nehlsen-Cannarella, JG Jacobson	27
1.1.2.	**The Current Application of Lung and Combined Heart and Lung Transplantation** SW Jamieson	32
1.1.3.	**Clinical Experience with Unilateral and Bilateral Lung Transplantation - The Toronto Group Experience** RJ Ginsberg, GA Patterson, R Grossman, M Goldberg, V Maurer, TR Todd, JD Cooper, FG Pearson	46
1.2.	**Tissue Immunology**	51
1.2.1.	**Preliminary Results of the Collaborative Heart Transplant Study** G Opelz, H Mollner, B Reichart, E Keppel	51
1.2.2.	**The Application of New Techniques in HLA Typing, with Special Reference to DRw6 in Clinical Transplantation** E du Toit, R Martell, M Oudshoorn	59
1.3.	**Immunosuppression**	64
1.3.1.	**Total Lymphoid Irradiation in Experimental and Clinical Transplantation** JA Myburgh	64
1.3.2.	**Clinical Application of Polyclonal Antibodies Antilymphocyte (ALG), Antithymocyte (ATG) Globulin in Heart Transplantation** B Reichart	79
1.3.3.	**The Use of Monoclonal Antibodies in Treating Cardiac Allograft Rejection: Our Experience with OKT-3** MS Sweeney, OH Frazier, JT Sinnott IV., JB O'Connell	82
1.3.4.	**The Monoclonal Antibody BMA 031 in Organ Transplantation** J Racenberg, R Zerban, R Kurrle, F Seiler	88
1.4.	**Rejection Monitoring**	92
1.4.1.	**Cyto-immunological Monitoring (CIM) for Differentiation between Cardiac Rejection, Viral, Bacterial or Fungal Infection; its Specificity and Sensitivity** C Hammer, D Klanke, P Dirschedl, C Lersch, BM Kemkes, M Gokel, H Reichenspurner, B Reichart	92

Table of Contents

Page

1.4.2.	**New Advances in Non-Invasive Rejection Diagnosis after Heart Transplantation** M Anthuber, BM Kemkes, H Reichenspurner, G Osterholzer, C Angermann, R Haberl, A. Weiler, B Reichart, A Hildebrandt, C Spes	98
1.4.3.	**Experimental Observations with Cytoimmunological Monitoring and Biochemical Rejection Markers after Pancreatic Transplantation and Immunosuppression with Total Lymphoid Irradiation and Cyclosporine** DF du Toit, JJ Heydenrych, B Smit	106
1.5.	**Heart Preservation**	120
1.5.1.	**Prolonged Ex-vivo Heart Preservation** E Solis, MP Kaye	120
1.6.	**Xenogeneic Transplantation**	127
1.6.1.	**Immunological Aspects and Recent Advances in Xenogeneic Transplantation** C Hammer	127
1.6.2.	**Recent Advances in Immunosuppression after Xenogeneic Heart Transplantation in Primates** H Reichenspurner, PA Human, DH Boehm, DKC Cooper, R May, AG Rose, P Zilla, R Fasol, B Reichart	137
1.6.3.	**The Virological Evaluation of Non-Human Primates for Xenotransplantation** PA Human, FJ van der Riet, DKC Cooper, SS Kalter, JE Fincham, HEM Smuts, H Reichenspurner, DL Madden, JL Sever, B Reichart	147
2.	**Artificial Heart**	153
2.1.	**Introduction: Mechanical Ventricular Assistance and Replacement** J Odell	155
2.2.	**State of the Art in Assisted Circulation** F Unger	158
2.3.	**Clinical Application and Patient Selection in the Use of a Total Artificial Heart as a Bridge for Transplantation - La Pitié Hôpital Experience 1986-1987** E Solis, C Muneretto, P Leger, I Gandjbakhch, A Pavie, V Bors, C Piazza, J Szefner, A Cabrol, C Cabrol	168
2.4.	**Clinical Experience with the Artificial Heart as a Bridge for Transplant** A Rokitansky, E Wolner, W Schreiner, U Losert	175
2.5.	**Skeletal Muscle Ventricles: Preliminary Results and Theoretical Design Considerations** CR Bridges Jr, JS Andersen, WA Anderson, RL Hammond, MA Acker, LW Stephenson	182
2.6.	**An Electromagnetic Actuator Using Recently Developed Rare Earth Permanent Magnets** MV Koroly, N Ida, LR Roemer	203
2.7.	**Blood Platelets during Experimental and Clinical Total Artificial Heart Replacement** MR Mueller, A Wohlfahrt, A Lee, P Zilla, R Fasol, E Wolner	206

Table of Contents

		Page
3.	**Endothelial Cell Lining**	213
3.1.	**Introduction: Endothelialization of Cardiovascular Prostheses** R Fasol, P Zilla, B Reichart	215
3.2.	**Basics of Endothelial Cell Lining**	218
3.2.1.	**Anticoagulant Properties of Vascular Endothelium** TC Vukovich, PN Knöbl	218
3.2.2.	**Heparin-Binding Growth Factors** T Maciag	229
3.2.3.	**Active Responses and Signal Transduction in Endothelial Cells** US Ryan	236
3.2.4.	**Immune Functions of Vascular Wall Cells** P Libby, SJC Warner, LK Birinyi	250
3.3.	**10 Years of Endothelial Cell Seeding**	270
3.3.1.	**The Tissue Culture Arterial Graft** AD Callow	270
3.4.	**Endothelial Cell Seeding and Sodding**	282
3.4.1.	**Technique and Experience with Clinical Endothelial Cell Seeding** P Örtenwall, H Wadenvik, J Kutti, B Risberg	282
3.4.2.	**Endothelial Cell Seeding of Synthetic Vascular Grafts - Evidence for a Systemic Effect on Early Patency** BM Bourke, TS Reeve, M Appleberg	295
3.4.3.	**Endothelial Cell Seeding with Microvessel Endothelial Cells - Animal and Human Studies** SP Schmidt, WV Sharp, MM Evancho, TR Pippert, SO Meerbaum, D Monajjem	310
3.5.	**Improved Harvest Technique**	323
3.5.1.	**Human Endothelial Cell Derivation Using the Neutral Protease Dispase** JC Stanley, BG Ruefer, WE Burkel, DW Haack, LM Graham, JL Fisher, NJ Sharber	323
3.6.	**Modification of Graft Surfaces**	332
3.6.1.	**Surface Modulation of Endothelial Cell Seeded PTFE Vascular Grafts** RB Patterson, RF Kempczinski	332
3.6.2.	**Surface Covering Precoating Procedures Enhance Adherence and Spreading of Seeded Endothelial Cells on PTFE Vascular Prostheses** J Kähler, P Zilla, R Fasol, M Deutsch	341
3.6.3.	**Cell Attachment Forces Regulating the Immediate Establishment of Endothelial Cell Monolayers** BE Jarrell, SK Williams, K Pratt, J Radomski, RA Carabasi	350

Table of Contents

		Page
3.7.	**In Vitro Lining**	360
3.7.1.	**In Vitro Lining of PTFE Grafts with Homologous Endothelial Cells** P Zilla, R Fasol, P Preiss, U Dudeck, J Odell, D Sanan, H Reichenspurner, B Reichart	360
3.7.2.	**Small Diameter Vascular Prosthesis with Highly Purified, Functional Autologous Venous Endothelial Cells** W Müller-Glauser, KH Lehmann, P Bittmann, U Bay, P Dittes, L von Segesser, M Turina	370
3.7.3.	**Cultivation of Human Endothelial Cells on Artificial Heart Materials** R Fasol, P Zilla, M Grimm, P Preiss, T Fischlein, O Krupicka	378
4.	**Laser Treatment**	387
4.1.	**Laser Treatment - Introduction** U von Oppell	389
4.2.	**The Physics of Laser Light and its Interaction with Matter** G Fasol	391
4.3.	**Coronary Artery Plaque Rapidly Induced by Local Electro-Magnetic Stimulation and Western Diet** H Breuer, J Fincham, P Hinrichsen, CJ Uys, H Weich, B Reichart	417
4.4.	**Excimer Laser - Tissue Interactions** G Wollenek, G Laufer, W Klepetko, F Grabenwöger, E Wolner	423
4.5.	**Peripheral Laser and Mechanical Angioplasty - The Stanford Experience** R Ginsburg	431
4.6.	**Percutaneous Atherectomy: A New Method for Non-Operative Vessel Reconstruction** B Höfling, A von Pölnitz, D Backa, G Bauriedel, L Lauterjung, KW Jauch, K Remberger	440
4.7.	**Contact Laser Surgery - A Study of Five Different Laser Probes** D Richens, MR Rees, DA Watson	451
4.8.	**Cardiovascular Applications of Laser Technology** RH Clarke, JM Isner	459
4.9.	**Endoscopically Guided Laser Angioplasty - A New Laser Angioscope** D Richens, MR Rees, DA Watson	469
4.10.	**Intraoperative Argon Laser Angioplasty in Coronary Arteries - First Clinical Results** FW Hehrlein, R Moosdorf	475
	Index	483

List of Authors

ACKER MA, MD	Harrison Department of Surgical Research, Department of Surgery, University of Pennsylvania, Philadelphia, Pennsylvania, USA
ANDERSEN JS, MD	Harrison Department of Surgical Research, Department of Surgery, University of Pennsylvania, Philadelphia, Pennsylvania, USA
ANDERSON WA, MD	Harrison Department of Surgical Research, Department of Surgery, University of Pennsylvania, Philadelphia, Pennsylvania, USA
ANGERMANN CH, PD, MD	Medizinische Klinik Innenstadt, University of Munich, FR Germany
ANTHUBER M, MD	Department of Cardiac Surgery, University of Munich, FR Germany
APPLEBERG M, MD	Department of Surgery, University of Sydney and Department of Vascular Surgery, Royal North Shore Hospital, Sydney, Australia
BACKA D, MD	Department of Medicinel, Klinikum Grosshadern, Ludwig-Maximilians-University, Munich, FR Germany
BAILEY LL, PROF	Department of Surgery, University of Loma Linda, California, USA
BAURIEDEL G, MD	Department of Medicine, Klinikum Grosshadern, Ludwig-Maximilians-Universität, Munich, FR Germany
BAY U, PhD	Clinic of Cardiovascular Surgery, University Hospital of Zurich, Switzerland
BIRINYI L, MD	Departments of Medicine and Surgery, Tufts University and New England Medical Center, Boston, Massachusetts, USA
BITTMANN P, PhD	Clinic of Cardiovascular Surgery, University Hospital of Zurich, Switzerland
BOEHM D, MD	Department of Cardiothoracic Surgery, University of Cape Town, South Africa
BORS V, MD	Department of Cardiovascular Surgery, Hôpital La Pitié, Paris, France
BOURKE BM, MD	Royal North Shore Hospital, Sydney, Australia

BREUER H, DR Phil Nat	Department of Cardiothoracic Surgery, University of CapeTown, South Africa
BRIDGES CR, MD, SCD	Harrison Department of Surgical Research, Department of Surgery, University of Pennsylvania, Philadelphia, Pennsylvania, USA
BURKEL WE, PhD	Department of Vascular Surgery, University of Michigan Medical School, Ann Arbor, USA
CABROL A, MD	Department of Cardiovascular Surgery, Hôpital La Pitié, Paris, France
CABROL C, PROF	Department of Cardiovascular Surgery, Hôpital La Pitié, Paris, France
CALLOW AD, PROF	Department of Surgery, Tufts University, Boston, Massachusetts, USA
CARABASI RA, MD	Department of Surgery, Jefferson Medical College, Philadelphia, Pennsylvania, USA
CLARKE RH, PROF	Department of Chemistry, Boston University, Boston, Massachusetts, USA
COOPER JD, PROF	Divisions of Thoracic Surgery and Cardiovascular Surgery, Department of Surgery, University of Toronto, Ontario, Canada
COOPER DKC, MD, PhD, FRCS	Oklahoma Transplantation Institute, Baptist Medical Center, Oklahoma City, USA
DEUTSCH M, PROF	Department of Cardiovascular and Thoracic Surgery, Wels, Austria
DIRSCHEDL P, MD	Institute for Statistics and Biomathematics, University of Munich, FR Germany
DITTES P, PhD	IMS - BIOPUR, Freienbach, Switzerland
DUDECK U, BS	Department of Cardiothoracic Surgery, University of Cape Town, Cape Town, South Africa
DU TOIT DF, PROF, PhD, FRCS	Department of Surgery, University of Stellenbosch, Medical School and Tygerberg Hospital, South Africa
DU TOIT E, MD	Provincial Laboratory for Tissue Immunology, Cape Town, South Africa
EVANCHO MM, BS	Vascular Research Laboratory, Akron City Hospital, Akron, Ohio, USA
FASOL G, PhD	Department of Physics, Cavendish Laboratory, University of Cambridge, United Kingdom

FASOL R, MD	Department of Cardiothoracic Surgery, University of Cape Town, South Africa
FINCHAM J, BVSC	Research Institute for Nutritional Diseases, Medical Research Council, Tygerberg, South Africa
FISCHLEIN T, MD	Department of Surgery, University of Vienna, and Department of Cardiovasclar and Thoracic Surgery, Wels, Austria
FISHER JL, PhD	Department of Vascular Surgery, University of Michigan, Medical School, Ann Arbor, USA
FRAZIER OH, MD	Division of Surgery, Texas Heart Institute, Houston, Texas, USA
GANDJBAKHCH I, MD	Department of Cardiovascular Surgery, Hôpital La Pitié, Paris, France
GINSBERG RJ, PROF	Mount Sinai Hospital, University of Toronto, Ontario, Canada
GINSBURG R, PROF	Center for Interventional Vascular Therapies, Stanford University, Medical Center, USA
GOKEL M, PROF	Institute of Pathology, University of Munich, FR Germany
GOLDBERG M, PROF	Divisions of Thoracic Surgery and Cardiovascular Surgery, Department of Surgery, University of Toronto, Ontario, Canada
GRABENWÖGER F, MD	Department of Surgery 2, University of Vienna, Austria
GRAHAM LM, PROF	Department of Vascular Surgery, University of Michigan Medical School, Ann Arbor, USA
GRIMM M, MD	Department of Surgery 2, University of Vienna, Austria
GROSSMAN R, PROF	Divisions of Thoracic Surgery and Cardiovascular Surgery, Department of Surgery, University of Toronto, Ontario, Canada
HAACK DW, PhD	Medical Products Division, WL Gore & Assoc, Flagstaff, Arizona, USA
HABERL R, MD	Medizinische Klinik I, Klinikum Grosshadern, University of Munich, FR Germany
HAMMER C, PROF	Institute for Surgical Research, University of Munich, FR Germany
HAMMOND RL, BS	The Harrison Department of Surgical Research, Department of Surgery, University of Pennsylvania, Philadelphia, Pennsylvania, USA

HEHRLEIN FW, PROF	Department Cardiovascular Surgery, Justus-Liebig-University, Giessen, FR Germany
HEYDENRYCH JJ, MSC, MMED	Department of Paediatric Surgery, University of Stellenbosch, Medical School and Tygerberg Hospital, South Africa
HILDEBRANDT A, MD	Department of Cardiacthoracic Surgery, University Cape Town, South Africa
HINRICHSEN P, BSc	Department of Medical Physics, University of Cape Town, South Africa
HÖFLING B, PROF	Department of Medicine, Klinikum Grosshadern, Ludwig-Maximilians-University, Munich, FR Germany
HUMAN P, MSC	Department of Cardiothoracic Surgery, University of Cape Town, South Africa
IDA N, MD	Department of Electrical Engineering, University of Akron, Akron, Ohio, USA
ISNER JM, MD	Department of Medicine, Tufts New England Medical Center, Boston, Massachusetts, USA
JACOBSON JG, MD	Department of Surgery, Loma Linda University, California, USA
JAMIESON SW, PROF	Heart and Lung Institute, University of Minnesota, Minneapolis, USA
JARRELL BE, MD	Department of Surgery, Jefferson Medical College, Philadelphia, Pennsylvania, USA
JAUCH KW, MD	Department of Surgery, Klinikum Grosshadern, Ludwig-Maximilians-Universität, Munich, FR Germany
KAEHLER J, MD	Department of Surgery, University of Vienna, Austria
KALTER SS, PhD	Department of Virology and Immunology, Southwest Foundation for Biomedical Research, San Antonio, Texas, USA
KAYE MP, PROF	Department of Cardiovascular Research, Minnesota Heart and Lung Institute, University of Minnesota, Minneapolis, USA
KEMKES BM, PROF	Department of Cardiac Surgery, University of Munich, FR Germany
KEMPCZINSKI RF, PROF	Department of Surgery, University of Cincinnati, Ohio, USA
KEPPEL E, MD	IBM Scientific Center, Heidelberg, FR Germany

KLANKE D, MD	Institute for Surgical Research, University of Munich, FR Germany
KLEPETKO W, MD	Department of Surgery 2, University of Vienna, Austria
KNÖBL PN, MD	Department of Medical Physiology, University of Vienna, Vienna, Austria
KOROLY MV, MD	Department of Vascular Research, Akron City Hospital, Akron, Ohio, USA
KRUPICKA O, MD	Department of Surgery 2, University of Vienna, Austria
KURRLE R, MD	Experimental Research, Behringwerke, Marburg, FR Germany
KUTTI J, MD, PhD	Department of Medicine, Ostra Sjukhuset, University of Goteborg, Sweden
LAUFER G, MD	Department of Surgery 2, University of Vienna, Austria
LAUTERJUNG L, PROF	Department of Surgery, Klinikum Grosshadern, Ludwig-Maxmilians-University, Munich, FR Germany
LEE A, MD	Department of Surgery 2, Ludwig Boltzman Institute, Vienna, Austria
LEGER PH, MD	Department of Cardiovascular Surgery, Hôpital La Pitié, Paris, France
LEHMANN KH, MD	Clinic of Cardiovascular Surgery, University Hospital of Zurich, Switzerland
LERSCH C, MD	Institute for Surgical Research, University of Munich, FR Germany
LIBBY P, PROF	Department of Medicine and Surgery, Tufts University, Boston, Massachusetts, USA
LOSERT U, MD	Department of Surgery 2, University of Vienna, General Hospital of Vienna, Austria
MACIAG T, PhD	Laboratory of Molecular Biology, American Red Cross, Maryland, USA
MADDEN DL, DVM, PhD	Infectious Diseases Branch, National Institute of Health, Bethesda, Maryland, USA
MARTELL R, FCP	Provincial Laboratory for Tissue Immunology, Cape Town, South Africa
MAURER V, PROF	Divisions of Thoracic Surgery and Cardiovascular Surgery, Department of Surgery, University of Toronto, Ontario, Canada

MAY R, MB, ChB	Provincial Laboratory for Tissue Immunology, Cape Town, South Africa
MEERBAUM SO, BS	Vascular Research Laboratory, Akron City Hospital, Akron, Ohio, USA
MOLLNER H, MD	Department of Transplantation Immunology, Institute of Immunology, University of Heidelberg, FR Germany
MONAJJEM D, BS	Vascular Research Laboratory, Akron City Hospital, Akron, Ohio, USA
MOOSDORF R, MD	Department of Cardiovascular Surgery, Justus-Liebig-University, Giessen, FR Germany
MUELLER-GLAUSER W, PhD	Clinic of Cardiovascular Surgery, University Hospital of Zurich, Switzerland
MUELLER MR, MD	Department of Surgery 2, University of Vienna, Austria
MUNERETTO C, MD	Department of Cardiovascular Surgery, Hôpital La Pitié, Paris, France
MYBURGH JA, PROF, ChM FRCS, FACS	Transplantation Research Unit, Department of Surgery, University of Witwatersrand, Johannesburg, South Africa
NEHLSEN-CANNARELLA S, PhD, MD	Department of Surgery, Loma Linda University, California, USA
O'CONNELL JB, MD	Division of Cardiology, University of Utah, Salt Lake City, Utah, USA
ODELL JA, PROF, FRCS	Department of Cardiothoracic Surgery, University of Cape Town, South Africa
OPELZ G, PROF	Department of Transplantation Immunology, Institute of Immunology, University of Heidelberg, FR Germany
OERTENWALL P, MD	Department of Surgery, Ostra Sjukhuset, Univesity of Goteborg, Sweden
OSTERHOLZER G, MD	Department of Cardiac Surgery, University of Munich, FR Germany
OUDSHOORN M, MSC	Provincial Laboratory for Tissue Immunology, Cape Town, South Africa
OWEN P, PhD	Ischaemic Heart Disease Research Laboratory, University of Cape Town, South Africa
PAOMSKI, J	Department of Surgery, Thomas Jefferson University, Philadelphia, USA

PATTERSON GA, PROF	Divisions of Thoracic Surgery and Cardiovascular Surgery, Department of Surgery, University of Toronto, Ontario, Canada
PATTERSON RB, MD	Division of Vascular Surgery, University of Cincinnati, Ohio, USA
PAVIE A, MD	Department of Cardiovascular Surgery, Hôpital La Pitié, Paris, France
PEARSON FG, PROF	Divisions of Thoracic Surgery and Cardiovascular Surgery, Department of Surgery, University of Toronto, Ontario, Canada
PIAZZA C, MD	Department of Cardiovascular Surgery, Hôpital La Pitié, Paris, France
PIPPERT TR, MS	Vascular Research Laboratory, Akron City Hospital, Akron, Ohio, USA
VON POELNITZ A, MD	Department of Medicine, Klinikum Grosshadern, Ludwig-Maxmilians-University, Munich, FR Germany
PRATT K, MS	Department of Surgery, Jefferson Medical College, Philadelphia, Pennsylvania, USA
PREISS P, MD	Department of Cardiothoracic Surgery and Medical Biochemistry, University of Cape Town, South Africa, and Department of Surgery 2, University of Vienna, Austria
RACENBERG J, MD	Clinical Research-Immunoloy, Behringwerke, Marburg, FR Germany
RADOMSKI J, MD	Department of Surgery, Jefferson Medical College, Philadelphia, Pennsylvania, USA
REES MR, MRCB	Cardiac Research Laboratories, Killingbeck Hospital, Leeds, United Kingdom
REEVE TS, MD	Department of Surgery, Univesity of Sydney and Department of Vascular Surgery, Royal North Shore Hospital, Sydney, Australia
REICHART B, PROF	Department of Cardiothoracic Surgery, University of Cape Town, South Africa
REICHENSPURNER H, MD	Department of Cardiothoracic Surgery, University of Cape Town, South Africa
REICHERT D, MD	Department of Cardiac Surgery, University of Munich, FR Germany
REMBERGER K, PROF	Department of Pathology, Klinikum Grosshadern, Ludwig-Maxlmilians-University, Munich, FR Germany

RICHENS D, FRCS	Cardiac Research Laboratories, Killingbeck Hospital, Leeds, United Kingdom
RISBERG B, PROF	Department of Surgery, University of Goteborg, Sweden
ROEMER LR	Department of Electrical Engineering, University of Akron, Akron, Ohio, USA
ROKITANSKY A, MD	Department of Surgery 2, University of Vienna, General Hospital of Vienna, Austria
ROSE AG, PROF	Department of Pathology, University of Cape Town, Medical School, South Africa
RUEFER BG, MS	Medical Products Division, WL Gore & Assoc, Flagstaff, Arizona, USA
RYAN US, PROF	Department of Medicine, University of Miami, Florida, USA
SANAN D, PhD	Department of Medical Biochemistry, University of Cape Town, South Africa
SCHMIDT SP, PROF	Vascular Research Laboratory, Akron City Hospital, Akron, Ohio, USA
SCHREINER W, MD	Department of Surgery 2, University of Vienna, General Hospital of Vienna, Austria
SEILER F, MD	Experimental Research, Behringwerke, Marburg, FR Germany
SEVER JL, MD	Infectious Diseases Branch, National Institute of Health, Bethesda, Maryland, USA
SHARP WV, MD	Vascular Research Laboratory, Akron City Hospital, Akron, Ohio, USA
SHARBER NJ, BS	Medical Products Division, WL Gore & Assoc, Flagstaff, Arizona, USA
SINNOTT IV. JT, MD	Division of Infectious Diseases, University of South Florida, Tampa, USA
SMIT B, MMED,	Department of Radiotherapy, University of Stellenbosch, Medical School and Tygerberg Hospital, South Africa
SMUTS HEM, PhD	Department of Medical Microbiology, University of Cape Town, South Africa
STANLEY JC, PROF	Department of Surgery, University of Michigan, Ann Arbor, USA

STEPHENSON LW, PROF	Division of Cardiothoracic Surgery, University of Pennsylvania, USA
SOLIS E, MD	Cardiovascular Research Laboratory, Heart and Lung Institute, University of Minnesota, Minneapolis, USA and Department of Cardiovascular Surgery, Hôpital La Pitié, Paris, France
SPES C, MD	Medizinische Klinik Innenstadt, University of Munich, FR Germany
SWEENEY MS, PROF	Division of Cardiovascular Surgery, University of South Florida, Tampa, USA
SZEFNER J, MD	Department of Cardio Vascular Surgery, Hôpital La Pitié, Paris, France
TODD TR, PROF	Divisions of Thoracic Surgery and Cardiovascular Surgery, Department of Surgery, University of Toronto, Ontario, Canada
TURINA M, PROF	Clinic of Cardiovasular Surgery, University Hospital of Zurich, Switzerland
UNGER F, PROF	Division of Cardiac Surgery, University of Salzburg, Austria
UYS CJ, MD	Department of Pathclogy, University of Cape Town, South Africa
VAN DER RIET FJ, BVSc, PhD	Department of Medical Virology, University of Cape Town, Medical School, Cape Town, South Africa
VON OPPELL UO, MD, FCS	Department of Cardiothoracic Surgery, University of Cape Town, South Africa
VON SEGESSER L, MD	Clinic of Cardiovascular Surgery, University Hospital of Zurich, Switzerland
VUKOVICH TC, PROF	Department of Medical Physiology, University of Vienna, Vienna, Austria
WADENVIK H, MD, PhD	Department of Medicine, Ostra Sjukhuset, University of Goteborg, Sweden
WATSON DA, FRCS	Cardiac Research Laboratories, Killingbeck Hospital, Leeds, England
WARNER SJC,	Departments of Medicine and Surgery, Tufts University and New England Medical Center, Boston, Massachusetts, USA
WEICH H, PROF	Department of Cardiology, University of Stellenbosch, South Africa

WEILER A, MD	Department of Cardiac Surgery, University of Munich, FR Germany
WILLIAMS SK, PhD	Department of Surgery, Jefferson Medical College, Philadelphia, Pennsylvania, USA
WOHLFAHRT A, MD	Department of Surgery 2 and Ludwig Boltzman Institute, University of Vienna, Austria
WOLLENEK G, MD	Department of Surgery 2, University of Vienna, Austria
WOLNER E, PROF	Department of Surgery 2, University of Vienna, Austria
ZERBAN R, MD	Clinical Research - Immunology, Behringwerke, Marburg, FR Germany
ZILLA P, MD	Department of Cardiothoracic Surgery, University of Cape Town, South Africa

Twenty Years Of Human Heart Transplantation

A Foreword

*B Reichart, H Reichenspurner, J Odell, U von Oppell,
P Human, R Fasol, P Zilla, DH Boehm*

*Department Of Cardiothoracic Surgery,
University Of Cape Town, Groote Schuur Hospital,
Cape Town, South Africa*

On December 3, 1967, Barnard and his team from Cape Town performed the first successful human heart transplantation (1). Although renal transplantation had been possible at that time for more than a decade, cardiac replacement was to become an epochal event. In order to commemorate its 20th anniversary, a congress on "Recent Advances in Cardiovascular Surgery" was held at Cape Town, from 7 - 9 December 1987. Four topics had been chosen - recent transplantation techniques, artificial hearts, endothelial cell lining, laser treatment - all of them now as new and on the brink of becoming a clinical method as heart transplantation was in 1967. This book provides a complete collection of the manuscripts of the talks given on the occasion in Cape Town.

The Development of Human Heart Transplantation since 1967

The following brief outline is added to the foreword rather than to the rest of the book, the logic being that cardiac replacement is now a standardized and clinical technique and does not belong any more to advances (which does not mean, of course, that paediatric heart transplantation is not still excitingly new).

The first human heart transplantation in Cape Town had a trigger function and 101 interventions were done the following year 1968. However, most of the transplants failed immediately, and these disappointing early results were a major reason why most units decided to stop their cardiac transplantation programme in the late sixties and throughout the seventies. During this time, the concept of heart transplantation was kept alive by groups from Stanford (Shumway who pioneered cardiac replacement in the laboratory (2) and started his programme in January 1968), Richmond (Shumway's co-worker Lower became Head of that Cardiosurgical Department), Paris (under the leadership of Cabrol) and Cape Town. In this crucial period, however, several notable advances took place, most of them initiated at Stanford University: endomyocardial biopsy for early and precise detection of acute rejection was introduced by Caves (3) in 1974; the use of rabbit antithymocyte globulin was reported at around the same time (Bieber, review in (4) and Copeland (5) described successful retransplantation). As a result, the one year survival rate at Stanford University, which had been 20% in 1968, gradually improved to be nearly 70% at the end of the seventies.

In 1973, heterotopic heart transplantation was successfully adopted for clinical use by Barnard and Losman at Groote Schuur Hospital (6).

The discovery and introduction of cyclosporine by Borel and his group from Basle (7), stimulated a world-wide renaissance in the field of cardiac transplantation in the early eighties. The function of cyclosporine is unique, since it blocks selectively the helper subset of the T-lymphocytes. Consequently only a few cytotoxic effector cells are produced, not enough to reject the transplanted organ. Cyclosporine, unlike corticosteroids, has no detrimental effect on the wound healing. Heart-lung transplantation became possible, first in primates, then in man (Reitz, Jamieson 8-10).

Since the beginning of the eighties, the number of heart transplantations per year has increased exponentially according to the Registry of the International Society for Heart Transplantation (11); in the year 1987, approximately 2100 heart transplantations were done. The availability of cyclosporine - together with increasing experience - improved the one year survival rate worldwide to nearly 90%. In addition, more sophisticated monitoring of acute rejection is being undertaken. Besides routine endomycocardial biopsies, non-invasive techniques like cytoimmunological monitoring have been employed in order to determine the number of activated T-lymphocytes of the peripheral blood (12).

In 1984, hormonal therapy of brainstem dead organs was initiated by Novitzky at Cape Town (13). By administering thyroid hormone T_3, cortisone and insulin, stability of the donor haemodynamics was usually achieved and explantation became more predictable - a fact which may prove crucial for difficult transplantations such as reoperations or heart-lung replacements.

The improved results after heart transplantation led to an extension of the operative indications: advanced age is no longer a contraindication, cardiac replacements are performed in the newborn (14) (see also the contribution of Bailey and his group from Loma Linda University in Chapter 1.1.1.). Patients with controlled diabetes mellitus are accepted for transplantation programmes. Various types of cardiac assist devices and even the total artificial heart are now utilized as a bridge to cardiac transplantation (15; see contribution of Solis and Cabrol from the Hôpital La Pitié - in Paris, Chapter 2.3.).

The Cape Town Experience

From December 1967 to December 1987, 110 heart and 12 heart-lung transplantations have been performed at the Groote Schuur Hospital. Sixty-one of the heart transplantations were heterotopic and 49 orthotopic procedures. Ten patients required retransplantation. These repeat procedures were necessary 8 times after heterotopic and twice after orthotopic transplantation. There were two third-time interventions.

The indications for the heart transplantations have been either dilated cardiomyopathy, or endstage ischaemic heart disease; rheumatic heart disease, endocardial fibrosis or rarely congenital malformations.

The results of heart-lung transplantation have recently been published and will not be discussed further (16).

For heart transplantation, three major immunosuppressive regimens have been utilized over the 20 years:

1. Group A
Conventional Immunosuppression

From 1967 to 1982 treatment consisted of a combination of 2-5 mg/kg/day azathioprine, 10 mg/kg/day methyl-prednisolone (tapered down to 1 mg/kg/day within three months, 0.25 mg/kg/day within one year) and 1-7 mg/kg/day IgG rabbit antithymocyte globulin.

2. Group B
High Dose Cyclosporine Therapy

From 1983 to 1984 patients received 18-10 mg/kg/day cyclosporine in combination with 1 mg/kg/day methylprednisolone (which was tapered down to 0.3 mg/kg/day within 3 months).

3. Group C
Low-dose Cyclosporine Therapy

This immunosuppressive medication has been used since 1984; 3-8 mg/kg/day cyclosporine A is administered in order to achieve whole blood trough levels of 300-500 ng/ml; 0-2 mg/kg/day azathioprine and 0.3-0.1 mg/kg/day methylprednisolone are added. Rabbit antithymocyte globulin is given for approximately 4 post-operative days, in order to decrease the peripheral T-lymphocyte count to less than 150 cells/mm^3.

Pulsed high dose methylprednisolone (1g i.v. for 3 consecutive days) was administered for acute rejection episodes, with rabbit antithymocyte globulin only in severe episodes of rejection.

There were 59 transplantations in 55 patients in group A (10 orthotopic and 49 heterotopic procedures), 16 interventions in 15 patients in group B (9 orthotopic and 7 heterotopic) and, finally, 35 operations in 30 patients in group C (30 orthotopic and 5 heterotopic). When the results of orthotopic and heterotopic transplantation were combined and compared for each group, the one and 2 years survival rates of group A and B revealed no significant difference: the one year survival rates were 48 and 42% respectively. At 2 years 38% of each group were alive.

In contraindication, group C had a significantly better one year survival rate of 78% (p<.05; Fisher's exact test). The results of group C within the last 12 months have been analysed separately, and the one year survival rate of these 19 patients (15 orthotopic and 4 heterotopic) is 94% (Figure 1).

When comparing orthotopic with heterotopic techniques, a similar survival rate of 70% was obtained after 6 months.

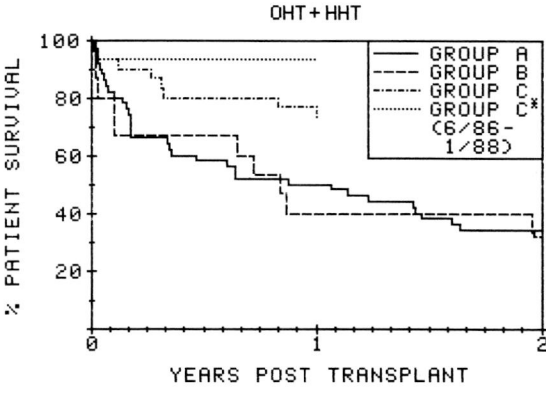

Fig. 1 One and two year survival rates within three different groups A, B and C.
(For explanation see text; Figure 1, thanks to the Southern African Medical Journal).

However, in the later follow-up period, the two groups differ significantly. After 2 years, 60% of the orthotopic transplant patients are alive, as opposed to 42% after hetertopic procedures (p<.05; Figure 2). However, one must mention that most of the heterotopic transplantations belonged to group A.

In summarizing, it may be truly stated, that the human heart transplantation is now an accepted and recommended treatment for end-stage heart failure, predominantly of coronary artery disease, dilated cardiomyopathy and certain congenital heart malformations without Eisenmenger reaction. The latest long-term results are excellent and compare favourably with those after renal transplantation.

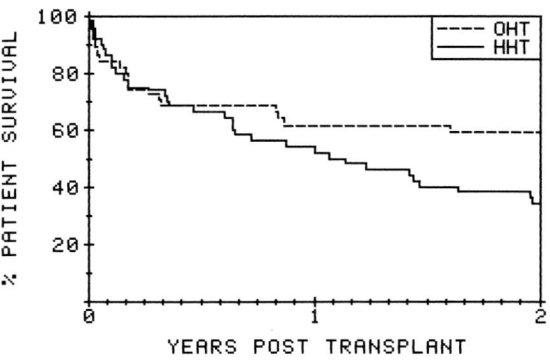

Fig. 2 One and two year survival rates of patients after either heterotopic or orthotopic heart transplantation. (Figure 2, thanks to the Journal of Heart Transplantation).

References

1. Barnard CN. The operation: a human cardiac transplant; an interim report of a successful operation at Groote Schuur Hospital, Cape Town. S Afr Med J 41, 1271, 1967.

2. Lower RR, Stofer RC, Shumway NE. Studies on the orthotopic homotransplantation of the canine heart. Surg Forum 11, 18, 1960.

3. Caves PK, Billingham ME, Stinson EB, Shumway NE. Serial transvenous biopsy of the transplanted human heart - improved management of acute rejection episodes. Lancet 1, 821, 1974.

4. Bieber CP. Pharmacokinetics of antithymocyte globulin (ATG) and cardiac transplant outcome. J Heart Transplant 1, 22, 1981.

5. Copeland JG, Griepp RB, Bieber CP, Billingham ME, Schroeder JS, Hunt S, Mason J, Stinson EB, Shumway NE. Successful retransplantation of the human heart. J Thorac Cardiovasc Surg 73, 242, 1977.

6. Barnard CN, Losman JG. Left ventricular bypass. S Afr Med J 49, 303, 1975.

7. Borel JF, Feurer C, Magnee C, Stahelin H. Effects of the new anti-lymphocytic polypeptide cyclosporine A in animals. Immunology 32, 1017, 1977.

8. Reitz BA, Burton NA, Jamieson SW, Bieber CP, Pennock JL, Stinson EB, Shumway NE. Heart and lung transplantation; autotransplantation and allotransplantation in primates with extended survival. J Thorac Cardiovasc Surg 80, 360, 1980.

9. Reitz BA. Heart-lung transplantation, a review. J Heart Transplant 1, 291, 1982.

10. Jamieson SW, Stinson EB, Oyer PE, Baldwin JC, Shumway NE. Operative technique for heart-lung transplantation. J Thorac Cardiovasc Surg 87, 930, 1984.

11. Kaye MP. The Registry of the International Society for Heart Transplantation; fourth official report - 1987. J Heart Transplant 6, 63, 1987.

12. Reichenspurner H, Kemkes BM, Osterholzer C, Reble B, Ertel W, Reichart B, Lersch C, Hammer C, Haberl R, Steinbeck G, Gokel J. Particular control of infection and rejection episodes after 4 years cardiac transplantation. Tex Heart Inst J 13, 5, 1986.

13. Novitzky D, Wicomb WN, Cooper DKC. Evidence of myocardial and renal functional recovery following hormonal therapy after brain death. Transplant Proc 18, 613, 1983.

14. Bailey LL, Nehlsen-Cannarella SL, Doroshow RW, Jacobson JG, Martin RD, Allard MW, Hyde MR, Dang Bui RH, Petry EL. Cardiac allotransplantation in newborns as therapy for hypoplastic left heart syndrome. N Engl J Med 315, 15, 1986.

15. Cabrol C, Gandibakhch I, Pavie A, Bors V, Cabrol A, Leger P, Vaissier E, Levasseur JP. Use of total artificial heart as a bridge to transplantation. J Heart Transplant 5, Programme Issue, 390, 1987.

16. Reichart B, Blaschke F, Cooper DKC, Novitzky D, Reichenspurner H, Odell JA, Rose AG, Kemkes BM, Klinner W. The transplantation of the heart and both lungs: initial experience of 12 operations in 10 patients. Clin Transplantation 1, 231, 1987.

1. Transplantation

1.1. Clinical Advances

1.1.1. Allogeneic and Xenogeneic Heart Transplantation in Infants

LL Bailey, S Nehlsen-Cannarella, JG Jacobson

Department of Surgery, Loma Linda University, Loma Linda, California, U.S.A.

Application of heart transplantation to neonates and young infants is gradually coming of age (1,2). It varies from heart transplantation in older children and adults in two important aspects:
1. it is usually done as corrective therapy for incurable structural heart disease, rather than for end-stage acquired myocardial disease, and
2. it is accomplished in the somewhat privileged milieu of the very young infant's less aggressive immune response (3,4).

This latter fact is exciting because it permits less ambitious early and late postoperative immunosuppression. Host growth and development may be expected to reach standard norms, and opportunistic infections are minimized. Finally, when implantation is accomplished perinatally, the possibility of acquired host immune tolerance to the heart graft exists.

The major limitation of successful organ transplantation in early life is the shortage of donor organs; this phenomenon is true for transplantation at any age. An estimated 10% of infants born with congenital heart disease have malformations too complex to be considered reparable (5). For these infants, performing palliative procedures frequently equates with postponing an inevitably poor outcome. Optimal therapy might very well consist of early diagnosis (even in utero) and expeditious heart or heart-lung replacement by means of transplantation. Selective xenografting, use of organs from anencephalic babies, and continued educational efforts to identify brain dead babies and encourage their parents toward organ donation, should all be explored as possible means to help narrow the donor-recipient gap. We are convinced that donor resources are available, if as yet only partially explored.

Xenografting the Neonate

A new era of cross-species organ transplantation was opened in October 1984, when a premature (36 weeks gestation) girl with hypoplastic left heart syndrome underwent implantation of a selected baboon heart (6,7). She was 12 days old at the time of transplantation and survived 3 weeks with the baboon graft. The infant recipient was found to be free of preformed antibody to baboons. She appeared to share Class I and Class II major histocompatibility common antigens with her baboon donor. Immunocyte reactivity in two-way mixed lymphocyte culture was significantly reduced against her particular donor in comparison to other donor panel baboons. In other words, the donor baboon utilized in the transplant surgery was selected on the basis of specific preoperative assays. We believe this selection process marked a significant advance in cross-species transplantation.

Historically, immunological selection had never been applied to xenografting. In this first clinical trial of the new era, the recipient was type 0. Therefore, using a baboon donor resulted in an ABO incompatibility, which, even in a premature newborn, resulted in death of disseminated hemagglutination on the 21st postoperative day. Her grafted heart, was one of the last organs to lose adequate function following the onset of renal, pulmonary, and cerebral dysfunction. Autopsy revealed virtually no cellular rejection of the graft, a fact which vindicated both the tissue selection process and the adequacy of T-cell function immunosuppression. Undoubtedly, ABO antibody played a role in direct myocardial injury. However, microcirculation in every organ system, including the graft, showed significant degrees of occlusion with distorted, agglutinated erythrocytes. This phenomenon, we believe, derived from the development of an ABO antibody directed against incompatible baboon blood antigens (expressed on graft endothelium) which then cross-reacted with host type O erythrocytes. The process was likely enhanced in the cross-species setting. Clearly, the cross-species donor selection equation must include ABO compatibility in all age groups. We are presently engaged in finalizing a protocol in which newborn recipients, for whom allografts cannot be identified, will be managed by selected cross-species transplantation as a bridge to eventual allografting. (Figure 3) To this end, we are now conducting a series of bridging xenotransplants in primates, later followed by allotransplants.

Use of Anencephalic Organs

When "live" born, an anencephalic (without cerebral hemispheres) infant is not technically brain dead by current statutes (8,9,10). Its functioning brain stem supports organic responses, such as respiration and other reflexes. At present, such infants are swaddled and provided with only passive care until death occurs, usually in the first 24 hours, and virtually always within the first 7 days. Death results from respiratory failure, bradycardia, infection, dehydration, or some combination of these problems. These infants, although of human conception, are not persons and have zero potential for personhood. They always lose residual organic function and die. Sadly, their organs die with them, usually to the chagrin and dismay of their parents.

Because anencephalic infants are of human conception and have varying degrees of organic brain stem function at birth, most countries have various social, ethical, and legal constraints preventing their utilization as organ donors. We have successfully utilized the heart from one anencephalic infant who met all established criteria for brain death. We would like to see a mechanism set in motion which would actively support these potential donors for a specified pe-

XENOTRANSPLANTATION PROTOCOL CURRENTLY UNDER REVIEW AT LLUMC

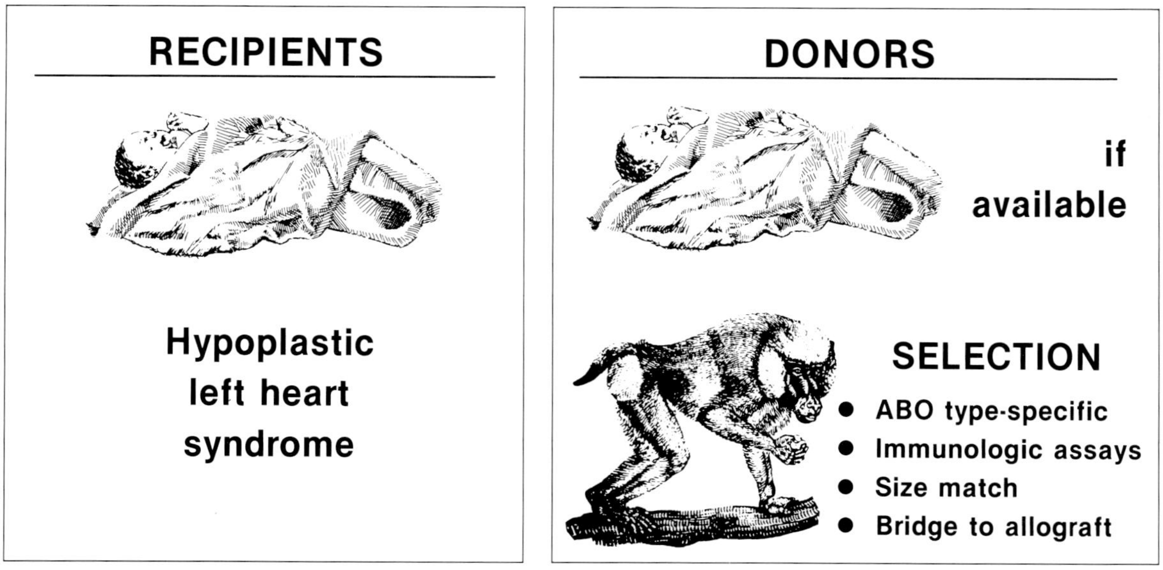

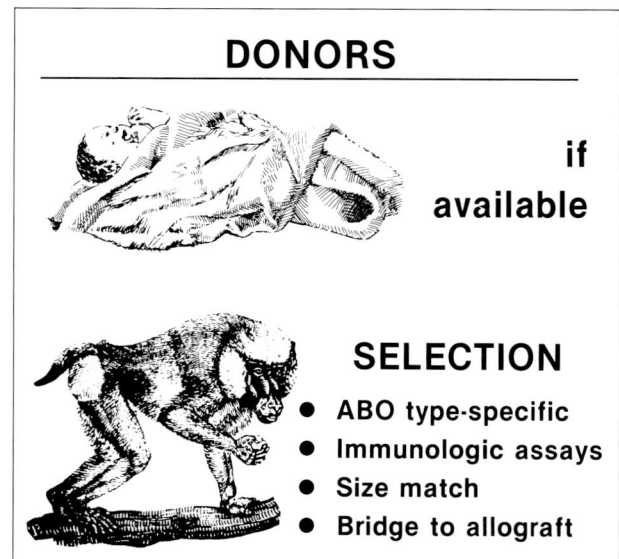

Fig. 3 An infant with hypoplastic left heart syndrome is a candidate for palliative reconstruction, orthotopic allotransplantation (if a human donor organ is available), or orthotopic xenotransplantation (as a bridge to allograft replacement), pending parental approval.

riod of time, during which current brain death criteria might be met (Figure 4). Such a mechanism could result in a considerably enhanced infant organ resource, improved parental contentment and satisfaction, and more positive social acceptance. It would not require changing the current legal definition of death. A commission, chaired by Dr. James Walters of Loma Linda's Center for Christian Bioethics, is presently formulating such a protocol.

Stimulating Public Awareness

Perhaps one of the most profound legacies of the initial cross-species infant heart transplantation has been a heightened public awareness of the need for infant donor organs. Public media are quite possibly the only effective means of disseminating this form of public education. Potential donor families must witness with their own eyes (in printed or video journalism) the joy of saving another infant's life by

---

BRAIN DEATH CRITERIA
FOR NEONATE AND SMALL INFANT DONORS

- Isoelectric EEG
- Coma
- Pupils fixed and dilated
- Absent oculocephalic reflex (doll's eyes)
- Absent gag and corneal reflexes
- Absent spontaneous respirations when $pCO_2 > 60$ Torr
- Normothermia
- No narcotics
- Barbiturate level below therapeutic levels

Fig. 4 Criteria currently accepted and utilized to confirm brain death in an infant organ donor. Serial examinations are done prior to declaration of death.

1. Transplantation

means of a transplanted organ. It is good and important news. Historically, the field of medicine has been cautious about public media attention. But in this new age of transplantation, in which donor resources are entirely dependent upon public awareness and confidence, media shyness is inappropriate, even destructive. Transplantation, for better or worse, has ushered in an era in which health professionals must learn to be media savy, media appropriate. The Loma Linda University program of infant heart transplantation has gained a measure of momentum which would not exist without the public awareness created by media interest. Hence, we have adopted a cooperative, rather than a resistant posture toward the public media with regards to transplantation. The symbiosis we believe is healthy and vital for continued awareness of the need for donor organs.

Pediatric Cardiac Transplant Program
Loma Linda University Medical Centre

Patient Number	Date of Tx	Current Age	Birthdate	Current Status
1	11/20/85	28 mos	11/16/85	Alive
2	01/23/86	26 mos	01/06/86	Alive
3	04/28/86	26 mos	01/10/86	Alive
4	06/10/86	22 mos	05/25/86	Alive
5	09/27/86	-	09/03/86	Died - 10/09/86
	COD: Perforated duodenal ulcer			
6	12/01/86	-	10/04/86	Died - 12/06/86
	COD: Graft failure unrelated to rejection			
7	02/07/87	16 mos	11/20/86	Alive
8	08/08/87	-	08/01/87	Died - 08/20/87
	COD: Necrotizing pneumonia			
9	10/16/87	5 mos	10/16/87	Alive
10	10/26/87	5 mos	10/15/87	Alive
11	11/20/87	7 mos	08/26/87	Alive
12	01/30/88	2 mos	01/12/88	Alive
13	02/14/88	5 wks	02/06/88	Alive
14	04/07/88	3 wks	03/17/88	Alive

(Abbr: COD = cause of death; TX = transplantation)

Table 1

Table 1 gives an account of 14 babies who have had heart transplantations at our institution over the past 2 years, the majority of whom are alive and well today. Many other infants could, and should have had similar therapy, had donor hearts been available. Our mandate is to ever broaden infant donor organ resources, and thus establish early transplantation as practical, rather than exceptional surgical therapy.

Addendum: At this printing, 21 additional neonates and infants (< 10 months old) have reeived autotopic cardiac allotransplantation. There has been only 1 additional peri-operative death and as yet, no late mortality.

References

1. *Bailey L, Nehlsen-Cannarella S, Doroshow R, Jacobson J, Martin R, Allard M, Hyde M, Bui R, Petry E. Cardiac allotransplantation in newborns as therapy for hypoplastic left heart syndrome. N Engl J Med 315, 949,1986.*

2. *Bailey L, Concepcion W, Shattuck H, Huang L. Method of heart transplantation for treatment of hypoplastic left heart syndrome. J Thorac Cardiovasc Surg 92, 1, 1986.*

3. *Stiehm ER, Fudenberg HH. Serum levels of immune globulins in health and disease: a survey. Pediatrics 37, 715, 1966.*

4. *Stiehm ER. Human neonatal immune capacity: the B, T, and monocyte/macrophage systems. In Hodes H, Kagan BM (eds). Pediatric Immunology, New York, Science and Medicine Publishing Co Inc, pp 75, 1979.*

5. *Penkoske P, Rowe R, Freedom R, Trusler G. The future of heart and heart-lung transplantation in children. Heart Transplant 3, 233, 1984.*

6. *Bailey LL, Nehlsen-Cannarella SL, Concepcion W, Jolley WB. Baboon-to-human cardiac xenotransplantation in a neonate. JAMA 254, 3321, 1985.*

7. *Bailey LL, Nehlsen-Cannarella S. Observations on cardiac xenotransplantation. Transplant Proc 18 (Suppl 2), 88, 1986.*

8. *Volpe J. Brain death determination in the newborn. Pediatrics 80, 293, 1987.*

9. *Ashwal S, Schneider S. Brain death in children: part I. Pediatr Neurol 3, 5, 1987.*

10. *Ashwal S, Schneider S. Brain death in children: part II. Pediatr Neurol 3, 69, 1987.*

1.1.2. The Current Application of Lung and Combined Heart and Lung Transplantation

SW Jamieson

*Cardiovascular and Thoracic Surgery,
Minnesota Heart and Lung Institute
University of Minnesota
Minneapolis, USA*

Introduction

It is now six years since the first successful combined heart and lung transplant was performed. The clinical applicability of this operation is now better understood, and enough patients have undergone operation to provide additional information on patient selection and long-term follow-up. Progress has been made in preservation of the lungs so as to allow safe long-distance transport, and the management of immunosuppression and the diagnosis of rejection are better understood.

It is now appreciated that successful transplantation of the lungs can take place without concomitant transplantation of the heart, and both single and double lung transplantation have found a place in clinical practice. This paper will address some of the lessons learned in the last six years, and focus on certain of the remaining problems in the transplantation of pulmonary tissue, with or without the heart.

Historical Review

Experimental heart and lung transplantation was first carried out by Demikhov (1), who performed transplants in dogs without the use of hypothermia or cardiopulmonary bypass, using a careful sequence of anastomoses to perform transplantation with a very short period of cerebral ischemia. Although only two of a total of 67 experimental animals survived for a maximum of five days, it was demonstrated that survival could be obtained after this operation.

Further experiments in dogs using central cooling and circulatory arrest led to survival periods of up to 22 hours following implantation of the heart and lungs (2,3). In dogs, the complete denervation of the heart and lungs following transplantation leads to an abnormal respiratory pattern incompatible with survival. However, in 1963 it was demonstrated that denervation of both lungs was compatible with a normal respiratory pattern in primates (4), and the ability of primates (but not dogs) to survive bilateral lung denervation was confirmed by Nakae (5). Subsequently Castaneda performed combined heart-lung autotransplantation in baboons and demonstrated prolonged survival (6,7).

The first human heart-lung transplant operation was performed in 1968 by Cooley in a two month old infant with an atrio-ventricular canal (8). The child had spontaneous respiration postoperatively, but died 14 hours after the operation of respiratory insufficiency. The second clinical heart-lung transplant was performed by Lillehei in 1970 in a 43 year old emphysematous patient who died of respiratory failure eight days postoperatively (9). In 1971, Barnard performed the third clinical combined heart-lung transplantation in a patient with chronic obstructive airways disease. The patient lived for 23 days (10).

The disappointing early clinical experience with both lung (11) and heart-lung transplantation confined further developmental work to the laboratory.

The discovery of cyclosporine A (12) provided the first real advance in immunosuppression for twenty years. Its use in the laboratory in 1978 showed that it was a powerful immunosuppressive agent for cardiac transplantation in primates (13). This led to the first use of cyclosporine in clinical cardiac transplantation in December 1980 (14).

Since cyclosporine differs from conventionally used immunosuppressive agents in allowing near normal healing of the tracheal anastomosis, it seemed appropriate to reinvestigate experimental combined heart and lung transplantation using this drug, since airway dehiscence would be less likely.

Using cyclosporine, extended survival was then reported in monkeys after auto- and allo- heart-lung-transplantation (15). A simplified operative method limited the number of anastomoses (16). Heart-lung transplantation was then reintroduced at Stanford University in 1981 with clinical success (17, 18). The first recipient in this series died recently of unrelated causes, five years after her operation.

This relatively new therapy has now been enthusiastically embraced by perhaps half a dozen centers, who combined have performed more than 150 operations (19). The experience of some of these centers has confirmed that this remains a difficult undertaking, both technically and in terms of post-operative management, and that extensive experience in cardiac transplantation is probably a requirement for success in this area.

Recipients

Classification of suitable recipients for heart-lung or lung transplantation can be conveniently divided into those with primarily cardiac disease who develop pulmonary hypertension, or those with primarily pulmonary disease who may not subsequently develop right heart failure ("cor pulmonale").

In the first category, those with Eisenmenger's syndrome form the biggest group. These patients cannot be treated with cardiac transplantation alone since the normal donor heart would fail when faced with the degree of irreversible pulmonary hypertension that had occurred during the patient's growth. Patients who develop pulmonary hypertension as a result of other cardiac disorders (e.g. end-stage valve disease) are usually beyond the suitable age limit for the operation once pulmonary changes occur. However, treatment for patients in these categories is only by combined heart and lung transplantation.

There are many patients with end-stage pulmonary failure, with or without cor pulmonale, who face certain death, and no other therapy is currently available except transplantation. It used to be thought that effective transplantation of pulmonary tissue could only be achieved with transplantation of the heart and lung block, but recent successful experience with clinical transplantation of either one or both lungs (20,21) has demonstrated that concomitant transplantation of the heart is not always necessary. Although heart-lung transplantation has been successfully undertaken in patients with chronic parenchymal lung disease, it may be that pulmonary transplantation is more suitable here if right ventricular failure has not occurred.

Since single lung transplantation has the disadvantage that one diseased lung will remain, this procedure should be reserved for the treatment of the pulmonary fibroses. This operation has the advantage of an easier surgical technique than either heart-lung or double lung transplantation, and the avoidance of concomitant cardiac transplantation. In addition, the operation can often be carried out without cardiopulmonary bypass. However, application of single lung transplantation is contraindicated where there is pulmonary sepsis (e.g. cystic fibrosis) since the remaining lung would persist as a source of infection after operation. Double lung transplantation is the operation of choice here, as it is for emphysematous conditions. In emphysema, single lung transplantation would result in disproportionate expansion of the remaining recipient lung and a subsequent ventilation-perfusion defect.

To what degree right ventricular failure would be reversible after lung transplantation remains unanswered. It is the author's opinion that moderate right heart failure will reverse, and that right ventricular dysfunction in the face of severe pulmonary hypertension should not necessarily be a contraindication to isolated pulmonary transplantation provided severe tricuspid regurgitation is not present.

Recipients for lung or heart-lung transplantation must have a severely restricted effort tolerance (New York Heart Association Class III or IV) leading to a poor quality of life, or a short life expectancy. Apart from cardiopulmonary impairment, the general physical condition of the recipient should be well maintained. Younger patients (less than 45 years old) without secondary renal or hepatic dysfunction are likely to have a lower morbidity, mortality and more successful rehabilitation, and in view of the great surfeit of suitable recipients for combined heart and lung transplantation compared with the available donors, this is probably a realistic upper age limit for recipient acceptance. The age limit for single lung transplantation may be higher, and, of course, criteria for acceptance in any program will ultimately hinge on the ratio of suitable recipients to available donors.

Previous extensive thoracic or cardiac surgery is associated with a higher mortality because of the increased risk of peri-operative bleeding; consequently patients with previous surgery are not currently accepted for operation. Other contraindications include poorly controlled diabetes mellitus, collagen vascular disease, active peptic ulceration, systemic sepsis, or a bleeding diathesis that cannot be reversed by administration of blood products. Careful psychological assessment should be performed.

Donors

The acquisition of suitable donors for heart-lung transplantation remains the most significant restriction to the wider application of this operation.

Most organ donors occur as the result of head trauma or vascular cerebral injury. Because of the necessity of ventilatory support, the lungs are prone to infection and atelectasis, but may also incur other complications such as neurogenic pulmonary edema and fat embolism. The tendency towards pulmonary edema is exacerbated by the difficulty of fluid balance in the presence of diabetes insipidus. In addition, urgent intubation may be necessary after fatal cerebral trauma, and this may be carried out in less than sterile conditions; the donor may have aspirated gastric contents; and subsequent management may not be optimal if it is clear to medical personnel that there is no likelihood of survival. Thus, the early onset of pneumonia is common in potential donors, eliminating their consideration for the transplantation of the lungs. This vulnerability to lung injury reduces the number of potential donors to a fraction of those used for liver, kidney, and heart donation.

In general terms, donors must meet the criteria of brain death and be free of cardiac or pulmonary impairment. Currently, selected donors are less than 45 years of age, and have no evidence of a penetrating chest injury or serious lung contusion. The chest radiograph and electrocardiogram must be normal. Short periods of ventilatory support are desirable in order to reduce the possibility of exogenous bacterial and fungal contamination of the trachea and bronchi, but donors ventilated for up to five days have been used successfully when pulmonary care has been optimal.

Peak inflation pressures on the respirator should be less than 30 cm H_2O with a minute ventilation of 15 cc/kg at eight breaths per minute. Adequate gas exchange is mandatory, with an arterial oxygen tension of more than 100 mmHg on an FiO_2 of 40%.

Matching of the donor is carried out by blood type and size. To match for size, measurement of the maximal thoracic diameter and the height of the thoracic cavity are compared between the chest radiographs of the donor and ABO compatible recipients. Although this matching technique for size is somewhat less objective, it is convenient and effective. Ideally, the donor thorax should be slightly smaller than that of the recipient to avoid postoperative atelectasis that would inevitably follow the inability of larger lungs to expand within a smaller chest cavity. Prospective cross-matching of donor lymphocytes against recipient serum is necessary for recipients who have tested positive against a random panel of lymphocytes.

Once the potential donor is deemed provisionally acceptable for heart-lung or lung donation, close liaison between the donating hospital and the transplant unit is continued, in order to maintain the donor organs in optimal condition. The potential heart-lung recipient is admitted to the hospital and prepared for surgery. Central venous and arterial pressure lines are inserted in the donor, who is placed on a warming blanket to prevent deterioration of cardiac function from hypothermia. The central venous pressure is kept as low as possible by fluid restriction and diuresis, provided hemodynamic stability is maintained. If excessive urine output occurs because of diabetes insipidus, vasopressin or desmopressin administration may be required. Fluid replacement should consist of Ringer's lactate at a volume to replace the previous hour's urine output, plus 30 to 50 cc's to cover insensible losses. Hemodynamic instability due to diuresis-induced hypovolemia should be partly corrected by fluid replacement and partly by manipulation of the peripheral vascular resistance using the alpha-adrenergic agonists phenylephrine or metaraminol.

In order to prevent the spill-over of gastro-esophageal contents or oropharyngeal secretions into the airways, a nasogastric sump tube is inserted and connected to low pressure wall suction. Careful attention is directed towards clearing pulmonary secretions with regular, gentle aspiration via the endotracheal tube. Retrieved aspirate is sent for culture and direct examination, and the results communicated to the recipient unit when available. The tracheal aspirate should not show gross contamination, particularly with candida.

Positive end-expiratory pressure of 3-5 cm H_2O is maintained to help prevent atelectasis, and the inspired oxygen fraction kept at 40% or lower to maintain a pO_2 greater than 100 mm Hg.

Pulmonary Preservation

Until recently, it was thought mandatory to bring the donor to the recipient site, as techniques for preservation of the lungs were unreliable. The restriction of donors that resulted from this requirement forced the use of preservation methods, and long-distant procurement is currently used by all major teams involved in heart-lung transplantation. However, this poses additional problems of timing of the recipient operation and ensuring a good size match, as well as the inability to thoroughly screen the donor before initiating the recipient operation.

The lungs are unique in having both a dual blood supply (pulmonary and bronchial arteries) and a connection to the atmosphere (bronchial tree). Because of the insulating nature of the alveolar structure, simple topical cooling is an ineffective method of cooling the substance of the lungs (22). Cooling via the airways has been demonstrated to be detrimental (23). Three methods of preservation have now been used clinically: flush perfusion of the pulmonary arteries, with subsequent static cold immersion (24, 25); cooling the donor systematically with cardiopulmonary bypass (bronchial artery and pulmonary artery cooling), with subsequent cold immersion (26); and the maintenance of a warm, ventilated preparation (the "Robicsek technique" (27), where the heart continues to beat in a closed circuit, with coronary sinus return being provided to the lungs (28).

All of these methods have produced satisfactory preservation for four hours or more, though attempted preservation at the present time for much longer periods would probably be unwise. No doubt, continued efforts will refine these techniques for the future, though it is likely that simplicity will be the key to the continued use of a certain technique. The simplicity of hypothermic flushing of the lungs via the pulmonary artery has led to the routine use of this technique at our institution.

The optimal composition of the pulmonary artery perfusate remains unclear. Cardioplegic type solutions, although satisfactory for myocardial preservation, are unsatisfactory in experimental lung preservation, and attention has centered around the use of a modification of Collins' solution that is used in renal allograft preservation. This solution, which has an intracellular type composition, is modified by the addition of 50% dextrose (65 cc/liter of solution) and magnesium sulfate (8 mEq) added to increase osmolarity and preserve membrane integrity (29). The resultant solution has been used clinically as a cold pulmonary artery flush, with successful results for ischemic times of up to four and one half hours.

Whole donor cooling, using cardiopulmonary bypass, is an alternative method of achieving lung hypothermia, with or without pulmonary artery flushing. Once cardiopulmonary bypass is established, cooling to around 12°C may be achieved within 15 to 45 minutes of the onset of bypass. At this temperature, the organs are harvested and stored in cold donor blood without further preparation. Preservation times of up to four hours again appear to be satisfactory using this method. This core cooling technique is attractive because experimental work suggests that cooling with normokalemic whole blood may be the most satisfactory solution for lung preservation (30), but the technique is noticeably more cumbersome than a simple pulmonary artery flush, requiring more personnel and additional equipment. In addition, the effect of core cooling on other organs being harvested remains unknown, and though it is unlikely to be detrimental, the technique is met with suspicion by many harvesting teams. In addition, the theoretical possibility exists that activation of complement by the polymers of the extracorporeal circuit (31) could lead to the sequestration of neutrophils within the pulmonary circulation and to lung injury (32).

Operation

There have been no new observations regarding the performance of the operation since the initial description of the technique (29). The salient features of the operation are the preservation of the vagus, phrenic and recurrent laryngeal nerves, and obtaining of.

All the technical challenge of the operation lies in the removal of the old organs. The diseased heart and lungs are excised separately in order to protect the phrenic nerves. The operation proceeds via a median sternotomy. Pleural and pericardial adhesions are divided prior to heparinization and the thymic fat pad excised, avoiding injury to the phrenic nerves, to expose the great vessels. Following the administration of heparin, cardiopulmonary bypass is established using bicaval cannulation and high ascending aortic return. The caval tapes are then snared, the aorta cross-clamped and the heart allowed to fibrillate. The excision of the heart is performed as for heart transplantation. A substantial atrial cuff is left in situ, the left atrial remnant of which is later excised during the bilateral pneumonectomy.

Attention is next directed to the left lung. The left atrium is divided vertically in the oblique sinus, allowing the separation of right and left pulmonary veins. An incision in the pericardium just anterior to the pulmonary veins, and posterior to the phrenic nerve frees the anterior aspect of the left pulmonary veins and the lung is removed following division of the left pulmonary artery and the pleural reflections. The left main bronchus is identified, the bronchial arteries are controlled by cautery or clips, the bronchus is stapled and divided, and the lung removed. The right lung is excised in a similar manner, leaving the tracheo-bronchial junction, aorta, and right atrium as the sites for subsequent anastomoses. Meticulous hemostasis of the posterior mediastinum is performed at this time, avoiding damage to the vagus nerve.

The donor operation is coordinated with other organ procurement teams. Following inspection of the heart and lungs through a median sternotomy incision, circumferential mobilization of the innominate vein, aorta and superior and inferior vena cavea is performed. The thymic fat pad is removed, and the pericardium is resected down to the level of the pulmonary veins, including the phrenic nerves. The trachea is exposed between the superior vena cava and ascending aorta.

The other organ procurement teams now mobilize the abdominal organs (liver, kidneys, pancreas) to be used for transplantation.

At the time of harvesting, heparin (3 mg/kg) is administered intravenously and infusion lines for the pulmonary artery flushing solution and for cardioplegia are placed in the main pulmonary artery and aorta respectively. The innominate vein and superior vena cava are ligated and divided. The inferior vena cava is clamped above the diaphragm and the heart allowed to empty. The distal ascending aorta is cross-clamped and cold cardioplegic solution (1000 cc) is instilled into the aortic root. Pulmonary artery flushing is commenced, using 60 cc/kg of modified Collins' solution infused into the main pulmonary artery over a period of four minutes with a roller pump. As soon as pulmonary artery flushing and instillation of cardioplegia commence, the tip of the left atrial appendage is amputated, and the inferior vena cava divided above the clamp to vent the heart. Additional topical cooling with copious amounts of 4°C cold Ringer's lactate solution aids the induction of hypothermia. Occasional manual ventilation is continued during pulmonary artery flushing, using unheated room air.

After completion of the infusions, the aorta is transected below the cross-clamp. The trachea is mobilized and stapled with the lungs held in a position of 50% inflation. Heart-lung harvesting is then completed by division of the posterior pleural reflections and pulmonary ligaments anterior to the esophagus. The organs are transferred to a container filled with cold Ringer's solution, which is then sealed and stored in a similar sterile box. This is then transferred into an insulated sealed transportation box containing cold 4°C electrolyte solution mixed with ice.

In the recipient operation room the donor organs are removed from their storage container and transferred to the operative field. Specimens for culture are taken from donor and recipient tracheas. The recipient trachea is trimmed one ring above the carina and the bronchial stumps excised. The donor trachea is divided at a similar level. The lungs are then placed into their respective cavities below the phrenic nerve pedicles, and the tracheal anastomosis performed, using a single continuous suture of polypropylene. During implantation, the heart and lungs are protected by continuous irrigation with cold electrolyte solution. The right atrial and aortic anastomoses are then completed, after opening the donor right atrium to accommodate the anastomosis and trimming the donor aorta to a suitable length.

Air is removed from the heart, ventilation recommenced, and the aortic cross-clamp removed. Upon completion of rewarming and the resumption of satisfactory cardiac activity, cardiopulmonary bypass is discontinued, with the patient ventilated on an FiO$_2$ of 40%, with 5 cm of positive end-expiratory pressure and an isoproterenol infusion to maintain the heart rate at 100-120 beats/minute. Following satisfactory hemostasis and the implantation of temporary pacing wires, the chest is closed with mediastinal and pleural drainage.

Immunosuppression

Various immunosuppressive protocols have been used in heart and lung transplantation, but at the present time we favor a triple therapy made up of steroids, cyclosporine VA and azathioprine. Perioperative steroids are administered as for heart transplantation, in a dose of 500 mgs i.v. immediately after releasing the aortic cross-clamp, then 125 mgs. every 8 hours for three doses. Further steroid therapy is withheld for two weeks, in order to allow healing of the tracheal anastomosis. After this time, immunosuppression with steroids is reinstituted at a dose of 0.2 mgs/kg given orally, and maintained indefinitely. Cyclosporine is given only orally, at an initial dose of 6mg/kg. Serum levels are then monitored, seeking to maintain trough levels of approximately 200 ng/ml for the first two weeks, then reducing this slightly if rejection has not been encountered. Intravenous administration of cyclosporine is not used at our center because of the potential added nephrotoxicity, more likely in these patients because of their pre-existing renal impairment as a result of venous congestion. Azathioprine is given orally at 2 mgs/kg, though this dose may need to be modified if leucopenia results.

Results of Transplantation

Immediately after transplantation, all afferent and efferent nerve supply is lost, lymphatic drainage disrupted, and the bronchial arterial supply served. Surprisingly little functional derangement results from this.

Because of the loss of lymphatic drainage the lungs readily develop pulmonary edema and a conscious effort must be made to minimize the administration of fluids until the patient has regained pre-operative weight. During surgery, pump priming volumes and intravenously administered fluids are kept to a minimum. Renal impairment is commonly seen in recipients preoperatively, and worsened postoperatively by cardiopulmonary bypass, and the toxic effects of cyclosporine. This may make fluid balance difficult to achieve, and plasma ultrafiltration with or without dialysis is often necessary early postoperatively and should be used aggressively.

In the first few days after operation, an impairment of gas exchange may be seen, accompanied by diffuse radiological opacity on the chest radiograph

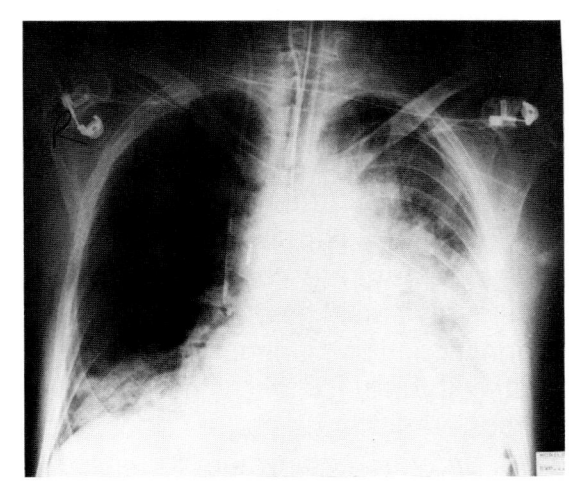

Fig. 5 Chest X-ray on the third post-operative day revealing an example of reperfusion reaction.

1. Transplantation

(Figure 5, 33). This is usually the result of fluid overload and the loss of lymphatics, but may be exacerbated by inadequate preservation. Once pulmonary edema is allowed to occur, subsequent removal of fluid may still result in a continued capillary leak syndrome manifesting itself in all ways similar to other types of adult respiratory distress, with the exception that it will resolve within a few days if supportive therapy can be maintained. Prolonged intubation and respiratory support will be necessary, administered with positive end-expiratory pressure less than 10 centimeters of water to protect the tracheal anastomosis. High peak inspiratory pressures may be experienced, and these may be minimized by rapid ventilation with lower tidal volumes. Fluid replacement is with colloid solutions or blood rather than crystalloids, and the hemoglobin is allowed to rise to the upper limits of normal so as to increase plasma oncotic pressure and oxygen carrying capacity.

Most patients are extubated on the first postoperative day and maintain satisfactory spontaneous ventilation. While intubated, pulmonary toilet is performed using soft suction catheters. Sputum accumulation in the denervated lung will not excite coughing, and chest physiotherapy is required to aid expectoration. After extubation, vigorous breathing exercises, supported by physiotherapy, are commenced. Daily chest x-rays must be obtained, and any suggestion of pulmonary edema treated rapidly. The pulmonary lymphatics regenerate after about ten days, and the requirement for rigorous fluid restriction then abates. Radiological opacity after approximately one week is usually the result of rejection,

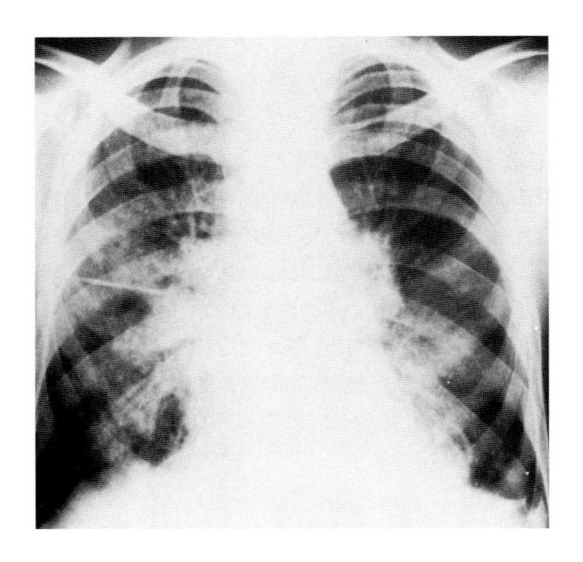

Fig. 6 Acute isolated lung rejection on the 12th post-operative day.

and accompanied by fever and leucocytosis (Figure 6). It is now well documented that the lungs may reject independently (34, 35, 36) and usually before the heart. Diagnosis of rejection is difficult because, unlike the heart, tissue for histological study cannot be easily obtained. Open lung biopsy provides substantial risk for the sick and immunosuppressed patient, and certainly cannot be performed repetitively. Biopsy by bronchoscopy may be helpful, though small specimens are obtained, and non-specific changes are often seen. We do not favor early bronchoscopy because of the risk of interference with the tracheal anastomosis. The diagnosis of rejection is therefore made by the time of onset of diffuse, often fluffy radiological opacities on chest radiograph, and by exclusion of infective causes. A hallmark of pulmonary rejection is that marked changes on the chest radiograph are accompanied by minor impairment, and are usually only slowly progressive.

Treatment of rejection depends on its severity and timing. Concern for the tracheal anastomosis encourages the avoidance of large dose bolus steroid therapy in the early postoperative period if possible, and initially attempts are made to optimize non-steroid immunosuppression by increasing the dose of cyclosporine to ensure adequate circulating levels and bringing forward the introduction of oral low dose prednisone (0.2 mg/kg). If these measures are not accompanied by rapid clinical improvement, bolus methylprednisolone (1 mg intravenously, daily times three) is administered. In refractory cases, antilymphocyte globulin may be added, with the aim of reducing the T-lymphocyte count to 5% of total lymphocytes.

Just as denervation of the heart is compatible with normal exercise, denervation of the lungs also appears to be without significance (37). Respiration continues in a normal pattern, and will increase in rate and depth with the demands of stress and activity. Regulation of respiration in the human apparently depends little on pulmonary afferent nerves, and early postoperatively is not related to blood gas levels. It is likely that chest wall receptors play a significant role in the regulation of respiration.

The loss of the bronchial arterial supply is also without apparent sequelae, and the tracheal anastomosis heals well, probably contributed to by the rich coronary artery-bronchial artery collateral circulation (18). We have not found it necessary to use omentum to reinforce the tracheal anastomosis in combined heart-lung transplantation where there is no source of arterialized blood to the donor airway (38) although the pulmonary artery supplies de-oxygenated blood to this site (39).

Broad-spectrum systemic antibacterial cover (we currently favor cephamandole and nafcillin) is commenced at anesthetic induction. Antibiotics are continued until the chest drains are removed. After extubation, oral nystatin and low dose cotrimoxazole are commenced in order to provide prophylaxis against oral candida and pulmonary pneumocystis infestation.

Late Postoperative Management

Following discharge from hospital, patients are reviewed twice weekly in order to adjust immunosuppression and to provide continued surveillance for infection and rejection. Frequent chest radiographs are performed, and renal function and cyclosporine levels monitored. By three months, patients tend to be well rehabilitated and, if stable, will be allowed to return to their homes.

In the early post-transplant period, pulmonary function tests show a restrictive ventilatory defect which improves slowly over the first 12 months. More ominously, a mixed obstructive and restrictive airway picture may develop at any time after six weeks following transplantation, signifying the development of a panbronchitis which can progress to an obliterative bronchiolitis and bronchiectasis (40). This condition, which is also a complication of bone marrow transplantation, but not of other organ grafts, is of unknown etiology, but may represent an abnormal response to viral infection, chronic rejection, or other host versus graft reaction. The most likely is injury by antibody.

Once established, the condition tends to deteriorate inexorably, although early diagnosis and treatment by high dose steroids may lead to its reversal or arrest (41). Symptomatically, patients present with a new cough or dyspnea. Examination reveals audible coarse crackles and occasional rhonchi. Hypoxemia and a mixed obstructive-restrictive ventilatory defect are found on pulmonary function testing. Chest radiography and sputum culture allow infection to be excluded. The chest radiograph is usually clear, although peribronchial thickening and lower zone micronodular opa-cities may be seen. Treatment of this condition is by augmentation of oral steroids. In late, irreversible disease, retransplantation may be necessary.

Other late complications, in common with heart transplantation, include hypertension, weight gain, opportunistic infections and progressive cyclosporin nephrotoxicity. Hypertension is managed by careful control of cyclosporin levels, diuretics and vasodilator therapy. Beta blockade is avoided because of its bronchospastic effects and negative chronotropy and inotropy.

Results

The International Registry of Heart Transplantation has collated data from 14 world centres that have performed a total of 163 combined heart-lung transplants (19). World-wide, an early operative mortality of 40% has been experienced. Early death is associated with prolonged periods of cardiopulmonary bypass and extensive hemorrhage. Previous extensive cardiac or thoracic surgery is associated with increased risk because of the presence of pleural and pericardial adhesions and subsequent major blood loss. Other deaths recorded in the registry are related to opportunistic infections, leading to systemic sepsis and multiple organ failure. Distant organ procurement appears to be associated with an increased mortality, probably related to inadequate lung preservation.

Fourteen single lung transplants have now been performed by the Toronto group. There were 11 operative survivors, and as of the time of this report, nine patients were alive, two having died of lymphoma and rejection respectively. (See also chapter 1.1.3.) Seven double lung transplants have been performed by the same group. Six of these patients remain alive, though follow-up is short.

Late Results

One year survival in the original Stanford series was 64%, falling to 55% at three years (41). Data from the International Registry for Heart Transplantation have shown an actuarial one year survival world-wide of 55.4%, falling to 51.9% at two years (19).

Of the patients surviving the perioperative period in the Stanford series, nearly $1/3$ developed late disability as a consequence of obliterative bronchiolitis (40,41). The etiology of this condition remains obscure. These late sequelae have included bronchiolitis obliterans, pulmonary vascular disease, and pulmonary fibrosis. Progressive intimal proliferation also occurs in the coronary arteries of the heart-lung transplant, and eventually cardiac failure and myocardial infarction can be anticipated in some recipients.

The precise etiology of these changes is unclear, though they are likely to be due to rejection. In the author's practice, immunosuppression for the last two years has been changed to the triple therapy outlined above, and although it is too early to make a definite statement, minimal late sequelae of the sort described above have been encountered since.

Future

Successful heart-lung transplantation has lead to a great improvement in the quality of life of recipients and the technique offers promise as a treatment of end-stage lung and heart disease. Further progress will be needed in a number of areas in order to reduce postoperative morbidity and mortality, and increase the application of this form of therapy.

Careful recipient selection will help to reduce perioperative mortality, by excluding patients with previous extensive cardiothoracic surgery and those with severe concurrent systemic disease. Wider application of the technique will depend upon the supply of donors. Increasing public awareness may increase the number of donors available but, more importantly, improvement in protection methods for the heart-lung bloc will enable maximal utilization of the present donor pool. The diagnosis of rejection and its differentiation from an infection or reimplantation process remains difficult. Studies of bronchial-alveolar lavage cell content are not sufficiently sensitive or specific at present, and further research is required into the diagnostic differentiation of the postoperative pulmonary infiltrate. An alternative to cyclosporine A is being sought to prevent the long-term nephrotoxic consequences of the use of this drug. Improved immunosuppression may prevent the late development of obliterative bronchiolitis.

References

1. *Demikhov VP: Some essential points of the techniques of transplantation of the heart, lungs and other organs. Medgiz State Press for Medical Literature in Moscow, 1960, translated from Russian by Basil Haigh, Consultant's Bureau, New York, 1962.*

2. *Neptune WB, Cookson BA, Bailey CP, Appler R, Rajkowski F. Complete homologous heart transplantation. Arch Surg 66, 174, 1954.*

3. *Webb WR, Howard HS. Cardiopulmonary transplantation. Surg Forum 8, 313, 1957.*

4. *Haglin J, Telander RL, Muzzal RE, Kiser JC, Strobel CJ. Comparison of lung autotransplantation in the primate and dog. Surg Forum 14, 196, 1963.*

5. *Nakae S, Webb WR, Theodorides J, Sugg WL. Respiratory function following cardiopulmonary denervation in dog, cat and monkey. Surg Gynecol Obstet 125, 1285, 1967.*

6. *Castaneda AR, Arnar O, Schmidt-Habelman P, Moller JH, Zamora R. Cardiopulmonary autotransplantation in primates. J Cardiovasc Surg 37, 523, 1972.*

7. *Casteneda AR, Zamora R, Schmidt-Habelman P, Hornung J, Murphy W, Ponto D, Moller JH. Cardiopulmonary autotransplantation in primates (baboons): late functional results. Surgery 72, 1074, 1972.*

8. *Cooley DA, Bloodwell RD, Hallman GL, Nora JJ, Harrison GM, Leachman RD. Organ transplantation for advanced cardiopulmonary disease. Ann Thorac Surg 8, 30, 1969.*

1. Transplantation

9. Lillehei CW. In discussion of Wildevuur CRH, Benfield RA. A review of 23 human lung transplantations by 20 surgeons. Ann Thorac Surg 9, 489, 1970.

10. Barnard CN, Cooper DKC. Clinical transplantation of the heart. A review of 13 years personal experience. J R Soc Med 74, 670, 1981.

11. Wildevuur CRH, Benfield RA. A review of 23 human lung transplantations by 20 surgeons. Ann Thorac Surg 9, 489, 1970.

12. Borel JF, Feurer C, Magnee C, Stahelin H. Biological effects of cyclosporine A: a new antilymphocytic agent. Ag Action 6, 468, 1976.

13. Jamieson SW, Burton NA, Oyer PE, Reitz BA, Stinson EB, and Shumway NE. Cardiac allograft survival in primates treated with cyclosporine A. Lancet 1, 545, 1979.

14. Oyer PE, Stinson EB, Jamieson SW, Hunt SA, Billingham M, Scott W, Bieber CP, Reitz BA, Shumway NE. Cyclosporine A in cardiac allografting: a preliminary experience. Transpl Proc 15, 1247, 1983.

15. Reitz BA, Burton NA, Jamieson SW, Bieber CP, Pennock JL, Stinson EB, Shumway NE. Heart and lung transplantation: auto-and allo-transplantation in primates with extended survival. J Thorac Cardiovasc Surg 80, 360. 1980.

16. Reitz BA, Pennock JL, Shumway NE. Simplified operative method for heart and lung transplantation. J Surg Research 31, 1, 1981.

17. Jamieson SW, Reitz BA, Oyer PE, Billingham M, Modry D, Baldwin J, Stinson EB, Hunt S, Theodore J, Bieber CP, Shumway NE. Combined heart and lung transplantation. Lancet 1, 1130, 1983.

18. Jamieson SW, Stinson EB, Oyer PE, Reitz BA, Baldwin J, Modry D, Dawkins K, Theodore J, Hunt S, Shumway NE. Heart-lung transplantation for irreversible pulmonary hypertension. Ann Thorac Surg 38, 554, 1984.

19. Heart Transplant Registry of the International Society for Heart Transplantation. 1987.

20. Dark JH, Patterson GA, Al-Jilaihawai, Hsu H, Egan T, Cooper JD. Experimental en-bloc double-lung transplantation. Ann Thorac Surg 42, 394, 1986.

21. Cooper JD, Pearon FG, Patterson GA, Todd TRJ, Ginsberg RJ, Goldberg M, Demajo WAP. Technique of successful lung transplantation in humans. J Thorac Cardiovasc Surg 93, 173, 1987.

22. Schuler S, Warnecke H, Hetzer R, Loitz F, Topalidis T, Borst HG. The limits of cold ischemia for preservation of the lung. J Heart Transpl 4, 70, 1984.

23. Haverich A, Scott WC, Jamieson SW. Twenty years of lung preservation - a review. J Heart Transplant 4, 234, 1985.

24. Jamieson SW, Starkey T, Sakakibara N, Baldwin JC. Procurement of organs for combined heart-lung transplantation. Transpl Proc 18, 616, 1986.

25. Starkey T, Sakakibara N, Hagberg RC, Tazelaar HD, Baldwin JC, Jamieson SW. Successful six-hour cardiopulmonary preservation with simple hypothermic crystalloid flush. J Heart Transplant 5, 291, 1986.

26. Hardesty RL, Griffith BP. Procurement for combined heart-lung transplantation: bilateral thoracotomy with sternal transection, cardiopulmonary bypass and profound hypothermia. J Thorac Cardiovasc Surg 89, 795, 1985.

27. Robicsek F, Tam W, Dougherty HK, Robicsek M. The stabilized autoperfusing heart-lung preparation as a vehicle for extracorporeal preservation. Transpl Proc 1, 834, 1969.

28. Ladowski JS, Kapelanski DP, Teodori MF, Stevenson WC, Hardesty RL, Griffith BP. Use of autoperfusion for distant procurement of heart-lung allografts. Heart Transplant 4, 330, 1985.

29. Jamieson SW, Stinson EB, Oyer PE, Baldwin JC, Shumway NE. Operative technique for heart-lung transplantation. J Thorac Cardiovasc Surg 87, 930, 1984.

30. Modry DL, Walpoth BW, Cohen RG, Seifert SC, Bleese NM, Warnecke H, Bieber CP, Billingham ME, Jamieson SW, Shumway NE. Heart-lung preservation in the dog followed by lung transplantation: a new model for the assessment of lung preservation. J Heart Transpl 2, 287, 1983.

31. Kirklin JK, Westaby S, Blackstone EH, Chenoweth DE, Pacifico AD. Complement and the damaging effects of cardiopulmonary bypass. J Thorac Cardiovasc Surg Vol 86, 845, 1983.

32. Till GO, Johnson KJ, Kunkel R, Ward PA. Intravascular activation of complement and acute lung injury. J Clin Invest 69, 1126, 1982.

33. Chiles C, Guthaner DF, Jamieson SW, Stinson EB, Oyer PE, Silverman JF. Heart-lung transplantation. The post-operative chest radiograph. Radiology 154, 29, 1985.

34. Scott WC, Haverich A, Billingham ME, Dawkins KD, Jamieson SW. Lethal lung rejection without significant cardiac rejection in primate heart-lung allotransplantation. J Heart Transpl 4, 33, 1984.

35. Jamieson SW. Recent developments in heart and heart-lung transplantation. Transpl Proc 17, 199, 1985.

36. McGregor CGA, Baldwin JC, Jamieson SW, Billingham ME, Yousem SA, Burke CM, Oyer PE, Stinson EB, Shumway NE. Isolated pulmonary rejection after combined heart-lung transplantation. J Thorac Cardiovasc Surg 90, 623, 1985.

37. Theodore J, Jamieson SW, Burke CM, Reitz BA, Stinson EB, Van Kessel A, Dawkins KD, Herran JJ, Oyer PE, Hunt SA, Shumway NE, Robin ED. Physiological aspects of human heart-lung transplantation: pulmonary status of the post-transplanted lung. Chest 86, 349, 1984.

38. Lima O, Goldberg M, Peters WJ, Ayabe H, Townsend E, Cooper JD. Bronchial omentopexy in canine lung transplantation. J Thorac Cardiovasc Surg 83, 418, 1982.

39. Ladowski JS, Hardesty RL, Griffith BP: Pulmonary artery blood supply to the supracarinal trachea. J Heart Transpl 4, 40, 1984.

40. Burke CM, Theodore J, Dawkins KD, Yousem SA, Blank M, Billingham ME, van Kessel A, Jamieson SW, Oyer PE, Baldwin JC, Stinson EB, Shumway NE, Robin ED. Post-transplant obliterative bronchiolitis and other late sequelae in human heart-lung transplantation. Chest 86, 824, 1984.

41. Jamieson SW, Dawkins KD, Burke C, Baldwin JW, Yousem S, Billingham ME, Hunt SA, Reitz BA, Theodore J, Oyer PE, Stinson EB, Shumway NE. Late results of combined heart-lung transplantation. Trans Proc 17, 212, 1985.

1. Transplantation

1.1.3. Clinical Experience with Unilateral and Bilateral Lung Transplantation - The Toronto Group Experience

RJ Ginsberg, GA Patterson, R Grossman, M Goldberg, V Maurer, TR Todd, JD Cooper, FG Pearson

Divisions of Thoracic Surgery and Cardiovascular Surgery, Department of Surgery, University of Toronto, Ontario, Canada

In 1951, Juvenelle et al (1) and Metras (2) both independently described pneumonectomy and successful reimplantation of a lung homograft in dogs. In 1954, Hardin and Kittle (3) used the dog model to confirm the feasibility of a single lung heterograft transplantation.

In 1963, Hardy (4) reported the first human single lung transplant. Although the patient survived for only 18 days, the feasibility of human single lung transplantation had been established. Subsequent to this, many centers performed single lung transplantation unsuccessfully.

The only moderate success was in 1971. Derom (5) transplanted a patient suffering from silicosis. That patient survived 10 months, the last two months out of hospital, only to die of chronic rejection and sepsis.

Prior to our first successful single lung transplantation in 1983, there had been at least 40 attempts without long-term clinical success.

The report of Reitz et al (6) of a successful heart-lung transplantation further demonstrated the fact that lung transplantation was feasible and would produce a functioning lung capable of normal gas exchange.

Our own efforts in lung transplantation began in 1963 with the development in our laboratories of a model to look at bronchial anastomotic healing, one of the major problems interfering with successful single lung transplantation. At that time, we demonstrated that normal bronchial revascularization takes up to six weeks in the dog model (7). Subsequent investigations demonstrated that this healing was adversely affected by corticosteroids (8). After a failure in our own center in 1978 (9) with a human single lung transplant patient due to sepsis and bronchial dehiscence, further efforts in our laboratories to accelerate bronchial revascularization developed the use of the omentum to protect the bronchial anastomosis (10). With the advent of newer immunosuppressive agents (cyclosporine and antilymphocyte globulin), early treatment with steroids was deemed not essential to the survival of the transplanted lung.

In 1982, we performed bilateral sequential lung transplantations in a patient suffering from acute paraquat poisoning and demonstrated that the use of omentum to protect the bronchial anastomosis would be successful.

While the patient died of chronic paraquat myopathy, both lungs survived and functioned normally (11).

With this experience in laboratory and human lung transplantation, we felt that a viable program could be developed for lung transplantation in highly selected patients with irreversible pulmonary disease. In 1983, we performed the first successful human lung transplantation to survive beyond 10 months (12).

Single Lung Transplantation

Recipient Criteria

Single lung transplantation is reserved for those patients with progressive pulmonary fibrosis. Such patients demonstrate desaturation on exercise, requiring chronic oxygen administration. The estimated survival for these patients is less than one year. These patients are fully assessed, both physically and psychologically. Significant complicating systemic disease or psychological imbalance frequently leads to rejection from the program. Patients requiring corticosteroid therapy are also rejected. The patient must be less than 60 years of age and have relatively normal cardiac function. A cardiorespiratory rehabilitation program is instituted once they are accepted for transplantation.

Donor Selection

The potential donor is screened for underlying disease, including diabetes, fulminating sepsis, pre-existing pulmonary disease, and hypertension. A match between donor and recipient with regards size is important (within 20 kg or 0.5 m^2). The estimated total lung capacity should match within 500 ml, as measured by the transverse chest diameter at the dome of the diaphragm and the vertical dimension from the apex to the highest part of the diaphragm. Histocompatibility matching is limited to ABO. Bronchoscopy and assessment of pre-existing infection is carried out. Antibiotics are given to the donor if required by gram stain analysis of bronchial washings and brushings. Gas exchange is estimated and a minimum of PaO$_2$ of greater than 30 torr at an FiO$_2$ of 100% on 5 cm H$_2$O PEEP is required. Prior to harvesting the lungs, all attempts are made to avoid pulmonary edema by restricting fluid administration.

Operative Procedure (13)

Early in our experience, the donors were transported to our center, both donor and recipient being harvested and transplanted in adjoining operating rooms. Presently, donor extraction is performed distantly. Initially, preservation of the organ was achieved simply by immersion in cold Collins' solution (4°C). Maximum allowable ischemic time is 4 hours. Recently, we have begun perfusing the lungs with PGE$_1$ and Euro-Collin's solution. The donor heart is extracted for a separate heart transplantation, before the lung is removed. Care must be taken to preserve a small cuff of left atrium on the donor lung.

For transplantation, we prefer the left lung, all things being easier. However, we have successfully transplanted two right lungs. An intrapericardial pneumonectomy is performed on the recipient, preserving length on the pulmonary artery, veins and bronchus. In most cases, one lung anesthesia is all that is required. However, if the recipient cannot tolerate one lung ventilation or clamping of the ipsilateral pulmonary artery, partial venoarterial bypass using femoral approach is instituted.

1. Transplantation

The transplant is completed by sequentially anastomosing the common atrial cuff, pulmonary artery and bronchus. The omentum, which previously has been harvested on a pedicle from the upper abdomen into the mediastinum, is then wrapped around the bronchial anastomosis.

Postoperative Care

Initial immunosuppression includes cyclosporine, azathioprine and antilymphocyte serum. Postoperatively, the patient is ventilated with early extubation, anticipated according to usual criteria.

Rejection is difficult to diagnose on clinical grounds. However, we rely mainly on chest X-ray (hilar flare), fever, and increasing hypoxemia as criteria for rejection. Infection is ruled out wherever possible. As yet, bronchoalveolar lavage or lung scans have not been of significant value. Rejection is treated by intravenous boluses of methylprednisone.

Ultimately, chronic immunosuppression includes: cyclosporine, azathioprine and prednisone.

Results

Since 1984, we have performed 14 single lung transplantations for pulmonary fibrosis. There have been three operative deaths. Two of these related to poor donor selection. One patient suffered a massive venous air embolism immediately following removal of a central venous catheter.

There have been two late deaths - chronic rejection and infection (1), lymphoma (1). The longest survivor has now lived for four years with a transplanted lung.

Serial pulmonary function studies do not demonstrate any significant loss of function in the transplanted lung. All survivors have returned to normal levels of activity without O_2. Two patients developed bronchial stenoses which required transbronchoscopic placement of an 8 mm, silastic endobronchial stent.

Double Lung Transplantation

Our program in double lung transplantation has been developed to accommodate patients with compliant lungs (emphysema), and bilaterally infected lungs (e.g. bronchiectasis, and cyctic fibrosis). Laboratory work demonstrated the ability to preserve the native heart and transplant both lungs using a left atrial, pulmonary artery and tracheal anastomosis in dogs and monkeys. Our clinical program began in 1986.

Recipient and Donor Selection

Recipient and donor selection is similar to that for single lung transplantation. The recipients must have normal or recoverable cardiac function. The exact role of double lung transplantation for primary pulmonary hypertension with a recoverable right heart function is yet unknown.

Operative Procedure

The technique of double lung extraction, preserving the heart for a second transplant, has been worked out in detail (14). In essence, the double lung specimen includes: trachea, a short cuff of main pulmonary artery, and a short cuff of left atrium. The recipient is placed on cardiopulmonary bypass after the omentum is mobilized. The lungs are extracted, one at a time, preserving the native pulmonary artery, atrium and trachea. The implantation occurs sequentially: tracheal, atrial and finally pulmonary artery anastomosis.

Postoperative Care

The immunosuppressive regimen in postoperative care is similar to single lung transplantation. Early extubation is anticipated. Rejection phenomena are monitored by chest X-ray, arterial saturation and temperature.

Results

We have performed seven double lung transplantations with one early death related to necrosis of the donor trachea and both main bronchi*. All other patients are surviving. One patient has a short ischemic stricture of the proximal left mainstem bronchus which required stenting.

Lung-Heart Transplantation

We have also had a limited amount of experience with lung-heart transplantation for pulmonary disease, mainly primary pulmonary hypertension. All of these patients have had concomitant pulmonary disease and right heart failure. Of 7 patients, we have had three postoperative deaths, and two late deaths due to progressive bronchiolitis obliterans. Two patients are alive at two years, both of whom have mild bronchiolitis obliterans.

Summary

The Toronto Lung Transplant Group has had experience with 28 transplantations for pulmonary disease. We are encouraged by the long-term survival of our single lung transplantation patients. The ultimate value of double lung transplantation is unknown, but our initial results are encouraging. The problem with bronchial healing has been partially resolved by the use of omentum. However, some of our patients have developped ischemia without dehiscence, requiring intralumenal stenting. Further methods of improving bronchial circulation in the early postoperative period are required before this problem can be completely resolved. Immunosuppression without steroids in the early postoperative period (except for bolus injections for rejection) is feasible, and helps to avoid problems of spesis and bronchial dehiscence.

---

*Editor's Remark: In a more recent presentation of the Toronto group, breakdown of the tracheal anastomosis seems to be a problem of bilateral lung transplantation, although omentum had still been used in all cases. Consequently, the group might change its policy to bilateral solitary lung transplantation, performing right- and left-sided bronchial anastomosis.

1. Transplantation

References

1. Juvenelle A, Citret C, Miles CE, Stewart JD. Pneumonectomy with reimplantation of the lung in the dog for physiologic study. J Thorac Surg 21, 111, 1951.

2. Metras H. Note préliminaire sur la graffe totale du poumon chez le chien. French Academy of Science 231, 1176, 1950.

3. Hardin CA, Kittle CF. Experiences with transplantation of the lung. Science 119, 97, 1954.

4. Hardy JD, Webb WR, Dalton ML, Walker GR. Lung transplantation in man. JAMA 186, 1065, 1963.

5. Derom F, Barbier F, Ringoir S, Versieck J, Rolly G, Berzsenyi G, Vermeire P, Vrints L. Ten months survival after lung homotransplantation in man. J Thorac Cardiovasc Surg 61, 835, 1971.

6. Reitz BA, Wallwork JL, Hunt SA, Pennock JL, Billingham ME, Philip MB, Oyer PE, Stinton EB, Shumway NE. Heart-lung transplantation successful therapy for patients with pulmonary vascular disease. N Engl J Med 306, 557, 1982.

7. Stone RM, Ginsberg RJ, Colapinto RF, Pearson FG. Bronchial artery regeneration after radical hilar stripping. Surgical Forum 17, 109, 1966.

8. Lima O, Cooper JD, Peters WJ, Ayabe H, Townsend E, Luk SC, Goldberg M. Effects of methylprednisolone and azathioprine on bronchial healing following lung auto-transplantation. J Thorac Cardiovasc Surg 82, 211, 1981.

9. Nelems JM, Rebuck AS, Cooper JD, Goldberg M, Halloran PF, Vellend H. Human lung transplantation. Chest 78, 569, 1980.

10. Morgan E, Lima O, Goldberg M, Ayabe H, Ferdman A, Cooper JD. Improved bronchial healing in canine left lung reimplantation using omentopedical wrap. J Thorac Cardiovasc Surg 85, 134, 1983.

11. Toronto Lung Transplant Group. Sequential bilateral lung transplantation for paraquat poisoning. J Thorac Cardiovasc Surg 89, 734, 1985.

12. Toronto Lung Transplant Group. Unilateral lung transplantation for pulmonary fibrosis. N Engl J Med 314, 1140, 1986.

13. Cooper JD, Pearson FG, Patterson GA, Todd TRJ, Ginsberg RJ, Goldberg M, Demajo WAP. Technique of successful lung transplantation in humans. J Thorac Cardiovasc Surg 93, 173, 1987.

14. Patterson GA, Cooper JD, Goldman B, Weisel RD, Pearson FG, Waters PF, Todd TR, Scully H, Goldberg M, Ginsberg RJ. Techniques of successful clinical double lung transplantation. Ann Thor Surg 45, 626, 1988.

1.2. Tissue Immunology

1.2.1. Preliminary Results of the Collaborative Heart Transplant Study

*G Opelz [1], H Mollner [1], B Reichart [2], E Keppel [3]
for the Collaborative Heart Transplant Study*

[1] *Department of Transplantation Immunology, Institute of Immunology,
University of Heidelberg, Heidelberg, FR Germany*

[2] *Department of Cardiothoracic Surgery,
University of Cape Town, Cape Town, South Africa*

[3] *IBM Scientific Center, Heidelberg, FR Germany*

Introduction

The Collaborative Heart Transplant Study was initiated in the spring of 1985 with strictly scientific aims. Through the voluntary collaboration of many transplant centers, data on a sufficiently large number of transplants were to be accumulated in order to identify immunological and other risk factors that influence graft outcome. At present (October 1987), 55 transplant centers are participating in this scientific effort. The current report is a first account of preliminary results. Transplantations done in 1985 and 1986 were analyzed.

Results and Discussion

The overall survival rates for transplants performed in 1985 and 1986 were identical. At one year, 78% of the grafts were still functioning (Figure 7).

That the patient's original disease leading to heart failure is an important variable for the prediction of graft outcome is illustrated in Figure 8. Whereas patients with cardiomyopathy, endstage coronary disease, or valvular disease had similar success rates of slightly better than 80% at one year, patients with congenital heart disease had a considerably lower success rate of 59%, and patients with primary pulmonary hypertension had the lowest graft survival rate of all groups: less than half of these patients survived at the 6-month-mark. The category "other" contains transplant recipients with various diseases for which the patient numbers were too small for meaningful individual analysis.

The influence of recipient age is shown in Figure 9 and that of donor age in Figure 10. Recipients younger than 20 had poorer results than recipients older than 20. Hearts from donors

1. Transplantation

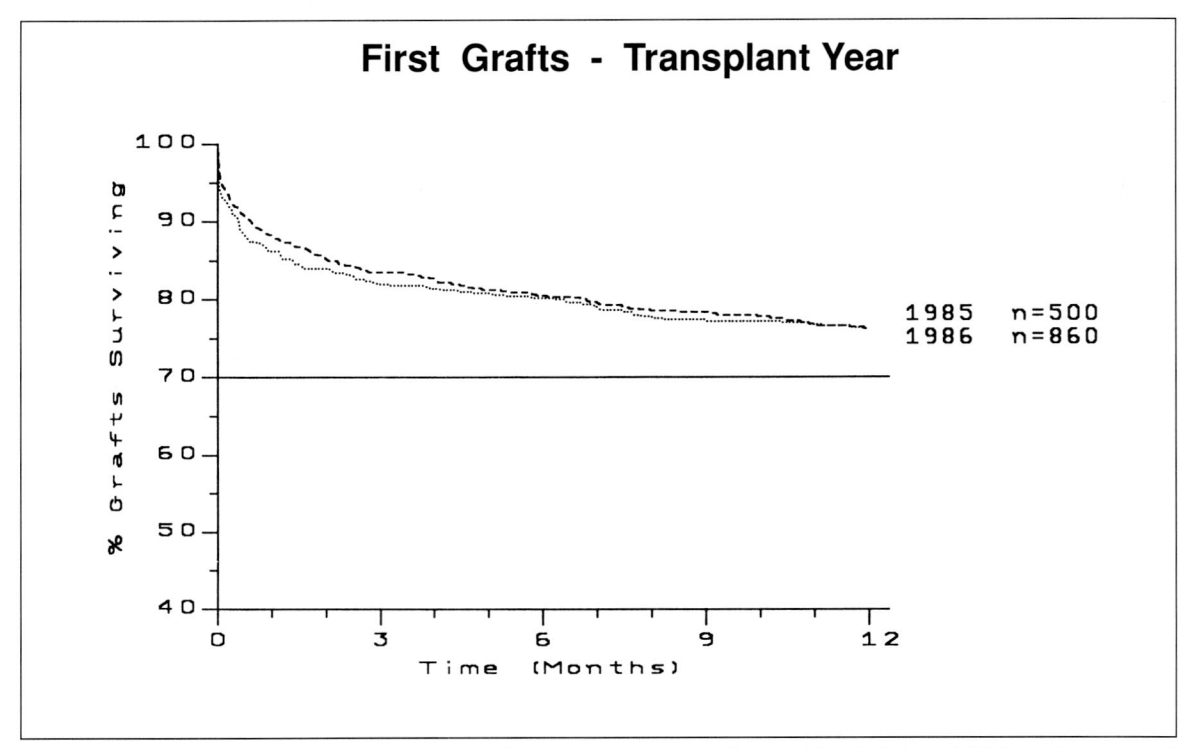

Fig. 7 Actuarial survival rates of first cardiac transplants performed in 1985 and 1986. Numbers of patients studied are indicated. The horizontal line at 70% was drawn to allow for better comparison with other figures. Note that the scales for graft survival in Figures 7-16 starts at 40%.

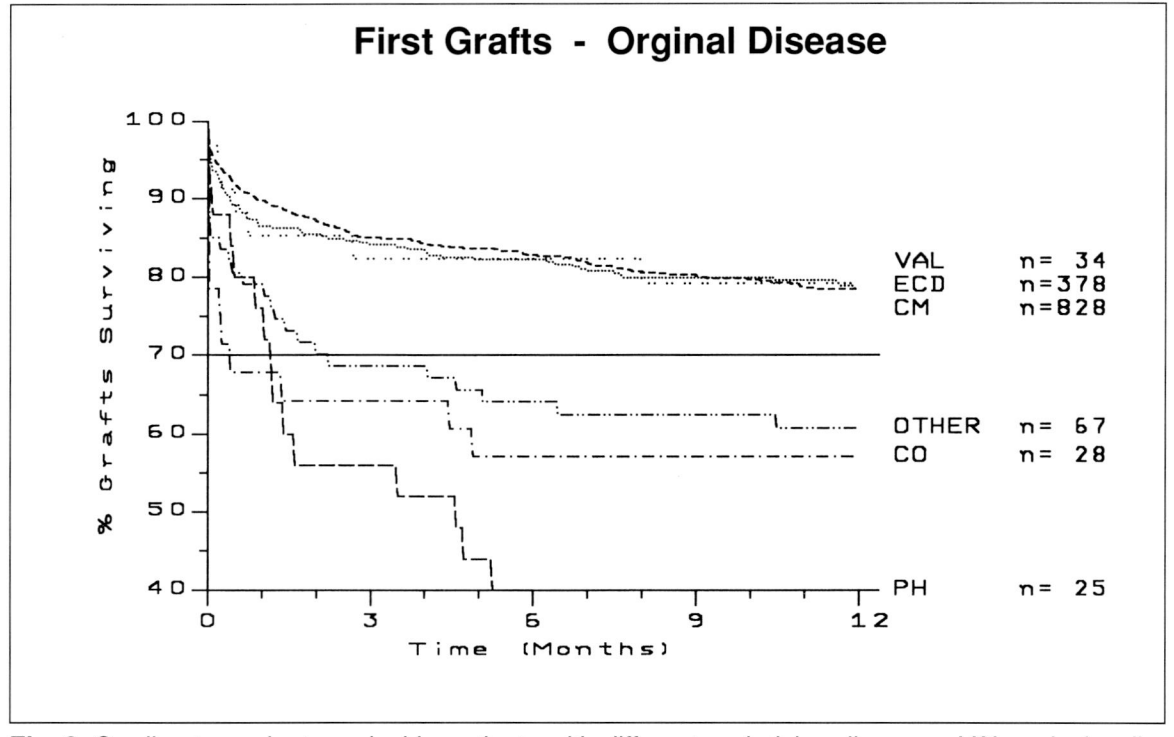

Fig. 8 Cardiac transplant survival in patients with different underlying diseases. VAL=valvular disease, ECD=endstage coronary disease, CM=cardiomyopathy, CO=congenital heart disease, PH=primary pulmonary hypertension.

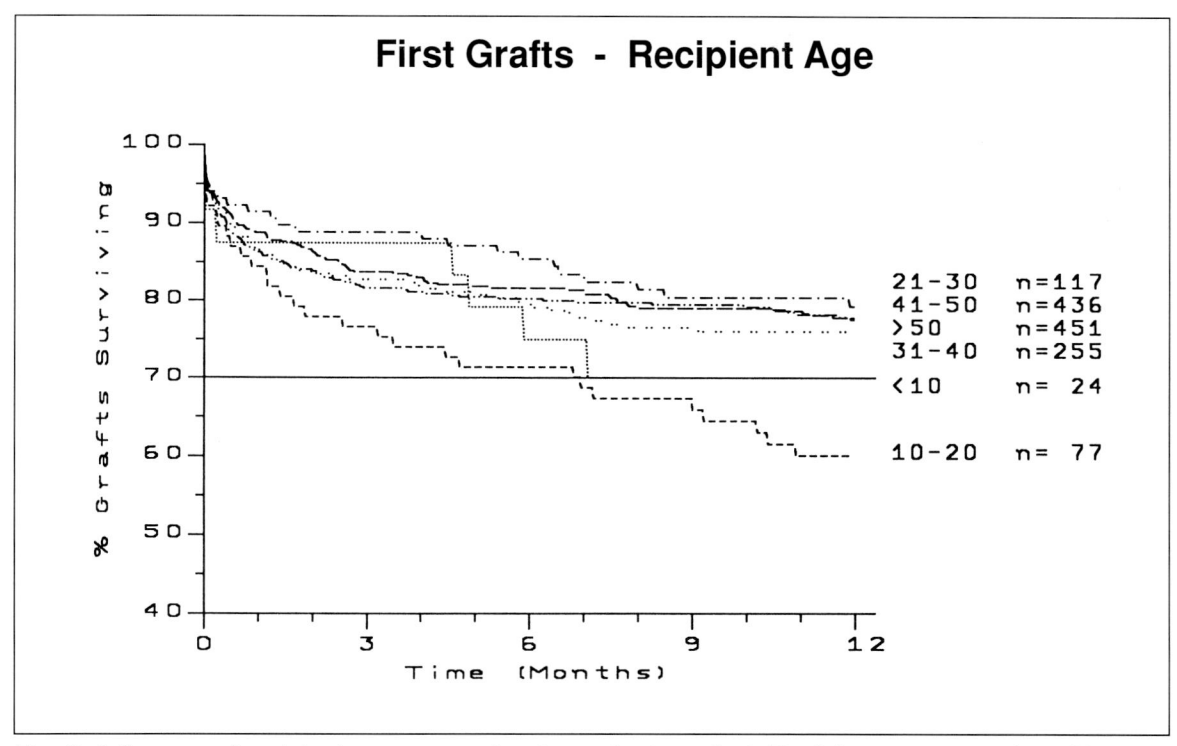

Fig. 9 Influence of recipient age on cardiac transplant survival. Recipients younger than 20 years had a lower success rate than recipients older than 20.

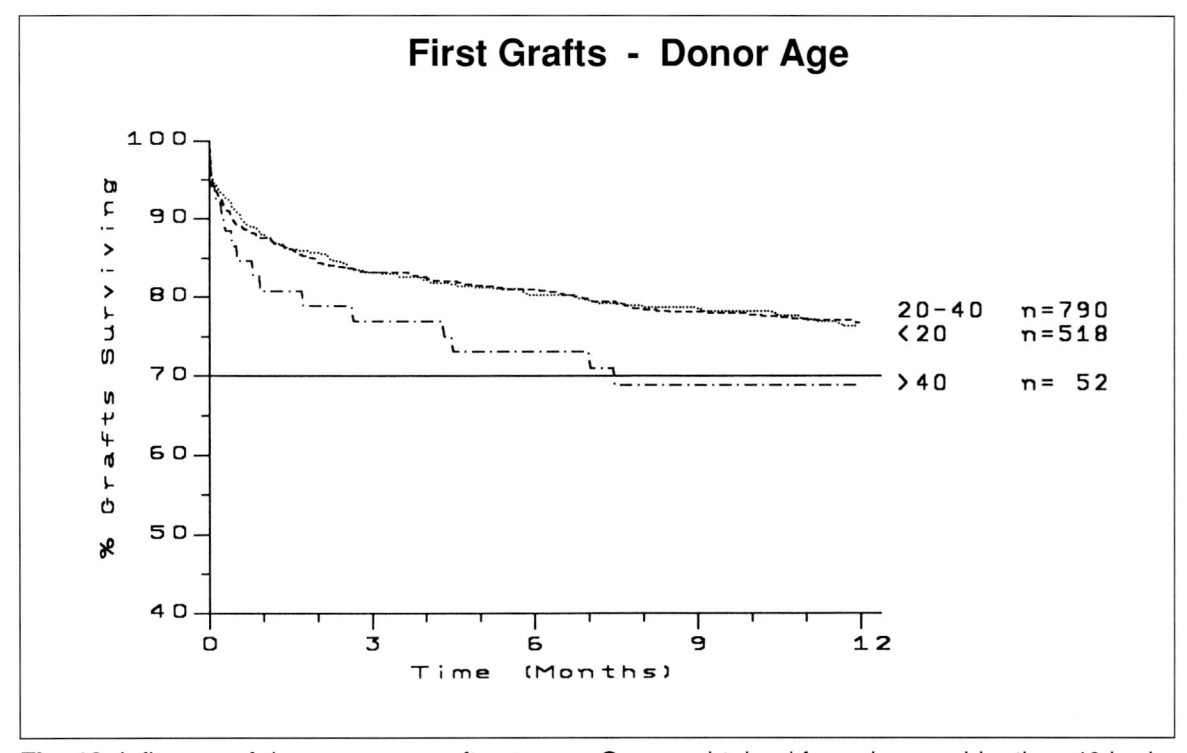

Fig. 10 Influence of donor age on graft outcome. Organs obtained from donors older than 40 had a 10% lower success rate at one year than organs from younger donors.

younger than 40 gave better results than those from donors over 40.

Recipient sex appeared to have an influence on graft survival. Male recipients did considerably better than female, with 1-year survival rates of 80% and 67%, respectively (Figure 11).

Figure 12 illustrates the influence of preservation time on graft survival. A trend toward lower success rates with increased ischemic times is evident.

The influence of HLA matching in cardiac transplantation is difficult to analyze. Because of the extreme polymorphism of the HLA system, the likelihood of an unmatched recipient and donor being HLA compatible is very small. Whereas in renal transplantation, kidneys are regularly shipped to the best compatible recipient, hearts, because of limited organ preservation time, are usually transplanted without consideration of HLA-matching. The analysis of HLA-matching in cardiac transplantation, therefore, suffers from an insufficient number of well-matched grafts. The vast majority of grafts are, in fact, mismatched in regard to HLA.

Figure 13 shows the retrospective analysis of matching for HLA-A and HLA-B antigens. There were only 66 transplants with zero or 1 mismatch, and they did marginally better than transplants with more mismatches. On the HLA-DR locus, there were 56 transplants with no mismatch, and they had an approximately 10% better graft survival at 1 year than was the case with mismatched grafts (Figure 14). The experience with renal transplants shows that matching for the combination of HLA-B and HLA-DR antigens gives a

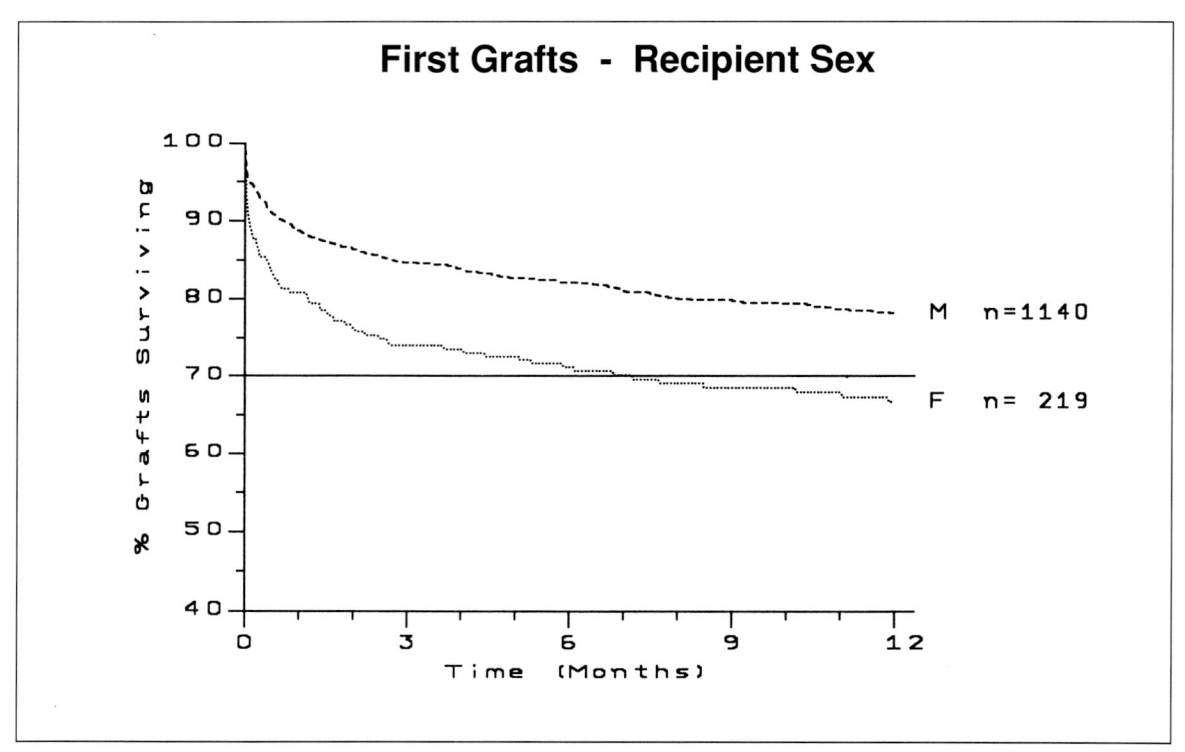

Fig. 11 Influence of recipient sex on graft outcome. Male recipients did noticeably better than female recipients. The proportion of female recipients was less than 20% of the total. M=Male recipients, F=Female recipients.

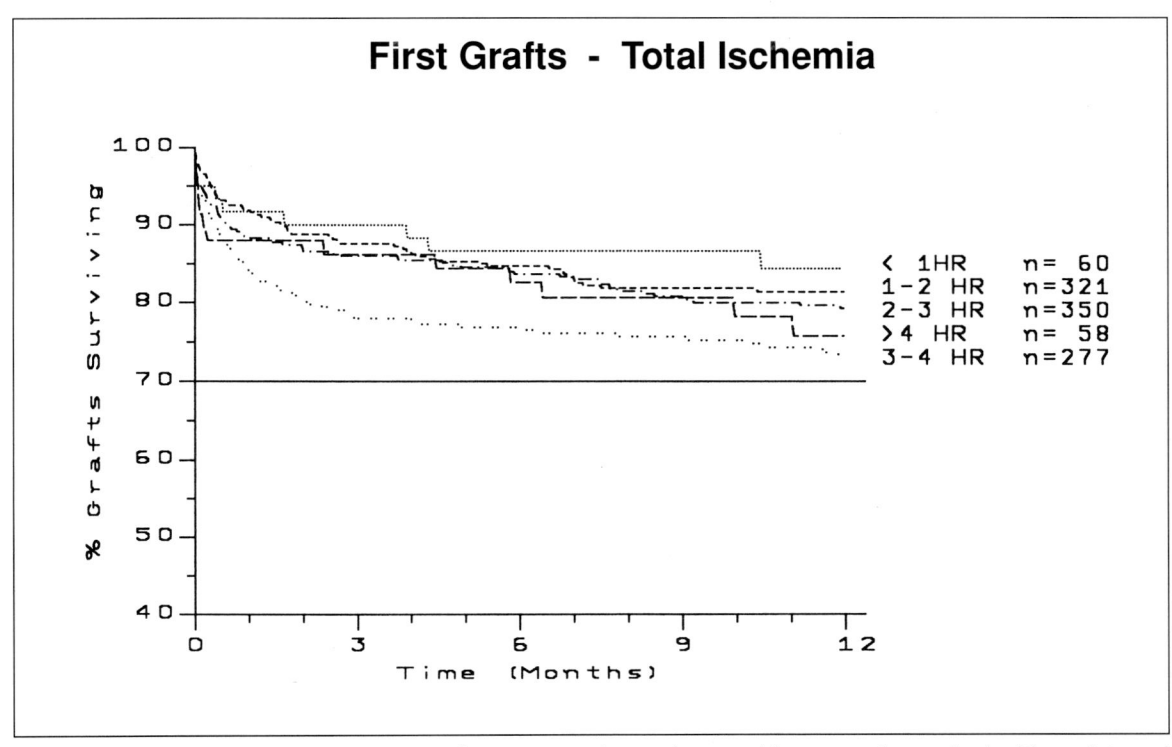

Fig. 12 Effect of ischemic time on graft outcome. A trend toward lower graft survival with prolonged ischemia is evident. Ischemic times in hours are indicated.

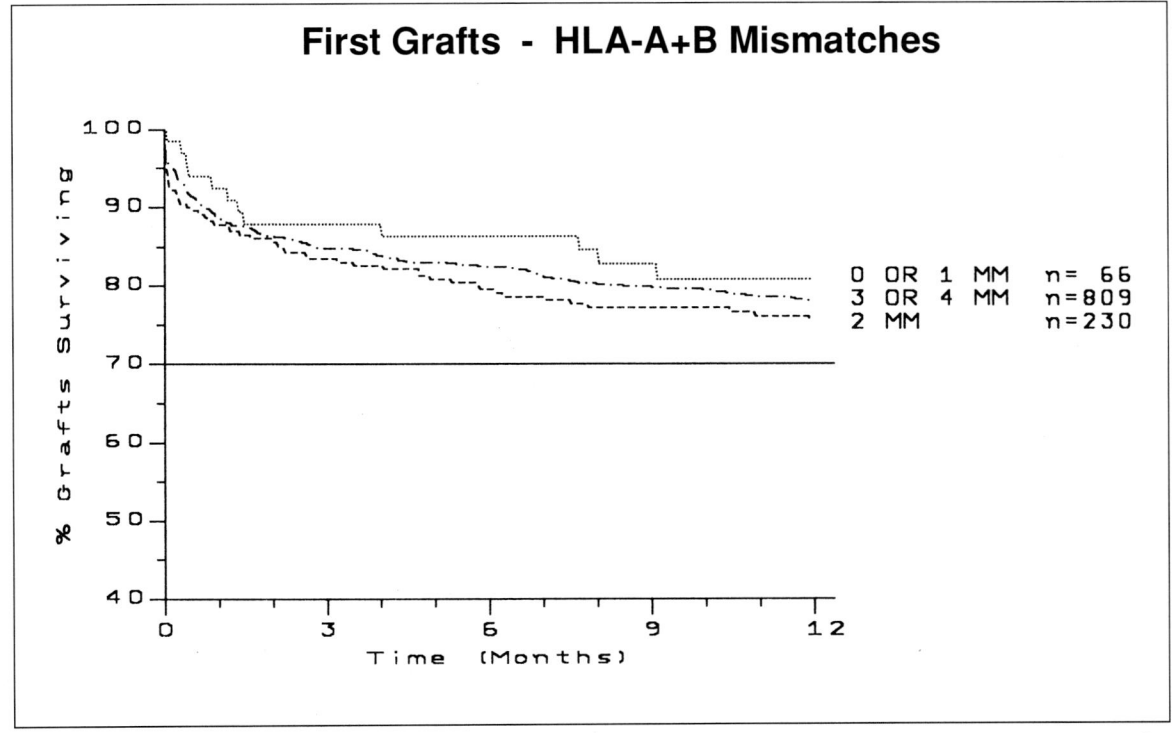

Fig. 13 Effect of matching for HLA-A, -B antigens on graft survival. Well-matched grafts (0 or 1 mismatch) did marginally better than poorly-matched grafts.

1. Transplantation

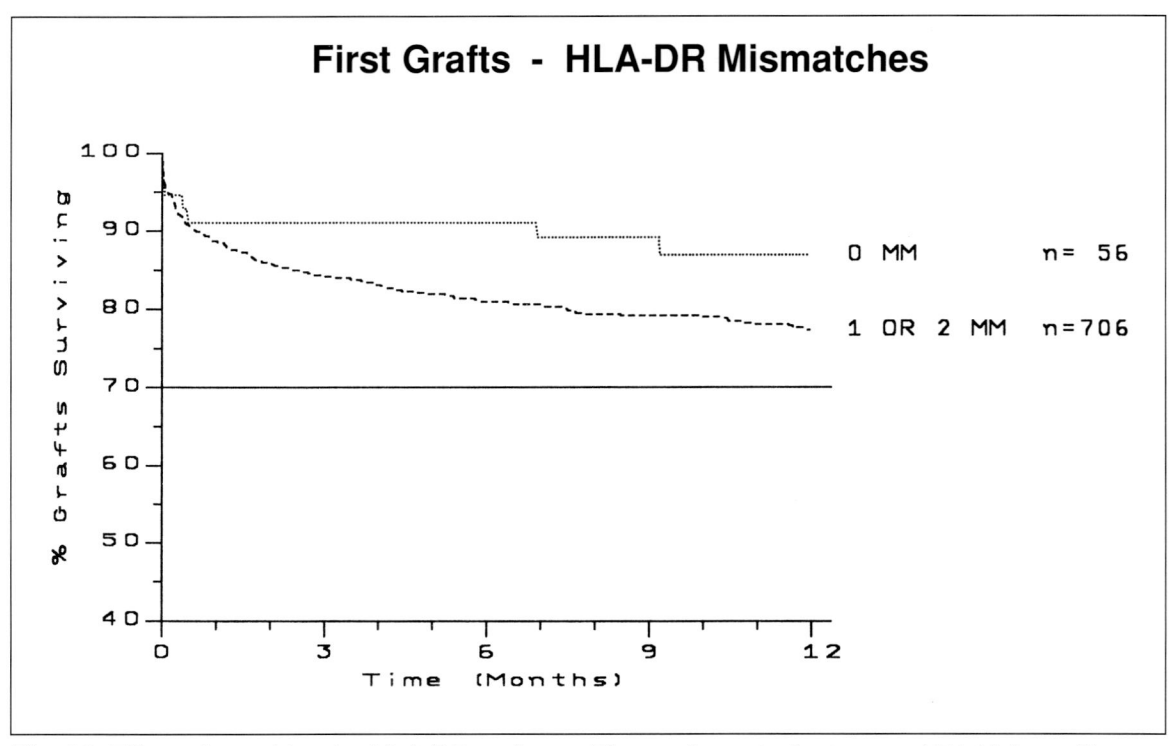

First Grafts - HLA-DR Mismatches

[Graph showing % Grafts Surviving vs Time (Months), with curves for 0 MM (n=56) and 1 OR 2 MM (n=706)]

Fig. 14 Effect of matching for HLA-DR antigens. The graft survival rate was 10% higher with zero mismatches than with 1 or 2 mismatches.

better correlation with graft survival than either the combination of HLA-A and HLA-B or that of HLA-DR alone (1). Although very few cardiac transplants were well matched for HLA-B and HLA-DR, grafts with 0 or 1 mismatch did exceptionally well (Figure 15).

However, because of the still small number of patients, all HLA data must be treated with reservation, and the analysis of a larger series of well-matched grafts should be awaited before conclusions can be drawn.

Finally, we would like to point out that the situation is further complicated by the fact that patients with different *a priori* risk are accepted for transplantation. On the basis of clinical risk factors, the patients were categorized at the time of reporting as "good", "moderate", or "poor" risks. Figure 16 shows that the risk categorization strongly correlates with graft outcome. Obviously, for increased accuracy, all analyses shown in Figures 8 through 11 should be carried out separately for these three risk categories. However, the number of patients is still too small for this to be meaningful.

In conclusion, this first report provides preliminary information on an international collaborative project, indicating that useful data can be gained through multicenter cooperation. Although we can speak only of trends, it is apparent that this method will eventually yield clinically relevant results. Complex factors, such as HLA matching, must be evaluated in large patient series. The time required for accumulating the necessary data can be shortened considerably if data from many centers are pooled. It is recognized that data pooling also carries a risk of increased heterogeneity. Nevertheless,

1. Transplantation

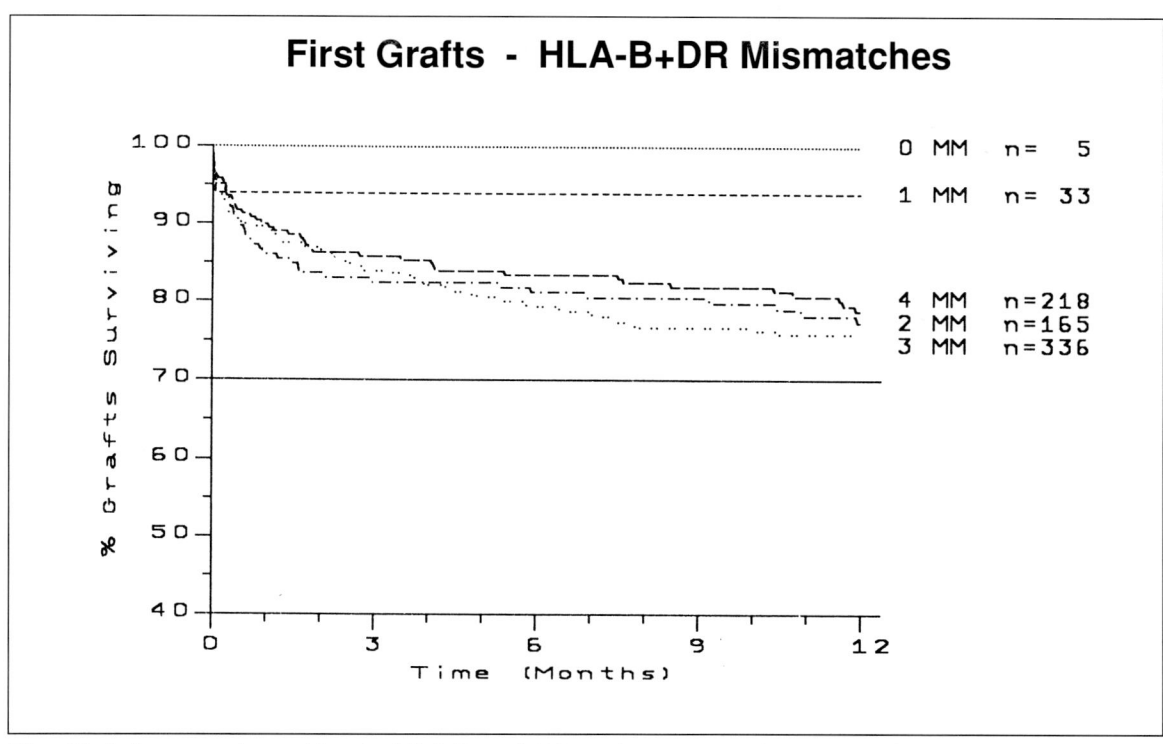

First Grafts - HLA-B+DR Mismatches

```
0 MM   n=  5
1 MM   n= 33
4 MM   n=218
2 MM   n=165
3 MM   n=336
```

Fig. 15 Influence of matching for HLA-B and -DR antigens on graft outcome. Number of mismatched antigens and number of patients studied is indicated for each curve. Only a small number of transplants were well matched. The striking difference in graft outcome needs to be followed up in a larger patient series.

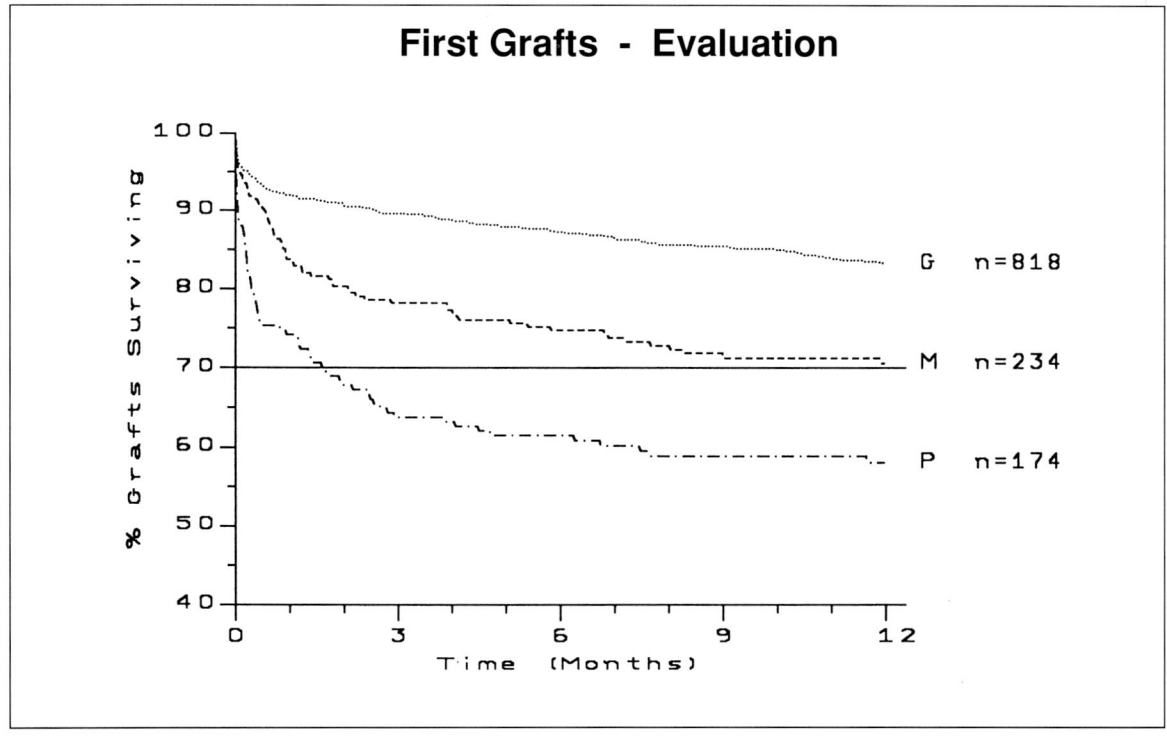

First Grafts - Evaluation

```
G   n=818
M   n=234
P   n=174
```

Fig. 16 Evaluation according to "general risk" at time of transplantation. G=good risk, M=moderate risk, P=poor risk. The difference in graft survival between good and poor risk patients was 25% at one year.

the example set by the Collaborative Renal Transplantation Study (1), as well as the preliminary data shown here, indicates that the collaborative approach is viable and useful. At the current level of activity of the study we can expect the data base to double within two years; this should allow for a much more complete and informative analysis.

Acknowledgments

The generous cooperation of 55 cardiac transplantation centers is gratefully acknowledged. We are also indebted to Erlinde Feisthammel and Deborah Back for maintaining the data files. Computer hardware and software support was provided by IBM Germany.

Reference

1. Opelz G for the Collaborative Renal Transplant Study. Effect of HLA matching in 10.000 cyclosporine-treated cadaver kidney transplants. Transplant Proc 19, 641, 1987.

1.2.2. The Application of New Techniques in HLA Typing, with Special Reference to DRw6 in Clinical Transplantation

E du Toit, R Martell, M Oudshoorn

Provincial Laboratory for Tissue Immunology, Cape Town, South Africa

Introduction

The HLA system in man is located on the short arm of chromosome 6 and consists of a complex of several genes, together with those encoding some of the complement proteins, 21-hydroxylase and tumour necrosis factor (Figure 17). The products of the HLA genes are glycoproteins, and have been divided into two groups, based on their molecular structure as well as their function. The Class I molecules, encoded by the genes in the HLA-A, B and C region, consist of a single glycoprotein chain non-covalently associated with β_2-microglobulin, and are present on all nucleated cells. Functionally, they are

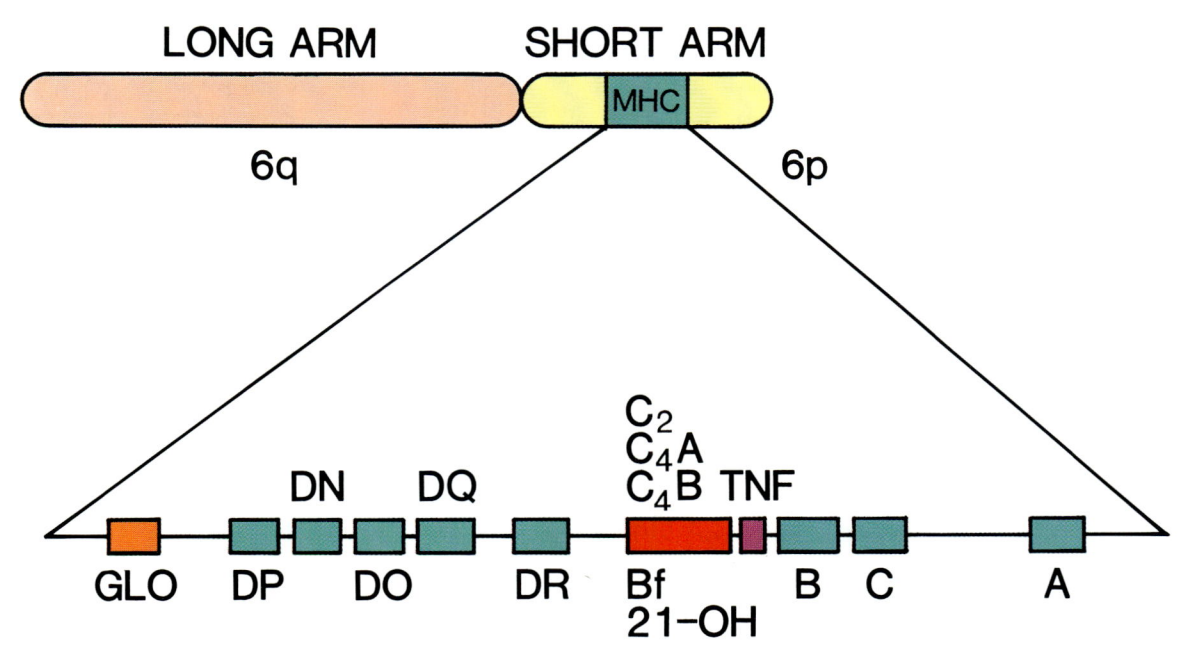

Fig. 17 Schematic diagram of chromosome 6 showing the arrangement of the genes of the Major Histocompatibility Complex (MHC). The complement loci (C2, Bf, C4A, C4B), the 21-hydroxylase gene (21-OH) and the gene for tumour necrosis factor (TNF) are located in this region between the HLA-B and DR loci. Glyoxylase I (GLO) is a polymorphic red cell enzyme marker situated in proximity to the Class II genes, and used to identify extended haplotypes. The entire MHC is approximately 3500 kilobases (kb), with the Class I genes occupying about 1,500 kb and the Class II genes about 1,000 kb.

1. Transplantation

thought to be responsible for presentation of foreign antigen to cytotoxic T-cells in the efferent limb of the cellular immune process. The second group, the Class II molecules, are encoded by a cluster of genes in the DR, DQ, DO, DN and DP regions. The DR, DQ and DP gene products are heterodimers, consisting of α and β glycoprotein chains, which are located on the surface of B-lymphocytes, macrophages, Langerhans' cells and activated T-lymphocytes. The DO and DN regions have no known gene product, but the DR, DQ and DP regions contain the A and B genes encoding the respective α and β peptide chains of the Class II molecules. These glycoproteins are responsible for presenting macrophage-processed antigen to the helper or inducer T-lymphocyte in the afferent limb of the cellular immune response.

Complexity of the HLA System

The HLA Class I and Class II glycoproteins are usually detected on the cell surface by allo- and monoclonal antibodies. The HLA typing is done according to a microlymphocytotoxicity technique (Figure 18). The killed lymphocytes take up the dye and are stained according to the colour of the dye added (Figure 19).

The genes of the HLA system show extreme polymorphism, and at the Tenth International Histocompatibility Workshop held in Princeton, U.S.A., in November 1987, the number of alleles recognised by serological techniques increased. There are now twenty A-locus alleles, forty-two B-locus alleles, ten C-locus alleles, sixteen DR-locus alleles, and seven DQ-locus alleles. The six DP-locus alleles were defined using a combination of serological and cellular techniques. The definition of

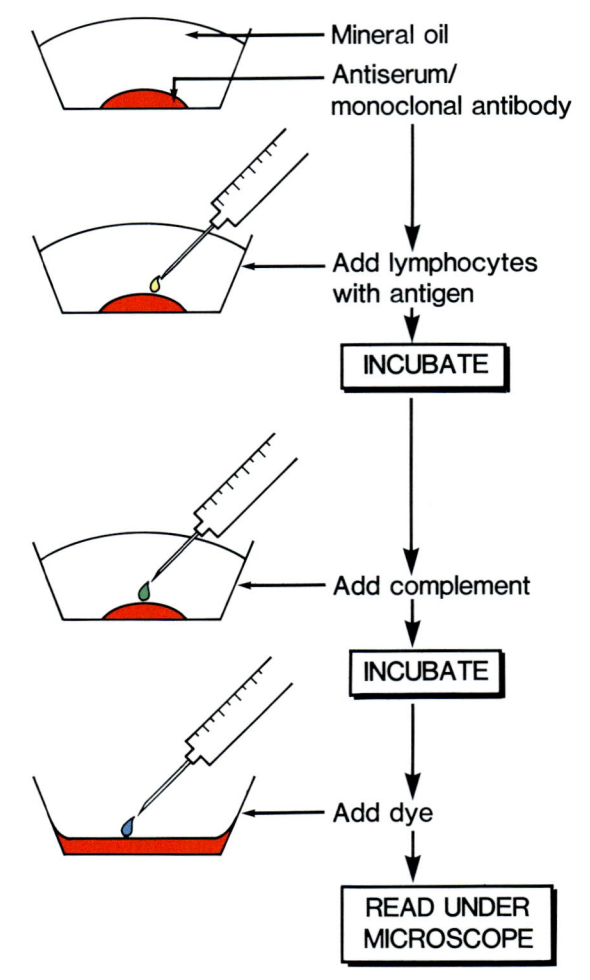

Fig. 18 A schematic presentation of the microlymphocytotoxicity test showing the basic principles. The antisera are dispensed into plastic trays containing sixty wells. The individual's lymphocytes are added to the wells with the antibody-containing serum under paraffin oil (to prevent evaporation) in the presence of complement. A solution of dye is added after incubation, and each well is examined under the microscope to see whether or not the cells have taken up the dye.

many of these alleles poses a particular problem in the various indigenous populations of Southern Africa, as a result of the many unique variants seen in the Negroid and Cape Coloured populations. For example, prior to the

Tenth International Histocompatibility Workshop, the DR3 allele was a single specificity mainly defined in Caucasoids. A subgroup of DR3 associated with Bw42 was defined by us in South African Negroes, using the Tenth International Histocompatibility Workshop reagents (1). This unique subgroup of HLA-DR3 has been named DRw18, and the original Caucasoid DR3 specificity was designated DRw17. The DRw6 antigen, which is often difficult to define in Caucasoid populations, due to a lack of specific antisera, appears to be even more complex in the local South African populations. Using the Tenth International Histocompatibility Workshop serological reagents, we recognised several variants which reacted with the DRw6 antisera plus other allo- and monoclonal antibodies which were specific for the alleles DRw8 and DRw12 (2,3). These variants of the DRw6 antigen were confined to the South African Negro and Cape Coloured populations that were studied, and were not seen in the South African Caucasoids. It is therefore apparent that the definition of the HLA antigens, particularly HLA-DRw6, remains problematic using the currently available serological methods.

HLA-DRw6 and Clinical Transplantation

These difficulties in the definition of the various HLA antigens are of considerable relevance, since HLA-matching of recipient and donor is still considered to be important in the transplantation of solid organs, even with cyclosporine as immunosuppressive therapy (4). It has been demonstrated that matching, especially at both the B and DR loci, has a significantly beneficial in-

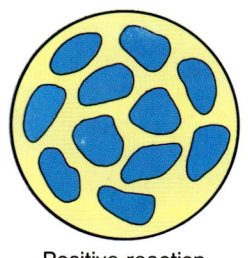

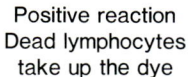

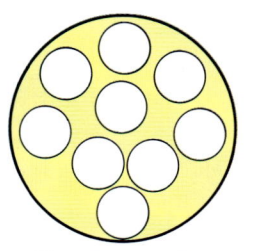

Fig. 19 The stained cells are the result of the uptake of a supravital stain such as trypan blue, when the cell membrane is damaged by the specific binding of complement-fixing antibody to the cell surface antigens.

Positive reaction
Dead lymphocytes take up the dye

Negative reaction
Live lymphocytes exclude the dye

fluence on graft survival (5). Furthermore, matching for the splits of HLA-A and B may produce a further significant improvement in graft survival in renal transplantation (G. Opelz, personal communication). With regard to HLA-DRw6, the Leiden group has published data emphasizing the importance of matching for this particular antigen, and the suggestion was made that recipients with DRw6 are more likely to reject the grafted kidney if there is a mismatch than recipients with any of the other DR antigens (6).

Application of Molecular Biology to the HLA System

In view of the complexity of HLA-DRw6 when recognised by serological techniques alone, we have further investigated the variants seen locally using Southern blot hybridization (Figure 20). The main advantage of this new HLA-typing technique is that there is now available a means of unravelling the serological complexity of the HLA system at the genetic level. Samples of DNA from genetically homozygous individuals and families with these unusual

1. Transplantation

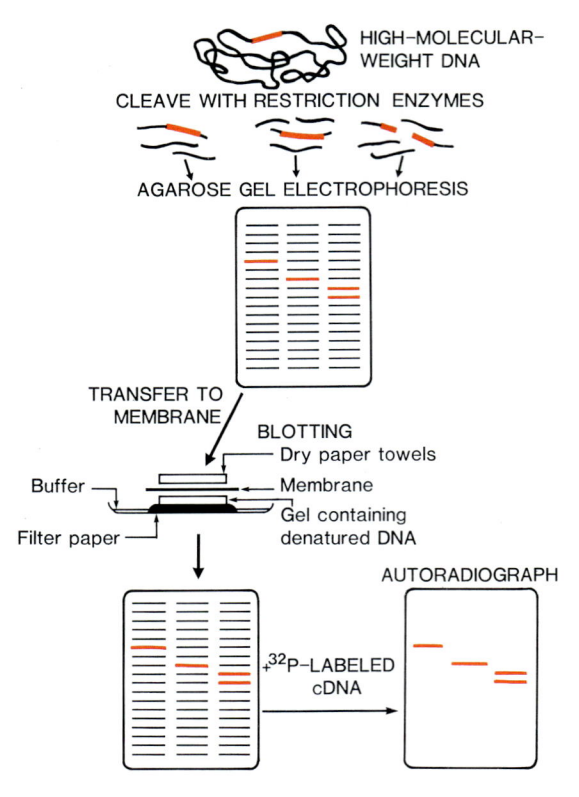

Fig. 20 Southern blot hybridization permits direct examination of an individual's HLA type at the genetic level. The essential stages in this technique are shown in this diagram.

DRw6 variants were digested with the restriction endonuclease Taq I, electrophoresed on agarose gel to separate the restriction fragments by size, and then transferred to a nylon membrane. A radio labelled piece of DNA (probe), which would hybridize with (or stick to) complementary sequences among the DNA fragments on the nylon membrane, was then added. Probes specific for the DRB, DQB, DPB and DQA genes were used for the hybridization, and their positions on the membrane were then detected by autoradiography. The restriction fragment sizes in kilobases (kb) were calculated by comparing them with standards of known molecular weight. This technique is thus a means of detecting distinctive variations within the A and B genes of the DR, DQ and DP regions. The patterns of restriction fragments that were observed in the homozygous individuals, or seen to segregate within the families, correlated with the serological findings, and appeared to represent unique restriction fragment length polymorphisms (RFLPs). These results are shown in Table 2, together with the RFLPs occurring in the classical DRw8, DRw12, DRw13 and DRw14 cells for comparison.

Using the DRB probe, the presence of a 9.7 kb-fragment, together with the ab-

Taq I RFLPs observed in the DRw6 variants, together with the classical DRw8, DRw12, DRw13 and DRw14 RFLPs for comparison

A plus (+) sign indicates that a fragment is present and a minus (-) indicates its absence

		DR Beta					DQ Alpha						DQ Beta		
DRw	Dw	11.3*	9.7	7.0	4.3	4.0	7.1	6.5	6.3	4.9	4.7	2.7	5.3	4.6	2.9
12	HERLUF	+	-	-	+	+	-	-	-	+	-	-	-	+	-
12x6	JOH	-	+	-	+	+	-	-	+	-	+	-	-	+	-
13	19	-	+	+	+	-	-	+	-	-	-	-	+	-	-
13	18	-	+	+	-	+	+	-	-	-	-	-	-	-	+
8x14	-	-	+	+	-	+	-	-	-	-	-	+	+	-	-
14	9	+	-	+	-	+	-	-	-	-	-	+	+	-	-
8	8	-	-	-	-	-	-	-	-	-	-	-	-	-	-

* Fragment size is indicated in kilobases (kb).

Table 2

sence of the 11.3 kb fragment seen in the homozygous DRw12 cell (Herluf), distinguish the DRw12x6 antigen from the classical DRw12 antigen. The 7.0 kb fragment seen in both the DRw13 and DRw14 cells is also absent in the DRw12x6 cell. Either a 6.3 or a 4.7 kb fragment was associated with the DRw12x6 antigen with the DQA probe. These fragments were not seen in association with the DRw12, the DRw13 or the DRw14 antigens.

The DRB RFLPs seen with DRw8x14 were similar to the DRw13 (Dw18) antigen, whereas the DQA and DQB RFLPs were the same as the classical DRw14 antigen. None of the RFLPs seen with the DRw8x14 antigens occurred in the homozygous DRw8 cell.

Conclusion

These results confirm the serological complexity of HLA-DRw6 and suggest that this antigen may consist of several subgroups, which may only be seen in the South African Negro and Cape Coloured populations. It is not surprising therefore, that we have been unable to detect any particular clinical effect of DRw6 in heart and kidney transplantations in these populations. These results also suggest that, prior to any further study of the effect of HLA-matching on graft survival in the populations of Southern Africa, the HLA antigens require clear and detailed definition at both the serological and genetic level, since several unique subgroups or splits of the broad antigens are now being recognised in these populations.

Acknowledgement

We wish to thank Valerie Myburgh, Medical Illustrator in the Department of Medicine, University of Cape Town, for the illustrations.

References

1. Oudshoorn M, Du Toit ED, Taljaard DG. A possible new negro HLA-DR3 variant. Tenth International Histocompatibility Workshop, Newsletter 1, 26, 1987.

2. Du Toit ED, Oudshoorn M. The HLA-DRw6 complex. Tenth International Histocompatibility Workshop, Newsletter 1, 2, 1987.

3. Du Toit ED, Oudshoorn M, Martell RW, MacGregor KJ. HLA-DRw6 and its complexity. In: Immunobioloy of HLA (ed. Dupont B) Springer-Verlag, New York, 1988, in press.

4. Cicciarelli J, Terasaki PI, Mickey MR. The effect of zero HLA Class I and II mismatching in cyclosporine-treated kidney transplant patients. Transplant 43, 636, 1987.

5. Opelz G. Effect of HLA matching in 10,000 cyclosporine-treated cadaver kidney transplants. Transplant Proc 19, 641, 1987.

6. Hendriks GFJ, Schreuder GMT, Claas FHJ, D'Amaro J, Persijn GG, Cohen B, Van Rood JJ. HLA-DRw6 and renal allograft rejection. Br Med J 286, 85, 1983.

1. Transplantation

1.3. Immunosuppression

1.3.1. Total Lymphoid Irradiation in Experimental and Clinical Transplantation

JA Myburgh

*Transplantation Research Unit, Department of Surgery,
University of the Witwatersrand
and the Johannesburg Hospital,
South Africa*

Despite the substantial improvement in the results obtained with renal, cardiac and hepatic transplantation in recent years, failures still occur in some cases, either because currently available immunosuppressive drugs, including cyclosporine, may fail to prevent irreversible graft rejection, or may be responsible for profound morbidity or even mortality. The fundamental goal in clinical transplantation still remains the production of immunolically specific, and operationally durable tolerance towards the graft without the need for permanent immunosuppressive drug therapy. This quest for the holy grail of transplantation has preoccupied many laboratories thoughout the world, including our own, for many years.

Slavin et al (1) first reported the exciting possibilities in this regard with the use of a modified method of total lymphoid irradiation (TLI) in a rodent model in 1977. We have studied this modality of potential tolerance production extensively in the baboon in the past decade, and have also applied it in clinical transplantation. We recently reviewed our experience with TLI in renal transplantation in baboons (2) and humans (3, 4). This report updates and extends this experience.

TLI in Experimental Transplantation

Pilot studies in baboon liver and kidney transplantation extablished that TLI is a remarkably potent graft, prolonging modality of treatment. However, it was also soon apparent that the irradiation protocol used successfully in mice and rats, namely a cumulative dose of 3400 cGy administered as 17 daily fractions of 200 cGy on 5 days each week, was associated with an unacceptable mortality rate. Accordingly, in the ensuing years, several factors of relevance to safe and effective potential clinical application were systematically studied in the baboon model. These included the cumulative dose of irradiation required to be administered, the fractionation regimen (including the dose per fraction, and frequency and number of fractions given), various field sizes of irradiation, the impact of delay between completion of irradiation and transplantation, and the necessity for donor bone marrow administration, which had been found to be essential for full tolerance production in skin grafts in mice and rats.

The results of several hundred transplantation experiments permitted the following conclusions:

Irradiation Protocol

The most effective and safest irradiation protocol for kidney or liver transplantation in baboons involves a cumulative dose of 800 cGy given as twice weekly fractions of 80 or 100 cGy each. With this fractionation protocol, the dose response curve appeared to be parabolic. Larger or smaller cumulative doses than 800 cGy were less effective.

Field of Irradiation

It was necessary to irradiate a wide field, substantially more extensive than the mantle and inverted-Y fields used in the treatment of patients with Hodgkin's disease, and similar to, although not quite as extensive as that used in the original rodent experiments. The field of irradiation required involved the whole torso from the base of the skull down to and including the bony pelvis, and also including the proximal ends of the humeri and femora. Supradiaphragmatic lungs and ribs could be shielded, but more extensive lateral abdominal shielding, including liver and spleen, which simulated the clinical Hodgkin's fields, markedly reduced efficacy. The field of irradiation therefore includes a major part of the haemopoietic bone marrow.

Donor Bone Marrow (BM) Injection

In contrast to the findings with skin grafting in rodents, the injection of donor BM was not essential for tolerance production, and the data even suggested that donor BM injection might be counterproductive. It was postulated that, in primarily vascularized organ grafts, sufficient transplantation antigen was released systemically to induce tolerance in a suitably conditioned host.

Delay between TLI and Transplantation

Of great potential relevance to the circumstances of clinical cadaver transplantation was the finding that organ transplantation did not have to be performed within a day or two of completion of TLI, as had been shown to be necessary in skin transplantation in mice and rats. There was no evidence that delays of up to 1 month affected tolerance production, and tolerance could be produced with delays of up to 4 months if monthly fractions of TLI were administered.

Frequency, Durability and Specificity of Tolerance

Operational tolerance may be defined as the indefinite survival of an allograft with normal function and without the necessity for the permanent administration of immunosuppressive drugs. At an immunological level, tolerance must be specific. The recipient must be unresponsive to the relevant allograft alone, and immunological responsiveness to third party grafts or other foreign antigens must be maintained or restored.

These criteria of durability and specificity have been realized with the use of TLI in baboon and kidney transplantation (5). Chronic rejection and loss of graft has occurred months after transplantation following TLI, but in 65 baboons with stable and normal graft function 1 year after transplantation, no grafts have subsequently been lost with observation periods of more than 8 years. In this model, the presence of normal graft function 1 year after transplantation can therefore be used as the criterion for the establishment of operational tolerance.

Immunological specificity of the tolerance has been demonstrated by in vitro and in vivo experiments. Baboons have been challenged with third party kidney allografts placed in the neck 1 year after renal transplantation. These grafts have been rejected in an unmodified acute fashion. The original kidney allografts were unaffected. In a more systematic study, baboons bearing kidney allografts were challenged with skin grafts at varying intervals up to 1 year after transplantation. All animals accepted permanently skin grafts from their original kidney donors. Third and fourth party skin grafts were rejected in a delayed fashion when placed 2 months after transplantation. By 4 months, third party skin graft rejection was only slightly delayed, and, between 7 and 10 months after renal transplantation, such grafts were rejected in an unmodified acute manner. A similar phenomenon was observed in appropriate mixed lymphocyte reaction (MLR) experiments. In the early months after transplantation, there was unresponsiveness or hyporesponsiveness to all allogeneic stimulating lymphocytes. With the passage of time, usually a year or more after transplantation, MLR to indifferent lymphocytes returns. MLR to kidney donor lymphocytes remains absent or low in some, but not all long surviving animals. The frequency with which tolerance has been established with the above-mentioned protocol of TLI has ranged between one third and one half of baboons in different groups. It has not yet been possible to predict, at the time of transplantation, which individual baboons will be rendered tolerant. All show the same degree of hypo- or non-responsiveness to polyclonal mitogens, and the level of pre-TLI MLR to the kidney donor has no bearing on the likelihood of tolerance induction. This has implications for the use of TLI in clinical transplantation, as will be discussed later.

Mechanism of Tolerance after TLI

As indicated above, tolerance after TLI and renal transplantation in baboons evolved in a matter of months from a broad, non-specific phase to a donor-specific phase. Earlier studies demonstrated that TLI produces a profound lymphopenia. This involves both T helper (Th, T4+) and T suppressor/cytotoxic (Tsc, T8+) subsets. After transplantation there is a rapid rise in the percentage of T8+ cells and a further fall in the percentage of T4+ cells. This persists for approximately 6 months, when there is a return to pre-TLI percentages, despite continuing normal graft function in the recipients. Furthermore, soon after transplantation both T4+ and T8+ subsets show evidence of activiation, as reflected by an abrupt rise in the percentage of Ia+ cells in the peripheral circulation. This evidence of immunological activation also wanes progressively in the ensuing months. The evolution of tolerance thus appears to be associated with intense immunological activity.

Evidence for a suppressor cell mechanism is readily obtained. An interesting finding in criss-cross MLR experiments

Effect of TLI on Stimulating Ability of Lymphocytes in MLR

Baboon Number	Pre-TLI Counts/2 min	S.I.	Post-TLI Counts/2 min	S.I.
1	5156 ± 472	19.9	855 ± 390	3.3
2	4370 ± 519	16.8	842 ± 580	3.2
3	7244 ± 1515	27.9	1504 ± 332	5.8
4	3861 ± 1021	14.9	775 ± 211	3.0
5	2560 ± 301	10.2	358 ± 17	1.4

MLR: Mixed lymphocyte reactivity.
S.I.: Stimulation Index.
Responder lymphocytes all derived from a single baboon.
All assays performed simultaneously with stored stimulator lymphocytes.

Table 3

Suppression of MLR by Post-TLI Lymphocytes

Responder Lymphocytes 2×10^5	Stimulator Lymphocytes 1×10^5	Add-in Lymphocytes 1×10^5	Counts per 2 mins	Stimulation Index	% Suppression
X	X	X	260 ± 16	–	–
X	A(pre-TLI)	A(pre-TLI)	7244 ± 1515	27.9	–
X	A(pre-TLI)	A(post-TLI)	3403 ± 1443	13.1	53
X	A(pre-TLI)	A(pre-TLI, RxT11)	11083 ± 4502	42.6	–
X	A(pre-TLI)	A(post-TLI, RxT11)	549 ± 95	2.1	92
A	A(post-TLI)	A(post-TLI)	1504 ± 332	–	–

X: Indifferent third party baboon.
RxT11: lymphocytes treated with OKT 11 and rabbit complement.

Table 4

was that lymphocytes harvested from animals after TLI stimulated allogeneic lymphocytes in MLR less vigorously than lymphocytes isolated from the same animals before TLI (Table 3). A possible explanation was found in coculture experiments (Table 4). The addition of post-TLI lymphocytes to MLR cultures between third party responders and pre-TLI lymphocytes from the same donors resulted in marked suppression. The suppressor cell was not a T-cell, as T-cell depletion with the monoclonal antibody OKT 11 abolished the suppression. This confirmed the non-T-cell, non-specific nature of suppression in the early stages after TLI. Oseroff et al have named these non-specific suppressor cells 'natural suppressor cells', and have suggested that they inhibit the generation of cytotoxic T-cells, but allow the emergence of antigen-specific suppressor T-cells (7). We have been able to demonstrate a late donor-specific T-cell mediated suppression in appropriate coculture experiments in some, but not all operationally tolerant baboons.

Modifications of TLI Protocol

In recent experiments we have assessed the effects of more frequent fractionation of the irradiation. The rationale was a possibly increased efficacy in terms of tolerogenesis, and a shortening of the total irradiation period required, with obviously beneficial logistic clinical implications. A variety of fraction sizes and frequency of administration were studied. Sixty of 70 cGy fractions administered 3 times a week to total dose of 840 cGy did not improve the tolerant fraction obtained, namely 2 of 12 baboons. However, 800 cGy administered as 10 fractions of 80 cGy each on 5 days per week - irradiation completed in only 2 weeks - produced tolerance in 3 of 6 baboons, thus confirming the safety and efficacy of a more abbreviated regimen. Further hyperfraction, 60 or 80 cGy fractions administered twice a day on 3 days per week, were counterproductive, with no tolerant baboons obtained in a group of 13, and a median graft survival of only 27 days.

In further groups of baboons, cumulative doses of 1200 and 1600, administered as 80 cGy fractions 5 days a week, resulted in reduced tolerogenic efficacy in both kidney and liver transplantation, thus confirming previous findings with a bi-weekly fractionation protocol. More irradiation is therefore not beneficial.

Immunological Manipulation after Transplantation

Further experiments were performed in attempts to increase the frequency of tolerance production after TLI.

Post-Transplant TLI

The administration of 2 fractions of TLI, 100 cGy each, in the second or third week after transplantation, the baboons having received 500 cGy before transplantation, virtually abolished tolerance production. Not only was tolerance achieved in only 1 baboon in a group of 15, but 9 animals rejected their kidney grafts in the first month, and median graft survival was reduced to 29 days.

Posttransplant Immunosuppressive Drug Therapy

Here too the results were disappointing. Six post-transplant doses of rabbit-anti-baboon thymocyte globulin did not increase the tolerant fraction obtained in 4 of 13 baboons. A 14 day course of post-transplantation cyclosporine after pretransplant TLI, at oral doses of 17.5 or 30 mg/kg/day, or intravenous doses of 2.5 or 5.0 mg kg/day, appeared to be counterproductive. Tolerance was attained in only 1 of 22 baboons. A post-transplantation course of prednisone lasting either 2 weeks or 3 months, had no significant effect on the tolerant fraction obtained. It remains to be seen whether different timing and/or duration of immunosuppressive drug treatment may alter this picture.

1. Transplantation

Donor Antigen Administration

Donor antigen administration after TLI, and at the time of renal transplantation, was studied in 3 groups of experiments. Donor blood, 100 ml, was infused during transplantation. Tolerance did not eventuate, and median graft survival was reduced to 23 days. Similar results were obtained with 3 transfusions from random donors in the interval between completion of TLI and transplantation. The administration of donor BM was re-evaluated following a 5 day fractionation protocol and a cumulative dose of 800 cGy. While previous studies suggested that donor BM administration was not essential for tolerance production, the present experiments showed a clear and dramatic deleterious effect on graft survival. Most grafts in a group of 11 animals studied were rejected in a virtually unmodified acute fashion, median graft survival was only 14 days, and no tolerant animals were obtained.

Previously published studies demonstrated a modest but significant prolongation of survival of liver allografts in otherwise untreated baboons following the administration of donor transplantation antigen prepared from spleen cells with either 3M KC1 or deoxycholate. More recently, Yasamura and Kahan reported similar results with 3M KC1 antigen in conjunction with cyclosporine in rats. We are currently studying the effects of administration of 3M KC1 donor antigen following TLI in baboon kidney transplantation. The experiment has not yet matured, but it is apparent that the results will be similar to those obtained with donor BM administration.

It may be concluded that the immunological status after TLI is conditioned for tolerance induction by a vascularized organ allograft. This may be a recapitulation of the state in the neonatal mouse. However, tolerance induction, which is an immunological active process, although poorly understood, may be impaired or abrogated by inappropriate immunological interventions.

TLI in Clinical Renal Transplantation

Results obtained with the use of TLI in clinical renal transplantation have been published previously (2, 3, 4, 10.). The questions to be answered refer to the overall efficacy of this modality of treatment and the prospects for achieving specific tolerance in the clinical context.

Patients

Fifty-two patients, who received their transplants at least 6 months previously, were evaluated. Four primary vascular failures have been excluded, leaving 48 patients who are immunologically evaluable (Table 5).

Immunologically Evaluable Patients	
Total number	: 48
Cadaver donor transplants	: 38
Related living donor transplants	: 10
Adult recipients	: 26
Paediatric recipients	: 22
First transplants	: 42
Second transplants	: 6

Table 5

The majority received cadaveric grafts, there were approximately equal numbers of adult and paediatric recients, and 6 patients received second cadaveric grafts.

1. Transplantation

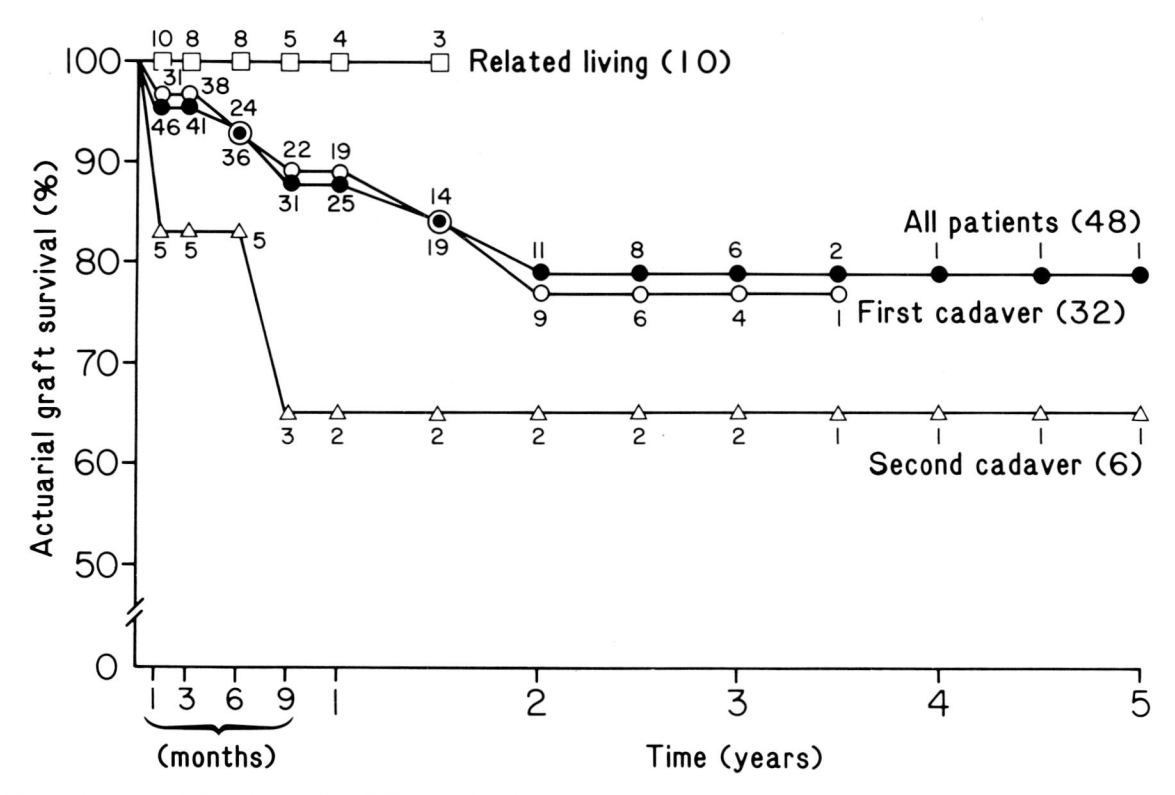

Fig. 21 Actuarial graft survival following TLI in clinical renal transplantation. Reproduced with the permission of the publishers of "Transplantation Proceddings" 1988, Vol XX No. 1 Suppl. 1.

Irradiation Protocol

The irradiation protocol was similar to that used in baboons. A basic course of 800 cGy was administered to a wide field, with shielding of supradiaphragmatic ribs and lungs, in 80 cGy fractions given twice a week. Booster fractions of 80 cGy were given at 3- or 4-week intervals if there were delays between completion of the basic course and transplantation. These delays ranged from 0 to 150 days, with a mean of 43 days. The irradiation schedule was interrupted if the peripheral blood white cell count fell below 1000/mm^3 or the platelet count fell below 35 000/mm^3. Such interruptions numbered from 0 to 4 and lasted 7 to 30 days.

Patient Survival

Patient survival is 98%. One patient died from a combination of myocardial infarction, haemorrhage from a duodenal ulcer and sepsis three months after transplantation.

Graft Survival

Overall graft survival is 85% (41 of 48 grafts). It is similar in paediatric and adult recipients. No grafts from living related donors have been lost, but 2 of 6 second cadaver transplants were rejected. Of the 7 graft losses, 1 was due to the death of the recipient, one was due to recurrence of the primary disease (oxalosis), and 5 grafts were rejected. Possible factors in the 5 graft losses from rejection were retransplantation in two, immunological evidence of presensitization in 3, problems of patient compliance in 3, and the immunosuppressive drug regimen used in 3 patients. These factors will be considered in more detail below. Actuarial graft survival is illustrated in Figure 21. For all patients it is 89% at 1 year and 79% from 2 to 5 years. The figures for first cadaver grafts are 89% and 77%, and 65% for second cadaver grafts.

Current Graft Function

Current graft function is normal (serum creatinine <130 μmol/l in adults and <100 μmol/l in children in 56% (27) of the patients). Serum creatinine is somewhat raised (mean 200±47 μmol/l), but satisfactory in 29% (14 patients).

possible that operational tolerance was being established.

The baboon studies described above indicated that the establishment of operational tolerance could be defined by the existence of stable and normal graft function one year after transplantation. Using this criterion in our patients, we analyzed 28 patients at risk for at least 1 year after transplantation.

Current Status of Patients at Risk for more than 1 Year with Normal Serum Creatinine Levels at Various Times after Transplantation

Current Status	Normal Serum Creatinine Levels at:			
	1 Month	3 Months	6 Months	1 Year
Normal Creatinine	10(63%)	9(60%)	10(63%)	9(90%)
Raised Creatinine	3(19%)	4(27%)	3(19%)	1(10%)
Graft Rejected	3(19%)	2(13%)	3(19%)	0(0%)

Table 6

Immunosuppressive Drug Therapy

Although the TLI protocol used was that which produced tolerance in one third to one half of baboons without the use of adjuvant immunosuppressive drug therapy, it was not possible to identify the individuals in whom tolerance would eventuate, as discussed above. For obvious ethical reasons, therefore, it was decided to use relatively low doses of post-transplantation immunosuppresive drugs in the human situation. Accordingly, all but 4 patients received 6 mg/kg/day of cyclosporine (CyA) and 20 mg/day of prednisone after transplantation.

These doses were tapered fairly rapidly, with the objective of ultimately withdrawing either or both if it appeared

It can be seen (Table 6) that, of patients with normal serum creatinines 1, 3, and 6 months after transplantation, approximately two thirds still have normal function more than 1 year after transplantation. However, of 10 patients with normal values at 1 year, all but 1 (90%) have maintained this status for $1\frac{1}{2}$ to $6\frac{1}{2}$ years after transplantation. By contrast, in patients with raised serum creatinines at 1 year (Table 7), two thirds have maintained this status, 13% (2 patients) have rejected their grafts and 3 patients (20%) currently have normal graft function.

Table 8 shows the current immunosuppressive drugs being received by these two groups of patients. Four pa-

1. Transplantation

Current Status of Patients at Risk for more than 1 Year with Raised Serum Creatinine Levels at Various Times after Transplantation

Current Status	Raised Serum Creatinine Leves at:			
	1 Month	3 Months	6 Months	1 Year
Normal Creatinine	3(27%)	4(33%)	3(30%)	3(20%)
Raised Creatinine	7(64%)	6(50%)	7(70%)	10(67%)
Grafts rejected	1(9%)	2(17%)	0(0%)	2(13%)

Table 7

Current Immunosuppressive Drug Therapy in Patients with Normal or Raised Serum Creatinine Levels 1 Year after Transplantation

Current Immunosuppression	Normal Creatinine at 1 Year n:mg/(kg)/day	Raised Creatinine at 1 Year n:mg/(kg)/day
Nil	1: -	0: -
Prednisone only	3: 3, 4 & 5	0: -
CyA + Prednisone	3: 2.2 + 5.8	6: 2.9 + 7.1
Azathioprine + Pred	2: 64 + 6.3	4: 100 + 9.4
CyA + Aza + Pred	1: 1.9 + 25 +	3: 2.6 + 25 + 12.5

Table 8

tients in the group with normal serum creatinine levels at 1 year are particularly noteworthy. One patient receives no immunosuppressive drugs and 3 receive very small doses (3, 4 and 5 mg/day) of prednisone only. In the first patient, prednisone was stopped $2^1/_2$ years after transplantation and azathioprine was stopped 3 years after transplantation. She retains normal graft function without any drug therapy $6^3/_4$ years after transplantation. Her lymphocytes show specific non-reactivity in cell-mediated lymphocytotoxicity assays against the lymphocytes of 3 HLA matched donors. Significant cell lysis occurred against the lymphocytes of 3 HLA mismatched donors (S. Strober, personal communication). She fulfils the criteria for durable and specific tolerance.

In the 3 patients receiving small doses of prednisone only, Cya was rapidly tapered and withdrawn 61 days, 69 days, and 1 year after transplantation, and they have now been followed for 3.3, 3, and 2 years respectively. Complete withdrawal of drugs has not been attempted in the group with raised creatinines. The current mean doses of CyA and prednisone or azathioprine are low in both groups, but particularly so in the group with normal creatinines at 1 year. Figures 22 and 23 show the serial mean

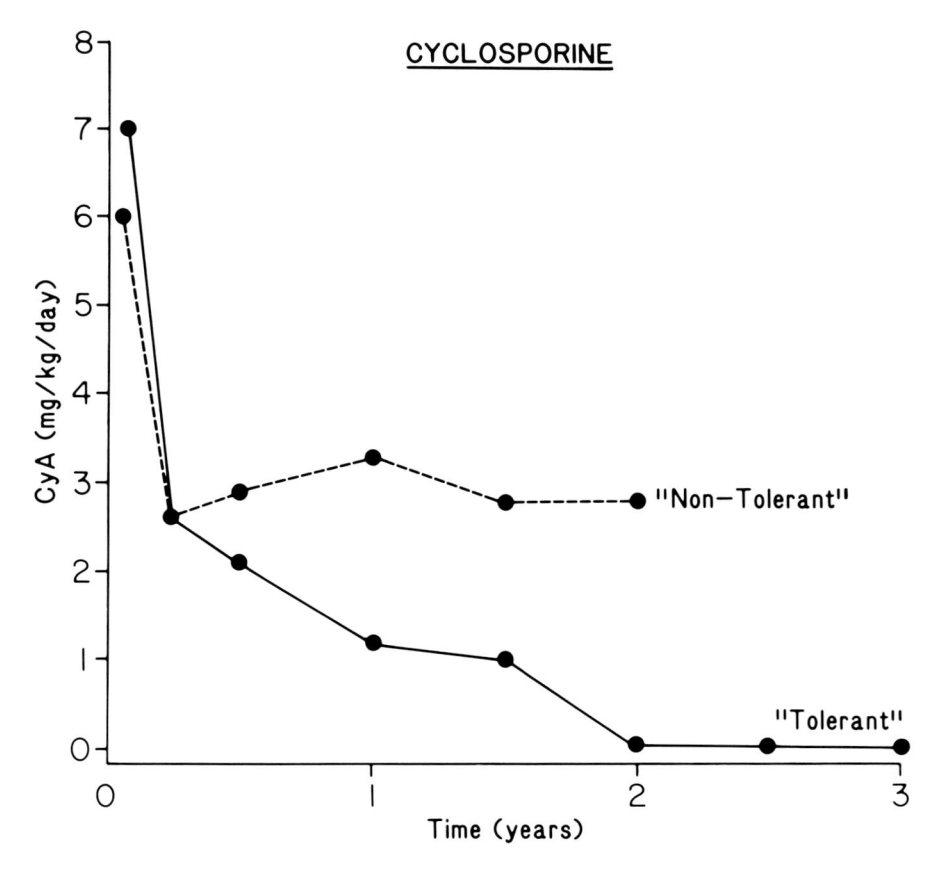

Fig. 22 Serial mean CyA doses in "tolerant" and "non-tolerant" groups.

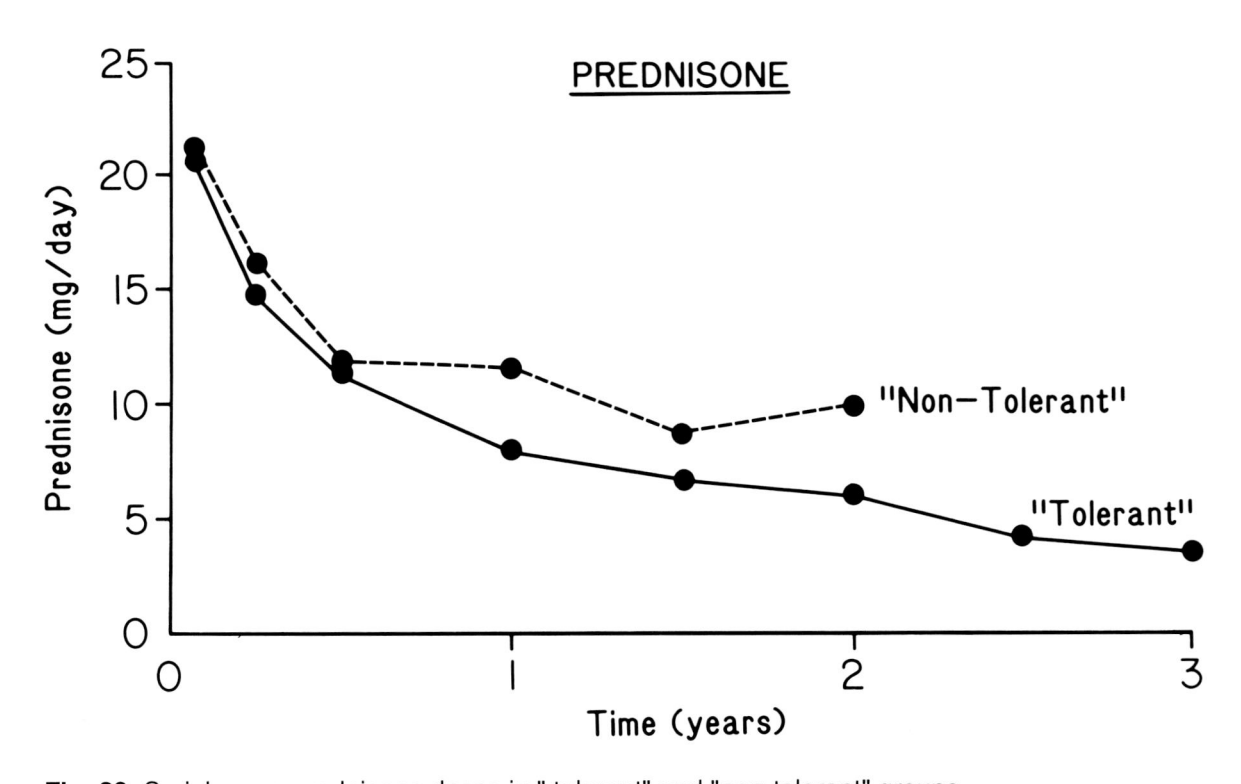

Fig. 23 Serial mean prednisone doses in "tolerant" and "non-tolerant" groups.

1. Transplantation

Presensitization Reflected by Panel Reactive Antibodies (PRA) in Patients with Normal or Raised Serum Creatinine Levels 1 Year after Transplantation

Panel Reactive Antibodies	Normal Creatinine at 1 Year (10)		Raised Creatinine at 1 Year (15)	
	Highest	Recent	Highest	Recent
All positive	9	7	13	9
50%	2	1	2	0
25-50%	3	1	5	2
<25%	4	4	7	7
Not done	1	1	-	-

Highest: highest levels at monthly screenings.
Recent: levels at most recent monthly screening.

Table 9

Rejection Episodes in Patients with Normal or Raised Serum Creatinine Levels 1 Year after Transplantation

Rejection Episodes	Normal Creatinine at 1 Year (10)	Raised Creatinine at 1 Year (15)
0	9 (90%)	4 (27%)
1	1 (10%)	2 (13%)
2	0	6 (40%)
3	0	2 (13%)
4	0	1 (7%)
Accelerated	0	6 (40%)
Slides	4 (40%)	6 (40%)

Slides: rises in serum creatinine requiring only minor adjustments of prednisone dosage.

Table 10

CyA and prednisone doses in the two groups indicated as "tolerant" and "non-tolerant".

Immunological Differences in the 'Tolerant' & 'Non-Tolerant' Groups

Panel Reactivity

Data concerning presensitization as reflected by the level of panel reactive antibodies are given in Table 9. Both groups show substantial, but not markedly different degrees of presensitization.

Rejection Episodes

Table 10 gives the details. Only 1 patient in the "tolerant" group experienced a rejection episode in the first year. By contrast, three-quarters of the patients with raised serum creatinine levels at 1 year experienced single or multiple rejection episodes, 40% of which were of the accelerated variety.

Donor Specific Presensitizaytion

All patients had negative dye exclusion crossmatches against their donors.

drawn early or not given at all at the time of transplantation (Table 12). Half the patients have done extremely well and have normal graft function on very low doses of immunosuppressive drugs from 2 years and 8 months to 3 years and 10 months after transplantation. In

1Cr Release Crossmatches in Patients with Normal or Raised Creatinine Levels 1 Year after Transplantation

51Cr crossmatch	Normal Creatinine at 1 Year (10)	Raised Creatinine at 1 Year (15)
Positive B Cell	4 (40%)	5 (33%)
Positive T Cell		
Historical	1 (10%)	4 (27%)
Recent	0 (0%)	3 (20%)
Positive LMC	0 (0%)	1 (7%)

LMC : lymphocyte mediated cytoxicity crossmatch

Table 11

However, with 51Cr release crossmatching (Table 11), only 1 patient in the "tolerant" group had a positive crossmatch (10% specific chromium release), and that with an historical serum only, but 27% of patients in the "non-tolerant" group had positive 51Cr release crossmatched with historical sera, and 20% were positive with recent sera. Positive "B-warm" 51Cr release crossmatches were present in similar proportions of the two groups.

The impact of these early events is graphically illustrated by the serial mean serum creatinine levels of the 2 groups (Figure 24).

The deleterious effect of donor presensitization is further illustrated by the course of events in a subset of 10 patients in whom CyA was either with-

the other 5 patients who either have functional grafts with abnormal function (2 patients) or who have rejected their grafts (3 patients), positive 51Cr release crossmatches were present in all, accelerated rejection episodes were seen in 2, and 2 were recipients of second cadaver grafts.

These findings are in keeping with previously published baboon data which showed that TLI was ineffective in producing tolerance in the face of donor-specific humoral presensitization, even though the tempo of rejection was somewhat slower.

Conclusions

TLI is a uniquely powerful method of producing durable and specific trans-

1. Transplantation

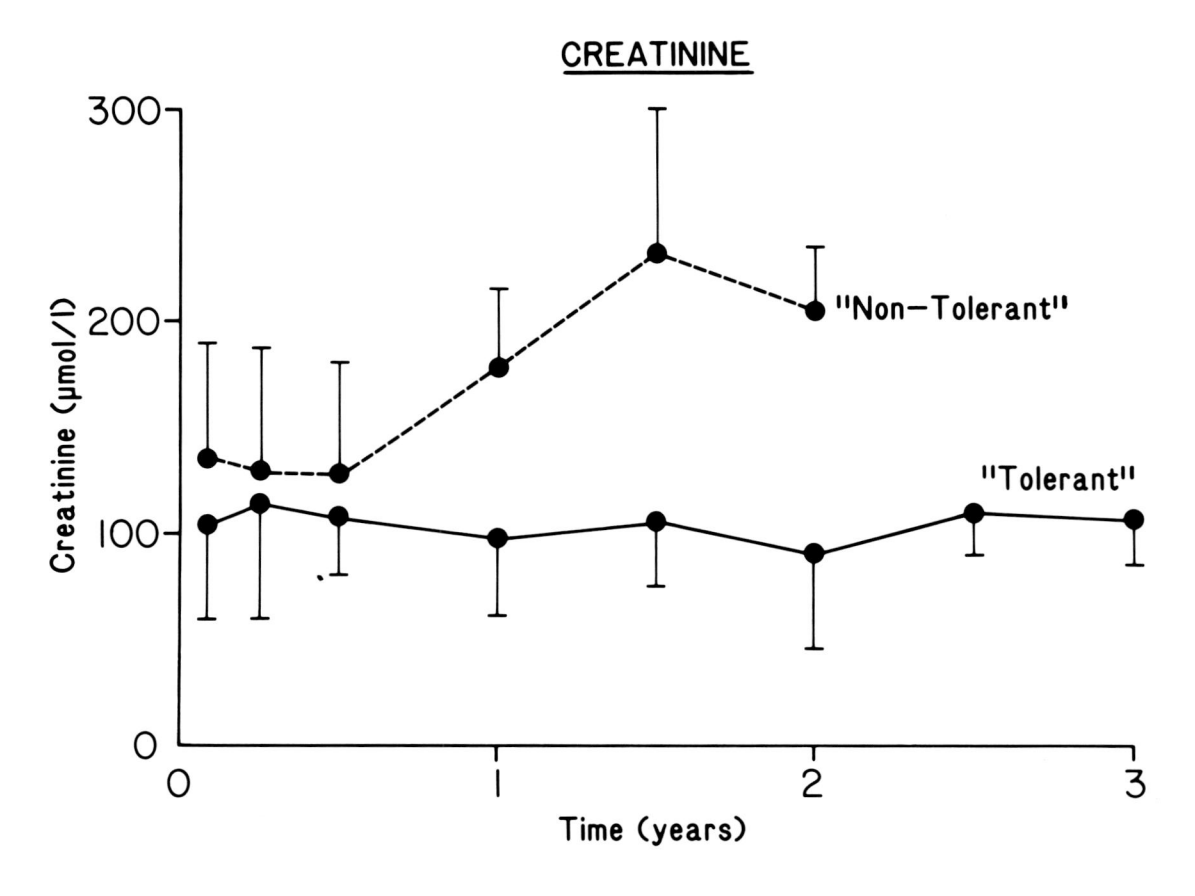

Fig. 24 Serial mean serum creatinine levels in "tolerant" and "non-tolerant" groups.

plantation tolerance in the outbred primate. With the currently optimal protocol which has evolved from many hundreds of experiments, tolerance production is, however, not universal, and is unpredictable in the individual. The evolution of specific tolerance after transplantation is gradual. Furthermore, it is an active immunological process which can be hindered or abrogated by inappropriate immunological manipulations in the form of either additional antigenic stimulation or additional post-transplantation immunosuppression. This poses problems in its clinical application, particularly with reference to the apparently counterproductive effects of post-transplantation CyA seen in the baboon.

Nevertheless, the clinical results are most encouraging. Specific tolerance has been obtained, and time will tell how frequently this will occur. If the criteria for operational tolerance delineated in baboon studies can be extrapolated to the clinical situation, the figure may turn out to be 32% (9 of 28), which is similar to that seen in baboons, although without adjunctive immunosuppressive drug therapy in the latter. A major factor militating against tolerance production is the presence of donor-specific humoral presensitization detected by 51Cr release crossmatching. In these circumstances, concomitant immunosuppressive drug therapy is clearly necessary, and permanently so.

It is important to note that even where tolerance has not eventuated, TLI has permitted the use of substantially lower

1. Transplantation

Current Status of Patients with Early Cya Withdrawal (8) or no Initial CyA (2)

Normal Creatinine (5):
Follow up : 2 yr 8 mo to 3 yr 10 mo
Creatinine : 113±11 μmol/l

Raised Creatinine (2):
Follow up : 2 yr 4 mo and 3 yr 2 mo
Positive ^{51}Cr crossmatch in both
Accelerated rejection in both

Grafts Rejected (3):
Rejection times : 7 days,
7 months,
22 months
Positive ^{51}Cr T cell crossmatch : 3 patients
Second cadavar transplants : 2 patients

Table 12

doses of immunosuppressive drugs, with a commensurate reduction in their untoward side-effects. CyA nephrotoxicity, for example, has not been seen, and steroid side-effects have been markedly attenuated. Alternative strategies of clinical management and basic immunological studies to promote greater understanding of the complex processes involved are clearly required, and are being pursued actively. There is no inherent reason why the attainment of the ultimate goal of clinical transplantation should not be available on a much wider scale in the future.

Acknowledgements

Thanks are due to all members of the Transplantation Research Unit, the medical and nursing staff of the Transplantation Service, and the Department of Radiotherapy. The work was supported by the South African Medical Research Council, the University of the Witwatersrand, and the Transvaal Provincial Administration.

1. Transplantation

References

1. Slavin S, Strober S, Fuks Z, Kaplan HS. Induction of specific tissue transplantation tolerance using fractionated total lymphoid irradiation in adult mice: Long term survival of allogeneic bone marrow and skin grafts. J Exp Med 146, 34, 1977.

2. Myburgh JA, Smit JA, Meyers AM, Botha JR, Browde S, Thomson PD. Total lymphoid irradiation in renal transplantation. World J Surg 10, 369, 1986.

3. Myburgh JA, Meyers AM, Botha JR, Thomson PD, Lakie R. Total lympoid irradiation in clinical kidney transplantation. Clin Transplant 1, 65, 1987.

4. Myburgh JA: Total lymphoid irradiation in transplantation. Transplant Proc 1988.

5. Myburgh, JA, Smit JA. Delineation, durability, predictability and specificity of operational tolerance with total lymphoid irradiation in baboon kidney transplantation. Transplant Proc 17, 1442, 1985.

6. Myburgh JA, Smit JA, Stark JH, Browde S. Total lymphoid irradiation in kidney and liver transplantation in the baboon: Prolonged graft survival and alterations in T cell subsets with low cumulative dose regimens. J Immunol 132, 1019, 1984.

7. Oseroff A, Okada S, Strober S. Natural suppressor cells found in spleens of neonatal mice and adult mice given total lymphoid irradiation. J Immunol 132, 101, 1984.

8. Little J, Myburgh JA, Austoker JL, Smit JA. Detergent solubilization of baboon histocompatibility transplantation antigens and their use is prolonging liver allograft survival. Transplantation 19, 53, 1975.

9. Yasamura T, Kahan BD. Prolongation of allograft survival by repeated cycles of donor antigen and cyclosporine in rat kidney transplantation. Transplantation 38, 418, 1984.

10. Myburgh JA, Meyers AM, Botha JR, Thomson PD, Smit JA, Browde S, Lakie R. Wide field low dose irradiation in clinical kidney transplantation. Transplant Proc 19, 1974, 1987.

1.3.2. Clinical Application of Polyclonal Antibodies Antilymphocyte (ALG), Antithymocyte (ATG) Globulin in Heart Transplantation

B Reichart

*Department of Cardiothoracic Surgery,
University of Cape Town, Medical School,
Cape Town, South Africa*

In contradistinction to the relatively new monoclonal antibodies, which are produced with the help of hybrid techniques and which react only with a certain leucocyte group, like the T-lymphocytes, antilymphocyte/antithymocyte globulins in current use consist of a variety of polyclonal antibodies; only approximately 10% of the drug actually reacts with T-lymphocytes. The following review should provide a brief update on antilymphocyte/antithymocyte globulins, presented at the end of 1987.

The characteristics of ALG depend on how it was produced; human lymphocytes (obtained from the thoracic duct), lymphoblast cultures, cells from the spleen or lymph nodes and thymocytes (lymphocytes originating from the neonatal thymus) may be used as antigens (review of the literature in 1,2). The cells are then washed and diluted to their final concentration. A certain quantity is injected intravenously into horses, sheep or rabbits for basic immunisation; booster doses are given at intervals of 4 weeks. The antibody fraction is extracted from the serum by a process of precipitation and adsorption and, finally, chromatography.

Since ALG contains foreign protein, all the risks involved in heterologous serum therapy apply.

Experience on ALG was first described by Woodruff and Anderson in 1963 (3) and introduced for clinical application by Starzl in 1967 (4). In West Germany, experiments were performed by Brendel, Pichlmayr and Land; they preferred horses for immunisation (5-7). Although the German authors were mainly involved in immunosuppression of renal-transplanted patients, Brendel was able to gain early experience in heart transplantation as well. In 1968 he and Barnard successfully controlled a severe acute rejection reaction in the second Cape Town patient, Dr Philip Blaiberg, and reported on this therapy in nine long-term survivors at the 2nd World Symposium for Heart Transplantation in Montreal a year later (8, 9).

While the Stanford group also experimented with horse ALG initially, rabbit serum was preferred after the early seventies (10). Thymocytes were used for immunization, which explains the name ATG (almost all heart transplantation centres now use rabbit-ATG). Also Stanford-specific are the alternating i.m.

1. Transplantation

and i.v. injections. It is their opinion that i.m. injections reach the lymphnode systems more directly.

The initial dose of ATG (like that of Fresenius, Gauting bei München, FRG) is 1.5-2.5 mg of IgG/kg/day, which results in a decrease of the peripheral T-lymphocyte count; the cells are thought to disappear into the reticuloendothelial system. Circulating lymphocytes become inactivated.

The resultant decrease in peripheral T-cells may be measured by performing the simple rosetting test (11, 12): T-lymphocytes, in contrast to B-lymphocytes, form spontaneous rosettes with sheep erythrocytes. Further control of ATG therapy is also achieved by using the test as a daily monitoring device. Ideally, the number of peripheral T-lymphocytes should fall from 4000 to less than 40 cells per mm^3. If the number of lymphocytes increases rapidly during treatment, a rejection reaction must be assumed and the ATG-dosage increased accordingly. After confirmation of acute rejection by endomyocardial biopsy, intravenous methylprednisolone treatment is added.

In the era of "classical" immunosuppression with azathioprine and steroids, ATG was given prophylactically for ten to fourteen days according to the Stanford regimen; treatment beyond five to six weeks was considered ineffective because of antibody formation. Since the introduction of cyclosporine, ATG has been used less frequently in order to prevent over-immunization and possible increased tumour neogenesis (13).

However, ATG usage has recently increased, but only for a short pre- and postoperative period. The Pittsburgh group is at present utilizing rabbit-ATG as additional therapy during severe acute rejection crises: if i.v. methylprednisolone in a total dose of 3g proves unsuccessful, treatment continues with additional ATG - "rescue therapy" which also proved effective in Cape Town.

In heart transplantation candidates in whom the prevailing disease is well advanced, conventional immunosuppression - including ATG - may be used initially in order to prevent the complication of postoperative oligo-/anuria caused by cyclosporine. After the patient is stabilised, ATG is replaced by cyclosporine.

In heart-lung transplantation, ATG is used according to the Stanford regimen during the first two weeks, and then replaced by corticoids. This is in order to obviate the unwanted steroid effects on tracheal healing.

1. Transplantation

References

1. Touraine JL, Malik MC, Traeger J. Antilymphocyte globulin and thoracic duct drainage in renal transplant, In: Salaman JR (ed), Immunosuppressive Therapy. MTP Press, Lancaster, p 55, 1981.

2. Cosimi AB. Antilymphocyte globulin - a final (?) look. In: Progress in transplantation, Morris PJ, Tilney NL (eds), Churchill Livingstone, Edinburgh, p 167, 1984.

3. Woodruff MFA, Anderson NF. Effect of lymphocyte depletion by thoracic duct fistula and administration of lymphocyte serum on the survival of skin homografts in rats. Nature 200, 702, 1963.

4. Starzl TE, Marchioro TL, Porter KA, Iwatsaki Y, Cerili GJ. The use of heterologous antilymphoid agents in canine renal and liver homotransplantation and in human renal homotransplantation. Surg Gynec Obst 124, 301, 1967.

5. Pichlmayr R, Brendel W, Zenker R. Production and effect of heterologous anti-canine lymphocyte serum. Surgery 61, 774, 1967.

6. Brendel W, Land W, Pichlmayr R. Intravenous treatment with horse antihuman lymphocyte (ALG) in organ transplantation and autoimmune diseases. In: Bertelli A, Monaco AP, (eds), Pharmacological treatment in organ and tissue transplantation, Excerpta Medica, Amsterdam, p 208, 1971.

7. Tidow G, Lauchart W, Pichlmayr R. Einsatz von Anti-Lymphozyten-Globulin bei Nierentransplantationen. Die gelben Hefte, Behringwerke 21, 108, 1981.

8. Brendel W. Intravenous use of high dosage of ALG. In: Heart Transplantation, Laval Press, Quebec, p 149, 1970.

9. Brendel W. Erste Muenchner Kontakte mit der Herztransplantation. Fortschr Med 101, 2007, 1983.

10. Bieber CP. Pharmacokinetics of antithymocyte globulin (ATG) and cardiac transplant outcome. J Heart Transplant 1, 22, 1981.

11. Jondal M, Holm G, Wigzell H. Surface markers on human T and B lymphocytes. J Exp Med 136, 207, 1972.

12. Lay WH, Mendes NF, Bianco C, Nussenzweig V. Binding of sheep red blood cells to a large population of human lymphocytes. Nature 230, 531, 1971.

13. Brumbaugh J, Baldwin JC, Stinson EB, Oyer PE, Jamieson SW, Bieber CP, Henle W, Shumway NE. Quantitative analysis of immunosuppression in cyclosporine-treated heart transplant patients with lymphoma. J Heart Transplant 4, 307, 1985.

1.3.3. The Use of Monoclonal Antibodies in Treating Cardiac Allograft Rejection: Our Experience with OKT-3

MS Sweeney [1], OH Frazier [2], JT Sinnott IV. [2], JB O'Connell [3]

*From the Divisions of Cardiovascular Surgery and Infectious Diseases,
University of South Florida, Tampa, Florida,[1]
the Division of Surgery, Texas Heart Institute, Houston, Texas, [2]
and the Division of Cardiology,
University of Utah, Salt Lake City, Utah.[3]*

Introduction

The treatment of allograft rejection is the most important consideration for a successful cardiac transplantation program. Such treatment is efficacious when it specifically targets the graft destruction process and reverses the rejection without intolerable sequelae. When baseline therapy of cyclosporine, azathioprine, and steroids (or some combination thereof) is overcome, some form of auxiliary support is needed, making these adjunctive immunotherapy protocols an important part of any treatment system. High dose steroid pulses or polyclonal antithymocyte globulins have often been used in this setting. Although these drugs can be helpful, they are not very specific to the graft destruction process, and are commonly associ-ated with side-effects when vigorous rejection demands their repeated or protracted administration.

The T-lymphocyte is central to the immune response, since its activation and the lymphokine recruitment that follows are the genesis of signals through which both antibody and cell-mediated immunity are sustained. The antigen recognition structures on the T-cell surface are associated with three polypeptide chains (the T-3 complex), which transduce the signal from the antigen and enable the T-cell to react, proliferate, and kill the foreign stimuli. A molecule that specifically reacts with the T-3 complex would therefore be capable of blocking the T-cell effector functions involved in cardiac allograft rejections.

This article reviews our experience with orthoclone OKT-3 in manipulating cardiac allograft rejections, both prophylactically and as "rescue" therapy for stubborn advanced rejection. This drug is a murine monoclonal antibody that is specifically directed against the T-3 antigen recognition structure of human T-cells, and as such is more selectively targeted for those lymphocyte functions that are important in clinical immunology. Our experiences confirm that orthoclone OKT-3 is a powerful and effective agent that is well tolerated and produces few side-effects that are difficult to manage.

Materials and Methods

OKT-3 as Treatment for Advanced Cardiac Allograft Rejection

The hospital records and follow-up clinical charts of 202 consecutive patients who received cardiac allografts between July 1982 and May 1987 were reviewed. All patients were treated primarily with cyclosporine, 14mg/kg/day administered orally, and prednisone, with cyclosporine levels regularly adjusted to maintain serum levels of 200 to 300 mg/ml. Failure of this baseline therapy was manifested by advanced rejection in 86 (43%) patients, as judged by endomyocardial biopsy. This group comprised 64 men and 22 women, ranging in age from 5 to 64 years (mean 46 years). Although human lymphocyte antigen typing was unavailable for many patients, each recipient and donor pair were selected on the basis of ABO-bloodgroup compatibility and a negative lymphocyte crossmatch. Indications for transplant included dilated idiopathic cardiomyopathy in 42 (49%) patients, ischemic cardiomyopathy in 38 (44%), endstage congenital disease in three (3.5%), and rheumatic heart disease in three (3.5%) patients. All recipients were selected according to standard criteria, and none had associated problems that were serious enough to predict extended hospitalization or require alteration of baseline immunotherapy.

Standard endomyocardial biopsies were performed regularly and interpreted using the McAllister scale (1), which assigns numerical objectivity to the degree of rejection. Advanced rejection is defined by a grade of 7 or more, in which perivascular aggregates and interstitial infiltrates of mononuclear cells are present, as well as multifocal cardiac myocyte degeneration of increasing frequency. At these levels of allograft rejection, an adjunctive immunotherapy protocol is required.

Pulse corticosteroid therapy was given to 82 patients for 101 advanced rejection episodes. Treatment consisted of 500 mg of methylprednisolone (solumedrol), administered intravenously every 8 hours, up to a total of 3 gms. In addition, the maintenance steroid (prednisone) dosage was increased and tapered slowly thereafter. ATG-therapy, 14 mg/kg/day in two divided doses, was given intravenously. Duration of therapy was modified by resolution of the rejection episode, by the development of significant drug side-effects, such as bone marrow suppression.

OKT-3 was used in 14 patients, who received a single 5mg/day intravenous bolus, with the average duration of therapy lasting 14 days. Prior to administration of the drug, a skin test (0.1ml of 1mg/ml solution given intradermally) was done to ensure that no performed antimurine antibodies existed. No patient had a skin test with positive results. In each patient a pretreatment regimen was administered before both the first and second dosages, when the physiological side-effects of systemic T-cell lysis generally occur. This pretreatment included an intravenous dose of 500 mg of diphenhydramine, both taken orally approximately 30 minutes in advance of the dose. Hydrocortisone (100 mg) was given intravenously 30 minutes after each of the first two dosages. Every effort was made to bring the patient's body weight to within 3% of his preoperative weight, and patients were given high doses of furosemide to achieve this if necessary. Routine pretreatment chest X-ray films were carefully examined for fluid overload, and vital signs were vigorously monitored once treatment had begun.

During the OKT-3 treatment course, daily blood work (sequential multiple analysis biochemical profile, complete blood count with differential) was obtained. In addition, both chest X-ray films and urine cultures were ordered every 3 days. For temperature elevations of 100.5°F, an infectious disease evaluation was performed, and a complete bacteriological and fungal surveillance was obtained. Pulmonary infiltrates were aggressively investigated with bronchoscopy, washings, and biopsy if necessary.

OKT-3 as Prophylaxis against Cardiac Allograft Rejection

The great majority of significant cardiac allograft rejections occur within the early (one month) post-transplant period. Because OKT-3 has been successful, not only in reversing rejection, but also, at least in theory, in modulating future immune responses, its use as an early, prophylactic, antirejection treatment was proposed. This philosophy has had its major proponents at the University of Utah, where 93 patients have recently been treated in this manner.

Treatment with OKT-3 has consisted of a daily 5 mg intravenous dose, given within 48 hours post-transplant. The pretreatment regimens and treatment schemes are otherwise similar to those outlined above. Three subsets of treatment regimens have been used in this series:

1) OKT-3 given daily for 14 days, with CY-A begun in standard doses on day 4,
2) OKT-3 given daily for 10 days, with CY-A begun on day 4, and
3) OKT-3 daily for 14 days, with CY-A begun on day 11. The first two of these subsets were changed in response to the transplant team's feeling that too much immunosuppression was aboard, and the third subset continues to be the preferred regimen at the University of Utah. Blood work and follow-up schemes were similar to those outlined in the "rescue" treated group above. The steroid regimen followed in the Utah OKT-3 prophylaxis group consisted of

a) 1mg/kg/day of prednisone while the OKT-3 course was underway,

b) 1mg/kg/day of prednisone for one week following the termination of the OKT-3, and

c) over the subsequent 2 weeks the steroids were tapered off completely.

Results

OKT-3 as Treatment for Advanced Cardiac Allograft Rejection

Of the 14 patients, 12 required treatment after failure of methylprednisolone pulse therapy, and two received OKT-3 as the initial augmentation treatment for advanced rejection. OKT-3 was successful as rescue therapy in 13 (93%) of these 14 patients. Other than infections, our OKT-3-treated group experienced minimal adverse medical sequelae, and in no instance was early interruption of therapy required.

In all 14 patients, overall T-cell counts decreased to zero within several hours of administration of the OKT-3 drug, and counts of T-cell subsets were similarly depleted. Pretreatment endomyocardial biopsy scores ranged from 6 to 9 (average 8.1). Biopsies were repeated near the termination of therapy (at approximately 10 to 15 days) and at approximately 1 month after the initial OKT-3 dose. The average biopsy score decreased to 4.1, a drop of four levels on the histologic grading scale. Moreover, a lasting effect was achieved in the majority of patients, as biopsy scores stayed within the mild to moderate rejection range thereafter and were matched by improved performance of the grafts.

Side-effects were experienced in fewer than half the patients and were well tolerated. Side-effects were manifested by chills (six patients), fever (six patients), nausea (three patients), headaches (three patients), and diarrhea (one patient). In those patients who experienced side-effects, they occurred within the initial 48 hours when lymphocyte destruction was greatest. In every instance these symptoms were either easily managed or went away without medical intervention.

Infectious complications were diverse and involved an array of bacterial pathogens. During the course of OKT-3 therapy, there were nine episodes of bacterial infections (bacteremia or positive urine cultures), five episodes of fungal diseases (oral candidiasis), six viral infections (5 oral contaminations of herpes simplex and 1 cytomegalovirus pneumonia), and no protozoal infection. In the subsequent month after therapy, five infectious processes were encountered; of these, three were bacterial, two were viral.

OKT-3 as Prophylaxis against Cardiac Allograft Rejection

With either a 10 or 14 day course of OKT-3 prophylaxis, the incidence of cardiac allograft rejection in the Utah series (to date) has been 1.5 - 1.6 episodes/pt over the initial 6 months following transplantation. This represents at least a 50% reduction in the rejection rate (episodes/pt over 6 months). The most common time for rejection to be seen was between 5 and 6 weeks post-transplantation. The reasons for this 5th-6th week "window" of vulnerability are not clearly understood, but some mild form of rebound from T-cell clone destruction is currently proposed. At any rate, the overwhelming majority of these rejection episodes have been easily treated with steroid pulses, manipulation of the cyclosporine doses, or by retreatment with OKT-3. Of the 8 patients who have required retreatment with OKT-3, 1 did not respond and died, 1 responded well but developed sepsis and died, and 6 were successfully treated and continue to do well. Infectious complications were generally similar to those experienced in the rescue treated group above, and, when present, were usually treated with ease. There was no difference in the infections experienced between the 10 day and 14 day OKT-3 prophylaxis subsets.

A major additional advantage in the "OKT-3-as-prophylaxis" group appears to be the limitation of steroids use. Fully 88% of the patients in the Utah series have required no maintenance steroids, which the Utah group feels contributed to a lessening of overall morbidity and mortality, a shorter hospital stay, and a reduction in medical expenses. Additionally, mean serum cholesterol levels in their patients were observed to be uniformly below 200, even after the OKT-3 course was completed. Whether this observation will result in any clinically practical benefits is unknown at present.

1. Transplantation

Summary

Interest in cardiac transplantation has surged with the ability to control rejection more predictably. Cyclosporine and steroids have become a major part of baseline immunotherapy, and this has appeared to result not only in better survival, but also in lower morbidity and shorter hospital stays. Despite well-monitered cyclosporine levels, almost 90% of serious rejection episodes in most series occur within 30 days of transplantation. It appears that, in addition to steroids and carefully regulated cyclosporine levels, some clue is required as to which patients are at risk for developing advanced rejection.

When advanced rejection is established, there are three potential treatment schemes currently used, namely:

1. high dose pulsed corticosteroids,
2. antithymocyte globulins (polyclonal), and
3. monoclonal antibodies.

Orthoclone OKT-3 is a murine monoclonal antibody that combines with a 20 000 Dalton molecule found only on mature T-cells and medullary thymocytes. It has no reactivity with B cells, platelets, macrophages, or granulocytes. The drug is produced by a genetic fusion of sensitized mouse lymphocytes with myeloma cells - a hybridoma. The fluid produced by implantation of this hybridoma into the peritoneum of a mouse has tremendous specificity, but is further purified before becoming the drug itself. The high degree of specificity and purity inherent in the production techniques no doubt accounts for the relative lack of systemic reactions when the drug is administered clinically.

When given intravenously, Orthoclone OKT-3 virtually eliminates all circulating T-cells within hours. In addition to specifically reacting with the T-cells population, the drug blocks their functions by the close association of the target molecule with the T-3 antigen recognition receptor on the cell surface. Although T-cells ultimately return to the circulation in numbers equivalent to pretreatment levels, the T-cells that reappear do not possess the OKT-3 reactive molecule. This phenomenon is called modulation, and explains the potential for continued immunosuppression after the initial treatment course.

Our data suggest that pulsed steroids as a front-line treatment for advanced rejection are often ineffective. Although pulses of methyprednisolone may be effective when used against less severe levels of rejection, they are not as effective when used against severe myocyte degeneration. Additionally, the use of multiple pulses of steroids within four to five weeks harbors potentially lethal hazards for the cardiac transplant patient.

Death and morbidity in heart transplant patients are caused by either unreversed rejection or opportunistic infections, and usually occur in patients who experience advanced rejection. ATG has been efficacous in the treatment of these patients, once serious rejection is established, and OKT-3 appears to be a very attractive therapy as well. The use of an OKT-3 course as early prophylaxis against rejection has worked extremely well in the hands of the University of Utah group,and gives much cause for thought in the quest for a safer, more successful approach to what will surely be an increasingly risky transplant candidate group over the next twenty years of medical progress.

1. Transplantation

Reference

1. McAllister HA, Schnee MJ, Radovancevic B, Frazier OH. A System for grading cardiac allograft rejection. Tex Heart Inst J 13, 1, 1986.

1. Transplantation

1.3.4. The Monoclonal Antibody BMA 031 in Organ Transplantation

J Racenberg [1], R Zerban [1], R Kurrle [2], F Seiler [2]

*[1] Clinical Research-Immunology,
[2] Experimental Research, Behringwerke,
Marburg, FR Germany*

Anti-CD3 monoclonal antibodies have been extensively used to analyse the role of the CD3 complex in the activation of human T-lymphocytes as well as in their effector functions.

Binding of anti-CD3 antigen may result in polyclonal T-cell proliferation, the modulation and internalization of the CD3 complex, in secretion of immunomediators such as IL-2 and in the appertaining expression of IL-2 receptor, as well as in the secretion of other immune factors such as gamma interferon and the haematopoietic growth factor GM-CSF. Further effects of CD3 monoclonal antibodies are the increase of Ca^{++} influx in anti-CD3 activated T-lymphocytes, the capability to induce T-suppressor cell proliferation, the inhibition of antigen-specific proliferation of T-helper cells, and the inhibition of the effector phase of cell-mediated cytolysis, as well as of the induction of cytotoxicity.

Which of the above-listed CD3 mediated reactions happens under physiological conditions, depends at least partly on the isotype of the anti-CD3 monoclonal antibody, as in most of these reactions the Fc-part of the antibody molecule is instrumental. Lymphocytes from nearly every donor respond to anti-CD3 monoclonal antibodies of IgG-2a isotype with a strong proliferation. In only 80% of the European population, however, does incubation of peripheral blood leukocytes with anti-CD3 monoclonal antibodies of IgG_1 isotype result in T-cell proliferation. When IgG-2b or IgM antibodies with specificity to the CD3 antigen-complex are used, mitogenic activity of such antibodies could be measured in less than 5 % of blood donors.

The molecular basis of antigen recognition, the human T-cell receptor(TCR), is a heterodimer of disulphide-linked alpha- and beta-chains, non-covalently associated with at least three chains of the CD3 antigen-complex. Over the last few years, our laboratories have isolated several monoclonal antibodies binding to the TCR/CD3 antigen complex. While BMA 030 antibody, isotype IgG-2a, binds to the chains of the CD3 complex, immuno-precipitation experiments confirmed the evidence that BMA 031, an IgG-2b isotype, recognizes epitopes within the constant part of the human TCR.

In Vitro Effects of TCR/CD3-Monoclonal Antibodies

	BMA 031 α/β-TCR; IgG2b	BMA 030 CD3; IgG2a
Induction of:		
Ca^{++}-influx	−	+++
Antigen-modulation	±	+++
Lymphocyte proliferation	+	+++
(day 3; optimal conc.)	≥10 ng/ml	0.001-1 ng/ml
Cyctotoxicity (CTL-clones)	+++	+++
Cytokine release/production		
Gamma-IFN	±	+++
IL-2	±	+++
GM-CSF	±	+++
Suppression of polyclonal B-cell activation	+ to +++	+ to +++

Table 13 (for abbreviations see text)

In Vitro Effects of BMA 031 and BMA 030

The immuno-regulatory capacity of BMA 031 has been analysed in numerous in-vitro experiments in comparison to the CD3 specific monoclonal antibody BMA 030 and other well-known anti-CD3 monoclonal antibodies.

The comparison of the in-vitro effects of BMA 031 versus BMA 030 is schematically listed in Table 13. This table clearly demonstrates that binding of BMA 031 to human T-cells, if at all, leads to T-cell activation only when applied in much higher concentrations than with BMA 030. This is reflected by the fact that mere binding of BMA 031 triggers neither calcium influx nor antigen modulation. On the other hand, BMA 031 acts with the same effectiveness as BMA 030 on cytotoxic T-cell clones and in the suppression of polyclonally induced immunoglobulin synthesis in-vitro. Of special importance, we be-lieve is the fact that after binding to T-cells, BMA 031 triggers the release of immuno-regulatory active substances such as IL-2 or GM-CSF to a much lesser extent than BMA 030. In addition BMA 031 induces only very low titres of gamma-interferon. This finding might be of clinical importance at least in situations where CD3 antibodies are used to prevent acute allograft rejection in organ transplantation. Clinical applications of high gamma-interferon doses are associated with side effects very similar to those observed after application of mitogenic anti-CD3 antibodies. In addition, gamma-interferon is able to increase the HLA-DR expression, an effect which, in contrast to the desired immuno-suppressive effect of anti-CD3 monoclonal antibody application, leads to augmentation of the allogeneic response.

1. Transplantation

First Clinical Experience

Based on the data of in-vitro experiments, we selected BMA 031 for clinical applications in immunosuppressive therapy. In ongoing phase 1 clinical trials, 33 patients have so far been treated with BMA 031. Nine patients were treated to overcome an acute steroid-resistant rejection crisis following kidney transplantation. Another 9 patients were treated prophylactically; in other words for seven days immediately following the kidney transplantation. These patients had preformed cytotoxic antibodies. Both studies are being carried out at the University Hospital of Munich and will be completed in February 1988.

Five patients were treated prophylactically for 7 days following heart transplantation at the University Hospital of Hanover. Ten patients have also been treated prophylactically following liver transplantation in Hanover.

The schedule for these trials is as follows: A few hours after the transplantation, the monoclonal antibody is administered daily for 7 days in dosages of 5 and 10 mg per day. Blood chemistry, human antimurine antibodies and the level of the monoclonal antibody in the blood, T-cell subsets, differential blood count, and physical examinations are carried out daily during the application course and on the scheduled days up to one year following the transplantation.

Table 14 demonstrates the reported side-effects and infections in the 33 treated patients. Undesirable effects occured in 4 patients. Three patients reacted with an acute rise in temperature, one of them during the first infusion; the treatment had to be stopped for this patient. Two others had a rise in temperature on the 2nd or the 5th day, and one patient had headache, bone-pain and backache following the infusion of the monoclonal antibody.

Two urinary tract infections following kidney transplantation were reported, as well as one gram-positive blood culture. One peritonitis following a multiple laparatomy was found, as well as one severe CMV-infection following liver transplantation. The five patients treated prophylactically following heart

---

Monoclonal Antibody BMA 031 (BI 51.013)
Preliminary Clinical Results

Low rate of undesirable effects
    4 / 33 patients
    3 patients with acute rise in temperature
    1 patient with headache, bone-pain, backache

Infections
    2 urinary tract infections following kidney transplantation
    1 gram-positive cocci in blood following kidney transplantation
    1 CMV infection following liver transplantation
    1 peritonitis after multiple laparotomy
    5 suspected CMV infection folloing heart transplantation

Table 14

transplantation had suspected (but not very severe) CMV-infection.

Summary

The murine monoclonal antibody BMA 031 of the IgG-2b isotype is directed to a monomorphic determinant in the alpha-beta chain of the human T-cell receptor. The IgG-2b isotype is unable to interact with the Fc-receptor of accessory cells. That means that IgG-2b monoclonal antibodies do not induce T-cell proliferation to the degree comparable to monoclonal antibodies of other IgG sub-classes. The monoclonal antibody has been used in 33 patients treated within 4 studies. The preliminary results show that there is a low rate of side-effects. The final dosage and hints on efficacy remain to be evaluated.

1. Transplantation

1.4. Rejection Monitoring

1.4.1. Cyto-immunological Monitoring (CIM) for Differentiation between Cardiac Rejection, Viral, Bacterial or Fungal Infection; its Specifity and Sensitivity

C Hammer [1], D Klanke [1], P Dirschedl [2], C Lersch [1], BM Kemkes [4],
M Gokel [3], H Reichenspurner [5], B Reichart [5]

*Institute for Surgical Research [1],
Institute for Statistics and Biomathematics [2],
Institute of Pathology [3] and Department of Cardiac Surgery [4],
University of Munich and Department of Cardio-Thoracic Surgery,
University of Cape Town [5]*

Introduction

For heart transplant patients, percutaneous transvenous endo-myocardial biopsies (EMB) introduced by Caves (1) and its evaluation according to Billingham (2) are still the standard methods for early detection of acute rejections, grading of the inflammation, and control of successful immunosuppressive therapy.

In order to reduce the frequency of this invasive tool, however, cyto-immunological monitoring was introduced (3). It is based on the observation that lymphocytes and their activated forms recirculate in the peripheral blood of heart transplant patients during various inflammatory episodes including acute rejection.

Material and Methods

CIM consists of two tests: A fast test which yields rough information about the activation of circulating white blood cells, and an extended test which allows a more sophisticated differential diagnosis.

Fast Test

Only 10 µl of peripheral blood are needed for a smear for differentiation of leucocytes; 40 µl for total leucocyte counting.

The mononuclear cells separated from 500 µl of heparinized peripheral blood over a Ficoll micro-gradient are spread on a slide using a cytocentrifuge. The smear is stained according to Pappenheim (30 min). All leucocyte populations and their activated forms are taken into consideration. As long as no signs of activation or other exceptional observations are found, an additional procedure is not necessary.

Extended Test

When any of the subpopulations are activated, the second test must be applied:

From 10 ml of heparinized peripheral blood, separated over a Ficoll gradient (d=1,077), the lymphocytes are counted using a cytofluorometer (4). All interesting subpopulations are distinguished by means of monoclonal antibodies. The most important lymphocytes are those labelled by CD4 and CD8 antibodies (5).

Immunosuppressive Therapy

All patients received cyclosporine with low-dose prednisolone as basic immunosuppression.

For statistical investigation of CIM, 72 out of 83 heart transplant patients were tested by various analyses. The eleven remaining patients were not included because three had received different immunosuppressive treatment and eight had died of early postoperative complications like organ failure and sepsis (6).

The aim of the study was to investigate the correlation between the established diagnosis of acute rejection by EMB and that given by CIM, and to determine the sensitivity and specificity of CIM relative to EMB (7).

As the simultaneous comparison of inter- and intra-individual data is not admissible for small sample sizes and by means of an unbiased selection of comparable data, the first inflammatory event was defined as the one to be investigated. This decision is also reasonable from a clinical point of view, for most of the therapy-resistant rejections occuring within the first two weeks.

Statistical Tests used:
- Estimation of reliability of lymphoblast counts (LB) of two raters
- The construction of a ROC-curve (Receiver Operating Characteristic curve) (8)
- A multiple logistic regression, i.e. discriminant analysis to select the best discriminating variables
- CART (classification and regression trees) (9)

Results

Evaluation

Activated lymphocytes (ALYs) and lymphoblasts (LBs) are the most important and indicative cells (Figure 25).

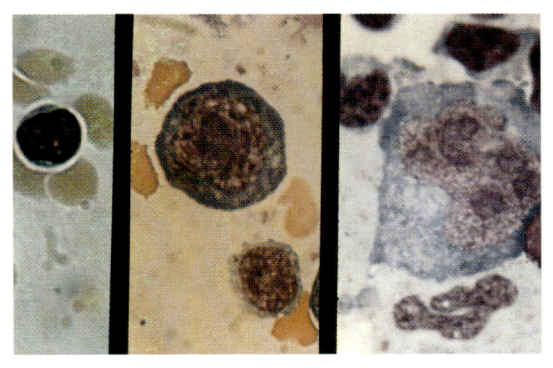

Fig. 25 From left to right, single lymphocyte, activated lymphocyte and lymphoblast for comparison. All cells shown at the same magnification (1 200 x). Note difference in size, basophilic plasma and structure of chromatin as well as number of nucleoli of the different cells.

A marked difference in size, basophilic plasma, structure of chromatin, and number of nucleoli exists, which makes the distinction of the lymphocytes possible. Three times 100 cells are differentiated according to a fixed scheme. The percentage is calculated and the CD4/CD8 ratio determined.

Acute Rejection

In a case of severe acute cellular rejection (AR), an activated mononuclear concentrate (MNC), including more than 7% blast cells or 20% activated lymphocytes, is found. The ratio of cells expressing the phenotypes CD4/ CD8

1. Transplantation

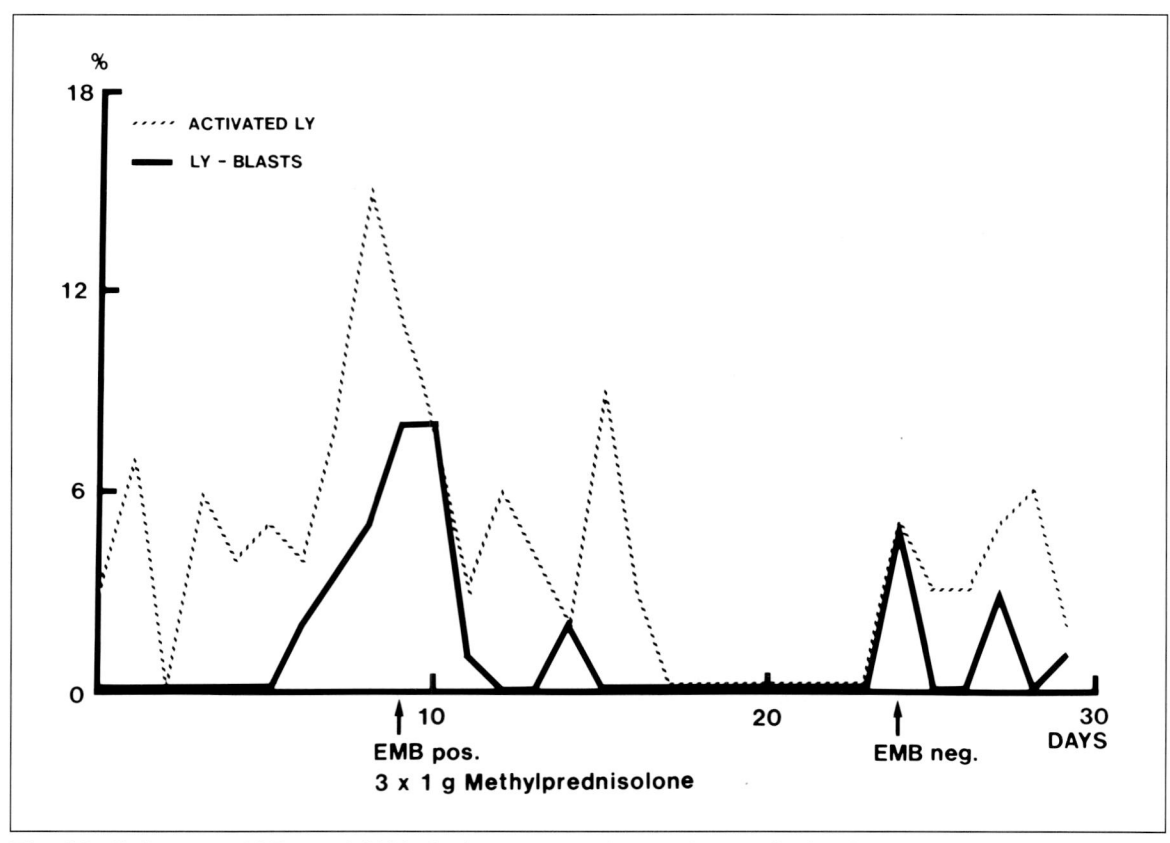

Fig. 26 Follow up of LBs and ALY of a heart-transplant patient suffering from acute rejection (day 7-10) and bacterial infection (day 25).

is approximately 1.5. B-cells numbers are lower than 15%.

Viral Infection

During viral infection, the activated MNC is of different consistence: The CD4/CD8 ratio is lower than 1.0. At the height of infection, the ratio is often as low as 0.1. The percentage of B cells remains unchanged or is slightly increased. So-called "large granular lymphocytes" (LGL), supposed to be natural killer cells, appear in high numbers, in most cases exceeding 5% of leucocytes; these LGLs sometimes comprise 40-50% of the lymphocyte population.

Bacterial Infection

Bacterial or fungal infections induce activation but no change in the CD4/CD8 ratio. A significant increase of B-cells and juvenile polimorphonuclear cells is found. Often this increase of promyelocytes makes the reading and distinction of cells of the lymphocyte line difficult. Beside CIM, other non-invasive methods such as Fast-Fourier-transformed ECG and echocardiography are applied. As soon as CIM together with another test is positive (CIM remaining the leading parameter) the patient is treated for rejection, and the process is then controlled by endomyocardial biopsies.

A typical follow-up of a patient (Figure 26) shows the behaviour of activated lymphocytes and blasts. An increase of ALYs and LBs at day 5 heralds a rejection sensitive to methylprednisolone. The peak at day 25, due to a bacterial infection, was negative in EMB.

1. Transplantation

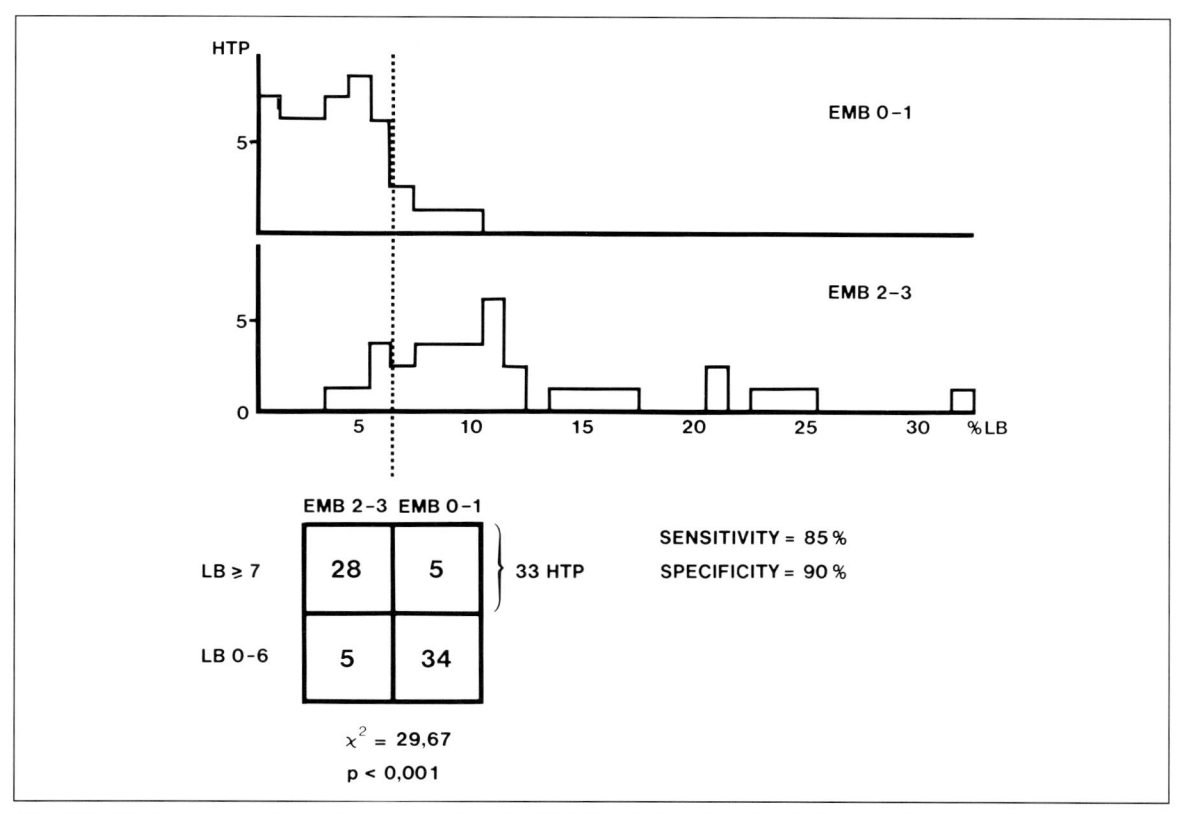

Fig. 27 Histogram and contingency table for % LBs during the first inflammatory event after cardiac transplantation.

Statistical Evaluation

The estimation of reliability, reflecting in this application an equivalent to the IRC (interrater correlation) for measurements, shows a nearly perfect concordance of LB-counts of two raters. The correlation coefficient of 0.99 supports this finding. The results of CIM were compared with those of EMB.

Histograms of LB and ALY were established and correlated to the histological findings, which were graded according to Billingham (2). To show the heterogeneity of LB classes in EMB groups, a cutpoint is set at LB <6 and LB >7. This comparison leads to a contigency table (Figure 27).

In 72 heart transplant patients, 33 CIMs and EMBs simultaneously diagnosed AR. In 5 cases CIM was positive without clinical correlate. In 39 cases, EMBs and CIMs were both negative, and in 5 patients, positive EMB was not accompanied by signs of activation in CIM.

According to this analysis the sensitivity of CIM is 85% and its specificity 90%, with a negligible error of first kind of $p < .0000001$.

The histogram of ALY shows a very low homogeneity, reflecting the insignificant information for diagnosis of rejection. By placing several cutpoints in the histograms and calculating sensitivity and specificity in each of them, a ROC-curve can be constructed (Figure 28).

In addition, this construction shows the decision point at LB >7, reflecting simultaneously the highest sensitivity and specificity. This indicated the optimal operation point at which to decide whether there is no/slight or moder-

95

1. Transplantation

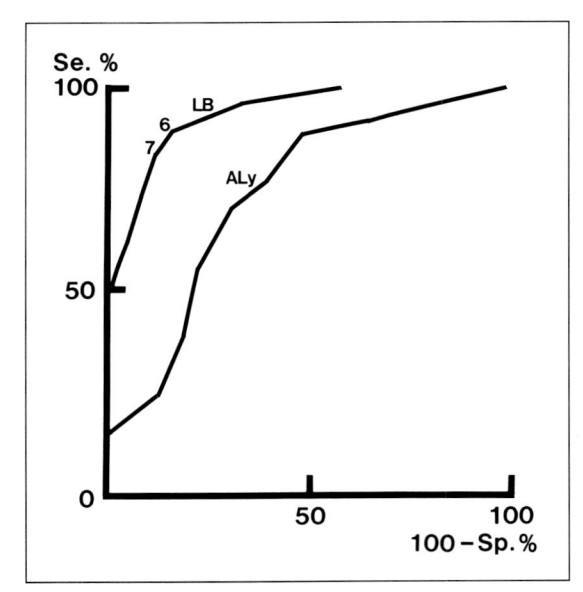

Fig. 28 ROC-curve for % LB and % ALys.

ate/severe rejection - the latter needing further immunosuppressive therapy.

The investigation of other variables in a logistic regression analysis allows testing for simultaneous effects and standardizes the multiple influence on AR. This analysis proves LBs to be the most valid criterion for AR, resulting in a chi-square of 42; that is, a measurement of inhomogeneity. As another variable, the increase of LBs from one day to the next (delta LB) with a chi-square of 27.5 seems to enhance the prognostic value of CIM.

As the distribution of variables is unknown, the use of parametric models, together with non-parametric analysis, is necessary to specify the underlying distribution. The method called CART has been shown to be asymptomatically efficient with respect to the error rates. CART supports the LBs to be the prognostic factor separating the groups best. According to the logistic regression CART, also proves that the daily increase of LBs gives additional information for the classification of the rejection stages (Figure 29).

Conclusion

The simple and atraumatic CIM method with a sensitivity of 85% and a specificity of 90%, was proved to be a valid and reliable method for diagnosis of acute rejection. EMB should therefore only be used to monitor the effect of medication during acute rejection.

CIM allows reduction in the frequency of EMB in the postoperative phase of HTP. The construction of a ROC-curve provides a preliminary definition of an optimal operational point at >7% of LBs in order to decide whether further or more potent therapy is necessary to control AR. Correlation with EMB indicated that this index coincides with the intramural inflammation episodes in the graft. Concerning the prognostic value of CIM, it is also useful to take the slope of acceleration of LBs

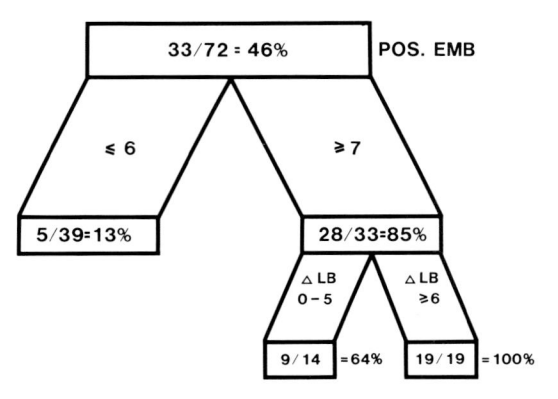

Fig. 29 Decision tree for acute rejection after cardiac transplantation, CART.

into consideration. The life table analysis supports the hypothesis that recipients undergoing a moderate/severe rejection as their first inflammatory event have the highest risk.

As these three different statistical analyses lead to the same result, it can be concluded that CIM, with its high sensitivity and specificity, provides good information about the extent of inflammation in the graft, thus providing an opportunity for early treatment and control of acute rejection.

References

1. Caves PK, Billingham ME, Stinson EB, Shumway NE. Serial transvenous biopsy of the transplanted human heart - improved management of acute rejection episodes. Lancet 11, 821, 1974.

2. Billingham ME. Diagnosis of rejection by endomyocardial biopsy. Heart Transplantation 1, 25, 1981.

3. Hammer C, Reichenspurner H, Ertel W, Lersch C, Plahl M, Brendel W, Reichart B, Uberfuhr P, Welz A, Kemkes BM, Reble B, Funcius W, Gokel M. Cytological and immuno logical monitoring of cyclosporine-treated human heart recipients. Heart Transplantation 3, 228, 1984.

4. Hammer C, Lersch C. Haematological cytology in transplantation p. 173-180. In : Surgical Research - Recent Concepts and Results. Springer Verlag, Berlin-Heidelberg, 1987.

5. Hammer C, Ertel W, Reichenspurner H, Brendel W. Immunologische Reaktionen nach Herztransplantation und ihr Nachweis. Fortschr Med 101, 2041, 1983.

6. Hammer C. Immunologisch-zytologische Überwachung herz-transplantierter Patienten. Z Kardiol, 75, Suppl 5, 121, 1986.

7. Klanke D, Hammer C, Dirschedl P, Kemkes BM, Reichart B, Gokel M, Krombach F. Sensitivity and specificity of cyto-immunological monitoring (CIM) in correlation to endo-myocardial biopsies (EMB) in heart transplanted patients. Transplant Proc 19, 3781, 1987.

8. Swets JA. ROC analysis applied to the evaluation of medical imaging techniques. Invest Radiol 14, 109, 1979.

9. Breiman L, Friedman JH, Olschen RA. In: Classification and regression trees, Belmond Edition, Wadsworth, 1984.

1.4.2. New Advances in Non-Invasive Rejection Diagnosis after Heart Transplantation

*M Anthuber, BM Kemkes, H Reichenspurner, G Osterholzer,
C Angermann, R Haberl, A Weiler, D Reichert, A Hildebrandt, C Spes*

*Department of Cardiac Surgery, University of Munich,
FR Germany*

After one unsuccessful trial of heart transplantation in 1969, cardiac transplantation was started again at the University hospital of Munich in August 1981. Up to now 84 heart- and 3 heart-lung transplantations have been performed.

Despite great advances and improved survival rates worldwide in recent years, acute rejections and infections are still the major complications after heart transplantation. An early diagnosis is mandatory both for rejections and infections, as in many cases a therapy can only be successful if started in time (1). Endomyocardial biopsy is the method which offers the most reliable result for diagnosis of acute rejection, but is an invasive method and cannot be performed on a daily basis (2,3). We therefore developped a program of non-invasive examination techniques to achieve three goals: Diagnosis of early onset of acute rejection; additional information for differential diagnostic considerations; and reduction of endomyocardial biopsies without jeopardizing the safety standard for the patient.

The non-invasive rejection monitoring in the first three to four postoperative weeks consists of daily examinations using the following three methods (Figure 30):
– Cyto-immunological monitoring (CIM) (4)
– Computerized frequency analysis of surface ECG by Fast-Fourier-Transformation (FFT) (5)
– Computer-assisted two-dimensional echocardiography (5,6)

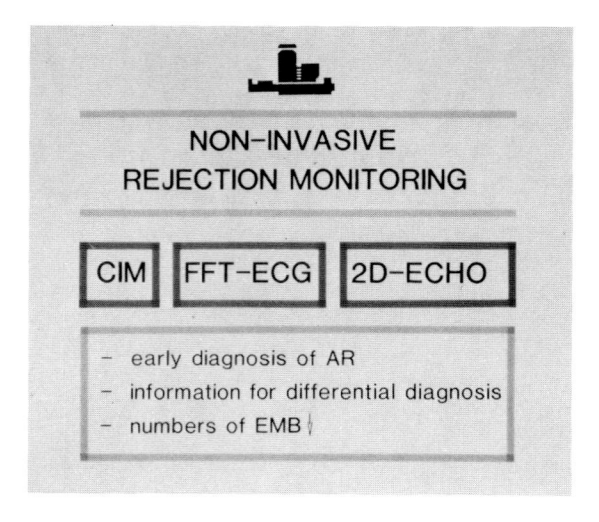

Fig. 30 Non-invasive methods for rejection-monitoring.

It is a great advantage that, in the hands of experienced examiners, performance and evaluation of each technique are easy and quick and all results are available in less than three hours if necessary.

1. Transplantation

Formerly, electrophysiological changes in the ordinary surface ECG, such as reduction of QRS-amplitude or arrhythmias were interpreted as a sign of acute rejection (9). But after the introduction of cyclosporine, this method lost most of its importance as a diagnostic tool.

A special surface ECG technique with high-gain, low-noise amplification analyses the frequency content of the QRS-complex and ST-segment by Fast-Fourier-Transformation (FFT). An analytic algorithm uncovers discrete changes in the frequency spectrum of the QRS-complex and ST-segment which are not visible in standard ECG-recordings (10). Any inflammatory process in the transplanted heart changes the electrophysiological qualities of the myocardium, and leads to different frequency spectra of the QRS-complex and ST-segment. Comparing examination series in transplanted patients and patients after coronary bypass surgery have proved that this special ECG technique is very sensitive in the detection of discrete changes which can be reliably correlated with acute rejection.

Until the patient is discharged, a daily ECG recording is performed and processed by a computer program. To reduce noise interferences from the surroundings, the preamplifier is placed inside the intensive-care unit, whereas the main amplifier and the computer system are outside the unit (Figure 31). The evaluation of the computer program produces the curves shown in Figures 7 to 10. On the x-axis, the frequency spectrum of the QRS-complex and ST-segment are marked respectively; on the y-axis, the relative portions of the different frequencies are depicted. The spectra of the 3rd, 4th, and 5th postoperative days

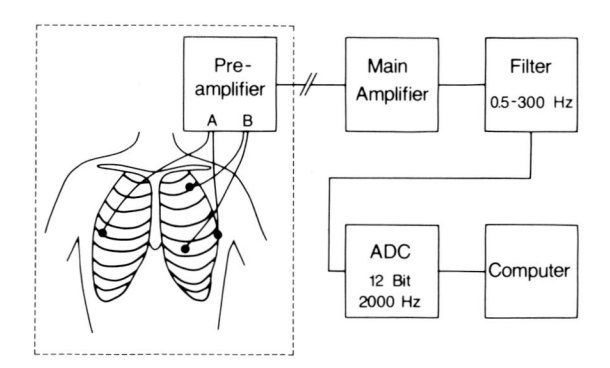

Fig. 31 Recording technique for FFT-ECG.

are nearly identical. On the 8th postoperative day, there is a distinct change that may be recognized as a shift of the distribution of the different frequencies of the QRS-complex and ST-segment. The frequency content of the QRS-complex has increased in the range between 70 and 100 Hz (Figure 32), while the frequency content of the ST-segment has, at the same time, decreased within the limits from 10 to 30 Hz (Figure 33). The endomyocardial biopsy, which was done simultaneously, revealed a moderate acute rejection.

The amplitude of the QRS-complex was also examined, but it turned out that a drop of more than 20% did not correlate significantly with bioptically proven rejections.

After rejection therapy, the frequency spectra returned to control values and remained constant for the following days (Figures 34 and 35). During 26 acute rejection crises in our last 32 patients which were diagnosed by biopsy or autopsy, corresponding alterations of the frequency spectrum were found in 24 cases (Figure 36). The false positive findings were, in one case, due to large pericardial effusion; in another due to mediastinitis.

These findings indicate that frequency analysis of QRS-complex and ST-seg-

1. Transplantation

FREQUENCY SPECTRUM OF QRS-COMPLEX AFTER HTx

O.T., ♂ 44 yrs.
—·— 3 rd p.o. day
--- 4 th
— — 5 th
—— 8 th

relative portion

frequency

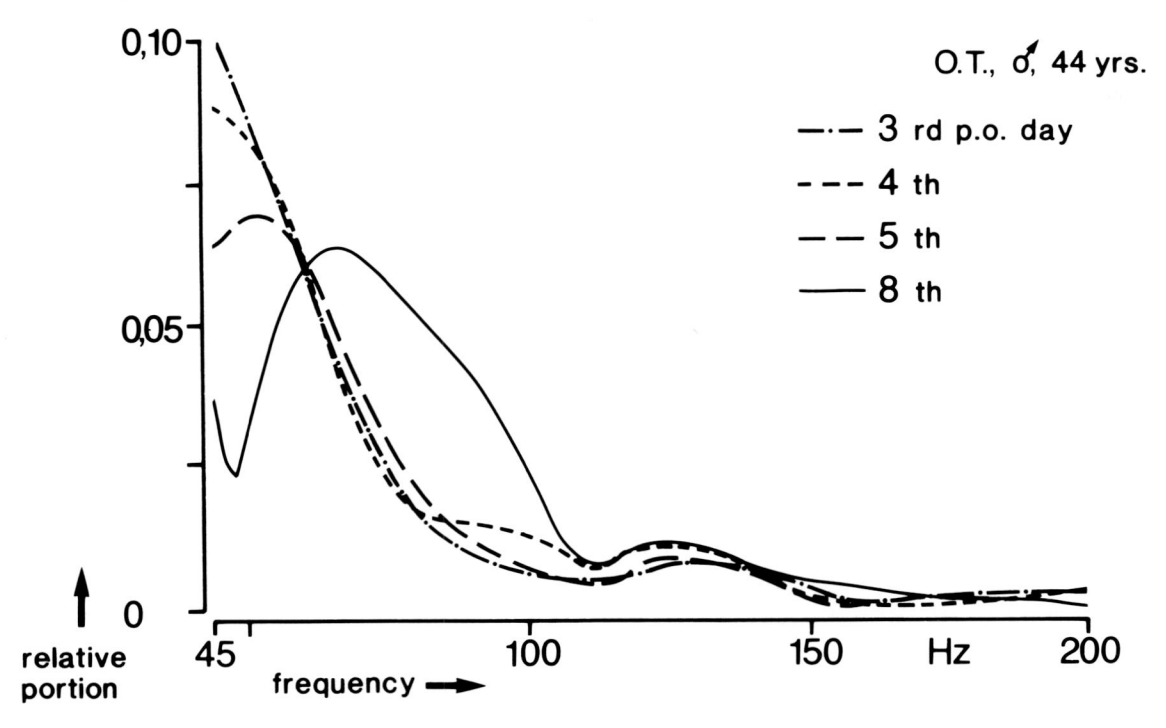

Fig. 32 (For explanation see Figure 33)

Frequency Analysis of ST-Segment after Heart Transplantation

—·— 3. day p.o.
— — 4.
--- 5.
—— 6.

FFT-Mag

Frequency

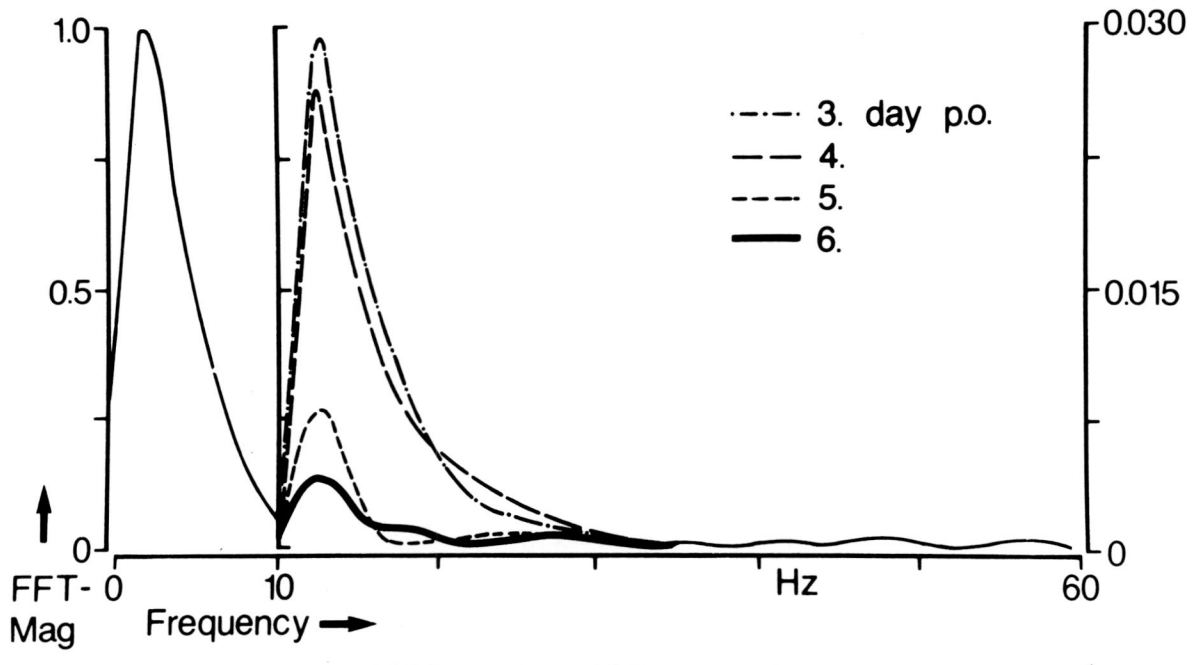

Fig. 33 Frequency spectrum of QRS-complex and ST-segment after heart transplantation; 8th postoperative day: acute rejection proved by endomyocardial biopsy, accompanied by an increase of frequency content of QRS-complex between 70 and 110 Hz and a decrease of frequency content of ST-segment between 10 and 30 Hz.

1. Transplantation

FREQUENCY SPECTRUM OF QRS-COMPLEX AFTER HTx

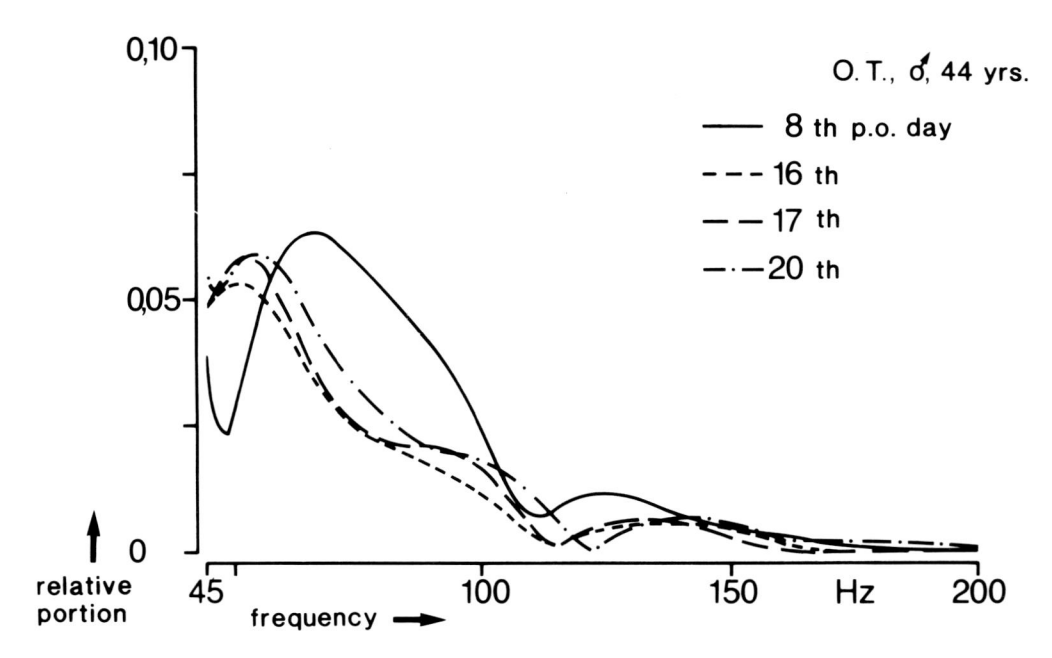

O.T., ♂, 44 yrs.
— 8 th p.o. day
--- 16 th
— — 17 th
—·— 20 th

Fig. 34 (For explanation see Figure 35)

Frequency Analysis of ST-Segment after Heart Transplantation

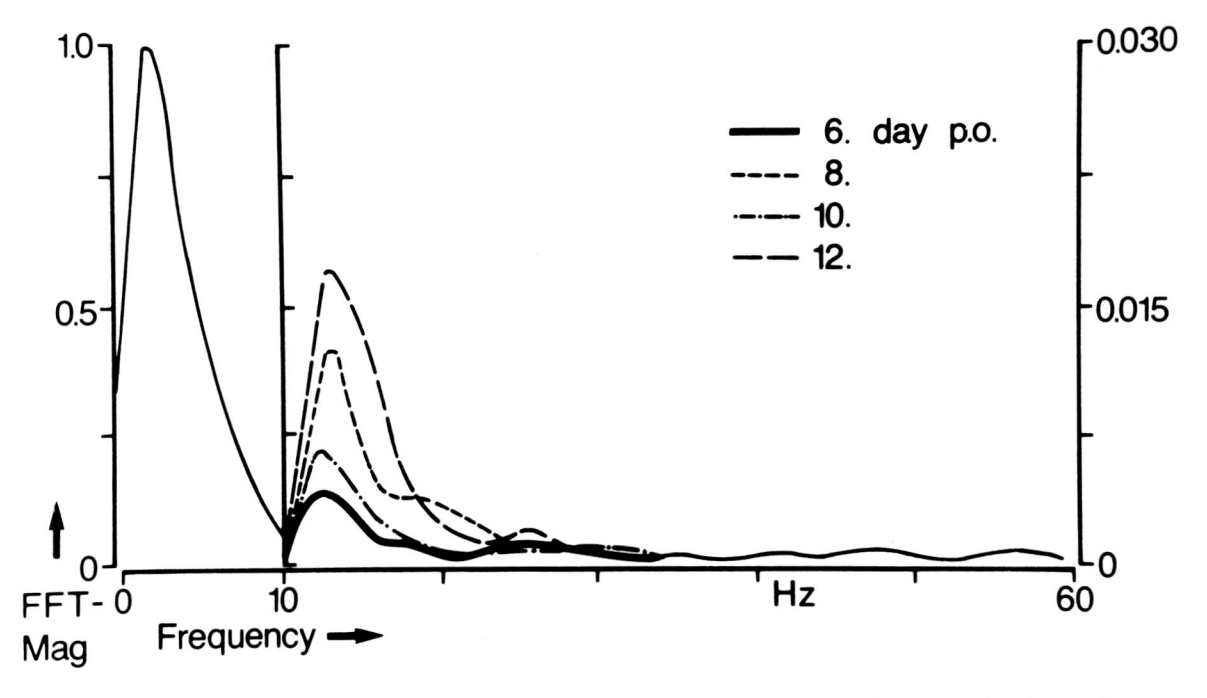

— 6. day p.o.
--- 8.
—·— 10.
— — 12.

Fig. 35 Frequency spectrum of QRS-complex and ST-segment returned to control values after rejection therapy.

1. Transplantation

Fast Fourier Transformation of Surface-ECG

7/85 – 3/87

Dept. of Cardiac Surgery, Univ. of Munich, FRG

patients n = 32

change	AR	∅AR
biopsy	26	–
FFT-Frequency content	24	2
Cytoimmunological Monitoring	26	6

Fig. 36 Results of Fast-Fourier ECG recordings in comparison to endomyocardial biopsy and cyto-immunological monitoring.

ment is a useful technique for early detection of acute rejection.

Echocardiography has reached great importance in the non-invasive diagnosis of cardiac diseases. It therefore seemed opportune to use echocardiography for short-term and long-term follow-up of heart-transplant patients. We routinely employ two-dimensional echocardiography as an additional tool for rejection monitoring. Up to now, 45 patients have been followed-up. Each examination is recorded and stored on video-tape in order to have chronological visual control of the cardiac function. Short axis cross-sections of the left ventricle are analyzed frame-by-frame for a whole cardiac cycle. Automated and computerized edge detection allows quantification of dynamic changes in systolic and diastolic function. The resulting curve of cross-sectional-area change resembles a ventricular volume curve, showing a decrease during systole and a fast increase during the diastolic rapid filling period (Figure 37). This curve changes in a typical way according to the performance of the heart. Figure 38 shows three different examples:

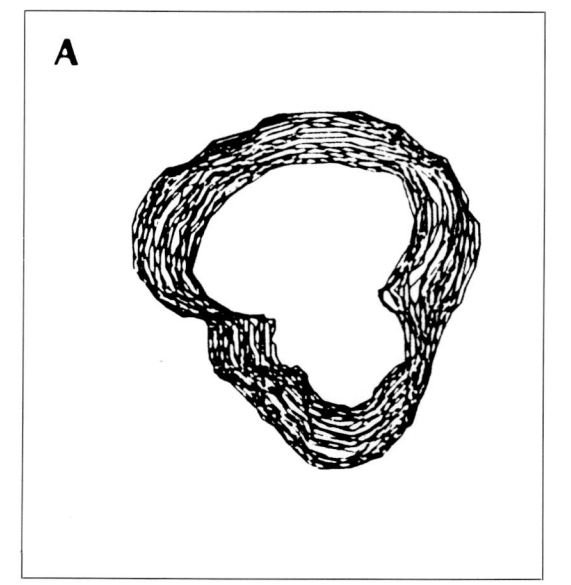

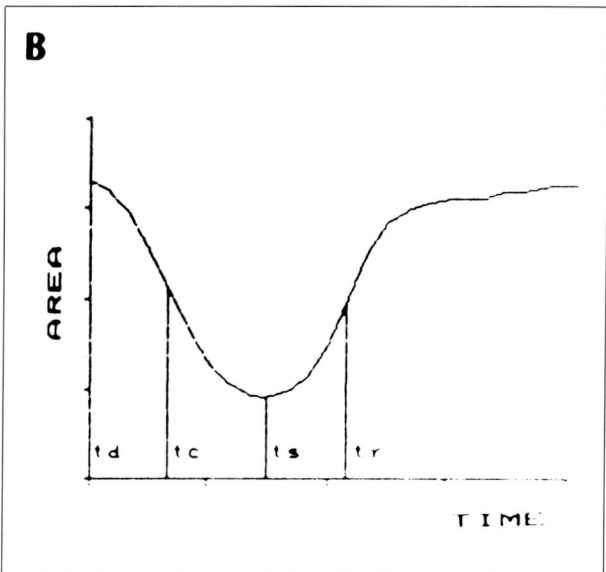

Fig. 37 Frame-by-frame computerized cardiac edge detection of left-ventricular function and left-ventricular area change during one cardiac cycle
    x-axis: QRS-complex time
    y-axis: area in cm²
    td =   enddiastolic
    ts =   endsystolic
    tc =   maximum velocity of systolic area change
    tr =   maximum velocity of diastolic area change.

1. Transplantation

(i) a cardiomyopathy;
(ii) a transplanted heart with good function; and
(iii) a transplanted heart with a restricted performance during acute rejection.

In the case of mild acute rejection, a significant increase in left ventricular wall thickness and, due to this, a decrease in left ventricular cross-sectional area, was found.

Moderate or severe acute rejections were characterized by a distinct increase in diastolic area, and a decrease in systolic area change and diastolic maximum velocity of area change (Figure 39).

Thirty-six acute rejection episodes were diagnosed by endomyocardial bi-

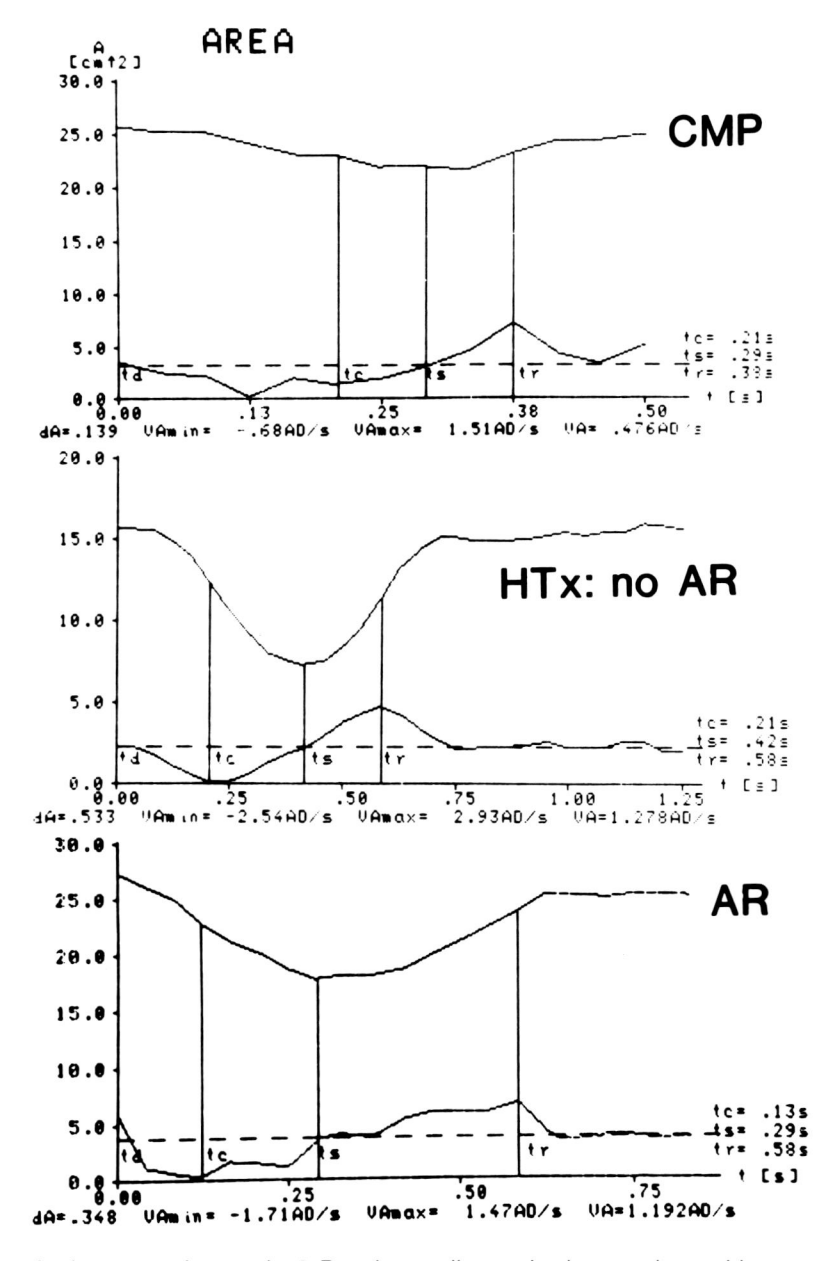

Fig. 38 Left-ventricular area change in 2-D echocardiography in a patient with severe dilated cardiomyopathy; after HTX without rejection and after HTX with moderate acute rejection.

1. Transplantation

REJECTION IN 2-D-ECHOCARDIOGRAPHY

- LV wall thickness ↑
- LV cross-sectional area ↓ } mild AR

- LV diastolic area ↑
- systolic area change ↓
- diastolic max. velocity of area change ↓ } moderate/severe AR

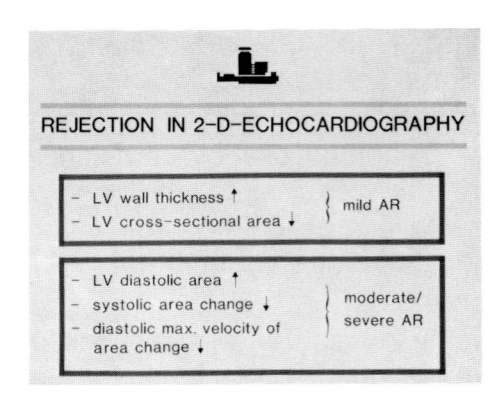

Fig. 39 Two-dimensional echocardiographic criteria for rejection diagnosis.

opsy in 47 patients during the observation period; of these, 32 caused measurable changes in two-dimensional echocardiography (Figure 40).

As a result of the particular rejection control with our non-invasive techniques, we were able to decrease the lethal rejection rate and, at the same time, the number of biopsies. At the moment we perform only 2 to 3 biopsies within the first three postoperative months. This means a reduction of biopsies of about 75% compared with former patient groups.

Conclusions

The combination of cyto-immunological monitoring, frequency analysis of surface ECG, and the two-dimensional echocardiography is an effective method of diagnosing the early onset of acute rejection. It helps to reduce the number of biopsies and yields more information for differential diagnostic considerations. But, if there is any doubt, because the non-invasive examinations do not allow a clear and definite diagnosis, we do not hesitate to perform an endomyocardial biopsy immediately. Furthermore, the success of rejection therapy has to be confirmed by a control biopsy, and it cannot be replaced by any non-invasive examination.

Our patients have been followed-up for only the first three to four postoperative weeks. Further studies will show whether these non-invasive examinations are also appropriate for long-term follow-up of heart transplantation patients.

ECHOCARDIOGRAPHY AFTER CARDIAC TRANSPLANTATION
8/85 - 3/87
PATIENTS n=47
0-65 months p op.

Changes in	Acute rejection	No rejection
MYOCARDIAL BIOPSY	36	—
ECHO (total)	32	2
Wall thickness LV	25	2
RV free wall	26	—
Syst. area change	27	—
Mean relaxation velocity	24	—
IVRT	20	—

Fig. 40 Results of two-dimensional echocardiography for rejection diagnosis.

1. Transplantation

References

1. Baumgartner WA. Infection in cardiac transplantation. Heart Transplantation 3, 75, 1983.

2. Billingham ME. Diagnosis of cardiac rejection by endomyocardial biopsy. Heart Transplantation 1, 25, 1981.

3. Caves PK, Stinson EB, Billingham ME, Rider AK, Shumway NE. The diagnosis of human cardiac allograft rejection by serial biopsy. J Thorac Cardiovasc Surg 66, 461, 1973.

4. Reichenspurner H, Ertel W, Hammer C, Lersch C, Uberfuhr P, Welz A, Reble B, Kemkes BM, Reichart B, Gokel M. Immunological monitoring of heart transplant patients under cyclosporine A immunosuppression. Transplantation Proc 16, 1251, 1984.

5. Reichenspurner H, Kemkes BM, Haberl R, Angermann CH, Weber M, Osterholzer G, Anthuber M, Steinbeck G. Frequency analysis of surface electrocardiogram and two-dimensional echocardiography for non-invasive diagnosis of rejection after heart transplantation. Transplantation Proc 19, 2552, 1987.

6. Angermann CH, Hart RJ, Spes CG, Struppler M, Marquart M, Schmidt DP. Automatic endocardial border detection in serial 2-D-echocardiograms of the short axis. Circulation 72, 353, 1985.

7. Reichenspurner H, Kemkes BM, Osterholzer G, Reble B, Ertel W, Reichart B, Lersch C, Gokel JM. Particular control of infection and rejection episodes after 4 years of cardiac transplantation. Texas Heart Inst J 13, 5, 1986.

8. Ertel W, Reichenspurner H, Lersch C, Hammer C, Plahl M, Lehmann M, Kemkes BM, Osterholzer G, Reble, B, Reichart B, Brendel W. Cyto-immunological monitoring in acute rejection and viral, bacterial or fungal infection following heart transplantation. Heart Transplantation 4, 390, 1985.

9. Haberl R, Weber M, Reichenspurner H, Kemkes BM, Osterholzer G, Anthuber M, Steinbeck G. Frequency analysis of the surface electrocardiagram for recognition of acute rejection after orthotopic heart transplantation in man. Circulation 76, 101, 1987.

1.4.3. Experimental Observations with Cytoimmunological Monitoring and Biochemical Rejection Markers after Pancreatic Transplantation and Immunosuppression with Total Lymphoid Irradiation and Cyclosporine

DF du Toit*, JJ Heydenrych, B Smit

Department of Surgery, Paediatric Surgery and Radiotherapy, University of Stellenbosch Medical School and Tygerberg Hospital, South Africa

* Supported in part by grants from the MRC and Harry-Crossley Fund; MRC Grant Recipient

Introduction

Experience from transplantation centres indicate that normoglycaemia can be consistently achieved in experimental models by segmental or whole pancreatic transplantation and in selected insulin-dependent diabetics with secondary complications (1-11). Since the introduction of cyclosporine (CSA) into clinical practice, the expected graft and patient survival rate at 1 year is 40 and 80% respectively, which indicates an improvement of overall results and attendant decline of patient mortality.

Improvement can be attributed to advances in immunosuppressive regimens, surgical technique, and better patient selection. Although major advances have recently been experienced with the introduction of newer immunosuppressive agents, such as CSA, surgical correction of diabetes by pancreatic transplantation remains controversial.

Despite the introduction of effective immunosuppressive agents such as CSA, technical complications related to the management of the pancreatic duct, together with rejection, have bedevilled implementation of pancreatic transplantation on a wider scale in man. In addition, early diagnosis of pancreatic rejection has been difficult due to insensitivity of pancreatic rejection markers. In practice, the occurrence of hyperglycaemia after successful pancreatic engraftment is usually associated with advanced histological rejection of the pancreas, and, at best, in only about one third of patients can reversal of rejection episodes be expected.

Pancreatic transplantation with urinary diversion of the exocrine secretion allows post-transplantation assessment of graft function by monitoring urinary amylase, the application of which has been encouraging but controversial (11-27). Results reported in the International Pancreatic Transplantation Registry indicate similar graft survival in patients undergoing pancreatic transplantation with enteric drainage.

This communication displays the data of our primate study after whole

1. Transplantation

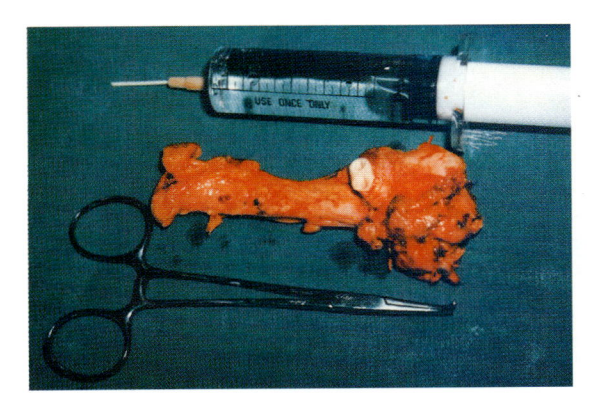

Fig. 41 Whole pancreatic allograft prior to transplantation.

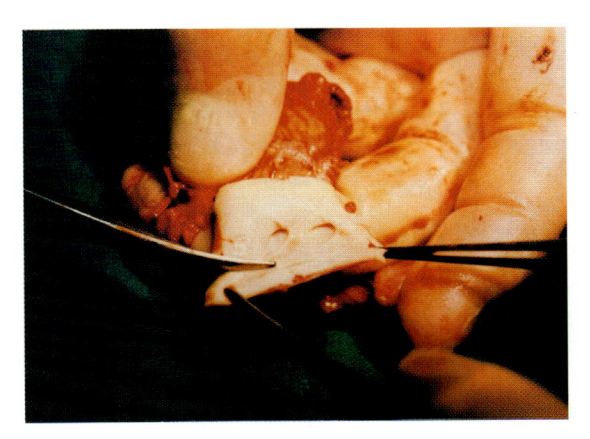

Fig. 42 Preparation of the cuff of the donor aorta showing orifices of the coeliac axis and superior mesenteric artery.

pancreatico-duodenal allotransplantation with bladder drainage, highlighting the utilization of cytoimmunological monitoring (CIM), together with urinary amylase determination as pancreatic graft rejection markers.

Material and Methods

Conditioned and disease-free, chacma baboons (Papio ursinus) of both sexes, weighing between 9 and 15 kg, were used. Primates were housed in squeeze cages, and all handling procedures were performed after administration of ketamine hydrochloride (Parke Davis) (5 mg/kg/imi). Tissue typing was not employed, and animals were only matched for major blood groups. Animals were kept under rigid laboratory conditions under supervision of a veterinary surgeon, and all experimental procedures had previously been approved by the Ethics Committee of the University of Stellenbosch. Recipients received a balanced, primate pellet diet supplemented with fresh fruit and vitamins (Labethica-B Complex).

(i) Technique of Transplantation

Heterotopic intraperitoneal engraftment of pancreatico-duodenal allografts (PDA) without spleen was achieved by vascular anastomosis between a cuff of donor aorta, including orifices of the coeliac axis, superior mesenteric artery, recipient aorta, donor portal vein cuff, and recipient inferior vena cava (Figures 41,42). There was no warm ischaemic time, as the grafts were removed from donors whose hearts were still beating. The cold ischaemic time was 1 hour, and the pancreas was stored on ice for 30 minutes at 4°C prior to transplantation. During harvesting of the pancreas, the duodenal ends were oversewn, and the graft vessels flushed at low pressure with 10 ml of heparinized saline at 4°C. Allograft recipients in this series were not heparinized, nor did they receive postoperative anticoagulants. The graft duodenal-conduit was anastomosed by side-to-side anastomosis to the dome of the bladder or the bowel, as previously described (27,28). Prolene was utilised to perform the anastomoses (Figure 43).

(ii) Irradiation of Primates

Two regimens were utilised. During irradiation, all animals were anaesthetised with intramuscular ketamine hydrochloride (5 mg/kg) for induction and in-

1. Transplantation

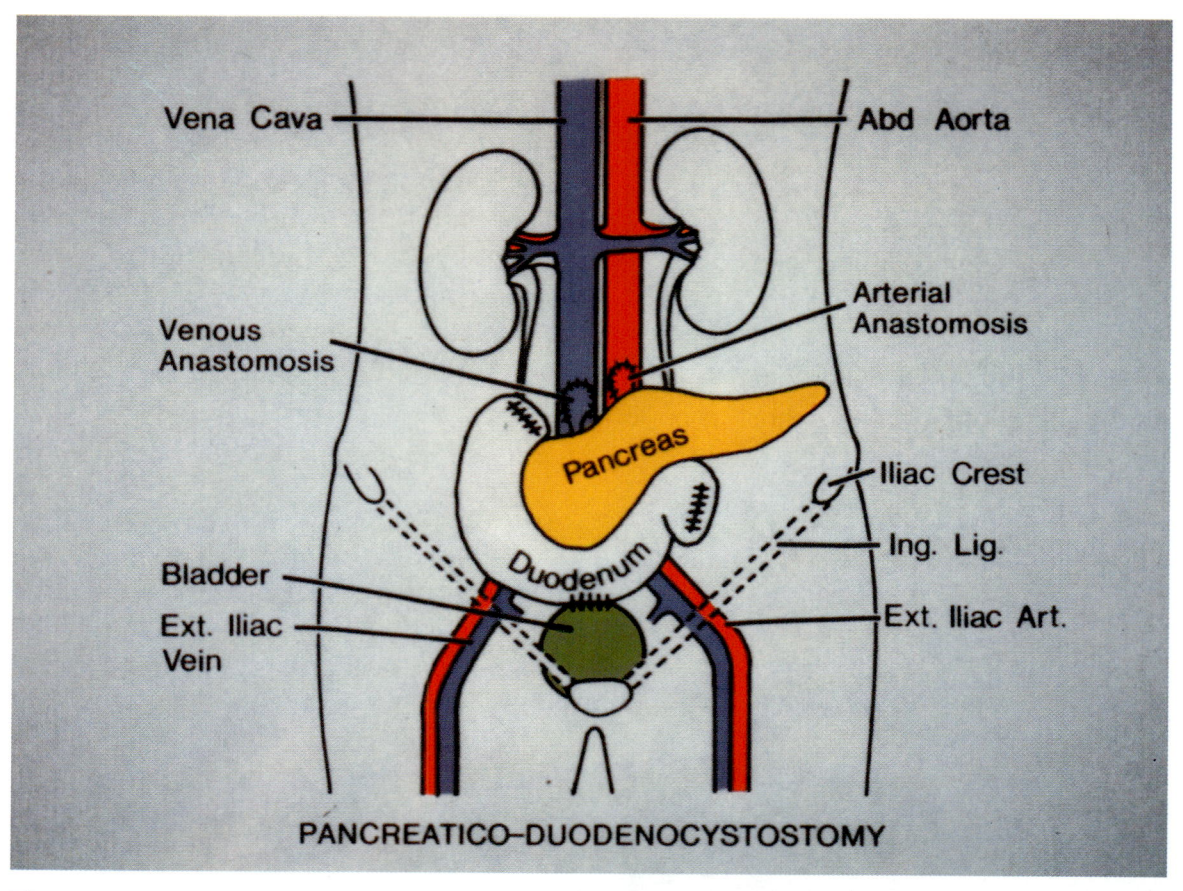

Fig. 43 Operative diagram showing pancreatico-duodenal allotransplantation with pancreatico-duodenocystostomy.

travenous sodium pentobarbitone (Sagatal; Maybaker - 10 mg/kg) for maintenance. Contrary to techniques previously utilised in man to treat Hodgkin's disease, primates in this study received modified fractionated, subtotal marrow irradiation with shielding of the head, arms and legs as previously described by Myburgh and co-workers (29,30,31). The fields included irradiation of the entire trunk below the base of the skull, thorax, abdomen, proximal femora, humeri, and tail (Figure 44). The fields utilised in this series were more extensive and amounted to near total body irradiation (9).

Regimen A: 100 RADS (1 GY) were administered weekly as photons from a 6 mv linear accelerator (Siemens Corp, Mevatron, Iselin. NJ. (Figure 45) USA) at 215 centimetre source-skin distance. The radiation rate was 2857 rad/hr and the exposure rate was 50 rads (0.5 GY) per 1.05 minutes. A total of 800 (8 GY) or 1000 rads (10 GY) were administered over 4 or 5 weeks (9).

Regimen B: 400 RADS (4 GY) total dose TLI was administered over 4 weeks (25 rads x 8 fractions) as photons from a Cobalt Source. The dose rate was 1000 rad/h (0.167 GY/ min) and administered as 50 rad (0.5 GY) over 1.5 minutes.

During irradiation, liver function tests, serum amylase determinations, and complete haematological profile, including peripheral smear, haemoglobin,

1. Transplantation

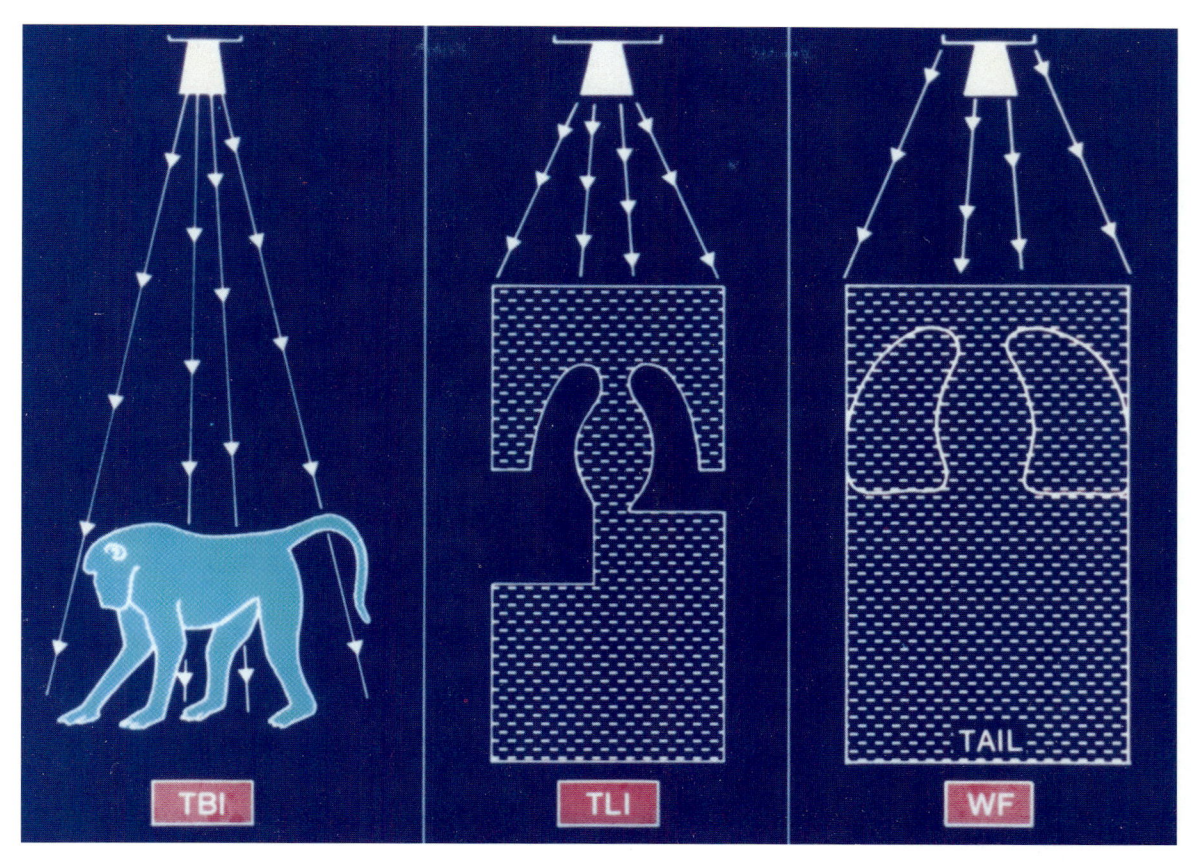

Fig. 44 Radiation fields previously studied include TBI and TLI, and WF (Wide-Field) currently used in this study.

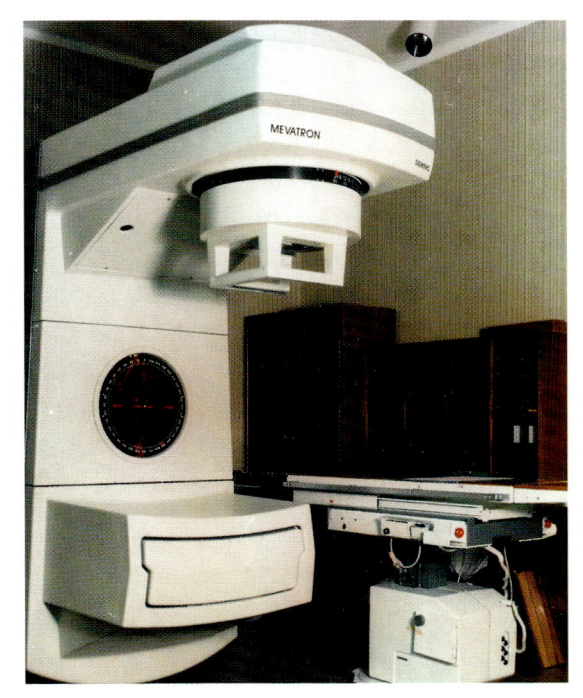

Fig. 45 Linear Accelerator (Mevatron, Siemens) utilised to administer irradiation.

white cell count, differential count, and platelet count were obtained.

(iii) Postoperative Immunosuppression

CSA administration commenced on the day of transplantation, and was given either orally (by gavage) or intramuscularly (Figure 46). In the majority of recipients, CSA was administered by gavage for 5 days (CSA 25 mg/kg/day - oral drinking solution / 100 mg/ml). Recipients on maintenance parenteral treatment received CSA (10 mg/kg/day) daily indefinitely. The intramuscular preparation consisted of CSA pow-der dissolved in alcohol and intralipid (4 grams CSA dissolved in 10 ml 75% alcohol and diluted in 20% intralipid). Daily blood specimens obtained after transplantation were assayed for CSA

1. Transplantation

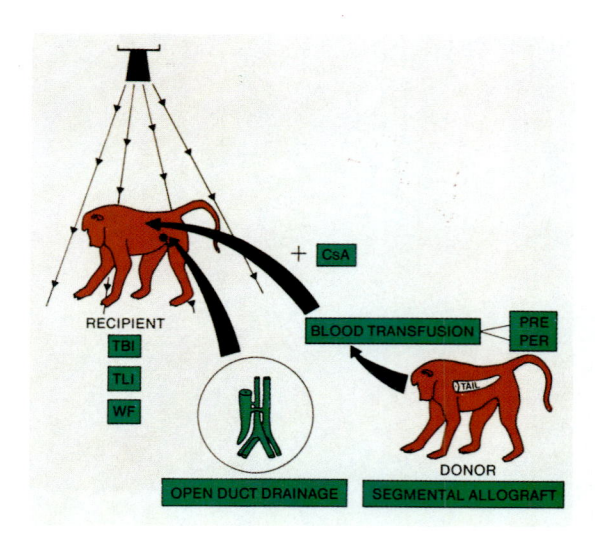

Fig. 46 Preoperative irradiation of recipient followed by transplantation (segmental or PDA) and immunosuppression with ST and postoperative cyclosporine.

levels by radioimmunoassay method (Sandoz RIA-Kit). Methyl Prednisolone (MP-Solumedrol-Upjohn) 50 mg was administered intravenously daily for 5 days after transplantation. Maintenance prednisolone (Deltacortril-Pfizer) 20 mg was given intramuscularly indefinitely daily, commencing on day 5 after transplantation.

(iv)Assays

Graft function was assessed postoperatively by fasting venous plasma glucose levels (PLG) and intravenous glucose tolerance tests (IVGTT).

Normoglycaemia was defined as PLG of less than 8 mmol/L and rejection of the graft was recognised when PLG rose above 8 mmol/L for 2 consecutive days. Glucose determinations were performed on peripheral venous blood, using the glucose auto-analyzer method (Beckman, Cal). Daily serum electrolytes (Na^+, K^+, Cl^-), pO_2, pCO_2, and bicarbonate measurements were done to assess the metabolic status.

Daily plasma and urinary amylase values were obtained after transplantation and determinations were based on the rate of hydrolysis of a soluble starch preparation at 37°C. Results are expressed in Street-Close units (S/C units). Daily immunomonitoring, using the method of Hammer, was utilised to assess acute pancreatic rejection (32-34). Peripheral blood samples were analysed daily, and white blood cells were counted and differentiated. A mononuclear concentrate was obtained by the Ficoll-Hypaque gradient centrifugation method, and cytocentrifuged onto slides. The cells were stained by the Giemsa method. Cell types were differentiated according to the degree of activation, i.e. either normal lymphocytes, lymphoblasts or prelymphoblasts. T cell subpopulations were studied in these primates with the use of anti-human monoclonal antibodies OKT11 (anti-total T cells), OKT4 (Th cells), and OKT8 (Tsc cells), as described by Myburgh and co-workers (29).

The Mann-Whitney U-Test was used for statistical comparison between groups, and the difference was considered statistically significant if $P<0.05$.

Experimental Groups
Group 1
Normal baboons provided the control values for blood glucose, plasma and urine amylase, urine pH, electrolytes and bloodgases, CIM, glucose tolerance and glucose degradation values (K-values), liver function tests, and haematological assessment.

Group 2
Total surgical pancreatectomy as a one-stage procedure. These primates received neither transplants nor exogenous insulin.

Group 3
Sham operated primates provided control values for plasma and urine amylase, IVGTT, K-values, and CIM.

Group 4
Radiation control: Fractionated TLI 800 rads (8 GY) (200 x 4 rads) administered over 4 weeks.

Group 5
Radiation control: Fractionated TLI 1000 rads (10 GY) (200 x 5 rads) administered over 5 weeks.

Group 6
Pancreatico-duodenal allografts with enteric drainage (PDA); TLI 800 RAD plus CSA 25 mg/kg/day (orally x 5 days); then maintenance CSA 10 mg/kg/day parenterally indefinitely.

Group 7
Pancreatico-duodenal allograft with vesical drainage; TLI 400 RAD plus CSA (as per group 6), MP (50 mg daily x 5 days), then maintenance CSA 10 mg/kg/day, and Prednisilone 20 mg/day parenterally.

Results

Normal primates (group 1) rendered mean fasting PLG of 5.6 ± 0.2 mmol/L (range 1.6-9.5 mmol/L), K value 2.4 ± 0.1 mmol/%/min (range 0.5-4.6). Mean plasma and urinary amylase levels were 807.9 Street-Close units (535-1713 S/C units) and 3184 S/C units (1535-6000) respectively. The mean urine pH was 5.6 (range 5.5-5.6), plasma sodium 145 mmol/L (142-146), and chloride 112 mmol/L (108-115). The acid-base status of controls yielded a mean pH of 7.42, plasma bicarbonate 28.3 (23.8-37.1) and base excess ranging from -2 to +8. Mean "activated" lymphocyte count was 1.92% (range 0.5-5%).

Apancreatic controls rendered significantly reduced K-values (0.3 ± 0.02 mmol/%/min) and insulin release during IVGTT. PLG rose immediately after pancreatectomy and remained elevated until termination of the experiment. Mean survival was 5 days (range 3-12 days).

T4 and T8 values of recipients subjected to 400 RAD TLI (group 7) increased from 31-39 (P=0.61) and 31-41% (P=0.1) respectively after TLI and OKT4/OKT8 ratios decreased from 1.0 to 0.95. (P=NS). T4 vs T8 ratio changes after TLI are reflected in Table 15.

Effect of TLI (WF) (400 RAD) on T4/T8 Ratios

Before TLI T4 : T8	After TLI T4 : T8
21 : 65	26 : 65
52 : 33	37 : 67
19 : 26	46 : 37
24 : 22	48 : 37
39 : 27	27 : 58
31 : 31.2 (1.00)	**39 : 41.2 (0.95)**
T4 (Th) 32	→ 39.2 (P=0.61)
T8 (Ts) 31.2	→ 41.2 (p=0.1)

Table 15

Recipients of PDA grafts with vesical drainage (group 7) sustained graft function between 10 and 35 days, a mean of 20 days (Table 16, Figure 47). Indefinite survival was not observed. Surgical technique was characterised by low morbidity and no operative mortality was recorded. Six of 10 animals rejected the graft on days 10, 12, 21, 21, 35 and 35

1. Transplantation

Survival Data after Pancreatico-Duodenal Allotransplantation with Enteric and Vesical Drainage*

Drainage Type	Survival (Normoglycaemic)	Mean (Days)
Enteric (800 RAD + CSA)	6,6,7,9,12,13,17,24,30,70,100, 101,102,102,104,105,110,122, (N=18)	57.8
Vesical (400 RAD + CSA)	10,10,12,14,21,21,21,21,35,35, (N=10)	20

Immunosuppression: TLI (800, 400 RAD) Plus CSA

Table 16

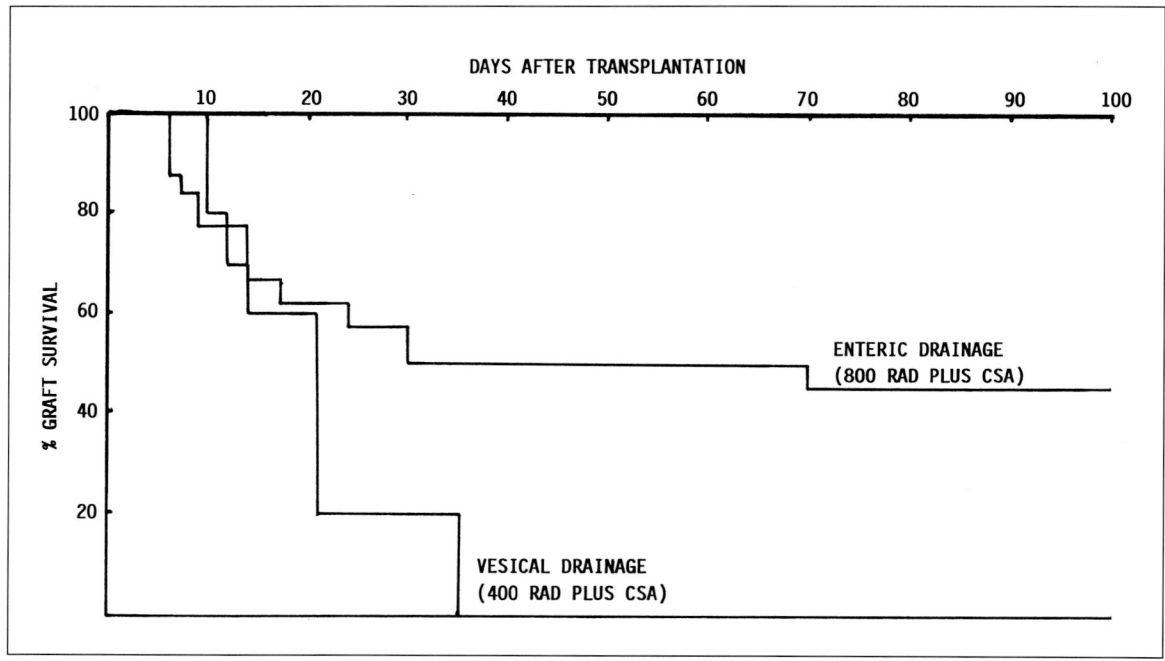

Fig. 47 Actual survival data of recipients with vesical drainage (400 RAD plus CSA) and primates with enterically drained pancreatic allografts (800 RAD plus CSA).

after transplantation, indicating suboptimal immunosuppression despite maintenance CSA and PRED administration. Urinary amylase increased from 27 366 to 44 700 units on day one posttransplant. A considerable variability in daily urine amylase values was observed in the respective recipients (Figure 48). In all recipients, urine amylase declined precipitously 2-3 days before the onset of hyperglycaemia (Figure 49). In this group the sensitivity and specificity of urine amylase as a rejection marker was 80 and 100% respectively. An absolute lower limit for urine amylase could not be established in this study - a decreasing

1. Transplantation

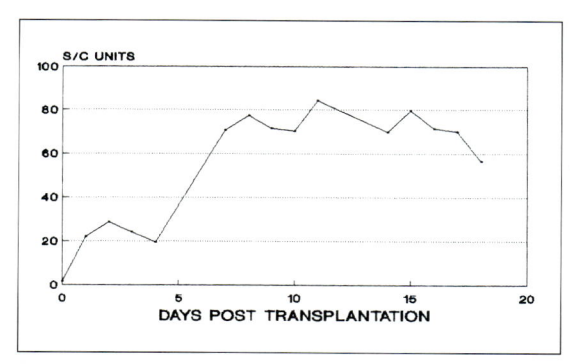

Fig. 48 Daily variation in urinary amylase values in a recipient with duodenocystostomy. No rejection was present.

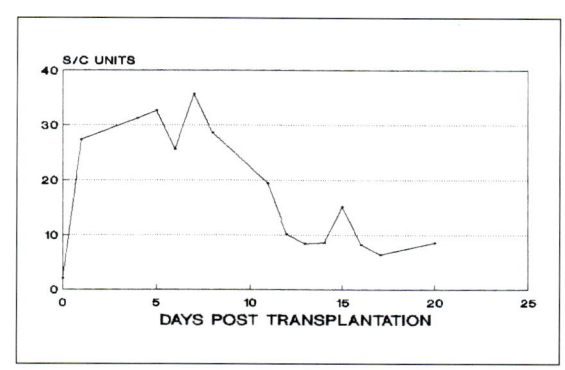

Fig. 49 Acute decrease in urinary amylase values indicating impending rejection of the pancreas.

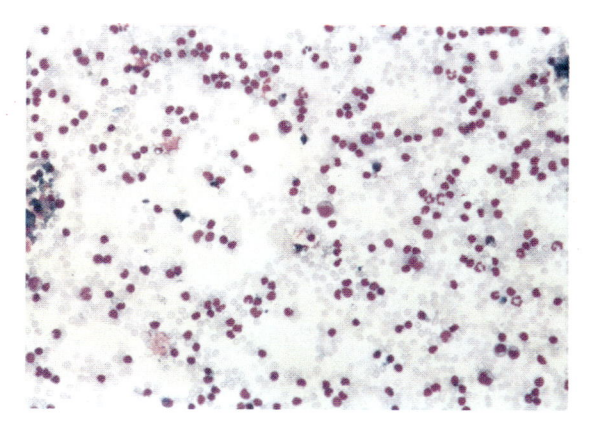

Fig. 50 CIM-Giemsa stain showing "activated" lymphocytes 10 days after pancreatic transplantation (Giemsa x 100).

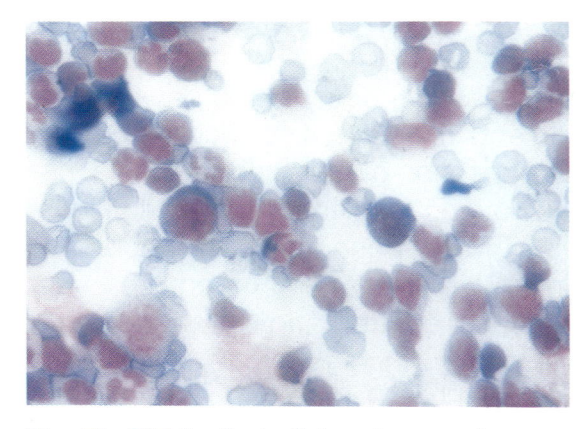

Fig. 51 CIM-"activated" lymphocytes in a recipient undergoing rejection of the pancreatic duodenal allograft (Giemsa x 400).

trend of urinary amylase on a daily basis was more suggestive of rejection than absolute levels. Rejection therapy was therefore instituted (ivi MP) at the earliest possible observation of a declining urinary amylase level. A temporary response was observed, and all grafts eventually rejected despite anti-rejection therapy.

Duodenocystostomy resulted in severe dehydration, persistent hypochloraemia, hyponatriaemia, and metabolic acidosis in all recipients. Four of 10 animals died thereof, despite intensive prophylactic intravenous bicarbonate administration. Typical findings reflected reduced pH (7.3 cf 7.4 grp 1), sodium (125-135 cf 140 grp 1), chloride (93-79 cf 112 grp 1), and plasma bicarbonate (14.2-23.5 cf 27 grp 1). The base excess was often reduced to -12. These changes became apparent approximately 10 days after transplantation when recipients were consuming a standard laboratory diet. Metabolic acidosis occurred in all recipients and varied from moderate to severe. Despite intensive supportive treatment with intravenous sodium bicarbonate, 4 of 10 animals demised on day 10, 14, 21 and 21. Metabolic acidosis occurred irrespective of the presence of underlying rejection.

In all the animals that rejected their grafts, the decline in urinary amylase

113

1. Transplantation

was accompanied by an elevation of "activated" lymphocyte count exceeding 5% (Figure 50, 51).

Sensitivity of 80% and specificity of 100% were observed in this small study. CIM provided early warning of impending rejection, together with a decline in urinary amylase (Figure 52). Increased "activated" lymphocytes above 5% also occurred in one recipient with a perforated duodenal conduit in the absence of rejection of the pancreas or duodenum, and also in the recipient with pyelonephritis, indicating the value of CIM in differentiating underlying bacterial infections from impending rejection (Figure 53). A moderate elevation of "activated" lymphocyte count was observed in the first 2-3 days after transplantation.

Recipients of PDA with enteric drainage (group 6) remained normoglycaemic between 10 and > 100 days with a mean of 57.8 days, which indicated a significant prolongation of graft survival (P<0.05) when compared to untreated allograft controls (mean survival 9 days) and recipients of vesical drainage (Table 16). Eight of 18 recipients had graft survival beyond 100 days. All recipients maintained normoglycaemia in the absence of metabolic acidosis, dehydration, and vesical complications. IVGTT confirmed moderate glucose intolerance when compared to sham operated controls and vesically drained recipients (Figure 54). K-values were reduced to 0.8 mmol/%/min. In 50% of recipients, well-preserved pancreatic architecture was present at autopsy, with atrophy of allografts varying from moderate to severe in the remainder. However, all recipients remained normoglycaemic, irrespective of the size of the graft at the time of performing the IVGTT. Histology of the allografts at 100 days, confirmed the presence of islets, together with a background of mononuclear cells, suggesting ongoing chronic rejection. Bone marrow biopsies after 100 days confirmed the presence of a moderately hypoplastic bone marrow.

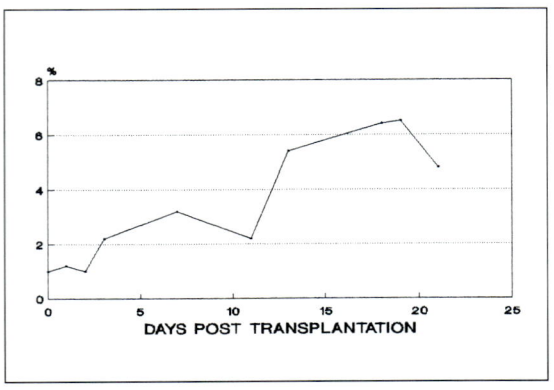

Fig. 52 PDA recipient with underlying rejection of the pancreas showing an elevation of CIM-"activated" lymphocyte count.

CSA serum trough levels of recipients showed moderate fluctuation from animal to animal receiving the same dose. Values fluctuated between 50 and 600 ng/ml.

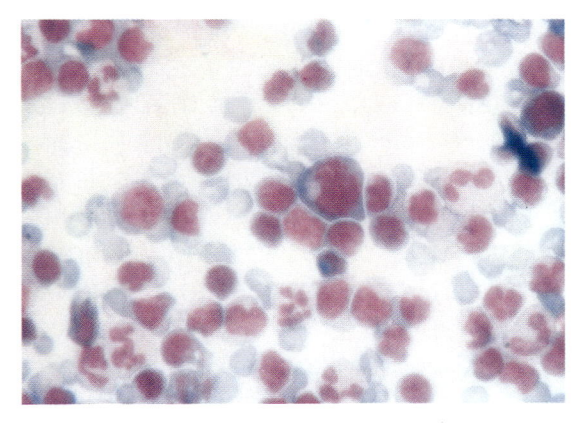

Fig. 53 CIM-"activated" lymphocytes present together with increased neutrophil count in recipient with underlying pyelonephritis.

Discussion

Since the introduction of CSA into clinical transplantation, the number of

1. Transplantation

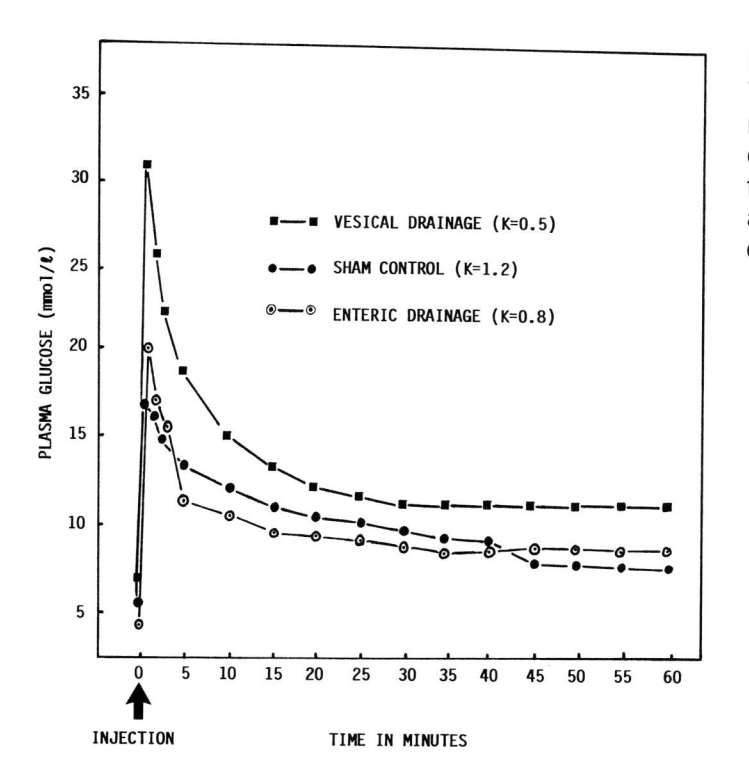

Fig. 54
VGTT showing glucose response, after vesical drainage (■ - ■), enteric drainage (○ - ○) and in sham operated control (● - ●)

pancreatic transplants performed yearly has increased significantly, and some units now report a 1 year graft survival rate of 75% (10). Although the results of pancreas transplantation have improved in recent years, a considerable number of grafts are still lost due to immunological rejection. Rejection of the pancreas remains a worldwide problem and is responsible for a considerable number of graft losses in the acute and late posttransplantation period. One important reason for this generally low success rate is the lack of sensitive markers to detect early rejection of the pancreas. This has particular relevance in recipients of pancreatic allografts without a kidney transplant in which the only sensitive parameter has been an elevation of the blood glucose level. Application of serum amylase determination has proved to be an insensitive and inconsistent marker of pancreatic rejection. Unfortunately, the recurrence of hyperglycaemia after pancreatic transplantation necessitating reinstitution of insulin is frequently associated with irreversible underlying rejection of the pancreas. This partially explains why only 30% of rejection episodes of the pancreas are successfully reversed with conventional antirejection therapy, if treatment is delayed until hyperglycaemia is present. In addition, pancreatic allograft recipients without simultaneous kidney transplant are at a relative disadvantage because rejection of the pancreas is not indirectly monitored by evaluating renal function/rejection by means of serum creatinine levels or renal biopsy.

This has practical implications in the clinical setting as pancreatic transplantation alone may well become standard treatment in non-uraemic diabetics with progressive nephropathy and other associated secondary complications of diabetes i.e. transplantation well before the development of end-stage renal failure.

1. Transplantation

In recent years drainage of exocrine pancreatic secretion via the ureter or bladder and utilization of urinary amylase as a sensitive rejection marker has been reported by numerous researchers in animal models and in man (12-22). The majority of reports indicate that urinary amylase can be used as a sensitive indicator of early pancreatic rejection. However, some researchers have pointed out the pitfalls of this pancreatic rejection marker (14). In a recent communication, the Minnesota Group showed in their dog pancreatic ductocystostomy model utilizing urinary amylase levels that impending pancreatic rejection could be diagnosed 9-10 days before elevation of the blood sugar occurred (13). However, despite a 5 day course of anti-rejection therapy loss of graft function ultimately occurred (13). The same group pointed out that a drop in urinary amylase is not necessarily a sign of rejection. On the other hand, other workers have indicated that a drop in urinary amylase levels similar to elevated blood glucose is a late manifestation of irreversible pancreatic rejection (14). Drainage of the pancreatic duct directly or via a duodenal conduit into the bladder is not without problems. Disadvantages of pancreatic juice drainage into the bladder include occurrence of persistent urinary tract infections (cystitis and urethritis) on the one hand, and development of intractable hyperchloraemic metabolic acidosis on the other (12,14,16). In some patients, metabolic acidosis was chronic and persistent, particularly when associated with rejection of the kidney in patients after synchronous pancreatic and renal transplantation. Despite these reports, some researchers have reported no pathological changes affecting the urinary tract in their animal models.

Results from our study show that pancreatico-duodenocystostomy is associated with significant structural changes to the bladder urothelium. Autodigestion of the bladder mucosa was a constant feature and all recipients developped microscopic haematuria. One recipient developped pyelonephritis. As in previous reports, metabolic acidosis occurred in all recipients in our study, irrespective of rejection. Despite intensive bicarbonate therapy by the intravenous route, 4 of 10 animals died thereof. Dehydration, weight-loss, and electrolyte imbalance also occurred due to uncontrollable, "uncycled" excretion of pancreatic juice via the pancreatico-vesical fistula. A recent modification to the transplant technique, including direct implantation of the pancreatic duct into the bladder, has abrogated the severe metabolic and structural abnormalities.

Despite these metabolic derangements following duodenocystostomy, measurement of urinary amylase proved to be an accurate marker of early pancreatic rejection and a mean decline of 11.4 days before elevation of blood glucose was recorded. Notwithstanding early recognition of rejection by this marker, anti-rejection therapy failed to arrest immunological destruction of the graft, and all recipients died of pancreatic rejection.

Our study indicates that cytoimmunological monitoring is a reliable tool for early detection of rejection of the pancreas. Impending rejection was diagnosed a mean of 10.2 days before elevation of blood glucose level commenced. Urinary amylase and CIM utilized as pancreatic rejection markers rendered a sensitivity and specificity of 80% and 100% respectively.

In summary, urinary amylase levels declined precipitously together with an elevation of "activated" lymphocytes during CIM before the onset of hyperglycaemia in primate recipients of whole pancreatic allografts with bladder drainage. These rejection markers accurately predicted impending rejection of the pancreas, but implementation of anti-rejection therapy could not entirely reverse the early rejection phase. Further studies remain necessary to ascertain whether or not the rejection process is reversible by the administration of anti-rejection therapy before the onset of hyperglycaemia.

Acknowledgements

The technical services of G Louw, T Zuurmond, D Els, M du Plessis, H Davids, LB du Toit, B le Roux, J Matthyse, W Wildeman, L Nieuwenhuis, M le Roux, and I Petersen are acknowledged. Cyclosporine was supplied by the Sandoz Corporation, Basle, Switzerland.

References

1. Du Toit DF, Reece-Smith H, McShane P, Denton T, Morris PJ. Prolongation of segmental pancreatic allografts in dogs receiving cyclosporine A. Transplantation 33, 432, 1982.

2. McMaster P, Procychyn A, Calne RY, Valdes R, Rolles K, Smith DJ. Prolongation of canine pancreas allograft survival with cyclosporine-A. Br Med J 280, 444, 1982.

3. Du Toit DF, Heydenrych JJ, Smit B, Louw G, Zuurmond T, Laker L, Els D, Weideman A, Wolfe-Coote S, Van der Merwe E, Groenewald W. Segmental pancreatic allograft survival in baboons treated with combined irradiation and cyclosporine: A preliminary report. Surgery 97, 447, 1985.

4. Du Toit DF, Heydenrych JJ, Louw G, Zuurmond T, Els D, Wolfe-Coote S, Laker L. Intraperitoneal transplantation of vascularised segmental pancreatic autografts without duct ligation in the primate. Surgery 3, 471, 1983.

5. Du Toit DF, Heydenrych JJ, Louw G, Zuurmond T, Laker L, Els D, Weideman A, Wolfe-Coote S, Davids H. Prolongation of intraperitoneal segmental pancreatic allografts in primates receiving cyclosporine-A. Surgery 96, 14, 1984.

7. Du Toit DF, Homan WP, Morris PJ. The effect of cyclosporine on experimental renal and pancreatic allografts in the dog. In Cyclosporine A (editor: DG White), Amsterdam, Elsevier Biomedical Press, pp 101, 1982.

8. Du Toit DF, Heydenrych JJ, Smit B, Zuurmond T, Louw G, Laker L, Els D, Wolfe-Coote S, van der Merwe E, Groenewald W. Segmental pancreatic allograft survival in pancreatectomised baboons treated with total body or lymphoid irradiation and pre-operative blood transfusions. Transplantation 16, 804, 1984.

9. Du Toit DF, Heydenrych JJ, Smit B, Zuurmond T, Louw G, Laker L, Els D, Weideman A, Wolfe-Coote S, Du Toit LB, Davids H, Groenewald WA, Van der Merwe E, Pistorius S. The effect of ionizing radiation on the primate pancreas. An endocrine and morphologic study. J Surg Oncol 34, 43, 1987.

1. Transplantation

10. Tyden G, Lundgren G, Ost L, Kojima Y, Gunnarsson R, Östman J, Groth CG. Progress in segmental pancreatic transplantation. World J Surg 10, 404, 1986.

11. Sutherland DER, Goetz FC, Najarian JS. One hundred pancreas transplants in a single institution. Ann Surg 200, 414, 1984.

12. Nghiem DD, Gonwa TA, Corry RJ. Metabolic effects of urinary diversion of exocrine secretion in pancreatic transplantation. Transplantation 43, 70, 1987.

13. Prieto M, Sutherland DER, Fernandez-Cruz L, Heil J, Najarian JS. Urinary amylase monitoring for early diagnosis of pancreas allograft rejection in dogs. J Surg Res 40, 597, 1986.

14. Munda R, Tom W, Firs M, Gartside P, Alexander J. Pancreatic allograft exocrine urinary tract diversion. Transplantation 43, 95, 1987.

15. Nghiem DD, Bentel W, Corry R. Duodenocystostomy for exocrine pancreatic drainage in experimental and clinical pancreatico-duodenal transplantation. Transplant Proc 18, 1762, 1986.

16. Tom W, Munda R, First M, Alexander J. Physiologic consequences of pancreatic allograft exocrine drainage into the urinary tract. Transplant Proc 19, 2339, 1987.

17. Tao L, Sutherland DER, Cavallini M, Najarian JS. Duct drainage in the bladder for management of exocrine secretions of segmental pancreatic grafts in dogs. Surg Forum 34, 376, 1983.

18. Nghiem D, Corry RJ. Technique of simultaneous renal pancreaticoduodenal transplantation with urinary drainage of pancreatic secretion. Amer J Surg 153, 405, 1987.

19. Sollinger HW, Kalayonglu M, Hoffmann R, Deierhoi M, Belzer FO. Experience with whole pancreas transplantation and pancreatico-duodenocystostomy. Transplant Proc 18, 1759, 1986.

20. Prieto M, Sutherland DER, Fernandez-Cruz L, Heil J, Najarian JS. Experimental and clinical experience with urine amylase monitoring for early diagnosis or rejection in pancreas transplantation. Transplantation 43, 73, 1987.

21. Gleidman M, Gold M, Whittaker J, Rifkin H, Sokerman R, Freed S, Tellis V, Veith F. Clinical segmental pancreatic transplantation with ureter-pancreatic duct anastomosis for exocrine drainage. Surgery 74, 171, 1973.

22. Nghiem D, Pitzen R, Corry R. Evaluation of techniques of controlling exocrine drainage after segmental pancreatectomy in dogs. Arch Surg 120, 1132, 1985.

23. Munda R, First M, Joffe SN, Alexander N. Experience with pancreatic allografts in renal transplant recipients. Transplant Proc 17, 353, 1985.

24. Powell C, Lindsey N, Nolan M, Boyle P, Wiley K, Beck S, Herold A, Fox M. Urinary amylase as a marker of rejection in duct to ureter drained pancreas grafts. Transplant Proc 19, 1023, 1987.

25. Toledo-Pereyra LH, Mittal VK. Complications of pancreas transplantation-effect on technique. Transplant Proc 19, 2319, 1987.

26. Toledo-Pereyra L, Mittal VK. Persistent urinary tract infections and wound infections after pancreatico-cystostomy. Transplant Proc 18, 1765, 1986.

1. Transplantation

27. Corry RJ, Schulak JA, Gonwa TA. Surgical treatment of diabetic nephropathy with simultaneous pancreatic duodenal and renal transplantation. Surg Gynecol Obstet 162, 547, 1986.

28. Hanto DW, Sutherland DER. Pancreas transplantation: Clinical considerations. Radiol Clin North Amer 25, 333, 1987.

29. Myburgh JA, Smit JA, Stark JH, Browde S. Total lymphoid irradiation in kidney and liver transplantation in the baboon: Prolonged graft survival and alterations in T cell subsets with low cumulative dose regimens. Immunology 132, 1019, 1984.

30. Myburgh JA, Smit JA, Browde S, Stark JH. Current status of total lymphoid irradiation. Transplant Proc 15, 659, 1983.

31. Myburgh JA, Smit JA, Browde S, Hill R. Transplantation tolerance in primates following total lymphoid irradiation and allogeneic bone-marrow injection. 1. Orthotopic liver allografts. Transplantation 29, 405, 1980.

32. Ertel W, Reichenspurner H, Lersch C, Hammer C, Plahl M, Lehmann M, Kemkes BM, Osterholzer G, Reble B, Reichart B, Brendel W. Cytoimmunological monitoring in acute rejection and viral bacterial or fungal infection following transplantation. Heart Transplantation 4, 390, 1985

33. Hammer C, Reichenspurner H, Ertel W, Lersch C, Plahl M, Brendel W, Reichart B, Uberfuhr P, Welz A, Kemkes BM, Reble B, Funccius W, Gokel M. Cytological and immunologic monitoring of cyclosporine-treated human heart recipients. Heart Transplantation 3, 228, 1984.

34. Hammer C, Lersch C, Klanke D, Reichenspurner H, Kemkes BM, Lehmann M, Krombach F, Brendel W. Early diagnosis of inflammatory complications in human heart recipients using monitoring of peripheral blood cells (CIM). JR Coll Surg Edinb 33, 28, 1988.

1. Transplantation

1.5. Heart Preservation

1.5.1 Prolonged Ex-vivo Heart Preservation

E Solis [1], MP Kaye [2]

[1]Department of Cardiovascular Surgery,
Hôpital La Pitié, Paris, France

[2]Department of Cardiovascular Research,
the Minnesota Heart and Lung Institute,
University of Minnesota,
Minneapolis, USA

Heart transplantation has become highly effective therapy for the treatment of end-stage heart disease. Even with the increasing survival rate and improvements in patients' quality of life, surgeons and patients still face two major obstacles: availability of donor organs and short time of safe preservation. The maximum safe time-limits of myocardial preservation have not been established; total ischemic time in clinical cases, has generally been limited to less than 4 hours (1-2). The International Society for Heart Transplantation has recently published (3) a relationship between donor heart ischemic time and 30 day mortality after transplantation. Early mortality increases up to 28.6% when the ischemic time is greater than 4 hours. Therefore, improvement in existing preservation techniques is essential to reduce mortality and expand the donor's pool.

To enhance availability and utilization of donor hearts we have developped a successful technique, that permits ex-vivo maintenance of a donor heart for at least 12 hours. It is the purpose of this manuscript to summarize our experience with this technique.

Technique

The perfusion system consists of a cylinder in which the heart is placed under cardioplegic arrest after a previous cannulation of the superior vena cava and brachio-cephalic artery. All the pulmonary arteries and veins are tied and severed with the exception of the right upper lobe pulmonary artery, which is left open for future drainage of blood returning from the coronary sinus and to permit the filling with blood of the cylinder to surround the heart. The blood coming from the venous return is extracted by the SVC cannula and from the cylinder drain into a 250 ml collapsible reservoir, a roller pump, a heat exchanger, a 0.4 m^2 membrane oxygenator, and a 27 micron final pore.

The aorta is perfused in a non-pulsatile retrograde fashion through the brachio-cephalic trunk. Aortic root pres-

1. Transplantation

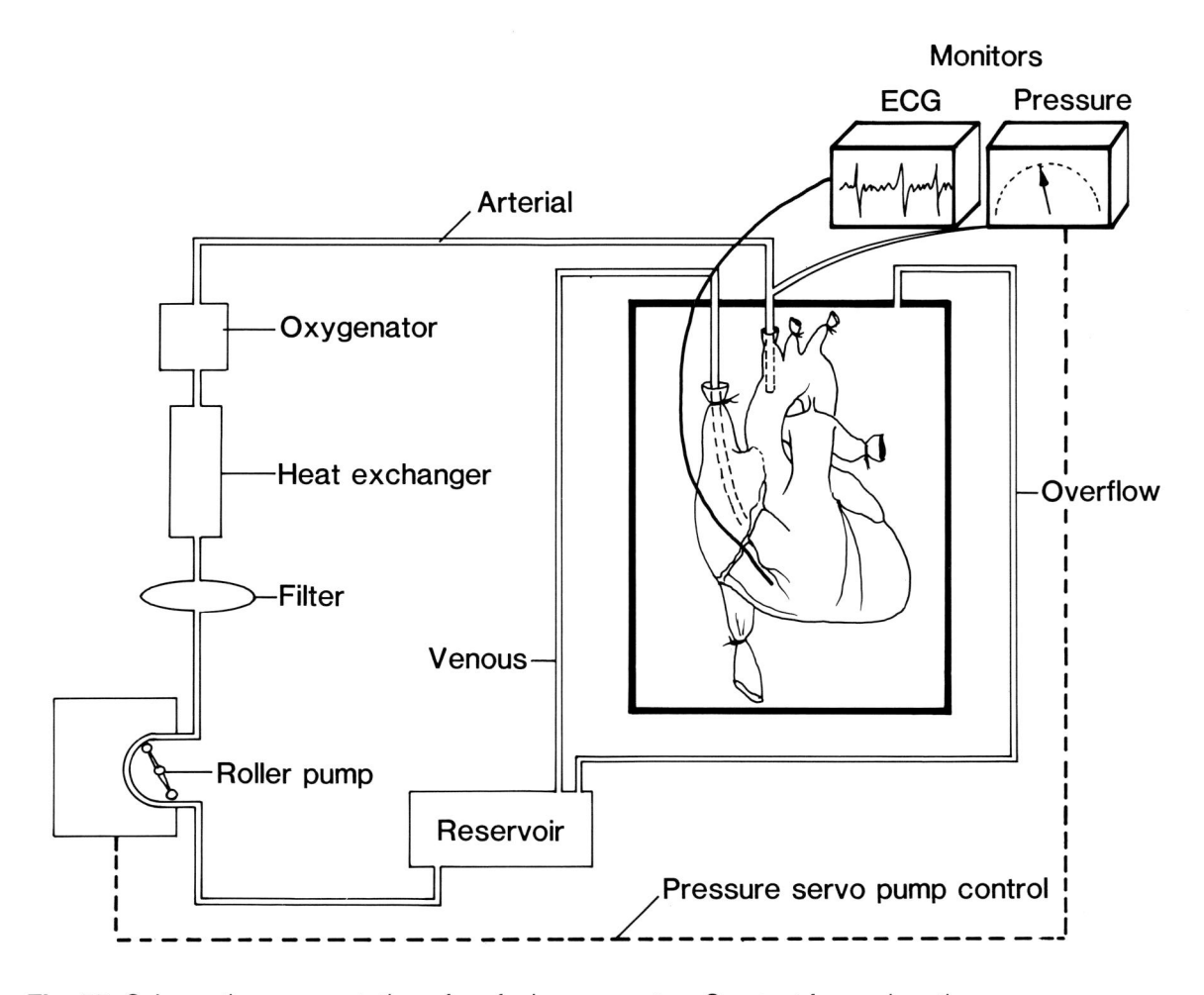

Fig. 55 Schematic representation of perfusion apparatus. See text for explanation.

sure is maintained at 85 mmHg by a servo-controlled roller pump. Perfusion is instituted at 37°C for the duration of the perfusion (Figure 55).

Blood glucose concentration is adjusted to 250-300 mg/dl and maintained by a continuous infusion of 14.25 mg/min. D-Rybose (250 mg/l) is added to the perfusate to accelerate adenine nucleotide the novo synthesis (9). Ibuprofen is added as an antiplatelet drug.

Blood gases, electrolytes, and pH are adjusted and maintained at physiological levels.

A continual exchange transfusion takes place, replacing the perfusate with fresh blood at a rate of 100 ml/hour.

A more complete description of the technique has been published previously (5,6,7,8).

Results

This technique has been evaluated by three independent studies (5,6,7).

In our initial study, 19 hearts were preserved for 24 hours. In 11 of them, light and transmission electron microscopy (TEM) were performed at three independent time intervals: At the end of the 24 hours preservation period and at 1 and 7 days post-orthotopic transplantation. Light microscopic examination of the perfused hearts revealed no cellular edema, myocytolysis, or necrosis.

121

1. Transplantation

Ventricular Function

	Denervated Hearts	Acute Orthotopic Transplantation	12 Hr Preserved Heart + Orthotopic Transplantation	P Value
	Group I n=6	Group II n=5	Group III n=6	
Heart Rate (beats/min)	124 ± 4	117 ± 10	117 ± 6	N.S.
Enddiastolic pressure (mmHg)	9 ± 1.7	8.5 ± 1.1	10 ± 2.1	N.S.
Endsystolic pressure (mmHg)	78 ± 6	64 ± 5	102 ± 9	0.05 vs GI & II
+dp/dt (mmHg/sec)	1495 ± 96	1118 ± 175	2097 ± 193	0.05 vs GI & II
-dl/dt (mm/sec)	26 ± 3	24 ± 1	36 ± 5	0.05 vs GI & II

Values expressed as mean ± SEM
all comparisons by unpaired t-test between groups

Table 17 Ventricular function of denervated hearts, acute ortotopic transplanted hearts and hearts preserved ex-vivo for 12 hours and ortotopic transplantation.

By TEM, no significant structural abnormalities of myocardial subcellular organelles were identified. The sarcotubular system was not dilate, and the mitochondria had no membrane disruption, mineral precipitation, or organelle swelling. Myocardial interstitium was lightly widened by apparent edema with good integrity of capillary endothelial cells and perivascular structures (7). 16 of these hearts were reimplanted in the orthotopic position, with 75% survival.

In a second study, the ventricular function of 17 hearts was evaluated, using sonomycrometric crystals, 24 to 48 hours post-operative. The systolic data obtained from acutely denervated hearts utilized as controls (GROUP I) were compared with 5 hearts subjected to immediate orthotopic transplantation (GROUP II) and with another group of 6 hearts subjected to 12 hours preservation plus orthotopic transplantation (GROUP III) (5).

During the 12 hours' preservation time, the initial coronary blood flow was 100 ± 12.6 ml/min as compared with 98 ± 17.2 ml/min after 12 hours of perfusion. Initial coronary vascular resistance was 0.824 ± 0.1 units as compared with $0,846 \pm 0.1$ units after 12 hours. Initial mean arterial lactate concentration was 5.8 ± 1.1 mM/l as compared with 3.7 ± 0.7 mM/l at the end ($p<0.04$). Changes in the blood components and blood gases were not significant during the perfusion period, but a marked reduction in phosphorous concentration was observed from 2 ± 0.37 mg/dl to 1.1 ± 0.93 mg/dl (p<0.05).

Table 17 summarizes the hemodynamic performance of these animals. Hearts orthotopically transplanted after 12 hours of ex-vivo preservation had a higher endsystolic pressure (peak +dp/dt and -dl/dt) than the denervated hearts (p<0.05) and the acutely orthotopically transplanted hearts (p<0.003). Left-ventricular hemodynamic performance utilizing the slope of endsystolic pressure dimension relationship, an index sensitive to changes in contractility but relatively insensitive to changes to preload and afterload, showed no significant difference between denervated hearts and hearts preserved for 12 hours, but the former showed a better preserved inotropic state (p= 0.04) than hearts preserved by hypothermic arrest (Table 18).

Finally, to complete the evaluation of this technique, myocardial metabolism was studied from five areas of the heart according to flow distribution by means of high energy phosphate levels and tissue catecholamine concentration (6).

Group I were 5 hearts arrested with 400 cc of cardioplegic solution used as control.
Group II were 6 hearts preserved for 2.5 hours in 2-4°C saline solution, as used in the standard technique for distant heart procurement before clinical transplantation and
Group III were 6 hearts preserved for 12 hours.

Table 19 summarizes the levels of myocardial high energy phosphates. The data demonstrate that only a slight but significant reduction (p<0.01) of ATP levels occurred during the 12 hour preservation period. Mitochondrial function of preserved hearts was adequately maintained, as evidenced by both high CP level and normal energy charge values. Heart preserved by cold ischemia had a reduction (p=0.03) of CP levels when compared with both control and 12 hour preserved hearts.

When these data were analyzed according to flow distribution, ATP and CP were equally distributed throughout the myocardium in all groups.

There were no significant differences in the concentrations of nor-epinephrine, epinephrine and dopamine used between groups.

Discussion

Since the beginning of organ transplantation in recent decades, one of the most difficult problems of the transplantation team has been the timely procurement, preservation, and transplantation of donated organs. In most situations, an organ transplantation is a race against the clock, as surgeons have a very limited time period available from explant to implant of the graft.

The current method for distant heart procurement is simple and easy, and has some advantages in transportation; but, unfortunately, the current method does not permit prolonged periods of preservation. Recent data (3) indicate that myocardial function declines directly as a result of ischemic time. While 30 day mortality is relatively low (4.9-6.3%) for ischemic periods from 0-2 hours, it begins to increase rapidly after two hours to 11.5%, 15.7% (at 3-4 hours), and 28.6% (at 4-5 hours). Therefore, improvement in the

1. Transplantation

Endsystolic Pressure/Internal Endsystolic Diameter

	Denervated Hearts	Acute Orthotopic Transplantation	12 Hr Preserved Heart + Orthotopic Transplantation	P Value
	Group I n=6	Group II n=5	Group III n=6	
Slope (mmHg/mm)	8.4 ± 3.1	9 ± 1.6	14.1 ± 2.1	P=0.04 GIII vs GII
Intercept (mm)	15.1 ± 5.1	23 ± 2.5	23.4 ± 4.6	N.S.
r-value	0.90 ± 0.008	0.89 ± 0.006	0.87 ± 0.01	N.S.

Values expressed as mean ± SEM
All comparisons by unpaired T test between groups
G = Group
N.S. = not significant

Table 18 Endsystolic pressure/internal endsystolic diameter relationship.

High Energy Phosphates

	ATP	CP	EC
Group I control n=6	5.8 ± 0.6	4.1 ± 1.6**	0.85 ± 0.01
Group II cold ischemic n=5	5.6 ± 0.2	2.4 ± 0.8** +	0.88 ± 0.001
Group III 12 Hr preserved hearts	4.6 ± 0.4*	10.6 ± 2.8	0.86 ± 0.008

* $p<0.01$ versus Groups I&II
** $p<0.01$ versus Groups III
** $p=0.03$ versus Group I

ATP = adenosine triphosphate
CP = creatine phosphate
EC = energy change

values expressed as mean ± SD

Table 19 Levels of myocardial high energy phosphates (mMol/mg wet weight).

existing preservation techniques is essential to reduce mortality.

When we started with our preservation technique, we believed that the stimulation of the conditions found in-vivo could allow a longer and better ex-vivo preservation, and that the utilization of this method could permit the evaluation of pre-implant function.

We chose total blood as perfusate, based on the idea that it is the most complete and perfect solution to perfuse an organ, and thinking that bloodless perfusates, in combination with hypothermia, although effective for short periods of time, are non-physiologic.

During the past seven years, we have developped a technique and a device which permits successful ex-vivo maintenance of a donor heart for at least 12 hours. This time period was chosen because we felt it was adequate to provide time for transport, tissue typing, and reimplantation anywhere within the USA.

We believe that we have documented the efficacy of this technique at the microscopic, functional, and metabolic level, and are currently making preparations for clinical application.

At the functional level our data shows 100% survival of recipients after 12 hours storage of the donor organ. Ventricular functional measurements done 24 to 48 hours following reimplantation with sonomicrometry and catheter tip transducers showed comparable results between 12 hours preserved hearts and denervated hearts. Furthermore, hearts preserved for 12 hours showed a better inotropic state than hearts preserved by hypothermic arrest (5).

Finally, at the metabolic level, ATP levels were found to be slightly reduced from control levels in the hearts preserved for 12 hours but the high CP level encountered in these hearts suggests that both the substrate and the mechanism necessary for production of high energy phosphate bonds are available (4).

The essential gain from storing the isolated heart is time. This includes time to transport the heart from donor to recipient, therefore expanding the geographic donor pool and the number of donors; time to do an elective operation, therefore reducing expensive and urgent procedures dictated by organ availability; time to tissue-type the heart and to find the best recipient, therefore increasing survival; time to gain anonymity of the heart and thus reduce undesirable publicity; and time, possibly, to resuscitate a heart damaged by ante-mortem changes, to transplant immediately.

1. Transplantation

References

1. Watson DC, Reitz BA, Baumgartner WA, Rancy AA, Oyer PE, Stinson EB, Shumway NE. Distant heart procurement for transplantation. Surgery 86, 56, 1979.

2. Thomas FT, Szentpetery SS, Mammana RE, Wolfgang TC, Lower RR. Long-distance transportation of human hearts for transplantation. Ann Thorac Surg 26, 344, 1978.

3. Kaye MP. The registry of the International Society of Heart Transplantation: fourth official report - 1987. J Heart Transplant 6, 63, 1987.

4. Solis E, Kaye MP. The registry of the International Society for Heart Transplantation: third official report - June 1986. J Heart Transplant 5, 2, 1986.

5. Solis E, Tago M, Kaye MP. Cardiac function following prolonged preservation and orthotopic transplantation. J Heart Transplant 4, 357, 1985.

6. Solis E, Tyce GM, Bianco R, Mahoney J, Kaye MP. High energy phosphates and catecholamine stores after prolonged ex-vivo heart preservation. J Heart Transplant 5, 444, 1986.

7. Tago M, Subramanian R, Kaye MP. Light and electron microscopic evaluation of canine hearts orthopically transplanted after 24 hours of extracorporeal preservation. J Thorac Cardiovasc Surg 86, 912, 1983.

8. Kaye MP, Tago M, Subramanian R. Prolonged preservation of the myocardium. Heart Transplantation 1, 12, 1981.

9. Paske MK, Spray TL, Pellom GL et al. Ribose enhances myocardial recovery following ischemic in the isolate working rat heart. J Thorac Cardiovasc Surg 83, 390, 1982.

1.6. Xenogeneic Transplantation

1.6.1 Immunological Aspects and Recent Advances in Xenogeneic Transplantation

C Hammer

Institute for Surgical Research, Klinikum Grosshadern, University of Munich, FR Germany

Organ availability is a continuing and increasing problem in transplantation. The shortage of human organs has stimulated trials for the use of organs from outside the human species. Highly potent immunosuppressive drugs and new immunomodulating methods have now pushed xenogeneic transplantation into a new era.

The pioneers of xenogeneic organ transplantation during the first era were Princeteau (1), Jaboulay (2), Unger (3), Neuhof (4) and Lexer (5), who tried to re-establish the function of organs of terminally-ill patients with grafts from animals. At that time their efforts were condemned to complete failure since rejection mechanisms were not understood, and the expression "transplantation immunology" did not even exist.

The classical experiments of Sir P Medawar during World War II, elucidating rejection mechanisms, stimulated once again the use of xenogeneic organs from non-human primates feasible. In clinical experiments Reemtsma et al (6) and Starzl et al (7) tried to win some time in desperate situations of organ failure with organs from chimpanzees and baboons as a temporary bridging measure.

Other results from animal experiments obtained during this second era of xenogeneic research showed that immunological events that followed certain rules and orders were the background of the mechanisms called "xenogeneic hyperacute rejection".

Preformed Natural Antibodies and Xenotransplantation

The limiting factor in the use of organs between distantly related species is the phenomenon of hyperacute xenograft rejection. The principal features are a rapid increase of the arterial resistance and subsequent cessation of renal blood flow within minutes. Extravasation of blood and haematuria is seen; urine production stops. The organ increases in size and changes in colour from pale red at the beginning of hemoperfusion, to dark blue after a few minutes. Although the exact mechanism of this dramatic phenomenon is not fully understood, the triggering mechanism is believed to be due to preformed natural antibodies (PNAB) directed against a great variety of tissue antigens (8/9).

Characteristics of Preformed Natural Antibodies

PNABs are found in numerous xenogeneic donor recipient systems. As a result of the observation that a correlation exists between survival time of xenotransplants, the zoological disparity of donor and recipient and the titre of PNAB sera of 48 species of mammals from 7 zoological orders were tested for their titres of PNAB. More than 8 300 combinations of serum samples and antigens of 111 individuals were tested for xenohaemagglutinins, xenoleukagglutinins, xenolymphotoxins, and complement fixing antibodies (10).

PNABs were found in all species against all antigens used. The choice of test methods had a significant influence on the titres, with the most reliable results revealed by haemagglutination. Age had a clear impact on the magnitude of titres.

The concentration of PNABs varies after birth in relationship to diaplacentaric immunoglobulin transport from mother to foetus or resorption of colostrum. Rabbits show an active transport of IGM-antibodies through the placenta. The maternal antibodies disappear in the newborn serum 2 weeks after birth, to be replaced after 8-12 weeks by the individual's own production. In other species, the content of IGM in newborns or very young individuals was negligible in comparison with adults.

The highest values of antibodies are reached in the first half of life, followed by a slow reduction with time. IGG-PNABs decrease with age to be replaced by IGM type antibodies.

Domestic animals showed higher levels of PNAB as compared with their wild counterparts. Wild rats have isoantibodies more frequently than inbred strains. No titre differences between males and females could be found in this study. In humans, however, women, mainly multiparous, showed higher titres of xenohaemagglutinins and isohaemagglutinins.

No biorhythm influence was found. Temperature and light showed no regularity in influence. Annual differences were found in humans, sheep and cattle, with a maximum of titres in late summer, and a low at the beginning of the year. This difference was shifted by 6 months in the southern hemisphere (11).

Chronically sick animals usually showed a decrease in titres with sometimes complete lack of PNAB of different types. Acute bacterial infections resulted in a slight increase of PNAB. Gnotobiotic animals, showing no PNAB, developed normal titres against all antigens tested within 2 weeks after being exposed to normal environment. One strain of bacteria was enough to induce PNAB against the whole panel of test xenoantigens.

Preformed natural antibodies against blood group antigens could be detected on several occasions. Blood group A was found only in chimpanzees, orangutans and in African subhuman monkeys. Antibodies against blood group A were found in gorillas, Rhesus-monkeys, zebras, and cattle.

An A-like substance exists in sheep (blood group R), cattle (blood group J), and pigs (blood group A). Four partial blood groups of A were described in dogs, pigs, sheep and goats (12). Blood group B, known to exist in orang-utans and gorillas, is lacking in chimpanzees

1. Transplantation

and most other monkeys tested. Anti-B-antibodies were found in humans, rabbits, guinea-pigs, and rats. Antibodies against red blood cells of blood group O were found in llamas, foxes, and horses.

Preformed Natural Antibodies and the Zoological System

Few references concerning this topic exist in literature. We found that the magnitude of titre correlates well with the zoological disparity, with the exception of isohaemagglutinins in primates and similar antibodies in ungulates. Within a zoological family, only low titres or no PNAB could be detected. They increase within the zoological order to reach values in widely-related species within the order as high as in extra-ordinal widely-divergent species. Closely related species like horses, donkeys, and zebras; wolves, dogs, foxes and dingos; cats, lions, and tigers; sheep and goats did not show preformed natural haemagglutinins against each other (Figure 56).

Species that show no PNABs are so closely related that hybridisation becomes possible in many cases. In combinations like sheep and goats, the hybrid embryos usually fail to survive beyond the 2nd month of gestation, probably due to a haematolytical disease (13).

The specificity of PNABs was tested in absorption studies. Exhaustive absorption by red blood cells (RBCs) eliminates all PNABs against RBC of the absorbing species; to a large extent against those PNABs that are directed against RBCs of closely related animals and, to a lesser extent, against other species. There seems to be a correlation between reduction of PNABs and the phylogeneic distance of the species involved (Figure 57).

serum / cells	primates	carnivores	equids	rodents	even-toed ung.
primates	10,0	17,8	20,0	2,2	34
carnivores	26,0	ø	ø	ø	1,4
equids	30,8	13,0	0,66	1,6	74
rodents	39,0	28,5	29,0	1,6	50
even-toed ung.	53,0	71,5	8,1	2,8	12,2

Fig. 56 Distribution of xeno-haemagglutinins in different zoological orders (titres expressed in a log).

1. Transplantation

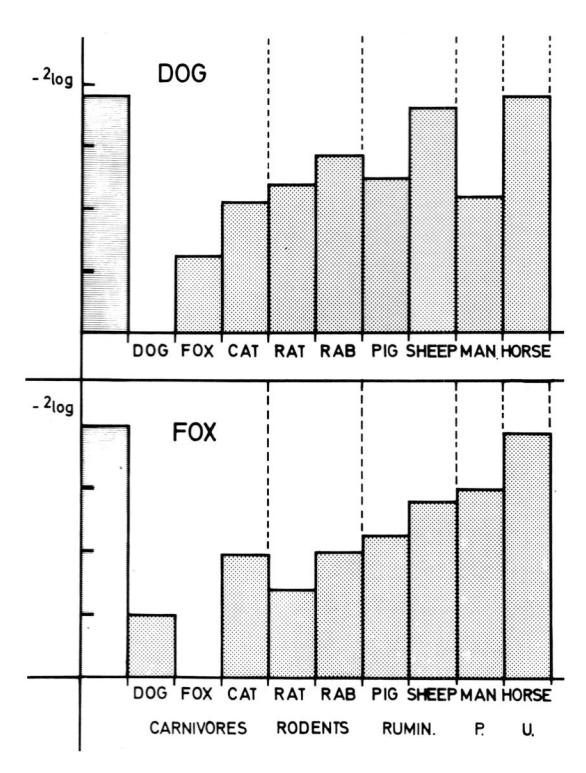

Fig. 57 Species specificity of xenohaemagglutinins as shown in absorption studies. PNAB from the horse, absorbing antigens of dog and fox RBC.

Fig. 58 Release of intracellular enzyme (LDH) after absorption of PNABs by xenogeneic kidneys.

PNAB in Xenotransplantation

Because PNABs are absorbed by the xenograft to a large extent (14), followed by signs of cell destruction (Figure 58) it is widely accepted that the hyperacute xenogeneic rejection depends on the effect of PNAB under cooperation of complement (15,16,17,18) and cellular blood-components mainly thrombocytes (19) and leucocytes (Figure 59). Masking of donor-specific antigens in the sense of "enhancement" (19), immunosuppression, inhibition of complement and coagulation (20), were introduced in order to modify hyperacute, xenogeneic rejection (21). The survival time of transplanted or ex-vivo haemoperfused kidneys or livers was, in terms of clinical application, not prolonged. A true function was never observed in widely divergent species, i.e. organs transplanted across the phylogeneic order or even the zoological family (22).

Elimination of PNABs

A new possibility of testing the action of PNAB was an active elimination of PNAB, complement and cellular blood components by isovolemic haemodilution, in combination with lymph-drainage or plasmapheresis. Extreme haemodilution to a haematocrit of 7% using Dextran was applied. Gamma globulins were reduced by 80%, complement by 90%, thrombocytes by 77%, and leucocytes by 45% compared with predilution values. Titres of xenohaemagglutinins were reduced from 1:64 to 1:2. Despite almost non-

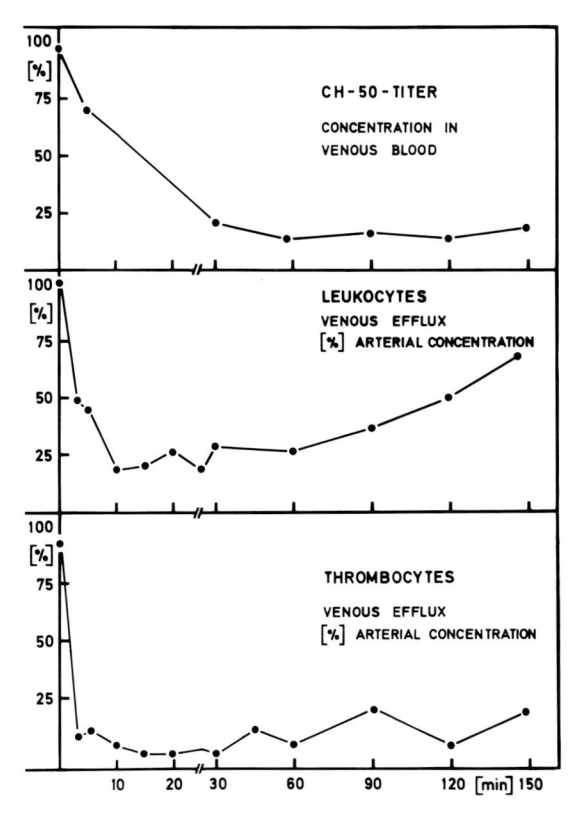

Fig. 59 Reduction of complement, leukocytes and thrombocytes during xenohaemoperfusion of pig kidneys with dog blood.

existing PNAB and extremely reduced viscosity of the blood, haemo-perfusion of pig kidneys by dogs ceased after 11 hours. Additional lymph drainage resulted in prolongation of perfusion by 14 hours (23).

No xenogeneic haemoperfused kidney was able to concentrate urine. Potassium and enzymes were significantly increased in the urine excreted. Histological investigation revealed typical damage on endothelial and mesangium cells, more expressed in the haemodiluted animals than in the controls.

Despite a significant improvement of renal blood flow and microcirculation in the transplant and an almost complete lack of PNAB, oxygen consumption of the transplant was not apparent. This indicates that incompatible enzyme systems might be one of the major reasons for the immediate collapse of transplant function. The large reservoir of PNAB and complement and their production in the dog during perfusion time could still be held responsible for later destructive events. Dogs surviving the perfusion showed total recovery of blood components between 1 and 2 days.

In vivo studies in which kidneys of widely divergent species were perfused with different serum fractions and combinations of serum fractions, together with cells, showed that leucocytes are not actively involved in hyperacute rejection mechanisms. Perfusion with antibody-free serum fractions led to the same type of hyperacute rejection. Disruption of white blood cells and thrombocytes led to deterioration of endothelial cells and haematuria when added to the perfusate. It was suggested that this was due to a release of lysosomal hydrolases from polymorphs, clearly proving non-specific immunological factors responsible for this xenogeneic reaction (24).

Xenotransplantation in Closely Related Species

Xenogeneic transplantation across families in closely related species within the zoological order resulted in survival times of hours up to a day. Despite low titres of PNABs, primary hyperacute rejections within minutes were rare. The delayed type of hyperacute rejection occurring still seems to be due to humoral mechanisms. It is not proven whether this action depends on the amount or specificity of PNABs. An influx of white blood cells and thrombocytes is probably induced by these humoral mechanisms (25-26). Elimination of the PNAB in this system has not been reported.

1. Transplantation

Second set transplantation of organs of closely related species underwent typical humoral rejections, indicating specific immunization in such extra-familial combinations. This specific sensitization induced hyperacute xenogeneic rejection because of specific antibodies and must be distinguished from unmodified xenogeneic rejections.

Xenotransplantation in Species of one Zoological Family

First encouraging clinical xenotransplantation was reported by Reemtsma et al (6) and Starzl et al (7), who grafted kidneys of nonhuman primates, phylogenetically related to man as closely as possible within a zoological family. Despite ABO incompatibility, the survival time achieved was of clinical interest (27-28). A few other less successful trials using hearts were reported.

In experimental studies, combinations within the zoological family like hare-rabbit (27), sheep-goat, mouse-rat, fox-dog (30) and wolf-dog were investigated. No PNABs were found. Survival times reached those reported in allogeneic systems. Rodents, ungulates, and canines develop xenogeneic anti-blood group and antileucocyte antibodies after transplantation specific enough to be used for blood group and tissue typing (29).

Good results were obtained when modern optimal immunosuppression was introduced. Using cyclosporine as immunosuppression in the fox-dog model, the usual survival time of 6.5 ± 1.2 days could be prolonged by 70%. ALG-treated dogs survived 13.4 ± 1.0 days after transplantation of fox kidneys. This is 124% longer than controls (32) (Figure 60).

ORGAN	IMMUNOSUPPRESSION	SVT(d)	N
HEART		8.4 ± 1.9	6
KIDNEY		6.5 ± 1.2	8
KIDNEY	ALG	13.4 ± 1.0	9
KIDNEY	AMS	15.8 ± 0.7	5
KIDNEY	ALG + AMS	17.7 ± 0.9	7
HEART	CSA + MP	20.2 ± 4.1	6
KIDNEY	CSA + MP	10.9 ± 3.0	7
KIDNEY	DEOXYSP.	13.0 ± 3.4	6

Fig. 60 Survival times of fox-organs transplanted into dogs using different types of immunosuppressive therapies.

Only modest cellular infiltrates of the graft could be detected by biopsy and fine needle aspiration cytology (FNAC), mainly consisting of monocytes. Fox hearts function 20.2 ± 4.1 days under cyclosporine A therapy, showing a type of rejection not dominated by cellular intergraft events but caused mainly by humoral immunological factors (31).

Wolf kidneys transplanted to non-treated dogs showed survival times longer than that of DLA incompatible dog kidneys, and approached survival times similar to those of DLA-identical littermate kidneys. ALG treatment improved the function time from 19.9 ± 2.4 days to 30.0 ± 2.7 days. Cyclosporine treated wolf kidneys reached maximum survival times up to 90 days with a mean of 58.0 ± 22.5 days (34).

Rejection mechanisms in these closely related systems are comparable to the allogeneic ones. After 3 days creatinine values rise. No major changes of mononuclear cells in the peripheral blood can be seen. Lymphocytes and monocytes, activated lymphocytes or blast cells invade the graft in the first 7 days, leading to rejection as proven by FNAC (32).

Interestingly enough, an increase in lymphocytes after day 4 is not as high in the xenograft as that seen in allografts. After 7 days, B-cells, also in the form of activated plasma cells, increase significantly in the xenograft but not in the allograft. Most observers therefore believe that here, humoral events overlap cellular rejection (32).

Advantages of Xenotransplantation

With regard to numerical problems, one must once again differentiate between closely related and widely divergent species.

In terms of discordant transplantation systems, many species with appropriate grafts are readily available.

In terms of concordant grafts, major problems exist. There is virtually no species of subhuman primates which is numerous enough to supply the lacking number of grafts. Baboons would be the only species accessible, but even these animals are limited if needed worldwide; specific breeding of non-human primates would be necessary. Under these circumstances, logistical problems would be easily solved since, for both types of xenogeneic transplantation, the animal could be farmed. Donors of appropriate size, organ, age, etc. could be culled at any time.

The question of transfer of virus disease has to be taken into consideration. Gnotobiotic or specific pathogen germ-free maintenance of the animals must be provided. Some of the viruses found in primates are known. However, little information exists about virus transfer from other species such as the pig, the sheep, or the dog, from which it is known that slow virus diseases may develop.

Routine xenotransplantation would open a totally new field of activity. Xenotransplantation could be applied on a large scale to treat congenital diseases, malformations or deficiencies like diabetes.

Ethical problems would exist mainly on the recipient side. However, one cannot foresee how society would react if xenotransplantation becomes a routine procedure.

Future Possibilities of Modulation of Xenogeneic Rejection

In discordant systems it appears as if depletion of preformed natural antibodies is of major importance.

As shown, isovolemic haemodilution was able to reduce the blood components - including the preformed natural antibodies - to almost zero. However, after 3 days most of the serum factors were brought back to their normal levels.

Clonal depletion of antibody-producing cells directed against the xenogeneic antigen has been proposed, a procedure as difficult as the induction of anti-idiotypic antibodies against PNABs.

Manipulation of the blood clotting system using anti-platelet aggregation factor and drugs inhibiting calcium-ion transport was suggested. Depletion of complement or inhibition of one specific part of the complement cascade has been described (33). With regard to cells or cultured cells, protection against immunological active components by membranes seems to be possible (34).

Thus it appears as if discordant transplantation in widely divergent species is a dream of the future. However, in the event of it becoming feasible, it would revolutionise medicine.

1. Transplantation

In concordant systems, total lymphoid irradiation (TLI) was used quite successfully by Bollinger et al (35-36) in a rat-hamster model. Together with potent immunosuppression, this could be a reasonable approach.

Induction of transplant tolerance or transplantation of bone marrow in order to produce xenogeneic chimeras should not be impossible and has already been shown successfully in rats and mice (37). Transplantation of cultured cells, depleted of passenger cells or class II antigens, should also be considered in xenotransplantation (38). Beside xenogeneic clinical transplantation, combination of closely related species might be used for pure scientific investigation of rejection mechanisms and as "hard models" to test, for example, new, more potent immunosuppressive drugs (39,40,41).

Thus, concordant transplantation has an immediate therapeutic future. Even now, by using the most powerful immunosuppressive strategies, xenotransplantation is available as a bridge in desperate situations for a time which is ethically justifiable (42,43,44).

References

1. *Princeteau M. Greffe renale. J Med Bordeaux 26, 549, 1905.*

2. *Jaboulay M. Greffe de rein au pli du conde par sondures arterielles et veneuses. Lyon med 107: 575-577, 1906.*

3. *Unger E. Nierentransplantation. 2. Mitteilung. Berl Klin Wschr 47, 573, 1919.*

4. *Neuhoff H. The transplantation of tissue. New York; Appleton & Co, 1923.*

5. *Lexer E. Die freien Transplantationen. Ferdinand Emke Verlag, Stuttgart, 1919.*

6. *Reemtsma K, McCraken BH, Schlegel JU, Pearl MA, Pearce CW, De Witt CW, Smith PE, Hewitt RI, Flinner RL, Creech O. Renal heterotransplantation in man. Ann Surg 160, 384, 1964.*

7. *Starzl TE, Marchioro TL, Peters GN, Kirkpatrick CH, Wilson WE, Porter KA, Ogden DA, Hitchkock CR, Wadden WR. Renal heterotransplantation from baboon to man. Experiences with 6 cases. Transplant 2, 752, 1964.*

8. *Rosenberg JC, Hawkins E, Rector F. Mechanisms of immunological injury during antibody-mediated hyperacute rejection of renal heterografts. Transplantation 11,151, 1971.*

9. *Rosenberg JC, Broersma RJ, Bullemer G, Mammen EF, Lenaghan R, Rosenberg BF. Relationship of platelets, blood coagulation and fibrinolysis to hyperacute rejection of renal xenografts. Transplantation 8: 152, 1969.*

10. *Hammer C, Chaussy CH, Brendel W. Preformed natural antibodies in animals and man. Eur Surg Res 5: 162, 1973.*

11. *Stone WH. The J substance of cattle, seasonal variation. J Immunol 77, 369, 1956.*

12. *Matousek J. Blood groups of animals. Ed: Czech Acad of Science, Prag, 1965.*

1. Transplantation

13. Gray A. Mammalian hybrids. Ed: Commonwealth Agricult Bureaux, Slough, England, 1971.

14. Clark DS, Gewurz H, Good RA, Varco RL. Complement fixation during heterograft rejection. Surg Forum 15, 144, 1964.

15. Hammer C, Fiedler L, Klövekorn L, Land W, Messmer K, Brendel W. Mitigation of the hyperacute xenogeneic rejection of kidneys in widely divergent species. Eur Surg Res 2, 112, 1970.

16. Hammer C, Land W, Pielsticker K, Brendel W. Experimentelle Xenotransplantation in entfernt stammesverwandten Speziessystemen. Res Exp Med 159, 124, 1972.

17. Winn HJ. Humoral antibody in allograft reactions. Transplant Proc 2, 83, 1970.

18. Giles GR, Boehmig HJ, Lilly J, Amemiay H, Takagi H, Coburg AJ, Hathaway WE, Wilson CB, Dixon FJ, Starzl TE. Mechanism and modification of rejection of heterografts between divergent species. Transplant Proc 2: 522, 1970.

19. Belitsky PH, Popovther M, Corman J, Launois B, Porter K. Modification of hyperacute xenograft rejection by intra-arterial infusion of disodium ethylenediaminetetra-acetat. Transplantation 15: 248, 1973.

20. Adachi H, Rosengard BR, Hutchins GM, Hall TS, Baumgartner WA. Effects of cyclosporine, aspirin and cobra venom factor on discordant cardiac xenograft survival in rats. Transplant Proc 19: 1145, 1987.

21. Messmer K, Hammer C, Land W, Fiedler L, Klövekorn WP, Holper K, Lob G, Merzel D, Brendel W. Modification of hyperacute xenogeneic kidney rejection. Transplant Proc 3, 542, 1971.

22. Fiedler L, Hammer C, Messmer K, Land W, Holper K, Klövekorn W, Pielsticker K, Chaussy C, Brendel W. Experimentelle Xenotransplantation in entfernt stammesverwandte Spezies- systemen. Res Exp Med 163, 137, 1974.

23. Hammer C, Land W, Brendel W. Experimentelle Xenotransplantation in entfernt stammesverwandten Speziessystemen. Res Exp Med 159, 239, 1972.

24. Land W, Corell J, Pielsticker K, Brendel W. Renale in Vitro-Xenohämoperfusion in verschiedenen Spezieskombinationen. Res Exp Med 159, 276, 1973.

25. Chaussy C, Hammer C, von Scheel J, Eisenberger F, Pielsticker K, Brendel W. Experimental xenogeneic kidney transplantation in closely related species. Res Exp Med 159, 266, 1973.

26. Hammer C, Chaussy D, Krebs G, von Scheel J, Brendel W. Experimental xenogeneic kidney transplantation in closely related species. Res Exp Med 160, 32, 1973.

27. Dieperink H, Steinbruchel D, Starklint H, Larsen S, Kemp E. Improvement in hare-to-rabbit kidney transplant survival. Transplant Proc 19, 1140, 1987.

28. Hammer C, Chaussy C, v Schell J, Pongratz H, Roscher E, Brendel W. Survival time of skin and kidney grafts within different canine species in relation to their genetic markers. Transplant Proc 7, 439, 1975.

29. Vriesendorp HM, Albert ED, Templeton JW, Belotsky S, Taylor B, Blumenstock DA, Bull RW, Cannon FD, Epstein RB, Ferrebee JW, Grosse-Wilde H, Hammer C, Krumbacher K, Leon S, Meera Khan P, Mickey R, Motola M, Rapaport FT, Saison F, Schnappauf H, Scholz S, Schroeder ML, Storb R, Wank R, Westbroek DL, Zweibaum A. Joint report of the second international workshop on canine immunogenetics. Transplant Proc 7, 289, 1976.

1. Transplantation

30. Böhm D, Krombach F, Hammer C, Gebhard F, Brendel W. Fine needle aspiration cytology in cyclosporin-treated xenogeneic kidney rejection. Transplant Proc 17, 2128, 1985.

31. Ertel W, Reichenspurner H, Hammer C, Welz A, Überfuhr P, Hemmer W, Reichart B, Gokel M, Brendel W. Heart transplantation in closely related species: A model for humoral rejection. Transplant Proc 16, 1259, 1984.

32. Krombach F, Hammer C, Gebhard F, Danko I, Scholz S, Gokel M. The effect of cyclosporine on wolf to dog kidney xenografts. Transplant Proc 17, 1436, 1985.

33. Zhang J, Munda R, Glas-Greenwalt P, Weiss MA, Pollak VE, Alexander JW. Prolongation of survival of a heart xenograft by defibrination with ancrod. Transplantation 35, 620, 1983.

34. Morris GE, Browse NL, Butler L. The latex isolator bag-an aid to intraperitoneal organ transplantation in the rat. Transplantation 44, 574, 1987.

35. Stuart J, Knechtle J, Edward C, Halperin C, Bollinger RR. Xenograft survival in two species combinations using total lymphoid irradiation and cyclosporin. Transplantation 43, 173, 1987.

36. Knechtle SJ, Halperin EC, Bollinger RR. Experimental xenografts. Transplant Proc 21, 1137, 1987.

37. Wade AC, Luckert PH, Tazume S, Niedbalski JL, Pollard M. Characterization of xenogeneic mouse-to-rat bone marrow chimeras. Transplantation 44, 88, 1987.

38. Chabot J, Weber C, Hardy MA, Rivera S, Bailey-Braxton D, Strausberg L, Wood M, Chow J, Pi-Sunyer FX, Reemtsma K. Synergy of ALS and UV-B in prolongation of primate-to-mouse islet xenograft survival. Transplant Proc 21, 1160, 1987.

39. Sadeghi AM, Robbins RC, Smith CR, Kurlansky RA, Michler RE, Reemtsma K, Rose EA. Cardic xenograft survival in baboons treated with cyclosporin in combination with conventional immunosuppression. Transplant Proc 21, 1149, 1987.

40. Lexer G, Cooper DKC, Wicomb WN, Rose AG, Rees J, Keraan M, Reichart B, Du Toit E. Cardiac transplantation using discordant xenografts in a nonhuman primate model. Transplant Proc 21, 1153, 1987.

41. Steinbruchel D, Kemp E, Starklint H, Dieperink H. Synergistic effect of cyclosporin A, cyclophosphamide, and steroids in rabbit-to-rat skin xenotransplantation. Transplant Proc 21, 1168, 1987.

42. Bailey LL, Nehlsen-Cannarella SL. Observations in cardiac xenotransplantation. Transplant Proc 18, 88, 1986.

43. Steinmüller D. Panel on xenografts. Transplant Proc 18, 98, 1986.

44. Veatch RM. The ethics of xenografts. Transplant Proc 18, 93, 1986.

1.6.2. Recent Advances in Immunosuppression after Xenogeneic Heart Transplantation in Primates

H Reichenspurner, PA Human, DH Boehm, DKC Cooper, R May, AG Rose, P Zilla, R Fasol, B Reichart

Departments of Cardiothoracic Surgery, Tissue Immunology and Pathology, University of Cape Town, Medical School, Cape Town, South Africa

Introduction

Since there is now a clearly perceptible need for organ replacement among patients in the early weeks and months of life, heart transplantation in neonates and infants is becoming increasingly necessary. Severe cardiac defects, such as hypoplastic left heart syndrome, do not have a good prognosis after conventional cardiac surgery, yet organ procurement within this age group is a major problem. The use of anencephalic donors still has ethical and legal restrictions (1); the only biological option to an allogeneic graft is therefore a xenogeneic donor heart.

Xenogeneic transplantation has become a more and more interesting field in research, the aim being to optimize the immunosuppressive therapy after xenogeneic transplantation. Cyclosporine, in addition to its well-known use in allogeneic transplantation, has also been described as prolonging graft survival after xenogeneic transplantation (2,3). The present study shows the influence of different immunosuppressive drug combinations with cyclosporine on xenograft survival, as well as occurrence and number of hyperacute and acute cellular rejection episodes.

Material and Methods

Vervet monkeys (2-6 kg b.w.) served as donors and Chacma baboons (Papio ursinus, 10-15 kg b.w.) as recipients. After premedication with ketamine (5 mg/kg b.w.), Morphine (0.25 mg/kg b.w.), Pancuronium bromide (0.2 mg/kg b.w.) and Atropin (0.5 mg), anaesthesia was maintained with a combination of halothane (1%) with oxygen, N_2O and room air as inhalation.

The operative technique was first described by Mann et al (4). After a median sternotomy, the pericardium was opened longitudinally in the donor animal. After ligation of both venae cavae and cross clamping of the aorta, the heart was perfused with cold cardioplegic solution according to Bretschneider. All pulmonary veins were ligated and the heart was explanted.

In the recipient animal, the carotid artery and internal jugular vein were prepared in the right neck. The donor's aorta was then anastomosed end-to-side with the carotid artery of the recipient and the donor's pulmonary artery with the right internal jugular vein. Thus, the donor heart was placed heterotopically in the neck of the recipient.

The heart was palpated every day to check the function, and every second day an ECG was read to control the electro-physiologic activity of the transplanted heart in comparison to the recipient's own heart. The rejection monitoring was based on daily cytoimmunological monitoring of the peripheral blood (5) and weekly transmyocardial biopsies. In case of cessation of graft function, the transplanted heart was explanted for autopsy.

Immunosuppressive Protocol

Depending on the immunosuppression, the following groups were formed:

Group 1 (n=8)
served as a control group and received no immunosuppressive medication.

Group 2 (n=5)
received cyclosporine given in a dosage of 20-40 mg/kg/day administered intramuscularly, depending on the whole blood trough level (between 400 and 600 ng/ml), cyclosporine was combined with azathioprine (2.5 mg/kg/day) and methylprednisolone (0.3 mg/kg/day).

Group 3 (n=6)
In addition to the regimen of Group 2, rabbit antithymocyte globulin (RATG, 9-15 mg IgG/kg/day) was given for postoperative days 1-5.

Group 4 (n=7):
In this group, cyclosporine, azathioprine and methylprednisolone were combined with 15-desoxyspergualine (15-DS, 3 mg/kg/day for post-operative days 1-5, and 2 mg/kg/day for post-operative days 6-10).

Acute rejection episodes were treated with 500 mg methylprednisolone intravenously for 3-5 consecutive days.

Histopathology of Acute Rejections

Acute rejection episodes were divided into 3 pathohistological groups:

- Acute cellular rejection: perivascular and interstitial mononuclear cell infiltration combined with interstitial oedema and/or the presence of myocyte necrosis (Figure 61).
- Hyperacute rejection: extensive interstitial oedema and haemorrhage combined with myocyte necrosis, usually occurring within the first 24 hours after implantation (Figure 62).
- Mixed rejection: this group represents a combination of the acute cellular and hyperacute type of rejection (Figure 63).

Cytoimmunological Monitoring

The cytoimmunological method of monitoring the peripheral blood has been described earlier (5).

Transmyocardial Biopsy

At weekly intervals, transmyocardial biopsies were performed. For this procedure, the animal was briefly anaesthetised and a small skin incision was made above the transplanted heart. The actual transmyocardial biopsy was performed using a prostatic gland bioptome and the sample sent for histological evaluation.

1. Transplantation

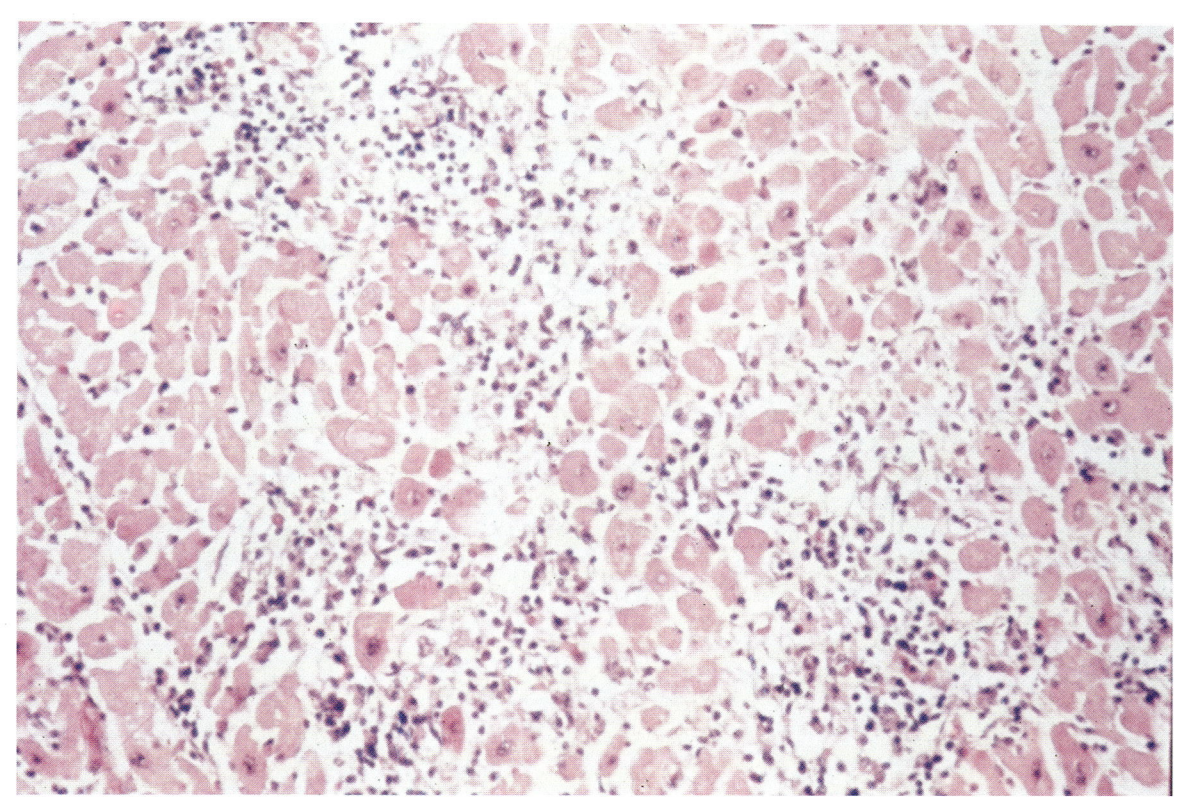

Fig. 61 Acute cellular type of rejection. Note the interstitial mononuclear cell infiltrate and myocyte necrosis.

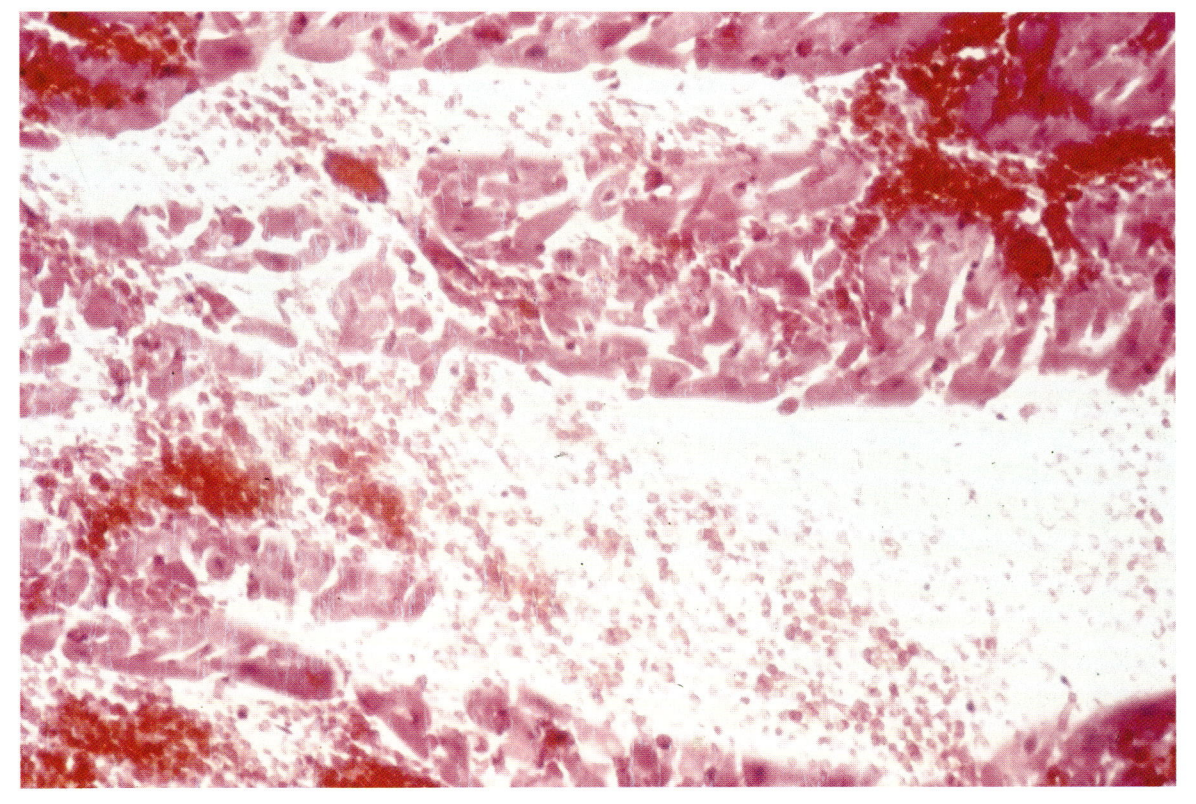

Fig. 62 Mixed type of rejection. Features of both the acute cellular and hyperacute rejection type are present.

1. Transplantation

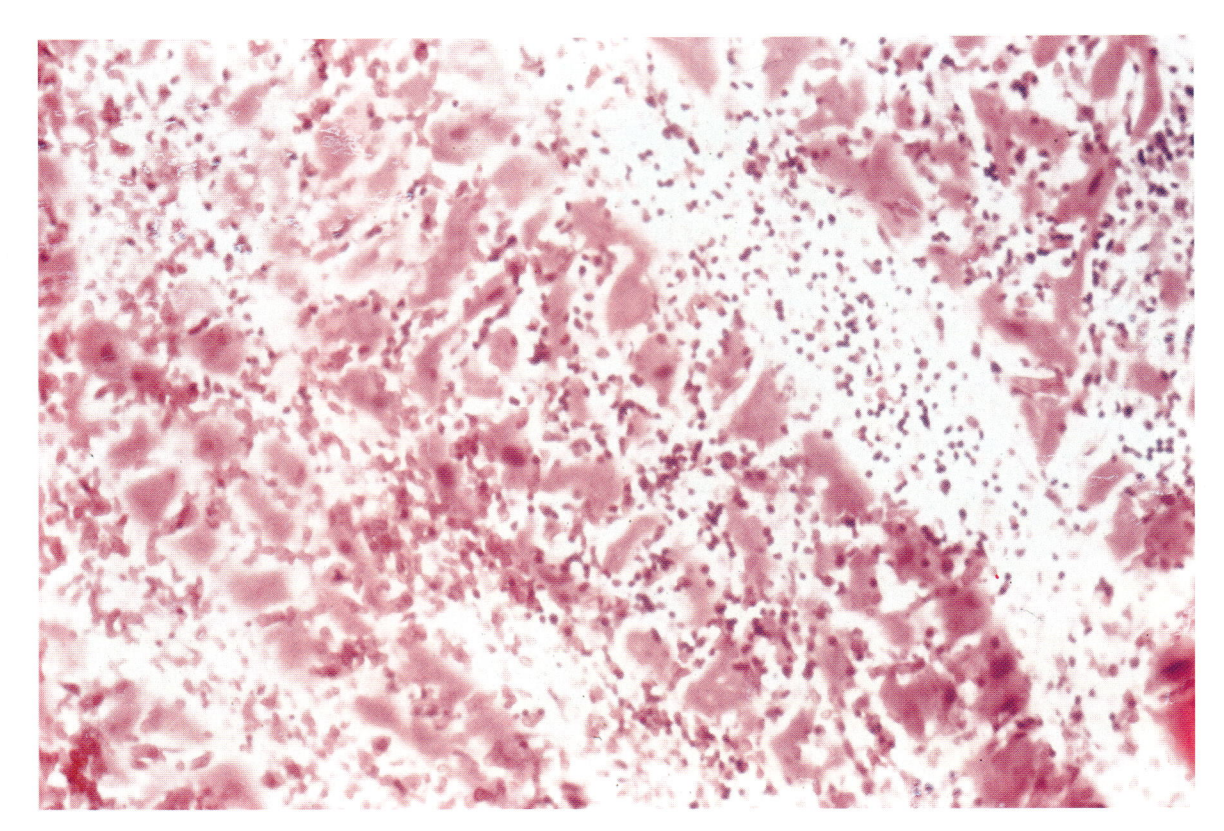

Fig. 63 Mixed type of rejection. Features of both the acute cellular and hyperacute rejection type are present.

Statistics

Statistical significance was calculated in accordance with the Log Rank analysis of the student's t-test.

Results

Survival rates

The survival rates for the different groups are listed in Figure 64. The control group had a mean graft survival of 10.3 ± 5.4 days. Group 2, with a survival rate of 19.0 ± 21.8 days, showed no significant difference from the control group. The survival rate of 43.3 ± 18.5 days in Group 3 was significantly better than in Group 1 or 2 ($p<0.005$). The longest living animal in this group lived for 83 days. In Group 4, the graft survival rate was also increased significantly to 20.1 ± 11.5 days ($p<0.05$) days as compared to Group 1.

Cause of Termination

In Groups 1 and 2, cellular and hyperacute rejections were the dominant causes of termination at 89% and 80% respectively (Figure 65). In Group 3, infections, diarrhoea and other complications, apart from rejections, were the

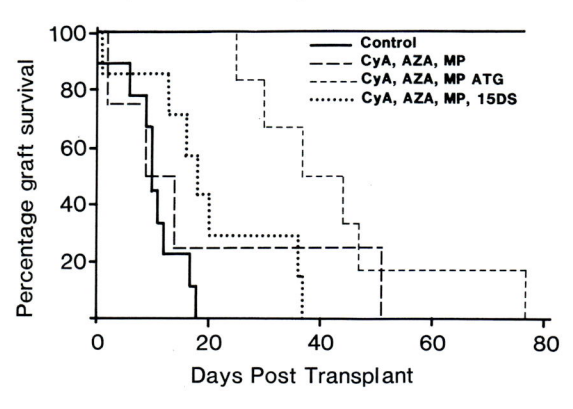

Fig. 64 Xenograft survival rates for the different treatment groups. The best graft survival rate was achieved with the combination of cyclosporine, azathioprine, methylprednisolone and ATG.

1. Transplantation

XENOGENIC HEART TRANSPLANTATION
CAUSE OF TERMINATION

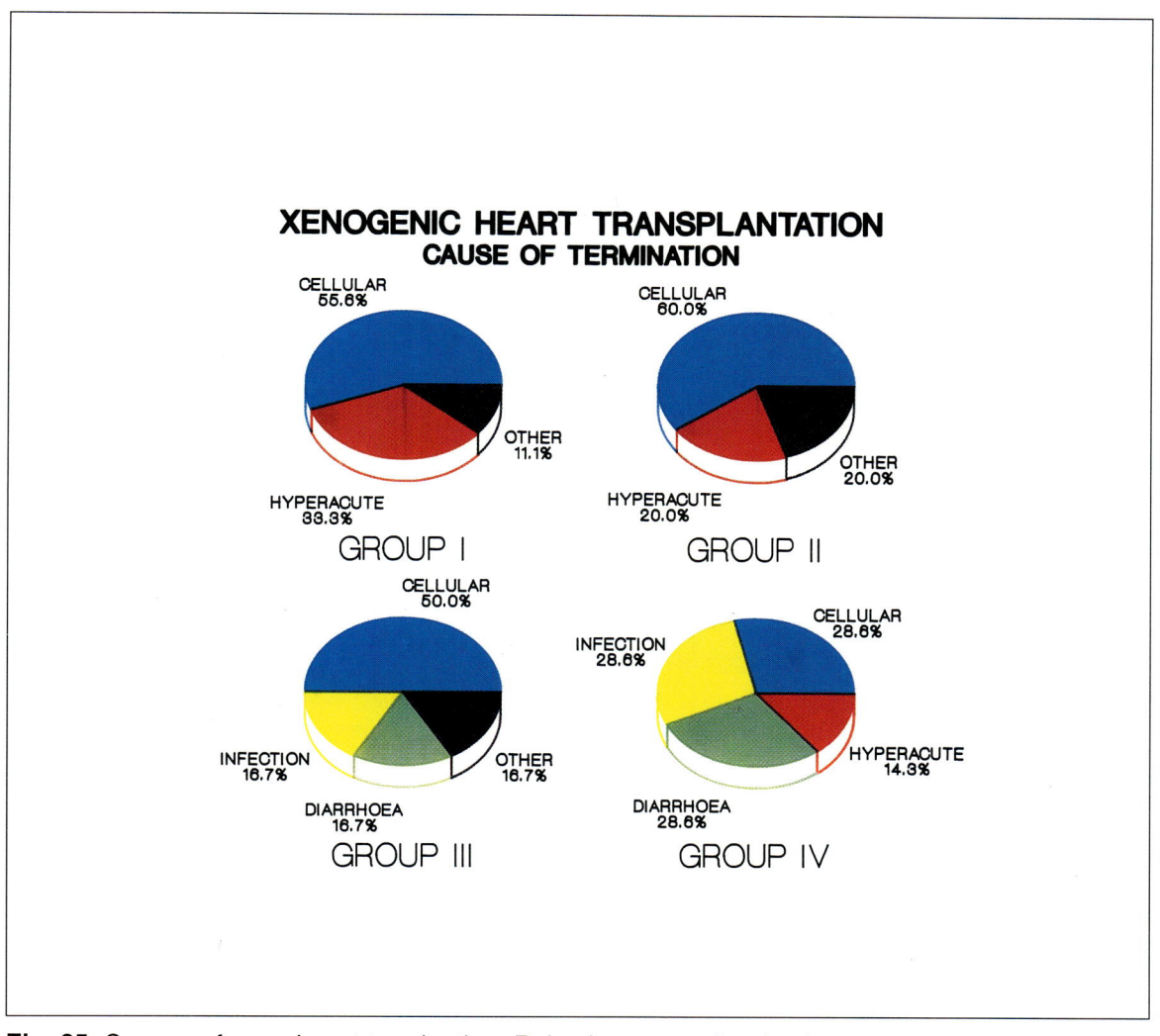

GROUP I: CELLULAR 55.6%, HYPERACUTE 33.3%, OTHER 11.1%
GROUP II: CELLULAR 60.0%, HYPERACUTE 20.0%, OTHER 20.0%
GROUP III: CELLULAR 50.0%, INFECTION 16.7%, DIARRHOEA 16.7%, OTHER 16.7%
GROUP IV: CELLULAR 28.6%, HYPERACUTE 14.3%, DIARRHOEA 28.6%, INFECTION 28.6%

Fig. 65 Causes of experiment termination. Rejections were the dominant causes in Groups 1 and 2, while infections and gastro-intestinal complications were major causes of termination in Groups 3 and 4.

cause of death in 50% of the animals. Acute cellular rejections terminated the graft function in the remaining 50%. In Group 4, infections and diarrhoea were the dominant causes of death in 57% of the animals. The remaining 43% of the experiments were terminated due to graft rejection (Figure 65).

Histopathology of Biopsies

In Group 1, hyperacute and mixed (hyperacute and cellular) rejection episodes were the dominant mode of graft rejection in 89% of the animals (Figure 66). In all treated groups, acute cellular type of rejection was the dominant one (67% of all rejections in Group 2, 87% in Group 3, and 71% in Group 4). In Groups 2, 3 and 4, hyperacute and mixed types of rejections occurred in 1 animal of each group. In Group 4, most of the biopsy findings (72,7%) were negative with regard to rejection, while in Group 3 only 18,5% of the biopsy results were normal.

Number of Rejection Episodes

The number of rejection episodes per group is listed in Table 20.

In the untreated Group 1 only one, but the graft function terminating rejection

1. Transplantation

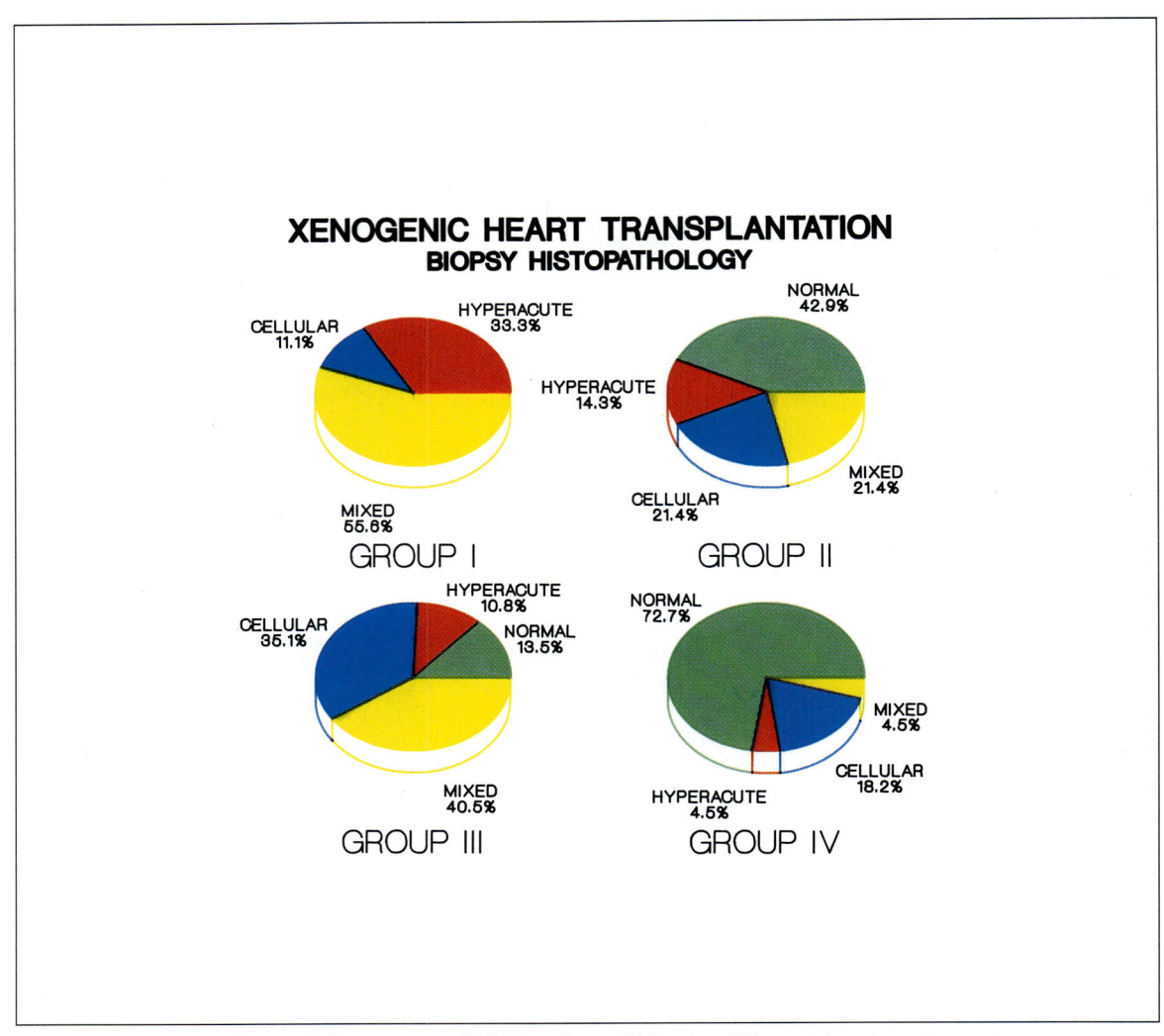

Fig. 66 Histopathology of the myocardial biopsies within the different treatment groups.

episode per animal occurred. In Group 2, an average of 1.5 rejection episodes per animal was observed. In Group 3, the group with the longest survival rate, 2.5 acute rejection episodes per animal were nevertheless observed.

Significantly different are the results in Group 4, where only 0.5 graft rejection episodes per animal occurred ($p<0.05$, Group 4 vs Groups 2 and 3).

Cytoimmunological Monitoring

Every second day, the peripheral blood of the animals was tested by cytoimmunological monitoring (5).

In all 3 treated groups a significant rise of activated lymphocytes per 100 lymphocytes was noted during rejection (Figure 67). In Group 2 from 2.5% to 4.6% ($p<0.012$); in Group 3 from 3.2% to 5.9% ($p<0.001$); in Group 4 from 2.0% to 4.4% ($p<0.007$). The decrease in the number of activated lymphocytes after successful rejection therapy did not show any statistical significance.

Discussion

Recent advances in clinical transplantation do not abolish the main limiting factor: the availability of organ donors. There is a constant waiting list of transplant candidates, many of whom still continue to die while waiting

Xenogenic Heart Transplantation
Number of Rejections

	Group I	Group II	Group III	Group IV
AR (n)	1.0	1.5	2.5	0.5+

+ p<0.05   Group IV vs Group III): Student T-test

Table 20 Number of acute rejections per animal in each treatment group. In Group 4, 15-desoxyspergualine led to a significant decrease in the number of acute rejections to only 0.5 acute rejections per animal.

for a suitable human graft. Human organs of all types are virtually unavailable for neonatal and infant recipients. Since organs from non-human species might be a solution, a great deal of research and clinical work has recently been done in this field.

In the present study, cross-species heterotopic hart transplantation was performed in primates, since these animals are immunologically very similar to humans and also have A, B, and AB blood group subtypes. AB-compatible pairs were used for transplantation, as previous experience in our own laboratory has shown that the risk of hyperacute rejection is increased in cases with blood group incompatibility (19).

Cyclosporine was used in different combinations to enhance the optimal immunosuppressive therapy with the lowest risk of rejection and treatment-related side effects. Graft survival rate, frequency, and types of rejection episodes were taken into consideration.

The combination of cyclosporine with azathioprine and methylprednisolone did not show a significant increase in xenograft survival rate. These findings have been confirmed by Sadeghi et al, who used a similar experimental model (20). A quadruple drug regimen with the addition of antithymocyte globulin (ATG) however, led to a highly significant prolongation of graft survival of 43.3 days as compared to 10.3 days in the untreated control group (p<0.005). Sadeghi et al did not confirm this finding, but the main difference between the two experimental models is that acute rejection was treated with cortisone therapy in our study to make the experiment as close to clinical transplantation as possible. The use of 15-desoxyspergualine instead of ATG also showed a significant increase in survival to 20.1 days which was, however, not as significant as under ATG treatment (p<0.05).

Graft rejection was the main cause of termination in the untreated control group, and in the cyclosporine, azathioprine, and methylprednisolone treated group 2 (89% and 81% respectively), which confirms the latter regimen as being insufficient (15). In Group 3 (33%) and particularly in Group 4 (53%) infections and gastro-intestinal complications, such as severe diarrhoea, were the main reasons for termination of the experiments. These problems might be due to the dosage and administration of 15-desoxyspergualine which was used in our model as reported from the company (Behring Inc, Marburg, FRG).

1. Transplantation

New treatment groups with changes in the dosages and administration of 15-desoxyspergualine will be necessary to demonstrate that these treatment-related side effects can be minimized. The most interesting finding in Group 4 was that 15-desoxyspergualine was able to reduce the number of hyperacute and acute cellular rejection significantly to only 0.5 rejection episodes per animal ($p<0.05$). This confirms studies after allogeneic transplantation in rats, where 15-desoxyspergualine even was able to reduce graft tolerance in animals after kidney transplantation (21).

The type of rejection episodes also showed different results for the 4 groups.

In the control group, hyperacute and mixed (hyperacute/acute cellular) rejections were mainly present (89%). In the 3 treated groups the acute cellular type of transplant reaction was predominant. In Groups 1, 3 and 4 only one hyperacute rejection episode occurred in one animal of each group. Thus, the decreased number and the histopathology of acute rejection were the most interesting findings in the 15-desoxyspergualine-treated group. These findings justified further studies with this drug with the aim of reducing the side effects of this treatment combination.

In concordance with Deodhar et al, it can be concluded:

An ideal immunosuppressive agent in the xenograft setting would be one

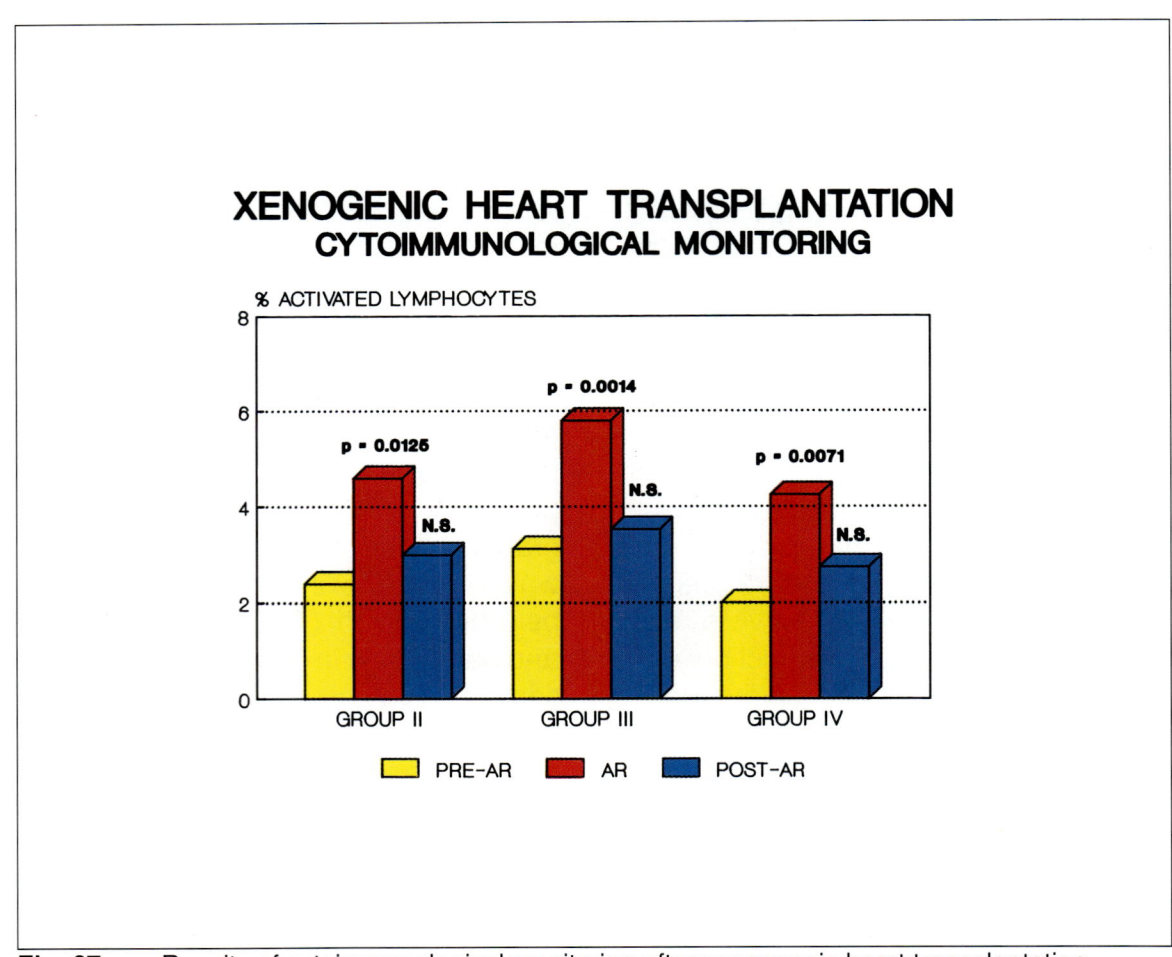

Fig. 67   Results of cytoimmunological monitoring after xenogeneic heart transplantation.

that would cause the recipient to accept a given xenograft as if it was an allograft (22).

Acknowledgements

We gratefully acknowledge the skilled technical assistance of F Barends, J Kloppers, P Madlingozi, J Place, F Snyders and F Tate.

Cyclosporine was generously supplied by Sandoz Ltd, Switzerland, for all experiments; RATG was supplied by Fresenius AG, Germany, and 15-desoxyspergualine by Behring-Werke, Germany.

References

1. Harrison MR. Organ procurement for children; the anencephalic fetus as donor. Lancet 2, 1383, 1986.

2. Homan WP, Williams KA, Fabre JW, Millard R, Morris PJ. Prolongation of cardiac xenograft survival in rats receiving cyclosporine A. Transplantation 31, 164, 1981.

3. Reichenspurner H, Ertel W, Reichart B, Peters D, Welz A, Uberfuhr P, Kemkes BM, Gokel JM, Hammer C. Xenogeneic and allogeneic canine heart transplantation: a model for cytologic and immunologic monitoring of rejection mechanism. J Heart Transplant 5, 471, 1986.

4. Mann FC, Priestley JT, Markowitz J, Yater WM. Transplantation of the mammalian heart. Arch Surg 26, 219, 1933.

5. Reichenspurner H, Kemkes BM, Osterholzer G, Reble B, Reichart B, Hammer C, Steinbeck G, Gokel JM. Particular control of infection and rejection episodes after 4 years cardiac transplantation. Texas Heart Inst J 13, 5, 1986.

6. Reemtsma K, McCracken BH, Schlegel JU, Pearl MA, De Witt CW, Creech O. Reversal of early graft rejection after renal heterotransplantation in man. JAMA 187, 691, 1964.

7. Starzl TE, Marchioro TL, Peters GN, Kirkpatrick CH, Wilson WEC, Porter KA, Rifkind D, Ogden DA, Hitchcock CR, Waddell WR. Renal heterotransplantation from baboon to man: experience with 6 cases. Transplantation 2, 752, 1964.

8. Hardy JD, Chavez CM, Kurrus FD, Neely WA, Eraslan S, Turner D, Fabian LW, Labecki D, Jackson M. Heart transplantation in man. JAMA 1132, 114, 1964.

9. Cooley DA, Hallman GL, Bloodwell RD, Nora JJ, Leachman RD. Human heart transplantation. Amer J Cardiol 22, 804, 1968.

10. Barnard CN, Wolpowitz A, Losman JG. Heterotopic cardiac transplantation with a xenograft for assistance of the left heart in cardiogenic shock after cardiopulmonary bypass. S Afr Med J 52, 1035, 1977.

11. Bailey L, Li Z, Lacour-Gayet F, Perier P, Killeen D, Perry J, Schmidt C, Roost H, Jolley W. Orthotopic cardiac transplantation in the cyclosporine-treated neonate. Transplant Proc 15, 740, 1983.

1. Transplantation

12. Dubernard JM, Bonneau M, Bomel J, Montagard J, Blitz M, Latour M, Blanc-Brunat N, Fries D, Brochard JC, Bansillon V, Bansillon G, Capodicasa G. Renal and skin xenografts from baboons to Macaques: effect of antilymphocyte globulins. Transplant Proc 3, 545, 1971.

13. Donawick WJ, Shaffer CF, Dodd DC, Buchanan JW, Fregin GF. Cardiac and skin heterograft rejection: suppression with antilymphocyte serum. Transplant Proc 3, 551, 1971.

14. Bailey LL, Jan J, Johnson W, Jolley WB. Orthotopic cardiac xenografting in the newborn goat. J Thorac Cardiovasc Surg 89, 242, 1985.

15. Sugimoto K, Shelby J, Corry RJ. The effect of cyclosporine on cardiac xenograft survival. Transplantation 39, 218, 1984

16. Hardy MA, Oluwole S, Fawwaz R, Satake K, Nowygrod R, Reemtsma K. Selective lymphoid irradiation: prolongation of cardiac xenografts and allografts in presensitized rats. Transplantation 33, 237, 1982.

17. Knechtle SJ, Halperin EC, Saad T, Bollinger RR. Prolonged heart xenograft survival using combined total lymphoid irradiation and cyclosporine. J Heart Transplant 5, 254, 1986.

18. Hyman PA, Cooper DKC, Rose AG, Reichenspurner H, Reichart B. Prolongation of cardiac xenograft survival in a concordant primate model with combined total lymphoid irradiation and immunosuppressive drug therapy. J Heart Transplant. Submitted for publication, 1988.

19. Cooper DKC, Human PA, Rose AG, Ries J, Keraan M, Reichart B, Du Toit E, Oriol R. The role of ABO blood group compatibility in organ transplantation between closely related animal species: an experimental study using the Vervet monkey to baboon cardiac xenograft model. Transplantation. Submitted for publication, 1988.

20. Sadeghi AM, Robbins RC, Smith CR, Kurlansky PA, Michler RE, Reemtsma K, Rose EA. Cardiac xenotransplantation in primates. J Thorac Cardiovasc Surg 93, 809, 1987.

21. Dickneite G, Schorlemmer HU, Walter P, Thies J, Sedlacek HH. The influence of ± 15-desoxyspergualine on experimental transplantation and its immunopharmacological mode of action. Behring Inst Mitt 80, 93, 1986.

22. Deodhar SD. Review of xenografts in organ transplantation. Transplant Proc 81, 83, 1986.

1.6.3. The Virological Evaluation of Non-Human Primates for Xenotransplantation

PA Human [1], FJ van der Riet [2], DKC Cooper [4], SS Kalter [5], JE Fincham [3], HEM Smuts [6], H Reichenspurner [1], DL Madden [7], JL Sever [7], B Reichart [1]

[1] Departments of Cardiothoracic Surgery,
[2] Medical Virology and [6] Medical Microbiology,
University of Cape Town Medical School, Cape Town,
[3] National Research Institute for Nutritional Diseases,
Medical Research Council, Tygerberg, South Africa,
[4] Oklahoma Transplantation Institute,
Baptist Medical Center, Oklahoma City,
[5] Department of Virology and Immunology,
Southwest Foundation for Biomedical Research, San Antonio, Texas
[7] Infectious Diseases Branch, National Institute of Health, Bethesda,
Maryland, United States of America

Introduction

Whereas their close phylogenetic relationship to man is a prioritous advantage in the field of clinical cross-species transplantation, the utilization of non-human primates as organ donors suffers the disadvantage of the strong likelihood of transmission of potentially pathogenic infectious agents.

The Chacma baboon (Papio ursinus) is a suitable candidate as 'organ donor' and we have therefore examined this species for serological evidence of selected viruses. In addition, we have examined a group of wild-caught and a group of first generation colony-bred African green monkeys (Cercopithecus aethiops) to test the hypothesis that, under proper management conditions, non-human primates bred in captivity might present with a reduced incidence of viral infection and therefore be more acceptable for transplantation into man.

Materials and Methods

Serum samples were collected from ten Chacma baboons, captured in the wild (Group A), from a group of ten African green monkeys (AGM), captured in the wild (Group B), and from a group of 14 first generation colony-bred AGM's selected on the basis of human T-cell lymphotropic virus type 1 (HTLV-1), Simian immunodeficiency virus (SIV_{mac}), Simian retrovirus type 1 (SRV-1), and human immunodeficiency virus type 1 (HIV-1) seronegativity (Group C).

Serological testing for the Herpes simplex type 1 (HSV-1), Varicella zoster (VZV), human cytomegalovirus (CMV), Epstein-Barr (EBV), Simian agent-6 (SA-6), Simian agent-8 (SA-8) and B-virus Herpesviridae, the SRV-1, Simian retrovirus type 2 (SRV-2) and Simian im-

1. Transplantation

munodeficiency virus (SIV$_{mac}$) Retroviridae, the Simian agent-11 (SA-11) rotavirus, the Marburg filovirus, the human influenza type A (H-Infl.A), human influenza type B (H-Infl.B), human measles and human mumps Myxoviridae, the lymphocytic choriomeningitis (LCM) arenavirus, and the human rubella togavirus was performed by a dot immunobinding assay (DIA) (1).

Results

Results of serological testing of the above three groups of non-human primates are presented in Table 21.

Results of Serological Screening for Selected Viruses in Non-human Primates

Results are expressed as a ratio of the number of seropositives against the number of animals tested.

Antigenetic Material	Group A	Group B	Group C
Herpesviridae			
B-virus	0/10	0/10	0/14
HSV-1	9/10	7/10	n.d.
VZV	7/10	n.d.	0/14
CMV	10/10	6/10	6/14
EBV	0/10	2/10	0/14
SA-6	10/10	7/10	7/14
SA-8	n.d.	7/10	0/14
Retroviridae			
SIV$_{mac}$ +	0/10	5/10	*
SRV-1	0/10	0/10	*
SRV-2	0/10	0/10	0/14 (**)
Reoviridae			
SA-11	8/10	2/10	n.d.
Filoviridae			
Marburg virus	0/10	0/10	0/14
Myxoviridae			
H-Infl.A	0/10	0/10	0/14
H-Infl.B	0/10	0/10	0/14
H-measles	0/10	n.d.	0/14
H-mumps	0/10	0/10	0/14
Togaviridae			
Rubella virus	0/10	0/10	0/14
Arenaviridae			
LCM	0/10	0/10	0/14

+ = suggests infection by the corresponding AGM strain (SIV$_{agm}$)
n.d. = not determined
* = seronegativity preselected
** = probable preselection due to close serological relationship to SRV-1

Table 21

Discussion

The high incidence of seropositivity with regard to the Herpesviridae in Group A is indicative of the ubiquity of this viral group amongst non-human primates (2). Additionally, it represents the high degree of serological cross-reactivity or 'biological overlapping' (3) associated with this family. Seropositivity of non-human primate sera with regard to antigenic material of a human virus, therefore, more likely refers to infection by a counterpart simian virus, and not necessarily to infection by species of clinical significance. This argument is demonstrated by the dual seropositivity in Group A with respect to CMV and SA-6. The former agent is characterized as being highly species-specific (4), and by its recognition as a potentially life-threatening pathogen in organ transplant recipients (5,6). The clinical relevance of the latter virus SA-6 is undetermined, although its designation as a cytomegalovirus-type simian virus is noteworthy.

Although occurring with relative frequency in Group A, and with high incidence amongst transplant patients, VZV infections are mostly benign in their effect (7). The association of VZV with myocarditis and life-threatening dysrhythmias in children, although infrequent, should, however, be realized (8).

HSV-1 occurs with high incidence in transplant patients, usually during the first post-operative month (7). These are more often the result of reactivation, rather than by primary infection, with the outcome very rarely proving fatal. Considering the marked serological prevalence of this virus within Group A, and the recognition of its potential for severe and extensive disease in immunosuppressed individuals (9), however, the utilization of non-human primates such as the baboon as donors in clinical cross-species transplantation should be conducted with the appropriate caution.

Although all animals of the above three groups proved seronegative for the Herpes B-virus, a previous study (unpublished) revealed a single AGM seropositivity. This animal was, however, also shown to be seropositive for both the HSV-1 and SA-8 herpesviruses, with the B-virus seropositivity being ascribed to a possible cross-reactivity of these two viruses, or at least to an antigenically related virus.

The failure to detect evidence of infection by the SIV_{mac} retrovirus in Group A has particular significance in the field of clinical xenotransplantation especially as a result of the recognition, in the last few years, of at least two etiological agents of the acquired immunodeficiency syndrome (AIDS), namely the exogenous HIV-1 and human immunodeficiency virus type 2 (HIV-2) viruses, and their relationship to SIV_{mac} (10,11,12). This finding has particular relevance after the report by Otha et al (13) of the isolation from healthy AGM's of simian retroviruses closely related to HIV-1. One of these, SIV[AGM-1] was obtained from a healthy HIV-1-seropositive animal and shown to have high sequence homology (60-75%) when compared to HIV-1.

Evidence for a possible HIV-1 infection in a non-human primate was forthcoming from a group of 138 wild-caught AGM's which we had examined previously (unpublished). In addition to being seropositive for both the HTLV-1 and SIVmac viruses, an individual animal was shown to be seropositive in western blotting tests, not only with the HIV-1 gag proteins p55, p17, and p24, but more importantly, with its envgene products, glycoproteins gp120 and gp160, thus suggesting possible infection with HIV-1 or a virus more closely related to HIV-1 than SIV_{mac}.

Although the serological prevalence of the Simian T-cell lymphotropic retrovirus type 1 (STLV-1) was not investigated in Group A, findings of an as yet unpublished investigation, in which HTLV-1 antigenic material was utilized (STLV-1 has been shown to be highly related to HTLV-1 (14)), suggested a high level of infection by STLV-1 in both the Chacma baboon (ca. 25%) and the wild-caught AGM (ca. 40%). Becker et al (15), however, suggest that infectivity of simian HTLV-1-related viruses for man may not be significant. They do nevertheless express the need to exclude animals with chronic simian retroviral infections if their tissues are to be used for transplantation.

The high incidence of the SA-11 rotavirus in Group A is noteworthy although the relevance of this simian virus, save the propensity of rotaviral species in general for inducing diarrhoea and gastroenteritis in humans (16), is as yet undiscovered in the immunosuppressed transplant patient.

The virological status of Group B, the group of wild-caught AGM's, was in essence similar to that of the Group A baboons, with the exception of the marked SIV_{mac} incidence and the low rate of EBV seropositivity. The overall reduced serological profile in Group C, the group of colony-bred AGM's, may hold promise in terms of xenotransplantation into man. The continued Herpesviridae prevalence involving CMV and its simian counterpart virus, SA-6, is nevertheless cause for concern. This viewpoint is further justified by the known oncogenicity of simian herpesviruses (17) and their pathogenic potential in secondary hosts, as is exhibited by the Herpes B-virus (2,18).

In terms of the Retroviridae, preselection against HIV-1, SIV_{mac}, SRV-1 and HTLV-1 (STLV-1) in Group C excluded the evaluation of colony breeding with regard to the prevalence of this viral family in non-human primates. With regard to SRV-1, however, to date no seropositive AGM's have been identified in the colony. The above selection criteria were adopted with the understanding that potential animal 'donors' would undergo at least the abovementioned retroviral screening. Our interest was therefore, at the time, directed towards the identification of other viral species associated with retroviral seronegativity. We are presently engaged in a study involving randomly selected animals to avoid this shortcoming, and hope to publish these findings in the near future. Data already in our possession do, however, suggest a reduction of both STLV-1 and SIV_{agm} infection in the AGM as a result of colony breeding.

In conclusion, the advantages of cross-species transplantation, namely that of providing a bridge to subsequent allotransplantation, especially with regard to cardiac transplantation in the neonate, and of it being possible to perform elective surgery, must be considered together with the disadvantage of the virological prevalence in the non-human primate. Admittedly, xenotransplantation offers to provide a 'last-resort' solution, and in this regard the requirement of a totally viral-free animal is debatable. We feel that screening for at least those viruses which are known to cause serious disease or death in man is, however, paramount. In this context, colony-bred animals offer a tempting compromise.

1. Transplantation

References

1. Heberling RL, Kalter SS. Dot-ELISA on nitrocellulose with psoralen inactivated Herpes virus. Abst Amer Soc Microbiol 85th Ann Mtg, Las Vegas 21, 510, 1985.

2. Kalter SS. Overview of simian viruses and recognized virus diseases and laboratory support for the diagnosis of viral infections. In: Primates. The Road to Self-Sustaining Populations. Benirschke K Ed Springer-Verlag New York, Chapter 46, 1986.

3. Kalter SS, Ablashi D, Espana C, Heberling RL, Hull RN, Lennette EH, Malherbe HH, McConnell S, Yohn DS. Simian virus nomenclature. Intervirology 13, 317, 1980.

4. Andrewes C, Pereira HG, Wildy P. In: Viruses of vertebrates 4th Edition. Bailliere Tindall, Chapter 15, 1978.

5. Rand KH, Pollard RB, Merigan TC. Increased pulmonary superinfections in cardiac transplant patients undergoing primary cytomegalovirus infection. N Eng J Med 298, 951, 1978.

6. Rakela J, Wiesner RH, Taswell HF, Hermans PE, Smith TF, Perkins JD, Krom RAF. Incidence of cytomegalovirus infection and its relationship to donor-recipient serologic status in liver transplantation. Transplant Proc 19(1), 2399, 1987.

7. Bateman ED, Forder AA. Infectious complications. In: Heart transplantation. Cooper DKC, Lanza RP (Eds). MTP Press Ltd, England, Chapter 13, 1984.

8. Woolf PK, Chung T, Stewart J, Liakos M, Davidian M, Gewitz MH. Life-threatening Dysrhythmias in Varicella myocarditis. Clinical Pediatrics 26, (9), 480, 1987.

9. Benenson AG (Ed). In: Control of communable diseases in man. Thirteenth edition. American Public Health Association, p 170, 1980.

10. Daniel MD, Letvin NL, King NW, Kannegi M, Sehgal PK, Hunt RD, Kanki PJ, Essex M, Desrosiers RC. Isolation of T-cell tropic HTLV-III-like retrovirus from Macaques. Science 228, 1201, 1985.

11. Chakrabarti L, Guyader M, Alizon M, Daniel MD, Desrosiers RC, Tiollais P, Sonigo S. Sequence of simian immunodeficiency virus from Macaque and its relationship to other human and simian retroviruses. Nature 328, 543, 1987.

12. Essex M, Kanki P. Reply to Kestler HW, Li Y, Naidu YM, Butler CV, Ochs MF, Jaenel G, King NW, Daniel MD Desrosiers RC. Comparisons of simian immunodeficiency virus isolates. Nature 331, 619, 1988.

13. Ohta Y, Masuda T, Tsujimoto H, Ishikawa K, Kodama T, Morikawa S, Nakai M, Honjo S, Hayami M. Isolation of simian immunodeficiency virus from African Green monkeys and sero-epidemiologic survey of the virus in various non-human primates. Int J Cancer 41, 115, 1988.

14. Guo HG, Wong-Staal F, Gallo RC. Novel viral sequences related to human T-cell leukemia virus in T cells of a seropositive baboon. Science 223, 1195, 1984.

15. Becker WB, Becker MLB, Homma T, Brede HD, Kurth R. Serum antibodies to human T-cell leukemia virus type I in different ethnic groups and in non-human primates in South Africa. S A Med J 67, 445, 1985.

16. Benenson AG (Ed). In: Control of Communicable Diseases in Man. Thirteenth Edition. American Public Health Association, p 148, 1980.

17. Ablashi DV, Easton JM, Guegan JH. Herpesviruses and cancer in man and subhuman primates. Biomedicine 24, 286, 1976.

18. Sabin AB, Wright AM. Acute ascending myelitis following a monkey bite, with the isolation of a virus capable of reproducing the disease. J Exp Med 59, 115, 1934.

2. Artificial Heart

2.1. Introduction: Mechanical Ventricular Assistance and Replacement

J Odell

*Department of Cardiothoracic Surgery,
University of Cape Town, Medical School,
Cape Town, South Africa*

Until 35 years ago, when the heart-lung machine was developped, cessation of the heart-beat was equated with death. Today, the heart is regularly stopped while cardiac surgery is being undertaken. In 1967 the replacement of a human heart by one from a brain dead donor captured the imagination of people throughout the world. Of similar dramatic impact was the replacement of the heart of Dr Barney Clark in December 1982 by an artificially developped heart. In this instance, diseased tissue was not repaired or replaced, nor was the diseased heart replaced by another natural healthy heart. Instead a man-made heart was implanted - an attempt had been made to emulate the creators' work. The success or failure of the device was eagerly awaited. Would it be the answer to the donor shortage? Would it be the forerunner of the totally implantantable device?

The point is that it was soon apparent that even though the driving console could be reduced to the size of a ladies' handbag that the patient still had limited quality of life because of the umbilical cord of tubing containing compressed air that connected his "heart" to "his machine."

Sadly, the most optimistic hopes proved to be unfounded. Barney Clarke died after 112 days. While he was able to talk he said that "it was worth it", it caused neither pain nor discomfort, nor did it interfere with his emotions or feelings towards his family. Other total artificial heart transplantations followed but none was truly successful - all patients developped cerebrovascular complications, probably the result of multiple embolic episodes. The enthusiasm for its permanent use rapidly declined, and a new term, "bridge to transplantation", was coined. The TAH was now to be used to support a patient until a suitable donor was found. Hopefully a donor would be found before the start of complications associated with the device. This was not a new concept - Cooley had, between 1969 and July 1981, supported three patients prior to cardiac transplantation - he termed it "staged cardiac transplantation". All three patients died of multiple organ failure and sepsis.

The concept of "bridge to transplantation" raises important questions that still need to be answered. The criteria to be used for implanting a TAH need to be defined. A healthy patient who, because

2. Artificial Heart

of a surgical mishap (or other reason) is unable to be weaned from bypass would be an obvious candidate. But would he have benefited from a left heart assist device and recovered? Approximately one-third of patients awaiting heart transplantation die because of lack of donors. The patient who is thought acceptable for transplantation and who deteriorates, may be considered the obvious candidate, but irreversible organ damage or sepsis may have occurred or be latent, and thus may compromise results. If a TAH is implanted in the belief that it is to function only as a bridge, one has already an implied commitment to that patient. This commitment to transplant should not obscure the fact that in the meantime the patient may have developped, for example, infected pulmonary oedema or renal and hepatic failure, and that to transplant and immunosuppress a patient under these circumstances will surely lead to failure. It is often very difficult to admit that one has made an error in selection (by missing infection). Instead, one hopes that difficulties will be sorted out later (which invariably does not happen). It then becomes difficult to switch off the machine in the case of a patient who is mentally alert.

Should a patient with a TAH in place become a more urgent candidate for transplantation than others? Are surgeons implanting the device knowing that from the limited donor pool the chances of doing the transplant are much better because the patient with a TAH has a greater priority? Is this going to improve their figures when compared with those of other transplanting surgeons? The other side of the coin is that it may be better to stabilize the patient and improve organ function with the TAH before transplantation, and so improve his chances. What is the role of bridging to transplantation in countries without computer donor matching, such as Australia, South Africa, New Zealand, and others? Is it justified to implant a TAH, knowing that the patient may be dependent on the device and be exposed to its complications for many months before a donor is found? These are all difficult questions to answer.

In this section, two papers deal with "bridge to transplantation". The paper of Dr Solis is one of the largest series in the world - 23 patients; Rokitansky's series is of 5 patients. The results confirm the concern raised in the previous paragraph. Patient selection is of prime importance, and any evidence of infection compromises results; it is concluded by Solis that patients already immunosuppressed - that is, patients with previous cardiac transplantation with rejection and severe cardiac failure, should not have implantation of a TAH. Rokitansky raises the interesting question whether the artificial heart stimulates the immune system as, in one patient rejection was particularly severe following transplantation, and was associated with high immunoglobulin levels. It is difficult to imagine how a mechanical device would do this - the Vienna group will surely investigate this possibility in the future.

Coagulation and bleeding, because of therapy to prevent coagulation complications, such as embolism, are significant problems. Muller, also from Vienna, discusses the coagulative and haemolytic changes associated with implantation of a TAH, and suggests that anti-aggregatory therapy may be worthwhile, but if used with other anticoagulants, may cause excessive bleeding (see Rokitansky's paper).

2. Artificial Heart

The umbical cord connecting the TAH to the controlling device is an anathema. It conjures up visions of inadvertently becoming disconnected or being deliberately switched off, of someone tripping over the pressure lines, or of being the source of infection. It remains therefore the goal of all involved in research with the TAH for the device to be totally contained within the body.

Two papers approaching this concept are discussed. Koroly discusses the feasibility of using an electromagnetic actuator, using recently developped rare earth magnets. Obviously, a lot more research into this possibility needs to be undertaken, but it does offer exciting possibilities for the future. Bridges and his associates have concentrated on using autogenous Latissimus dorsi muscle conditioned by a pacemaker to act in a similar fashion to heart muscle. Obvious advantages are that it is contained within the body, is autogenous and unlikely to stimulate rejection, and is readily available. The methodology of its use needs to be determined. Should it be used to wrap the heart and squeeze it during systole, or should it function in similar fashion to an intra-aortic balloon pump - to contract and obstruct the descending thoracic aorta during diastole? We eagerly await further developments in this field, as it theoretically has exciting possibilities.

2. Artificial Heart

2.2. State of the Art in Assisted Circulation

F Unger

*Cardiac Surgery Salzburg
St John's Hospital,
Salzburg, Austria*

Abstract

The possibilities to mechanically support a failing heart in the post-operative course, or after an acute myocardial infarction, has changed tremendously during the last 30 years since Dennis (1951) and Harken (1958) defined "assisted circulation". Since 1967, the year of the first clinical application of the intraaortic balloon pump (IABP), approximately 400 000 of such devices have been implanted. The indication is still myocardial infarction and cardiac failure after open heart surgery. However, the latter incidence has declined due to improved techniques, including those of myocardial protection, from 10% in 1975 to 1% in 1987, and this in spite of the overall increase in extracorporeal circulation (by 1987, 370 000 cases worldwide).

The left- and right-ventricular (LVAD, RVAD) and bi-ventricular (BVAD) assist devices with pulsatile pneumatic driven chambers and non-pulsatile impeller pumps were designed in the late 1960s. In contrast to the IABP, these assist devices can maintain the whole heart function. Since 1975, 345 cases (LVAD, RVAD, BVAD) using various blood pumps have been implanted. The overall outcome is encouraging, keeping in mind the desperate clinical status of the patients; 34% could be weaned and 15% were discharged.

Assist devices were also used as a bridge towards transplantation in 18 cases with endstage cardiomyopathy.

Since 1982, 8 total artificial hearts (TAH) have been used. The longest implantation has been 427 days with a pneumatic driving system. The TAH recipients are exposed to a high degree of infection and thromboemboli, and because of this, the indication for TAH changed completely towards the concept of bridging to transplantation in patients with endstage cardiomyopathy. Until December 1987, 86 patients have temporarily received an artificial heart. In 52 cases, a consecutive transplantation could be performed; 39 patients (75% of the total) could be discharged and are alive.

For permanent heart substitution, mechanical-electric devices with integrated monitoring systems need to be developped.

Introduction

Assisted circulation has changed tremendously within the last 30 years. Initially the main focus was to overcome cardiac failure following cardiopulmonary bypass, which occurred in 10-15% of the open heart patients (1). Due to improved techniques in cardiac surgery, and especially the introduction of cardioplegic solutions, the incidence of post-operative cardiac failure decreased to 1% of the pump cases (2). Half of these patients can be treated successfully with modern catecholamines. The remaining half - or 0.5% of total - need additional support either by means of the intra-aortic balloon pump (IABP) (3), left-, right-ventricular (LVAD, RVAD), bi-ventricular assist devices (BVAD), or total artificial replacement of the heart (TAH).

Assisted circulation may further be indicated after myocardial infarction and in endstage cardiomyopathy. In selected patients this technique has become a bridge toward a consecutive cardiac transplantation (4).

After open heart surgery, it is assumed that there is a worldwide need of cardiac assist devices in approximately 2 000 cases. After myocardial infarction, the number would be roughly 200 000 (5). Accordingly, increasing clinical applications of cardiac assist devices of various types are being observed.

Intra-Aortic Balloon Pump (IABP)

Beside prolonged extracorporeal circulation, intra-aortic balloon pumping was the earliest clinically applied concept. Although the relative numbers are declining, the absolute figures increase. The IABP which works in series with the heart, is the most beneficial in unloading the left ventricle and in increasing the coronary blood flow as a result of the augmented diastolic pressure. The device is driven pneumatically according to the patient's ECG.

However, the advantages of the IABP is limited by ventricular fibrillation; it is not beneficial in patients with severe cardiac failure. The IABP is accepted in the CCU, in patients with cardiac failure after myocardial infarction (6,7) and in those with dilated cardiomyopathy (16).

Assist Devices

Left-ventricular, Right-ventricular and Bi-ventricular Assist Devices (LVAD, RVAD AND BVAD)

Left-, right- or bi-ventricular mechanical devices are indicated in patients where it is not possible to achieve and to maintain a sufficient circulation despite the IABP. Presently, pulsatile systems driven pneumatically, and *non*-pulsatile electrical ones, are being clinically investigated. Since 1975, 345 implantations have been reported, mainly with pulsatile mechanical devices. However, the number is incomplete due to the fact that non-pulsatile assist devices do not require registration for clinical investigation.

Left-ventricular assist devices work parallel to the heart. An inflow cannula collects blood which is returned by the artificial ventricle to the aorta (Figures 68 and 69). The site of the inflow cannulation is under discussion. It is possible to insert the cannula into the left atrium

- via the left atrial appendage
- via the right superior pulmonary vein
- or via the roof of the left atrium (between the superior vena cava and the ascending aorta).

This just-described technique represents an atrio-aortic bypass. The advantage is the easy approach, the disadvantage is the uncontrolled filling of the left ventricle. As the aortic valve

2. Artificial Heart

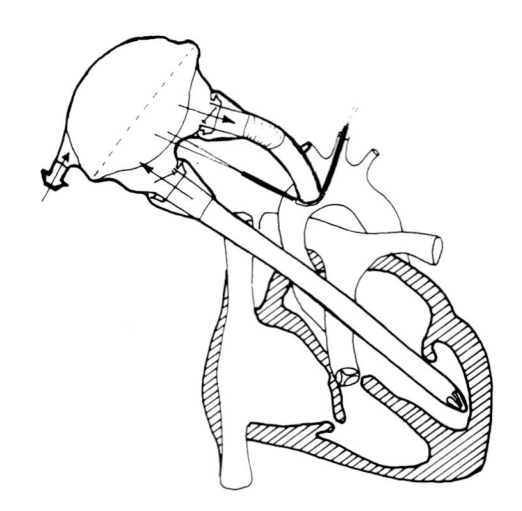

Fig. 68 Implantation sites of a left ventricular assist device.

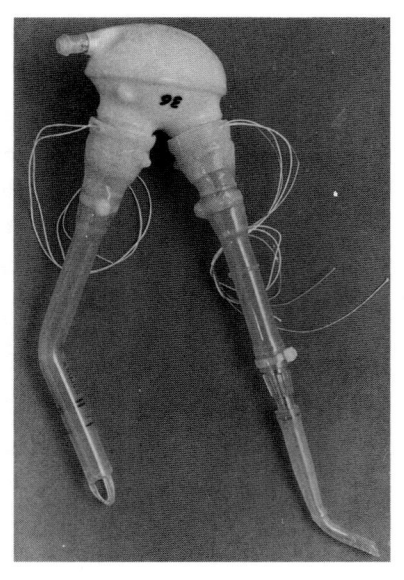

Fig. 69 Ellipsoid heart adapted with cannulas for a left ventricular assist device or right ventricular assist device.

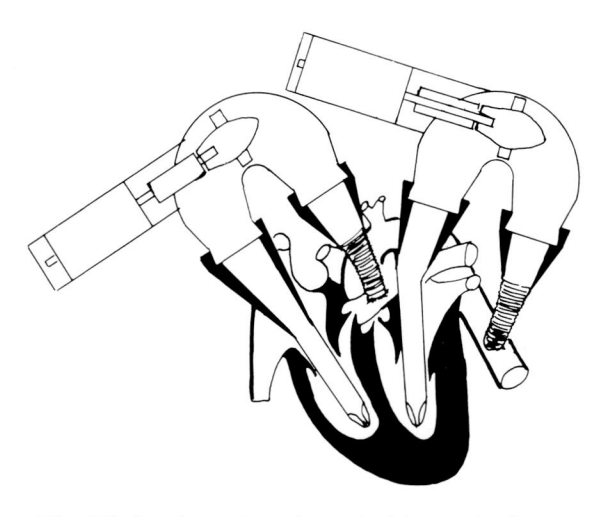

Fig. 70 Implantation sites of a bi-ventricular assist device (with 2 impeller pumps).

of the left ventricle. As the aortic valve remains closed, it is possible that the ventricle can overfill and result in additional cardiac disability.

The superior technique represents a ventriculo-aortic bypass. The left ventricle can be cannulated
- via the apex (17)
- or via the left atrium and mitral valve.

The transapical cannulation should be avoided or used only in patients who are candidates for a heart transplant (18), as the left ventricular apex is damaged by implantation of the cannula. An inflow cannula into the left atrium is thus preferred via the right superior pulmonary vein (Figure 68).

At present, 7 different mechanical pulsatile devices (Bernhard, Norman, Portner, Unger, Pierce, Atsumi, Buecherl) have been implanted in 345 patients since 1980 (19) (Table 22). In 118 instances (34%) the patient was successfully weaned and in consequence 52 (15%) are alive. In another 52 patients (15%) a heart transplantation has been performed, of these, 39 could be discharged, (11% of total or 75% of the transplant group). In total, 91 patients (26%) could be discharged.

In 188 patients, a LVAD was sufficient, 73 patients could be weaned and 34 were discharged. 20 patients received a consecutive heart replacement; 16 of these patients were discharged.

Impaired cardiac function may be a result of isolated right heart failure. A right ventricular assist device (RVAD)

2. Artificial Heart

Clinical Implantations of Assist Devices since 1980

	no	W	D*	HTX	D**
LVAD	188	73 (38%)	34 (18%)	20 (10%)	16 (80% or 8.5% of total)
RVAD	35	14 (40%)	7 (20%)	1	1
BVAD	122	31 (25%)	11 (9%)	31 (25%)	20 (64% or 16.5% of total)
	345	118 (34%)	52 (15%)	52 (15%)	39 (75% or 11% of total)

W = weaned off
D = discharged
HTX = heart transplantation
LVAD = left-ventricular assist device
RVAD = right-ventricular assist device
BVAD = bi-ventricular assist device

* after implantation of assist device alone
** after assist device and HTX

Table 22

can then help. The implantation of a RVAD is analogous to the LVAD: The inflow cannula is implanted via the right atrial appendage, via the tricuspid valve into the right ventricle and the pump returns blood to the pulmonary artery. Of 35 patients, 14 could be weaned, 7 of whom were discharged. One patient received a donor heart and survived.

If both devices are inserted, this is termed a bi-ventricular assist device (BVAD) which replaces the function of the heart completely (Figures 70, 71).

In 122 patients mentioned so far worldwide (Table 22), the use of a LVAD alone was not effective because of additional right heart failure, so that an additional RVAD was required. 31 patients

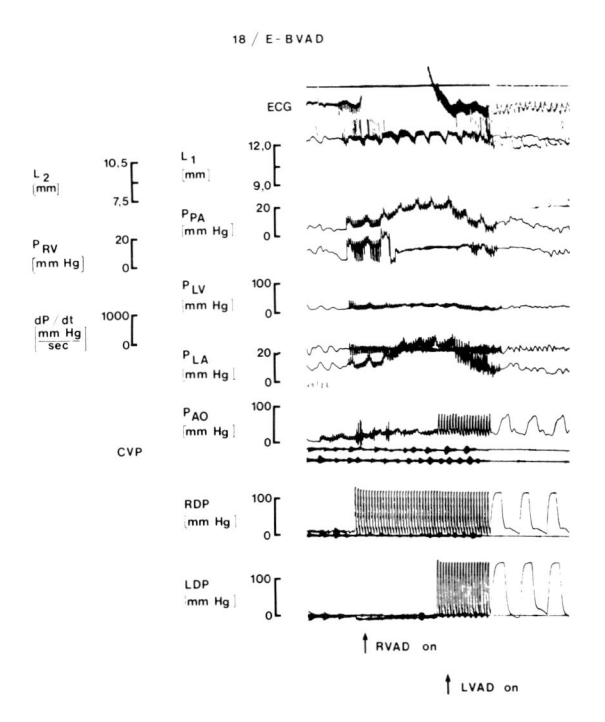

Fig. 71 (left)
Haemodynamic responses to a pulsatile bi-ventricular assist device during ventricular fibrillation. On the left the LVAD and RVAD are off, on the right both are working.
P_{PA} = pulmonary artery pressure
P_{LV} = left-ventricular pressure
P_{LA} = left-atrial pressure
P_{AO} = aortic pressure
RDP = right driving pressure
LDP = left driving pressure
CVP = central venous pressure

2. Artificial Heart

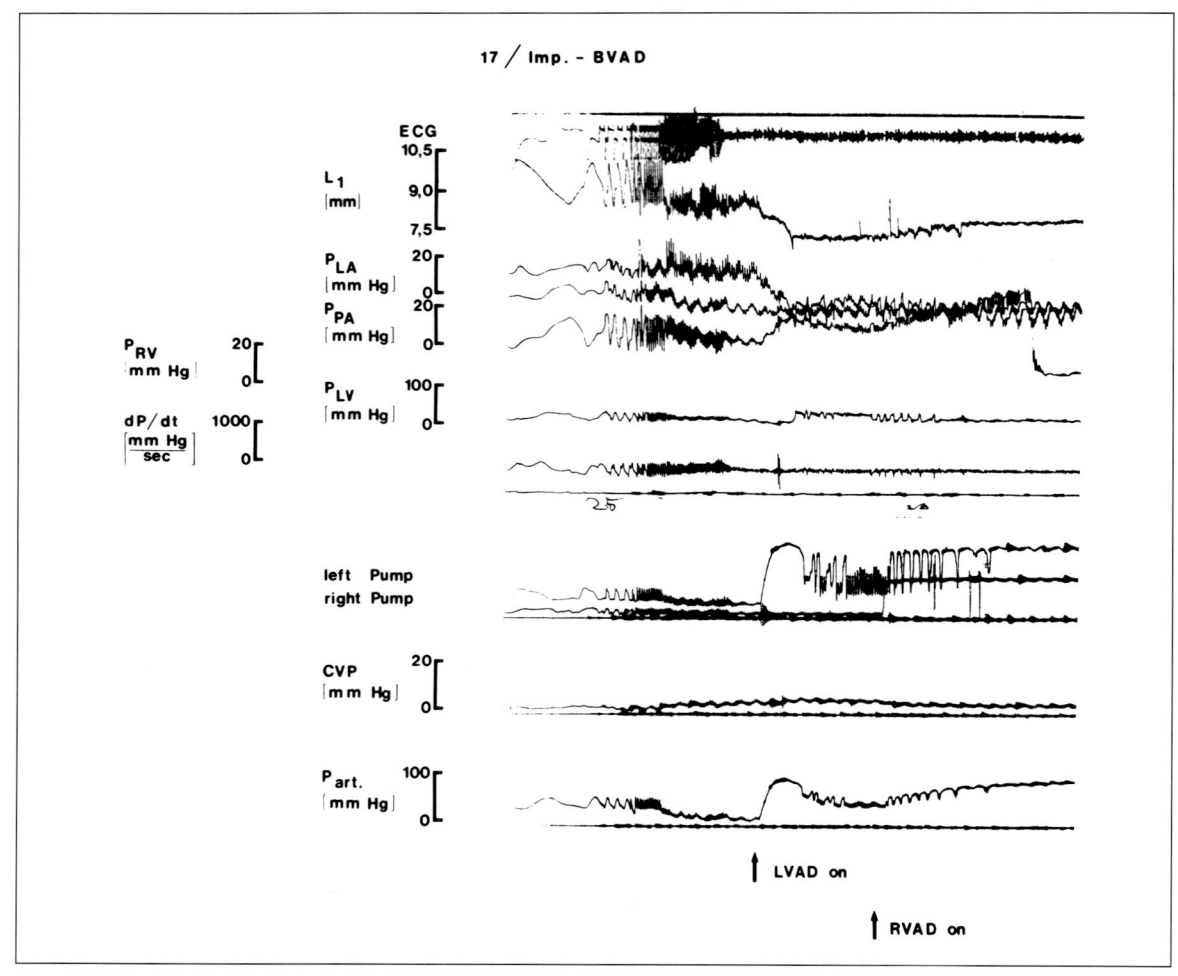

Fig. 72 Haemodynamic response to a non-pulsatile bi-ventricular assist device during ventriular fibrillation. On the left both pumps are off, on the right both pumps are on (for abbreviations see Fig 71; P_{art} = aortic pressure).

could be weaned, 11 are presently alive. 31 patients were transplanted, 20 of whom are alive.

The main indication for the various assist devices was cardiogenic shock after open heart surgery. (The use of these devices in relation to cardiogenic shock after myocardial infarction needs to be evaluated). Complications were: bleeding, requiring a second thoracotomy in 48% of the patients, renal failure in 33%, emboli in 15% (patients with pulsatile mechanical assist devices need full anticoagulation with heparin or coumadine), infection in 30%, and neurological disorders in 15%. Of importance was the fact that pump failure, rupture of the membrane and failure of the driving systems did not occur as complications.

Lately, non-pulsatile blood flow is preferred (1). The number used is uncertain, as these cheap devices do not require special registration. (There exists a rough estimation of 40 000, but few precise reports are available). It may also be used to replace a heart totally (BVAD) (Figures 70, 72) (19, 20). Non-pulsatile blood pumps like the ones made by Biotest have been designed to replace the roller pump, and can be applied with low doses of heparin.

2. Artificial Heart

in patients with cardiogenic shock after myocardial infarction since the systems can easily be inserted percutaneously (21).

The results are similar to pulsatile blood pumps: 48% of the patients could not be weaned, 32% could be discharged, and 20% died after being weaned. However once again, these results should be interpreted cautiously because of the limited numbers reported. Main complications were traumatic hemolysis, renal failure, and thromboembolism.

There are attempts to design implantable devices and to replace the heart totally (22, 23), (Figure 73).

Total Artificial Heart

The total artificial heart driven pneumatically (Fig 74) has now a definite role as a bridge toward transplantation. A potential candidate therefore needs to be eligible for heart transplantation. TAH may also be used to control severe irreversible rejection episodes. There are currently 6 devices in use (Berlin, Brno, Jarvik, Kolff, Pierce, Unger).

The implantation technique is now established (11), (Figures 75, 76, 77).

Since 1969, 94 patients received a TAH (3, 10), in 8 as a permanent substitute and in 86 as a bridge (on average for 16 days) toward transplantation. 53% of the latter patients' group could eventually be discharged. Complications were bleeding, emboli (patients need to be anti-coagulation), and severe infections which originated mainly around the drive lines (12). No device failure was reported. However, in one case a valve cracked.

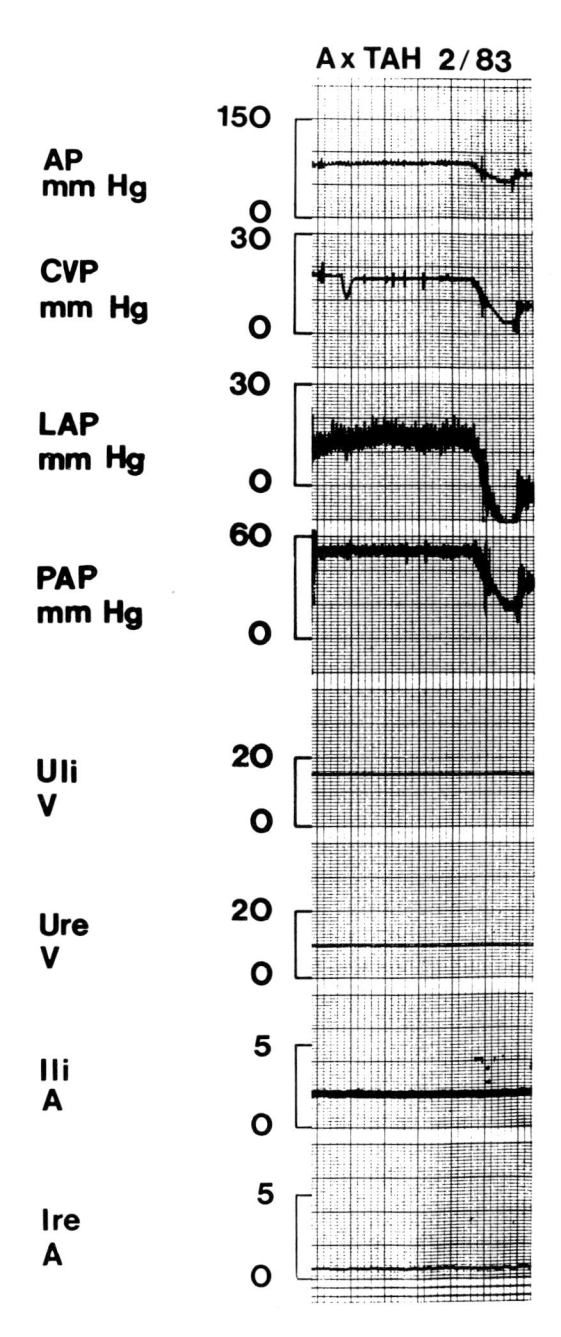

Fig. 73 Haemodynamic in a calf with a total non-pulsatile electrically driven artificial heart. Aortic pressure, central venous pressure, left atrial pressure, pulmonary artery pressure.
- Uli = Voltage left
- Ure = Voltage right
- Ili = Ampere left
- Ire = Ampere right

The indications for these devices are similar. However, they may be utilized

2. Artificial Heart

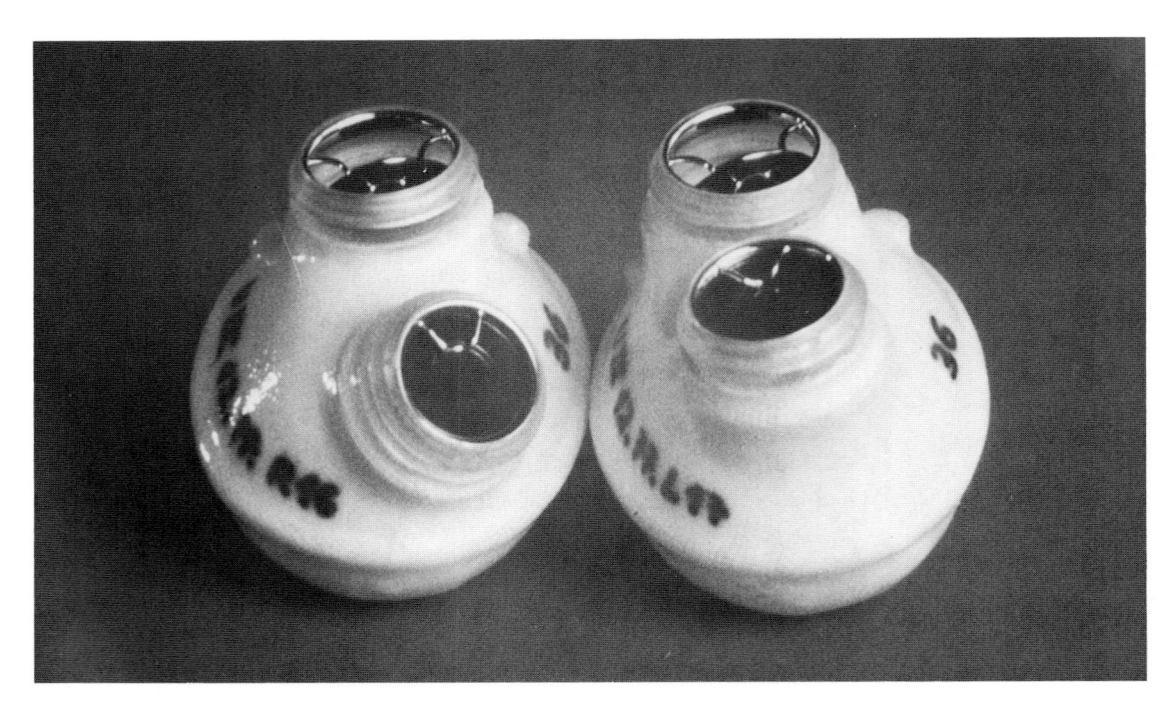

Fig. 74 Ellipsoid heart for total heart replacement.

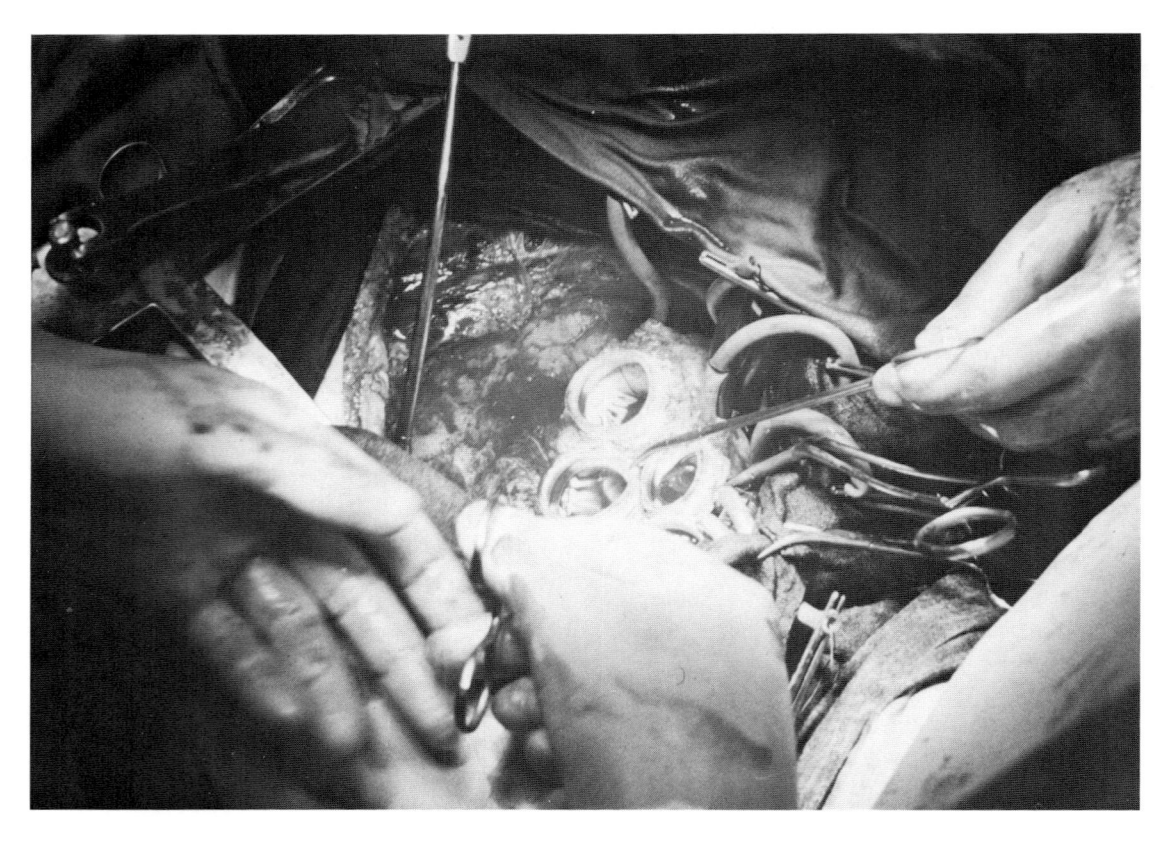

Fig. 75 Pericardial sac without the natural heart. On the atria and large vessels so called quick adaptors are sutured to allow a connection to the artificial heart.

2. Artificial Heart

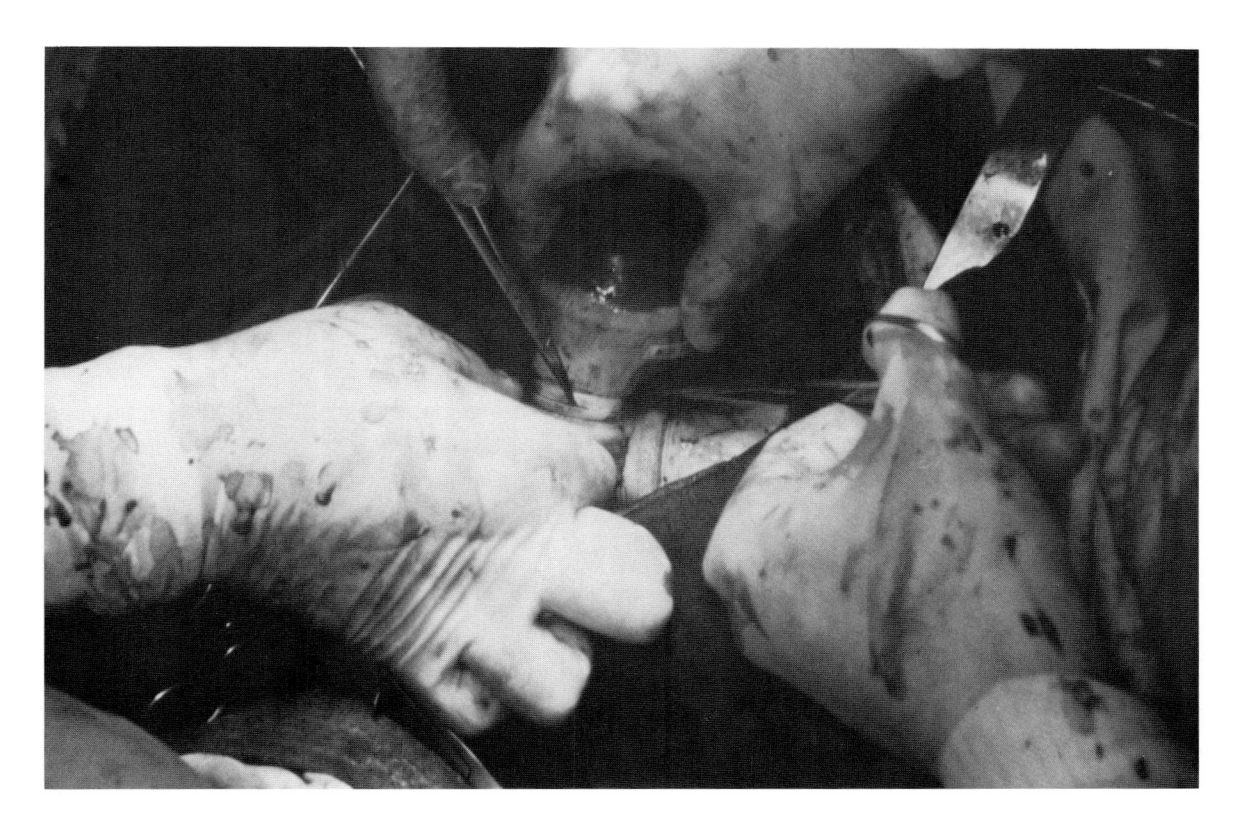

Fig. 76 Implantation of a TAH. The left heart is already in place, the implantation of the right sided device is in progress.

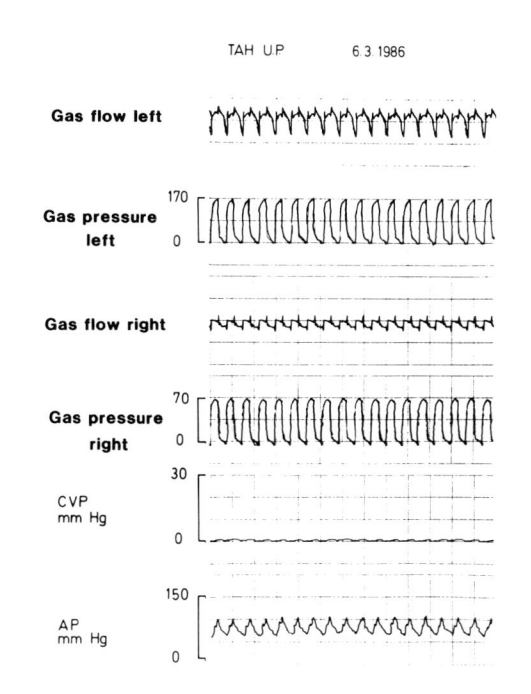

Fig. 77 Haemodynamics of a total artificial heart recipient.
CVP = central venous pressure
AP = aortic pressure
Driving parameters of the TAH.

Thrombus formation within the artificial ventricles is still an unsolved main problem (whether endothelial cell lining is able to solve that problem must be awaited; see contribution Chapter 3.7.3.). Thrombus formation takes place at suture lines, valves, valve support rings, and, finally, the heart chamber itself.

The construction of an artificial heart encompasses a housing and a moving membrane separating the blood from the driving chamber. In the junction between the two, thrombi are formed. This obstacle can be overcome by designing the membrane of circular shape at cross section (Figure 78). It is then always rinsed during the cardiac cycle (1,2).

The use of a permanent substitute is presently remote (13). A possibility is to

2. Artificial Heart

design mechanical blood pumps driven electromechanically (14).

Conclusion

Assisted circulation has a definite role and is complementary to heart transplant programs. Until December 1987, 345 patients have received Assist Devices and 94 total artificial hearts. Left-ventricular, right-ventricular and bi-ventricular assist devices were most important after difficult cardiac- surgical interventions. In comparison, the total artificial heart has its place predominantly around cardiac transplantation.

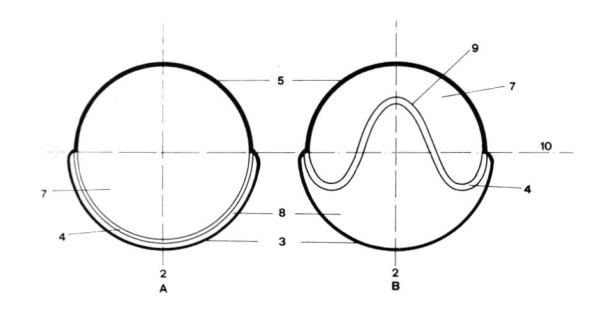

Fig. 78 Cross-section of the Ellipsoid heart (original description for patent application).

References

1. Unger F. Assisted Circulation. Springer-Verlag Berlin, Heidelberg, New York 1979.

2. Unger F. Assisted Circulation. Springer-Verlag Berlin, Heidelberg, New York 1984.

3. Norman J. Effect of intra-aortic balloon pump on right ventricular function. J Thorac Cardiovasc Surg 90, 152, 1985.

4. Olsen DB, Riebman JB, De Paulis R, Durrant G, Nielsen STD. Registry and tabulations of orthotopic total artificial hearts in humans. ASAIO 33, 182, 1987.

5. Unger F. Coronary Artery Surgery: Demand for the Nineties. Report for WHO - Regional Office for Europe, Salzberg, 1985. Heidelberg: Springer, 1986.

6. Sanfelippo PM, Baker NH, EwY HG , Moore PJ, Thomas JW, Brahos GJ, Vicker RF. Experience with intra-aortic balloon counterpulsation. Ann Thorac Surg 41, 36, 1986.

7. Corrall CH, Vaughn CC. Intra-aortic balloon counterpulsation: an eleven-year review and analysis of determination of survival. Tex Heart Inst J 13, 39, 1986.

8. Pennington DG, Bernhard WF, Golding LR, Berger RL, Khuri SF, Watson JT. Long-term follow-up of post-cardiotomy patients with profound cardiogenic shock treated with ventricular assist devices. Circulation 72 (Suppl II), 217, 1985.

9. Birnbaum PL, Henderson MJ, Weisel RD, Benak AM, Madonik NM, Mickleborough LL, Williams WG, Scully HE, Goldman BS, Baird RJ. Extracorporeal Circulatory Assist Devices. ASAIO 33, 190, 1987.

10. Cooley DA. Heart substitution: transplantation and total artificial heart. The Texas Heart Institute experience. Artif Organs 9, 12, 1985.

11. De Vries WC. Artificial heart still holds promise: De Vries says, program continues. Med News 253, 2807, 1985.

2. Artificial Heart

12. Mc Bride LR, Ruzevich SA, Pennington DG, Kennedy DJ, Kanter KR, Miller LW, Swartz MT, Termuhlen DF, ASAIO 33, 201, 1987.

13. Taylor KD, Gaykowski R, Keate KS, Winters S, Price RR, Topaz SR. Explant analysis of thirty-three bridge to transplant J7 total artificial heart devices. ASAIO 33, 738, 1987.

14. Kolff J, Deeb GM. Artificial heart and left ventricular assist devices. Surg Clin North Am 65, 176, 1985.

15. Watson JT. The present and future of cardiac assist device. Artif Organs 9, 138, 1985.

16. Gaul G, Blazek G, Deutsch M, Laczkovics A, Mohl W, Heeger H, Wolner E. Chronic use of an intra-aortic balloon pump in congestive cardiomyopathy. Assisted Circulation 2. Berlin, Heidelberg, New York, Tokyo: Springer-Verlag 28, 1984.

17. Portner PM, Oyer PE, Jassawalla JS, Chen H, Miller PJ, Laforge DH, Green GF, Shumway NE. A totally implantable ventricular assist device for end-stage heart disease. Assisted Circulation 2. Berlin, Heidelberg, New York, Tokyo: Springer-Verlag, 115, 1984

18. Richenbacher WE, Wisman CB, Rosenberg G, Donachy JH, Landis DL, Pierce WS. Ventricular assistance: clinical experience at the Pennsylvania State University. Assisted Circulation 2. Berlin, Heidelberg, New York, Tokyo: Springer-Verlag, 70, 1984

19. Unger F, Genelin A, Hager J, Kemkes BM, Koller I, Schistek R. Functional heart replacement with non-pulsatile assist devices. Assisted Circulation 2. Berlin, Heidelberg, New York, Tokyo: Springer-Verlag, 163, 1984

20. Park SB, Liebler GA, Burkeholder JA, Maher TD, Benckart DH, Magovern GJ Jr, Christlieb IY, Kao RL, Magovern GJ Sr. Mechanical Support of the Failing Heart. Ann Thorac Surg 42, 627, 1986.

21. Philips SJ, Ballantine B, Slonine D, Hall J, Vandehaar J, Kongtahworn C, Zeff RH, Skinner JR, Reckmo K, Gray D. Percutaneous initiation of cardiopulmonary bypass. Ann Thorac Surg 36, 223, 1983.

22. Unger F. Current status and use of artificial hearts and circulatory assist devices. Perfusion 1, 155, 1986.

23. Unger F. The artificial heart - assisted circulation. Annal of Cardiac Surgery 1987, Gower Academic Journals, 45, 1987.

2. Artificial Heart

2.3. Clinical Application and Patient Selection in the Use of a Total Artificial Heart as a Bridge for Transplantation
La Pitié Hôpital Experience 1986 - 1987

E Solis, C Muneretto, P Leger, I Gandjbakhch, A Pavie, V Bors, C Piazza, J Szefner, A Cabrol, C Cabrol

Department of Cardio Vascular Surgery, Hôpital La Pitié, Paris, France

Presently, the total artificial heart is indicated for use in patients unable to be weaned from bypass, for use in transplant candidates when death is judged imminent, and in cardiogenic shock patients where no additional conventional therapy is applicable (1). Major complications associated with the use of this device in desperately ill individuals include sepsis, multi-organ system failure, hepatic dysfunction, pulmonary oedema, and renal failure.

Between April 1986 and October 1987, 23 patients underwent orthotopic implantation of a total artificial heart (TAH) (Jarvik 7) at La Pitié Hôpital. An analysis of factors that can influence mortality and survival of these implantations is presented.

Patients and Methods

Our 23 patients were 20 men and 3 women with a mean age of 37.6 ± 11 years (range 19 - 56 years).

The clinical indications for the implantation of the TAH were: non-obstructive idiopathic cardiomyopathy in 9 patients, 4 of them with sudden cardiac decompensation and 5 with chronic terminal failure.

Seven had ischaemic heart disease, five with terminal chronic dysfunction and the remaining two had acute myocardial infarction. Two women had acute irreversible post partum cardiomyopathy and another patient had terminal valvular disease. Four patients had severe rejection 5 and 10 years, 86 and 29 days after heart transplantation. All patients were desperately ill, with low cardiac outputs, renal insufficiency, and hepatic insufficiency.

The device implanted was the total artificial heart (Jarvik 7), the 70 ml in 11 patients (mean weight 66,6 ± 5,4 kg) and the 100 ml in 12 patients (mean weight 69 ± 10 kg).

For analysis of the mortality the patients were separated into two groups: acute decompensation and chronic disease. Acute decompensation was considered when terminal heart failure developped within one month of the implantation of the artificial heart. Further evaluation by age was also analysed. Immunosuppressed patients were ex-

2. Artificial Heart

Patient	Age	Sex	Sudden Decomp.	Chronic Disease	Diagnosis	Time in Support (days)	Type of Art. Heart	Outcome
1	25	M		*	HF + DVR	13	J-70	Died of septicemia
2	56	M		*	ICM + PH	14	J-70	Died of sepsis and MOF
3	22	M	*		ICM + viral myocarditis	13	J-100	Transplanted, died of Kaposi's sarcoma 476 days post-transplant
4	40	M		*	ICM	14	J-100	Transplanted, alive
5	34	M	*		ICM	13	J-70	Transplanted, alive
6	19	M		*	RAT (1982)	2	J-100	Died of MOF
7	33	F	*		PPC	2	J-70	Transplanted, alive
8	39	M		*	ID	2	J-70	Transplanted, died 20 days later of an anoxic coma
9	36	M	*		ICM	12	J-100	Transplanted, alive
10	20	M		*	ICM	26	J-100	Transplanted, alive
11	47	M		*	ID	16	J-100	Died of MOF
12	27	F	*		PPC	5	J-70	Died of sepsis & MOF
13	45	M	*		ID	21	J-100	Transplanted, died of fulminant hepatitis 18 days post-transplant
14	31	F		*	RAT (1977)	5	J-70	Died of MOF
15	47	M		*	ICM	9	J-100	Died of pulm. embolism
16	43	M	*		ICM	20	J-100	Died of septicemia
17	46	M		*	ICM + transp. (failed)	7	J-100	TAH-thorax missmatch, died of MOF
18	54	M		*	ID	8	J-70	Died of septicemia
19	55	M	*		ID + AMI	13	J-70	Transplanted, alive
20	37	M		*	ID + transp. (failed)	31	J-100	Transplanted, alive
21	28	M		*	RAT 29th day	16	J-70	Died of septicemia
22	51	M		*	RAT (86 days)	42	J-70	Died of septicemia
23	30	M		*	ID	12	J-100	Transplanted died of mediastinitis 10th day

Table 23 Total experience at La Pitié Hôpital in the use of a total artificial heart as a bridge to transplantation.

    M = Male, F = Female
    PH = Pulmonary Hypertension
    MOF = Multiple Organ Failure
    HF = Heart Failure
    DVR = Double Valve Replacement
    ICM = Idiopathic Cardiomyopathy
    RAT = Rejection After Transplantation
    PPC = Post Partum Cardiomyopathy
    ID = Ischemic Disease
    AMI = Aute Myoardial Failure

2. Artificial Heart

cluded from the overall analysis and considered as an independent group.

Results

Our total experience is summarized in Table 23. Of the 23 patients treated, 11 (47.8%) had adequate support and were successfully transplanted; of these 7 are alive and well. Twelve patients (52.2%) died during circulatory support. Causes of death were sepsis in 6 patients, multiple organ failure in 4 patients, and a combination of both in 2 patients.

Mean CPB time for the implantation of the artificial heart was 153 ± 34 minutes. Mean time of mechanical support was 13.7 ± 9.6 days with a range of 2 to 42 days. Our total experience in TAH implantation is 316 days under mechanical support. There was no clinical evidence of thromboembolic complication during this time. In only one patient did a mismatch in size between the TAH and the thorax occur.

Table 24 summarizes the influence of age on the outcome of patients with TAH support. Patients younger than 40 years have an 81.8% chance of successful transplantation, compared with a 25% chance in the older group.

Table 25 summarizes the influence of the duration of the disease before the implantation of the TAH, as a predictor of the outcome of these patients. Patients with acute failure had a 75% successful transplantation, compared with 45.4% in patients with chronic disease.

Table 26 shows age and duration of the disease considered together. Young patients with acute disease have an 80% chance of successful transplantation in comparison with 66.6% in the older group. Young patients with chronic disease have an 83.3% chance of success, compared with no survival in the older group. Therefore young patients with an acute or chronic disease, and older patients with acute disease, benefit most by this procedure.

Influence of Age on the Outcome of Patients in TAH (n=19)		
	<40 years n = 11	> 40 years n = 8
Died during TAH support	2 (18.2%)	6 (75%)
Transplanted alive	6 (54.5%)	1 (12.5%)
Transplanted, died; cause *not* related to TAH	2 (18.2%)	1* (12.5%)
Transplanted, died; cause related to TAH	1** (9.1%)	-
Overall success in being transplanted	9 (81.8%)	2 (25%)

* Patient died 18 days post-transplant of fulminant hepatitis
**Patient died 10 days post-transplant of mediastinitis and sepsis, due to pseudomonas.

Table 24   Influence of age on the outcome of patients with TAH. Overall group of patients separated in A: 40 years of age or less and B: more than 40 years of age. Immunosuppressed patients were analysed in a separate group.

Influence of the Duration of the Disease on the Outcome of TAH Patients

	Acute decompensation n = 8	Chronic disease n = 11
Died during TAH support	2 (25%)	6 (54.5%)
Transplanted alive	4 (50%)	3 (27.3%)
Transplanted, died; cause *not* related to TAH	2* (25%)	1** (9.1%)
Transplanted, died; cause related to TAH	–	1*** (9.1%)
Overall success in being transplanted	6 (75%)	5 (45.4%)

*   One patient died 18 days post-transplant of fulminant hepatitis, the other of a Kaposi's sarcoma due to azathioprine treatment 476 days post-transplant
** Patient died 20 days post-transplant of an anoxic coma
*** Patient died 10 days post-transplant of a mediastinitis due to pseudomonas.

Table 25 Influence of the duration of the disease on the outcome of TAH patients. One group of patients with an acute decompensation of less than one month before the implantation of the total artificial heart and another group of patients with long lasting chronic cardiac disease (immunosuppressed patients again not included).

Of the 12 patients that died during mechanical support, 7 had sepsis. The origin of the infections was the lung in 3 cases, non-specific in 3 cases, and a purulent peritonitis originating from the colon in one. The drive lines and the TAH were not, in any case, found to be the origin of the infection.

Mean follow-up time in the 11 transplanted patients is 257 ± 189 days, for a total follow-up time of 2 833 days.

Five of the transplanted patients developped an infection in the immediate post-transplant period. Three of these infections were successfully treated with antibiotics. Two patients died, one 10 days post-transplant from mediastinal sepsis, the other patient died 18 days post-op of a fulminant hepatitis. Another 2 patients died during the follow-up period of causes not related to the TAH support, one of a Kaposi's sarcoma secondary to his azathioprine treatment 476 days post-transplant, the other died of an anoxic coma 20 days post-transplant. To date, 7 patients remain alive and well.

Our experience with the implantation of the TAH in immunosuppressed patients is summarized in Table 27.

Discussion

Total artificial heart implantation for temporary use in combination with transplantation has become a clinical reality. Practical aspects in the decision for the selection of patients have not been entirely worked out. In our initial review (2), we concluded that the best indication of the use of an artificial heart as a bridge to cardiac transplantation was in young patients (less than 40 years) in recent, acute intractable cardiac failure with reversible organ dysfunction.

2. Artificial Heart

The Influence of Age and Duration of the Disease in the Outcome of TAH Patients

Duration of Dis. Age	Chronic <40 years n = 6	Chronic > 40 years n = 5	Acute <40 years n = 5	Acute > 40 years n = 3
Died with TAH support	1 (16.66%)	5 (100%)	1 (20%)	1 (33.3%)
Transplanted alive	3 (50%)		3 (60%)	1 (33.3%)
Transplanted, died; cause *not* related to TAH	1* (16.66%)	–	1*** (20%)	1**** (33.3%)
Transplanted, death related to TAH ;	1** (16.66%)	–	–	–
Overall success in being transplanted	5 (83.3%)	0 (0%)	4 (80%)	2 (66.6%)

*   Patient died 20 days post-transplant of anoxic coma
** Patient died 10 days post-transplant of a mediastinitis due to pseudomonas
*** Patient died 476 days post-transplant of a Kaposi sarcoma due to azathioprine

Table 26 The combined influence of age and duration of the disease on the outcome of TAH patients.

TAH Experience in Immunosuppressed Patients

Diagnosis	Age (years)	Time of Support (days)	Outcome
RAT (1982)	19	2	Died of MOF
RAT (1977)	31	5	Died of MOF
RAT (29 days)	28	16	Died of sepsis
RAT (86 days)	51	42	Died of sepsis

Table 27 Group of immunosuppressed patients in which a total artificial heart was used as a bridge to transplantation (n=4).

RAT = Rejection after Transplantation
MOF= Multiple Organ Failure

2. Artificial Heart

As evidenced in this analysis, young patients (40 years of age or less) in whom an artificial heart has been implanted as a bridge for transplantation show a greater success (81.8%) of being transplanted than older patients (25%) (Table 24). In the same way, patients that suffered from an acute decompensation did better (75% success) than patients with long standing cardiac failure (45.4% success) (Table 25). Young patients, as well as patients that developed an acute decompensation, should be in better condition in comparison with older patients or patients that suffer a more chronic evolution of the disease. The influence of age on the outcome of the patients with a chronic disease after transplantation is apparent - no survivor if older than 40, an 83.3% survival in those younger than 40 (Table 26). This finding is not so obvious when the analysis is made of patients that developped an acute decompensation younger than 40 years (80%) with those older than 40 years (66.6%).

Young patients and patients with an acute decompensation should have a greater reserve and/or be able to reverse the damage created by the circulatory collapse more readily when compared with older patients and patients in a terminal stage of a chronic disease.

During mechanical support, the clinical condition of the survivors improved, with correction of the pulmonary edema, improvement in lung function, reversal of the renal and/or hepatic insufficiency, and improvement in the nutritional status. In those that died, the main complications were related to the poor condition of the patients in the preoperative period. These patients are too weak to support a major surgical procedure, and the damage produced by the long-lasting cardiac failure in other organs might be irreversible.

Early infection after transplantation occurred in 45% of the patients in whom a TAH was used. These infections were resolved with the use of antibiotics in 60% of the patients, but proved to be fatal in 40%. Therefore the risk of infection should be carefully considered, especially when temporary total assist devices are used in patients who will be rapidly subjected to a second operation and are, or soon will be, immunosuppressed.

Pulmonary function is critical in the patients receiving a TAH, because a prolonged intubation period pre-disposes to infection. In our experience, more than 30% of TAH patients had pulmonary infections, and the lungs were the origin of generalised sepsis in more of 35% of the cases. Preoperative pulmonary status and mechanical compression by artificial ventricles (especially left sided athelectasis) may be related to the high rate of infections in these patients.

Our experience in immunosuppressed patients (Table 27) made us conclude that the use of an artificial heart is contraindicated in these patients, due to the high risk of infection.

In conclusion, of the 23 patients treated with TAH as a bridge to transplant, 11 (47.8%) had adequate support and were successfully transplanted; of these, 7 (63.4%) are today alive and well. The high early infection rate associated with the use of this device, is in our opinion, related to the combination of three factors: the implantation of the device; a second operation in a short period of time; and the immunosuppression of the patients.

2. Artificial Heart

References

1. Jarvik, RK. Clinical application of the total artificial heart. Presented in the 2nd International Symposium on Cardiac Surgery, Rome Italy 1987. D'Alessandro KG, Rome: Scientifica International, 1987.

2. Cabrol C, Gandjbakhch I, Pavie A, Bors V, et al. Total artificial heart as a bridge for transplantation. La Pitié 1986-1987. Submitted for publication. J Heart Transplantation.

2.4. Clinical Experience with the Artificial Heart as a Bridge for Transplant

A Rokitansky, E Wolner, W Schreiner, U Losert

*2nd Surgical Department, University of Vienna,
General Hospital of Vienna, Austria*

Introduction

The continuously rising number of heart transplantations has increased the demand for donor organs, and patients' registries have had to be created as a consequence. In our clinic it takes about 25 days ±18 days (shortest time: 1 day / longest time: 84 days) until a donor heart can be found via Eurotransplant. According to our records covering 69 HTX patients, 33% of the patients die while awaiting transplantation. This unsatisfactory situation could be improved by using temporary circulatory assistance, such as TAH bridging or VAD implantation.

The following groups of patients are potential candidates for temporary mechanical circulatory support: (a) HTX candidates developing acute cardiac failure; (b) transplanted patients developing acute rejection; and (c) patients who cannot be weaned off extracorporal circulation (ECC) after open heart surgery. For these patients, the temporary orthotopic implantation of a total artificial heart (TAH) or a ventricular assist device (VAD) can be a lifesaving intervention, which maintains circulation and improves organ function during bridging to transplant.

Up to now, clinical TAH-bridging has been performed by 19 teams in 7 countries (USA, Canada, France, Germany, Great Britain, Sweden, Austria); 8 different devices were used (1). Since the TAH performed by Cooley in 1969 (2), until March 1987, 77 artificial hearts have been implanted; 62 patients underwent subsequent transplantations, 36 of whom are still alive (3). Considering all TAH patients, the largest number is recruited from the groups with ischaemic and idiopathic cardiomyopathy and TX-rejection.

Complications and problems related to TAH-bridging are difficulties in positioning, bleeding, thrombus formation and thromboembolism, infection in partial implantable systems, device dysfunction (e.g. valve breakdown or kinking of the drive lines), and possible immunoreactions interfering with the subsequent HTX. Using the new (and smaller) designs (like Jarvik 7-70, Utah 100 etc.), most of the difficulties in positioning as well as device dysfunctions seem to be controlled (4).

Patients

Since May 1986, 5 patients of our department suffering from endstage cardiomyopathy in 4 cases, and coronary heart disease in one case, underwent TAH implantation as a bridge to transplant (5).

Devices

On three occasions the "Ellipsoid Heart" was used, and twice the "Berlin Heart". Both systems work with membrane pumps connected to an external driving unit by transcutaneous tubes and have been previously described (6,7).

Implantation

The implantation itself was done under total extracorporeal circulation, after removing the patient's own heart along the atrio-ventricular border, preserving as much atrial and arterial tissue as possible. Connectors for the TAH-ventricles were then anastomosed to the residual atria, the aorta and the pulmonary artery by running sutures. Using a fibrin glue (Tissucol), the sutures were sealed.

The Dacron coated tubes for the driving gas were led through the abdominal wall. Following completion of all connections, pumping was started. After decannulation, the median sternotony was closed.

Pumping Mode

The pumping mode of the artificial heart can be adapted by changing the driving pressure, the vacuum, the systolic duration, and heart rate. Filling of the blood compartment is performed by deflation and vacuum suction of the gas compartment, which moves the membrane towards the tube connection, and causes the inflow valves to open. Ejection of blood is performed by rapid filling of the gas compartment, moving the driving membranes (and thus the blood) towards the valves. The "Berlin Heart" ventricles were driven in a partial filling-full ejection mode according to the Frank-Starling mechanism. On the contrary, the "Ellipsoid Heart" ventricles were operated in a full filling-partial ejection mode so as to minimize membrane stress in endsystolic position.

With both types of ventricles, the left pump was adjusted so as to maintain a sufficient cardiac output (CO). As a criteria for CO demand, the oxygen tissue utilisation was calculated from arterial and venous blood gas analysis. Cardiac output was considered sufficient if the oxygen tissue utilization was below 25%. The ejection of the right ventricle was adjusted on the basis of left atrial pressure to provide optimal filling of the left pump. Since the filling pressure of the right pump is determined by central venous pressure, it was regulated by fluid substitution or diuresis (8). Given a certain CO (required to keep oxygen utilisation low) the resulting arterial pressure was kept within the physiological range by adjusting the peripheral resistance with vasoactive drugs.

Results

Since 1984, we performed 69 orthotopic cardiac transplantations. Survival has improved with time. Two patients had to be retransplanted because of acute rejection. Since April 1986, we have used immunosuppressive triple therapy consisting of azathioprine, cyclosporine and corticosteroids. This resulted in an one-year survival rate of 84%, and, since then, no patient has been lost as a result of acute rejection.

Considering the improved prognosis for HTX and the incidence of acute, irreversible biventricular insufficiency in

2. Artificial Heart

patients still on the waiting list, the necessity to establish TAH implantation in our department became evident.

Our first patient (O. in Figure 79) to be bridged was 48 years old and suffering from cardiomyopathy (CMP). Due to his severe cardiogenic shock, the decision for artificial heart implantation was made. He received the "Ellipsoid Heart" for 9 days. Elevating his cardiac output from 3.6 l/min to 7.5 l/min by TAH pumping with a frequency of 77.7 ± 9.8 beats/min his organ functions recovered significantly. The free haemoglobin was 3.9 ± 2.6 g/dl. After 9 days the patient fulfilled all criteria for HTX and was successfully transplanted on the 10th day. Unfortunately, after closing his thorax under stable haemodynamic conditions, he died from intrapericardial bleeding caused by a rupture of the pulmonary artery running suture.

The second patient (P. in Figure 79), 49 years old, suffered from an acute cardiac insufficiency superimposed on CMP. Keeping the oxygen utilisation at about 25% and the CO between 5.6 and 10 l/min, a pumping frequency of 82 ± 5.3 beats/min was used. The mean free hemoglobin was 5.4 ± 4.4 g/dl. He was supported for 10 days with the "Ellipsoid Heart" and underwent successful transplantation. 10 days later he could be discharged from the ICU. Despite immunosuppressive therapy with cyclosporine (serum level: 260-320 ng/ml), azathioprine (2-4 mg/kg/day), methylprednisolone (0.2 mg/kg/day), anti-human T-lymphocyte globulin (ATG), and specific T-lymphocyte surface-antigen (OKT-3, 5 mg/day) he developped acute unresponsive rejection after 40 days, and died thereof.

The third patient (D. in Figure 79) was also hospitalized because of CMP. Ad-

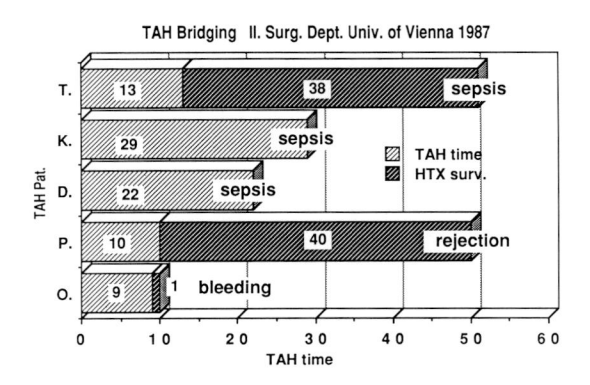

Fig. 79 Days of TAH pumping and bridging duration in our 5 patients.

ditionally, he showed pulmonary embolism due to thrombosis of the pelvic veins. He developed an infected infarction of the left lower lung lobe and his cardiac functions decreased rapidly. Despite infection being a contraindication, we made the decision for TAH implantation, since the patient was only 36 years old. Simultaneously with the implantation, the infected lung was resected. He developped septicaemia (blood cultures contaminated with staphylococcus epidermidis, pseudomonas aeruginosa, cand. albicans). The patient could not be weaned off the respirator. Despite administration of antibiotics and pumping a CO of max 10.2 l/min (with a free haemoglobin of 6.2 ± 4.4 g/dl) he developped multiple organ failure with impairment of neurological functions. TAH pumping was stopped after 22 days.

The fourth patient (K. in Figure 79) with a cardiac index of 1.9 l/min/m^2, due to CMP, received the "Berlin Heart". Again, implantation was successful, but the patient developed recurrent bleeding episodes during the pumping period of 29 days and had to undergo repeated explorations. Resistant infection (cand. albicans in urine and tracheal fluid, contamination of the blood with staphylo-

2. Artificial Heart

coccus epidermidis, meningo-encephalitis) caused death after 29 days.

The last patient (T. in Figure 79) had severe three vessel coronary disease and developed acute infarction of the anterior left wall with subsequent cardiogenic shock. As no donor heart was available and coronary revascularisation proved to be impossible, the "Berlin Heart" was implanted for 13 days, and he was transplanted successfully thereafter. After TX he developped an infection (pseudomonas aeruginosa and staphylococcus epidermidis were found in blood and cand. albicans in the tracheal fluid). Although the patient received Optocillin, Curacel, Anearobex, Mycostatin, Dakatrin, and Ofloxacine, the infection persisted, and he died 38 days after HTX.

Anticoagulation

After the first postoperative day, heparin was administered in a dosage between 200 and 1000 IE/h, depending on the thrombin time. One patient – no. 4 – additionally received 2g acetylsalicylic acid, but developed bleeding which could be stopped by conservative measures.

Discussion

In a cardiac transplantation unit, the implantation of mechanical circulatory support devices (VAD or TAH) can be a lifesaving intervention. Five HTX candidates who had developped acute biventricular insufficiency, received TAH implantation. In all five patients it was possible to reestablish and to maintain the circulatory function as well as to improve the patients' organ functions. Three patients fulfilled the criteria for HTX, which was performed after periods of 9 and 13 days of bridging. The main TAH-related complications were difficulties in positioning, bleeding, infection, thrombus formation, thromboembolism, and device dysfunction.

Positioning

The Jarvik 7-100 cc device should be limited to patients weighing more than 75 kg and having an anterior vertebral to posterior sternal distance of at least 13 cm (9). Using the "Ellipsoid Heart" and the "Berlin Heart" in our patients weighing between 60 and 85 kg we had no problems in closing the thorax. In three patients, however, the left pleural space had to be opened and the left ventricle was positioned laterally and partially intrapericardially. Lateral positioning is a remedy for these problems. Due to compression of the left lung in the first two patients (pumped with the "Ellipsoid Heart"), left inferior lobe atelectases and left pleural effusions occurred. Other positioning problems, like kinking of the drive lines or irritation of the phrenic nerve, were not observed. Nowadays smaller TAH designs with improved implantation characteristics, like the mini Jarvik 7-70 ml or the Utah 100, are available (4).

We designed a new artificial heart, smaller than most of the other devices available. This new design also fits into a normal-sized pericardium. Ejection volume is 87 cc for the left and 75 cc for the right ventricle. This new heart is still under experimental investigation, and up to now it has been implanted in 10 calves. Pumping with a frequency of about 115 beats/min, a cardiac output around 7 l/min could be obtained. After extensive experimental tests, the new Viennese heart will be implanted clinically.

Bleeding

In the early postoperative period, bleeding is a significant problem. Because of haemorrhage, 10 of 27 patients reported required reoperation (1). In our five patients, a major hemorrhage requiring reoperation occurred in patient no. 4. The bleeding hazard in TAH patients is increased by a reduced number and activity of the platelets (10). Therefore, exact surgical haemostasis is required for successful bridging. In contrast to the reported cases from the USA (11) we use fibrin glue (Tissucol) to seal the anastomotic sites.

Anticoagulation, Thrombus Formation and Thromboembolism

In order to prevent thrombus formation and embolism during TAH pumping, various drugs for anticoagulation and antiaggregation (heparin or heparin and dipyridamole) were used. For short-term implantations thromboembolism prevention was also achieved, using low molecular macrodex only (11). For anticoagulation we used heparin in a dosage of 200 to 1000 IU/h. On one occasion, we additionally administered i.v. 2g acetylsalicyclic acid and induced bleeding, which could be stopped by conservative measures. Considering the irreversible damage of platelet function caused by acetylsalicyclic acid, it seems to be dangerous to use both drugs simultaneously.

In none of the patients did we observe clinical signs of arterial embolism. However, in patient 5, a thrombus had developped in the inflow connector of the left "Berlin ventricle". In patient 3 there was a small embolic infarction in the anterior lobe of the left cerebral hemisphere, but no thrombotic growth could be found in the "Ellipsoid Heart" after explantation. A relationship between infection and thrombus formation on the inflow connectors has been described experimentally (12).

Besides contact with artificial surfaces, slow blood flow is an additional factor for thrombus formation. In the new small designs, driven with frequencies around 110 beats/min, there is an improved "wash out" and thus a reduced susceptibility for thrombotic growth.

Infection

Because of transcutaneous driving lines, catheters and intracorporeal artificial surfaces, the risk of infection during TAH pumping is high. Most of the patients on TAH who could not be transplanted, suffered from incurable infections (2,3). Two of our patients on TAH died from sepsis and did not reach transplantation. In patient 5, infection started after HTX. Since we lost 2 patients because of sepsis while still on TAH, we consider that infection during bridging is an incurable and lethal complication. The septic course of patient 3 underlines that infection is a clear contraindication for TAH implantation.

Immunology

The fatal course of patient 2 raised the question whether the artificial heart stimulated the immunological system. In our experience with 69 heart transplantations we never experienced such a severe acute incurable rejection. Stelzer et al (14) from the University of Louisville reported increased complement concentrations in total artificial heart recipients. In our patients 2 (P.) and 5 (T.), we observed low C3 concen-

2. Artificial Heart

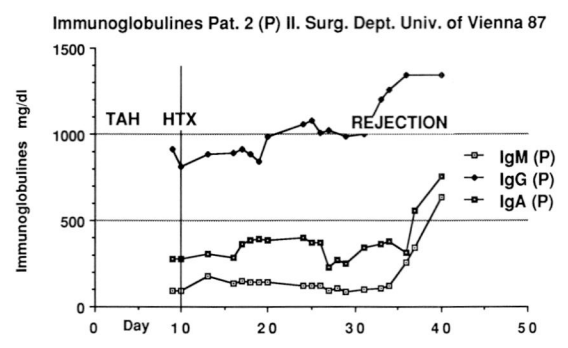

Fig. 80 Blood concentrations of the immunoglobulins (IgM physiological value (pv): 60-320 mg/dl; IgA pv: 70-320 mg/dl; IgG pv: 640-1350 mg/dl) in patient 2, who developed an incurable rejection after HTX.

trations before TAH implantation, which increased to physiological values during TAH pumping. After HTX in patient 2, C3 values remained normal whereas in patient 5, who acquired an infection, they decreased again. In both patients elevated C3 levels could not be found. The decreased C3 levels may be due to a disturbed liver function or an infection-related complement consumption. Contrary to patient 5 (T.), patient 2 revealed a drastic increase of the immunoglobulins IgM and IgA synchronously with his severe terminal rejection (see Figure 80). Related to the aggressive immunosuppressive therapy, he developped a leucopenia (2.4 cells/nl) at that time. A viral infection (cytomegalovirus, herpes or varicella) was serologically excluded. The cause of the fatal rejection is still unclear, but a TAH related stimulation of the humoral immunologic defence mechanisms should be kept in mind. Considering the reported cases of successful bridging, we report that TAH related immunologic stimulation leading to an incurable rejection is possible.

VAD versus TAH

The question may arise, if preference should be given to total artificial cardiac replacement or to the ventricular assist device. In our opinion, the TAH implantation is indicated in patients with irreversible bi-ventricular cardiac insufficiency. Patients with reversible cardiac disease should preferably be treated with the ventricular assist device.

2. Artificial Heart

References

1. Joyce LD, Jhonson KE, Pierce WS, De Vries WC, Semb BK, Copeland JG, Griffith BP, Cooley DA, Fraizer OH, Cabrol C, Kenon WJ, Unger F, Buecherl ES, Wolner E. Summary of the world experience with clinical use of total artificial hearts as heart support devices. J Heart Transplant 5, 229, 1986.

2. Cooley DA, Liotta D, Hallmann GL, Bloodwell RD, Leachmann RD, Hilan JD. First clinical implantation of a total artificial heart. Trans ASAIO 15, 68, 1969.

3. Olsen DB. ISAO International Registry, TAH-bridge to transplant experience; patient status as of June 30, 1987. Latest data periodically published in Artif. Organs or directly available via the Institute of Biomedical Engineering, University of Utah, Salt Lake City, USA.

4. Joyce LD, Pritzker MR, Kiser JC, Nicoloff DM, Kersten TE, von Rueden TJ, Eales F, Jhonson KE, Jorgensen CHR, Gobel FL, van Tassel RA. Use of the mini Jarvik 7 total artificial heart as a bridge to transplantation. J Heart Transplant 5, 203, 1986.

5. Trubel W, Losert U, Schima H, Rokitansky A, Spiss CHK, Coraim F, Laczkowics A, Wolner E. Total artificial heart bridging: a temporary support for deteriorating HTX-candidates. Thorac Cardiovasc Surg 35, 277, 1987.

6. Unger F. Konstruktion und tierexperimentelle Befunde mit einer neuen Form des künstlichen Herzens: Das Ellipsoidherz. Wien Klin Wschr 89/3, Suppl 65, 1977.

7. Akutsu T, Jarvik RK, Zartnack S. Blood pumps, Proc. 2nd world Symp. Artif. Heart; Vol 1 ed. by E Buecherl. In: Adv. System Analysis, Vieweg Verlag, Braunschweig - Wiesbaden, 59, 1986.

8. Rokitansky A, Trubel W, Coraim F, Schima H, Laczkovics A, Mueller MR, Buxbaum P, Schreiner W, Losert U, Haider W, Wolner E. Clinical TAH-bridging in Vienna: haemodynamics and regulation. Artif Organs (in print).

9. Griffith BP, Hardesty RL, Kormos RL, Trento A, Borovetz HS, Thompson ME, Bahnson H. Temporary use of the Jarvik 7 total artificial heart before transplantation. N Engl J Med 316, 130, 1987.

10. Mueller MR, Wohlfahrt A, Lee A, Trubel W, Zilla P, Fasol R, Wolner E. Observations on human thrombocytes during TAH replacement. Artif Organs (in print).

11. Magovern JA, Pennock JL, Campbell DB, Pae WE, Pierce WS, Waldhausen JA. Bridge to heart transplantation. The Penn State experience. J Heart Transplant 5, 196, 1986.

12. Weidemann H. Künstlicher Totalherzersatz - Korrelation klinischer, hämodynamischer und morphologischer Befunde in 4 Entwicklungsphasen 1972-84; Kap. 3, p. 91f: Klinikum Charlottenburg der Freien Universität Berlin, Eigenverlag, 1985.

13. Cole HM. Four years of replacing ailing hearts: Surgeons assess data, questions remain. JAMA 256, 292, 1986.

14. Stelzer GT, Ward RA, Wellhausen SR, McLeish KR, Jhonson GS, De Vries WC. Alterations in select immunologic parameters following total artificial heart implantation. Artif Organs 11, 52, 1987.

2. Artificial Heart

2.5. Skeletal Muscle Ventricles: Preliminary Results and Theoretical Design Considerations

CR Bridges Jr, JS Andersen, WA Anderson, RL Hammond, MA Acker, LW Stephenson

The Harrison Department of Surgical Research, Department of Surgery, University of Pennsylvania, Philadelphia, Pennsylvania, USA

Introduction

Skeletal muscle is capable of transforming chemical energy into mechanical work with an efficiency unparalleled by man-made engines. Recently, there has been considerable interest in the use of skeletal muscle to assist the circulation. This is because of the high mortality of patients who present with irreversible congestive heart failure. Their prognosis has changed little despite advances in medical therapy, cardiac transplantation, and improvements in mechanical assist devices. Autogenous skeletal muscle has several advantages as a source of mechanical energy to assist the failing heart. Since it is autogenous, it does not provoke an immune response. There is no shortage of donors, and no requirement for a cumbersome external power source. In addition, autologous skeletal muscle has the potential for growth which may make it applicable for correction of certain complex congenital cardiac defects.

We have shown that skeletal muscle ventricles (SMVs) or pumping chambers constructed from canine latissimus dorsi muscle are quite capable of continuous cardiac work for periods of up to 11 weeks (1-3). The stroke work of these skeletal muscle ventricles (SMVs) is intermediate between that of the animal's left and right ventricles (1-7). Given the demonstrated feasibility of using skeletal muscle ventricles as cardiac assist devices, we have applied the principles of solid mechanics to develop a detailed mathematical model of the SMV. This model predicts that optimal design of an SMV from a single latissimus dorsi muscle will result in a power output similar to that of the left ventricle.

Historical Perspective

In laboratories worldwide, two approaches have been developed in attempts to utilize skeletal muscle to augment cardiac function. Skeletal muscle grafts have been applied directly to the beating heart in hopes of improving the collateral blood supply to ischemic myocardium, and to bolster cardiac contractile function (8-26).

The other avenue of investigation has been the formation of skeletal muscle pouches or ventricles which provide their own pumping function when stimulated to contract. A number of investigators have constructed pumps from skeletal muscle (27-30), but until the recent work in our laboratory (1-7), these muscle pumps were commonly plagued by the problem of rapid fatigue.

Spotnitz found that pumps constructed from rectus muscle were less compliant than the heart (30). These pouches required unusually high filling pressures of 50 - 160 mmHg to attain peak pressures during contraction. We have noted that the latissimus is also less compliant than cardiac muscle. However, through the application of mathematical modelling to analyze skeletal muscle ventricle mechanics, we show that it should be possible to design efficient pumping chambers with the desired pressure and volume characteristics.

Cardiac and Skeletal Muscle: A Comparison

Both cardiac and skeletal muscle convert chemical energy into mechanical work. Their basic ultrastructure is similar: the longitudinal orientation of the myofibrils, and the basic contractile unit - the sarcomere - is essentially identical in the two types of muscle. Both cell types have an sarcoplasmic reticulum, and similar transverse tubular systems (31).

The differing metabolic demands of skeletal and cardiac muscles, however, dictate differences in the design of these biologic engines. Cardiac muscle must contract rhythmically and relentlessly throughout an entire lifetime without developing fatigue. Skeletal muscle generally is required to perform mechanical work for relatively short periods of time, with intervening periods of rest. Cardiac muscle has a highly developed aerobic metabolism, and the cardiac cell contains approximately 30% mitochondria by volume (sceletal muscle from 2 to 5%; 31). Mitochondria are the organelles primarily responsible for replenishing ATP via oxidative phosphorylation.

Cardiac muscle functions as an electrical syncytium since current flows between cells. Intercalated disks are thought to facilitate the flow of current. This accounts for the nearly simultaneous contraction of all cardiac muscle cells, as well as the "all or none" response of the heart to electrical stimulation. Skeletal muscle cells are organized into motor units, each containing its own nerve endings. A given stimulus applied to the motor nerve may be sufficient for the contraction of some, all, or none of the motor units. The strength of contraction is dependent upon the number and rate of fiber recruitment.

Therefore, while stimulation of the heart via direct muscle electrodes is relatively simple, optimal stimulation of skeletal muscles via their motor nerves is complex. A single muscle twitch generated by a single electrical stimulus does not yield optimal power generation for cardiac type work. The work of Chiu, Dewar and associates (16,32), and our own laboratory (1-4), indicates that burst stimulation leads to mechanical summation and generation of substantially greater force. The parameters that define burst stimulation are burst frequency, pulse duration, pulse amplitude, and burst duration. For a given muscle, these parameters govern the force and duration of contraction. Investigators in our laboratory and others have shown that chronic burst stimulation does not generally cause muscle or nerve damage (1,2,32-37).

Skeletal muscle cells, in contrast to relatively uniform cardiac muscle cells,

2. Artificial Heart

can be divided into two basic types. Slow or type I fibers, like cardiac muscle cells, are relatively fatigue resistant. They utilize aerobic metabolism even during prolonged periods of stimulation, possess a large mitochondrial volume, a relatively small sarcoplasmic reticulum, and a specific complement of "slow" isoforms of myosin and other contractile proteins. Muscles composed of primarily type I fibers are usually postural in function. Type II fibers are characterized by brisk tension development, aerobic metabolism during rest, and rapid conversion to glycolytic metabolism, even during brief exercise periods. They have an extensive sarcoplasmic reticulum, a small mitochondrial volume, and an analogous complement of "fast" isoforms of myosin and other contractile proteins. Typical predominantly fast muscles, such as the extraocular muscles, are ideally adapted for intense episodic activity, but fatigue rapidly (31). The muscles that have been used for cardiac augmentation including the diaphragm, rectus, pectoralis, and latissimus, of which all are mixed fiber type muscles.

Skeletal Muscle Conditioning

The relationship between training (or *conditioning*) and fatigue resistance of skeletal muscle is well-known to the endurance athlete. Similarly, fatigue resistance skeletal muscle used for augmentation or replacement of myocardium has been achieved through extensive work in the area of electrical conditioning (33,38-53). The inherent plasticity of skeletal muscle has a biochemical and ultrastructural basis. In 1960, Buller et al anastomosed the motor nerve of a fast-twitch muscle to the motor nerve of a slow-twitch muscle and vice versa. Eventually after the terminal axons regenerated, each muscle was transformed to the opposite type (54). In 1969, Salmons and Vrbova determined that it was actually the pattern of stimulation of the motor nerve which governed the muscle fiber type (52). When a fast-twitch muscle was stimulated for several weeks at 10 hz, the fibers were converted to slow, type I fibers. These transformed, fatigue-resistant fibers more closely resemble cardiac muscle fibers than ordinary type I fibers (Table 28), both in terms of mitochondrial content and oxidative enzyme complements (51,53,55).

The sequential changes in skeletal muscle in response to chronic low frequency stimulation begin with an increase in capillary density in the first week. In the second week, there is an increase in the volume fraction of mitochondria, an increase in oxidative enzymes, and a reciprocal decrease in glycolytic enzymes. By three weeks time, there is a marked reduction in the calcium transport ATPase activity of the sarcoplasmic reticulum. By six to eight weeks, histochemical myosin ATPase stains indicate a complete transformation of the type II fiber to a type I fiber (51,53,56).

Working in our laboratory, Macoviak et al showed that direct electrical conditioning of canine diaphragm at 10 Hz for five weeks resulted in a nearly complete transition to a uniform population of type I fatigue-resistant fibers (46). Armenti et al showed that a similar fiber type transformation could be achieved by stimulation of the diaphragm via the phrenic nerve at 2 Hz, a frequency similar to the dog's own heart rate (41). Acker et al showed near complete transformation of latissimus

Comparison of Enzyme Activities (mol/kg/hr)

Enzyme	Fast-Twitch	Slow-Twitch	Myocardium	Conditioned
Glycolytic				
PFK	31	3	6	6
LDH	208	52	30	47
Phosporylase	30	4	2	5
GS	0.5	0.4	0.2	0.4
Oxidative				
MDH	8	14	36	42
Citrate Synthase	3	4	16	18
BOAC	2	6	18	20
Hexokinase	0.2	0.4	1.3	2.4

Table 28 Glycolytic and oxidative enzyme activities of canine skeletal muscle are altered during electrical conditioning. Comparison of a fast-twitch muscle (tibialis anterior) with electrically conditioned muscle (conditioned tibialis anterior), slow-twitch muscle (soleus) and myocardium reveal the transformation that occurs. There is a reduction in the enzyme activity of glycolytic pathway and a concomitant increase in the enzyme activity of oxidative pathways. The enzyme activities of conditioned fast-twitch skeletal muscle and slow-twitch skeletal muscle are similar to those of cardiac muscle. PFK, 6-phosphofructokinase; LDH, lactate dehydrogenase; GS, glycogen synthase; MDH, malate dehydroegnase; BOAC, B-hydroxyacyl CoA dehydrogenase (see reference #55 for myocardial enzyme activity). We thank Dr Patti M Nemeth from the Dept of Neurology, Washington University School of Medicine, St Louis, Missouri, for providing enzyme activity for fast-twitch, slow-twitch and conditional skeletal muscle.

dorsi muscles after several weeks of stimulation using a 25 Hz burst frequency (312 msec ON, 812 msec OFF) (2). In these experiments, the latissimus dorsi muscle was configured as a skeletal muscle ventricle (SMV). These SMVs were conditioned while simultaneously performing stroke work intermediate between that of the left and right ventricles for up to nine weeks.

Acker and Clark (39) from our laboratory have studied the bioenergetics of skeletal muscle using phosphorus nuclear magnetic resonance. Both electrically conditioned and contralateral control muscle were studied during vigorous exercise tests. For control muscles, the tension-time index reached a plateau level while Pi/PCr continued to increase. In contrast, the increase in Pi/PCr was relatively small for the conditioned muscle. Even when the conditioned muscle was being stimulated at 25 Hz for 800 ms of every 1100 ms cycle, there was no evidence that a plateau level had been reached. These studies indicated that the conditioned muscle had a capacity for oxidative phosphorylation which rivalled that of the heart itself,

2. Artificial Heart

while the non-conditioned muscle fatigued rapidly (Figures 81a, 81b).

In a complementary study (40), oxygen consumption was studied in electrically conditioned and contralateral control muscle during a similar vigorous exercise test. This study showed that transformed muscle is also more efficient than control muscle. Conditioned muscle generates as much internal work as control muscle, or more, while consuming less oxygen per gram of tissue. Isometric tension is maintained by turnover of actin-myosin cross-bridges without relative movement of the filaments. The rate at which these cross-bridges cycle determines the energy cost for the maintenance of tension. The fact that cross-bridge cycling is more rapid in fast muscle than in slow muscle reflects differences between the rates of ATP hydrolysis of the fast and slow isoforms of myosin (57,58). Since the conditioned muscle in these experiments were homogeneously slow, a given isometric tension could be maintained at the expense of less ATP hydrolyzed. It seems, therefore, that less oxygen should be consumed by the electrically conditioned muscle for the same amount of isometric tension developped. Therefore, increased fatigue-resistance of conditioned muscle is a result of its increased capacity for oxidative phosphorylation and its greater efficiency of oxygen utilization.

The above biochemical, ultrastructural and mechanical adaptations to chronic electrical stimulation, are also accompanied by an approximately 30% reduction in fiber size and peak tetanic tension development (47,51, 53). In addition, there is a variable degree of accumulation of intracellular

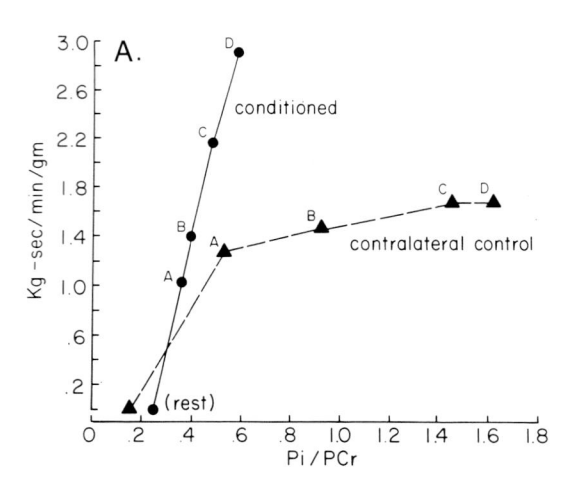

Fig. 81 a) Graph combining the results of physiological and ^{31}P-NMR spectroscopic measurements for control and conditioned muscles. The tension-time index (kg-sec x min^{-1} x g^{-1}) is plotted against Pi/PCr, calculated from NMR spectra. Pi is inorganic phosphate and PCr is phosphocreatine. Points A through D correspond to increasing duration of burst stimulation at 25 Hz for 200, 300, 500 and 800 msec of an 1100 msec duty cycle, respectively.

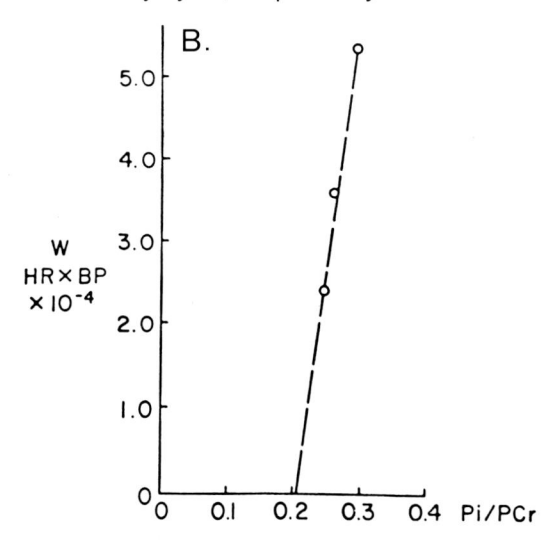

Fig. 81 b) Pi/PCr vs. heart rate blood pressure product (W) for the canine left ventricle. (We thank Dr BJ Clark of Children's Hospital of Philadelphia for this figure.)

connective tissue in muscles subjected to chronic electrical stimulation. These potentially adverse responses to conditioning - if progressive - would limit the long-term utility of skeletal muscle as a myocardial substitute. To investigate this possibility, Acker et al stimulated canine diaphragm at 2 Hz or 4 Hz for one year (38). At the termination of this study, there was no evidence of muscle damage, and the fiber size and intracellular connective tissue density reached a stable equilibrium by about six weeks.

Skeletal Muscle Ventricles

The latissimus dorsi is frequently used for cardiac assistance since it is large, supplied by a single motor nerve, and in close proximity to the heart. As discussed above, previous attempts to use skeletal muscle to construct skeletal muscle ventricles (SMVs) were typically characterized by initial success followed by muscle fatigue, often within minutes (13-16,29,30,59).

SMV Construction

Our current technique for construction of SMVs requires a flank incision with ligation and division of the collateral blood vessels to the latissimus (1-7). The muscle is completely mobilized from its attachments so that only the thoracodorsal nerve artery and vein connect the muscle to the body of the dog as illustrated in Figure 82. The muscle is then wrapped around a Teflon mandrel of a given size and shape, and sutured to a felt collar attached to the mandrel. Construction of SMVs of a variety of shapes using this technique is demonstrated in Figure 83. A specially modified Medtronic electrode is placed around the proximal thoracodorsal nerve and connected to a permanent implantable pacemaker.

Although the neurovascular pedicle supplies adequate circulation to prevent muscle necrosis, division of the collateral blood supply during ventricle construction renders the canine latissimus dorsi muscle ischemic, and ablates the exercise-induced increase in blood flow. A three-week vascular delay period, however, allows recovery of normal resting and exercise-induced blood flow (4,34). The combination of both a vascular delay and electrical preconditioning allows construction of fatigue-resistant

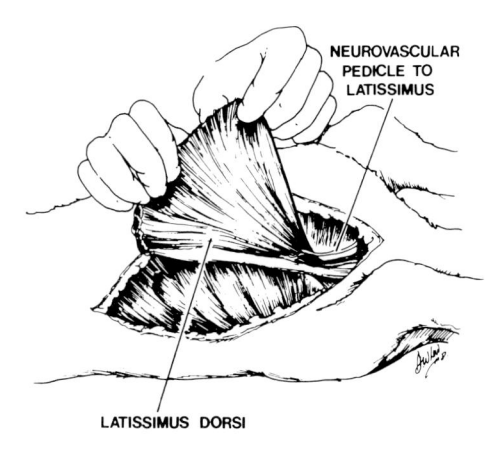

Fig. 82 The mobilized canine latissimus dorsi muscle, attached by the neurovascular pedicle containing the thoracodorsal artery vein and nerve.

SMVs (4). Using labelled microspheres, we have demonstrated that all layers of the SMV receive substantial blood flow while the ventricles are pumping in the circulation (5).

Skeletal Muscle Ventricles in Mock Circulation

In earlier studies, SMVs were constructed as described above using a 17cc cone-shaped mandrel. These SMVs underwent a three-week vascular delay period followed by six weeks of electrical preconditioning. The SMVs were then connected to a totally im-

2. Artificial Heart

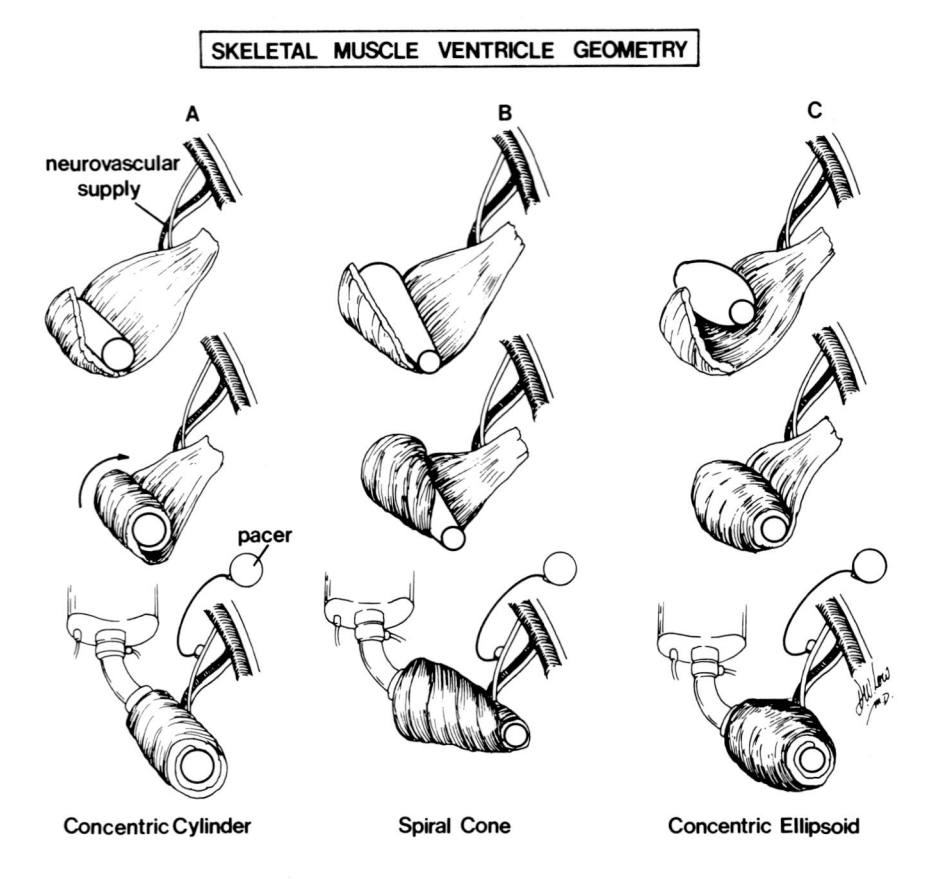

Fig. 83 Skeletal muscle ventricle (SMV) geometry. Three possible configurations for SMV design are illustrated.

plantable mock circulation device developed by Acker and Hammond (1). This device allowed control of both preload and afterload, and measurement of SMV output. No wires or tubes crossed the animals' skin barrier. The animals were able to move about freely with no apparent discomfort or physical impairment. The muscles were stimulated via the thoracodorsal nerve with a 25 Hz burst frequency (312 msec ON, 812 msec OFF), resulting in 54 contractions per minute. These SMVs pumped continuously against an afterload of 80 mmHg with a preload of 40 to 50 mmHg. At the initiation of pumping, mean systolic pressure was 134 mmHg, and flow was 464 ml/min. After two weeks of continuous pumping, systolic pressure was 104 mmHg and flow was 206 ml/min.

Two SMVs pumped for five and nine weeks respectively.

In a subsequent study (2), SMVs were constructed with a vascular delay period, but without preconditioning. These SMVs were connected to the mock circulation system and stimulated via the thoracodorsal nerve at a 25 Hz burst frequency, as in the previous study. Preload and afterload were again set at 40 mmHg and 80 mmHg, respectively. After two weeks of continuous pumping, the mean stroke work of the SMVs was 0.4×10^6 ergs. The stroke work of these SMVs, as shown in Figure 84, was intermediate between that of the canine left and right ventricles. Two dogs continued to produce significant stroke work after two months. Stevens and Brown have also measured similar

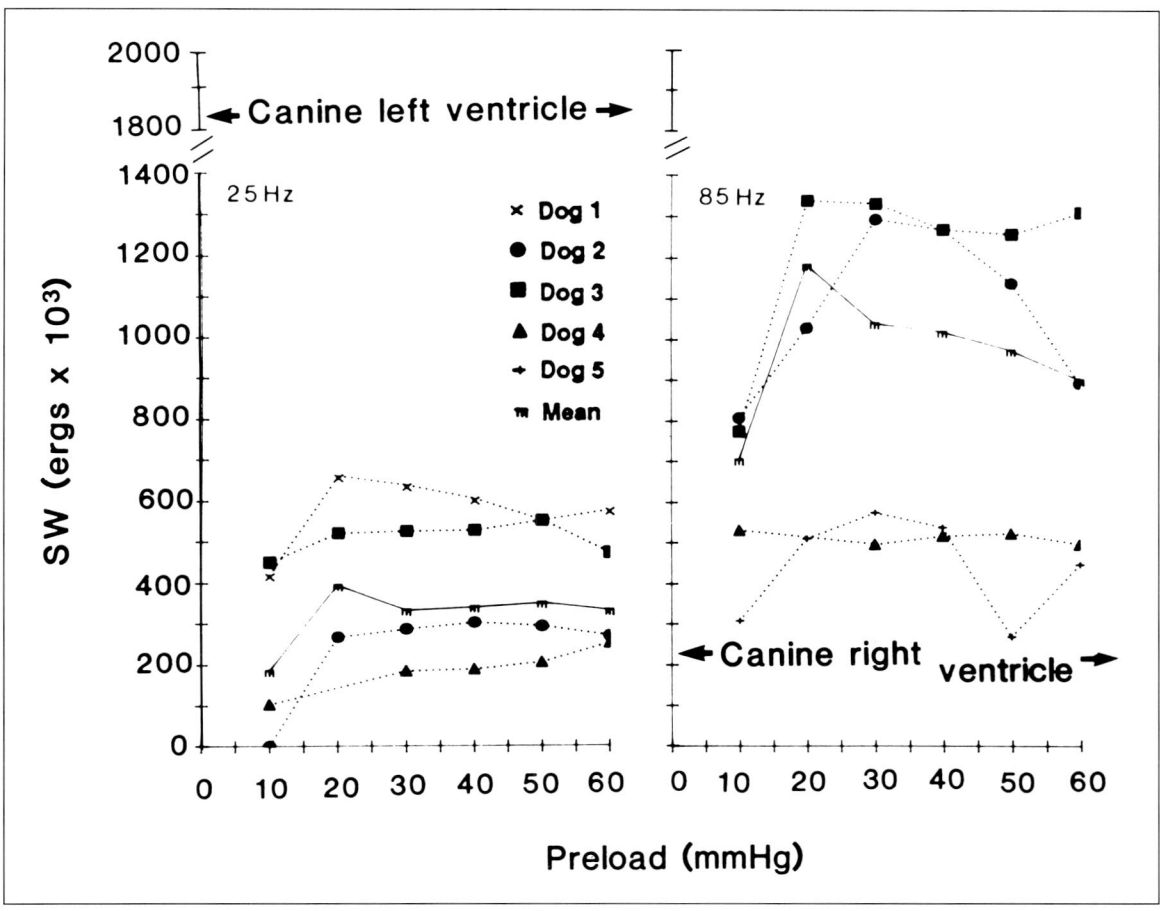

Fig. 84 Stroke work (SW) plotted against preload (filling pressure) for SMVs of five dogs after two weeks. Values are intermediate between the stroke work of the canine left and right ventricles.

heart and SMV work outputs using canine rectus abdominus muscle (60).

Skeletal Muscle Ventricles as Arterial Diastolic Counterpulsators

Working in our laboratory, Mannion et al showed that SMVs constructed in this fashion were able to function in the circulation for up to fourteen hours as diastolic counterpulsators in the descending aorta (7). Properly conditioned muscles with a vascular delay were generally functioning well for many hours. SMV function eventually deteriorated, however, due to anemia, hypoxia, hypotension, and other complications inherent in prolonged acute experiments of this type. The stroke work of these SMVs was 0.68×10^6 ergs after four hours, roughly three times the stroke work of the right ventricle and nearly one half the left ventricular stroke work. These acute studies documented the ability of an SMV to do useful work in the circulation, while the mock circulation studies demonstrated the ability of SMVs to function for up to two months pumping against physiological afterloads. Neilson and associates showed an improvement in the subendocardial viability ratio during acute studies when SMVs were used in circulation as diastolic counterpulsators (32,61). Taken together, these studies suggested that a chronic circulatory as-

2. Artificial Heart

sist device could be constructed from skeletal muscle.

Acker et al (3) subsequently constructed skeletal muscle tube ventricles (SMTVs) in five mongrel dogs. The SMTV differed from the ventricles constructed in previous experiments, since these ventricles had a cylindrical geometry with both inflow and outflow conduits as depicted in Figure 85. The SMTVs functioned chronically in the circulation as diastolic counterpulsators. The SMTVs were connected to the systemic circulation after a three to four week vascular delay period but without electrical preconditioning. The SMTVs were stimulated to contract during diastole, generally with a synchronization ratio of 1 : 2 or 1 : 3, depending on the heart rate. A totally implantable Medtronics pacemaker was used to stimulate the SMTVs via the thoracodorsal nerve. This pacemaker delivered burst stimuli at 25 Hz to 85 Hz, with a burst duration of 185 to 240 msec and a 240 msec delay from the onset of the R-wave. These animals were tether-free in that no tubes or wires crossed the skin. They moved about freely with no apparent discomfort or impairment.

Two-dimensional short axis echocardiograms of the SMTV obtained from one dog after twelve days of continuous counterpulsation are shown in Figure 86. During these measurements, the burst frequency was altered from the chronic setting of 25 Hz to 43 Hz and 85 Hz. These echocardiograms demonstrate a 70%, 90%, and 100% decrease in cross-sectional area at the midpoint of the SMTV at 25 Hz, 43 Hz, and 85 Hz, respectively, during SMTV contraction. Pulsed Doppler blood flow measurements just distal to the outlet end of the SMTV during a normal cardiac cycle were compared with those during an as-

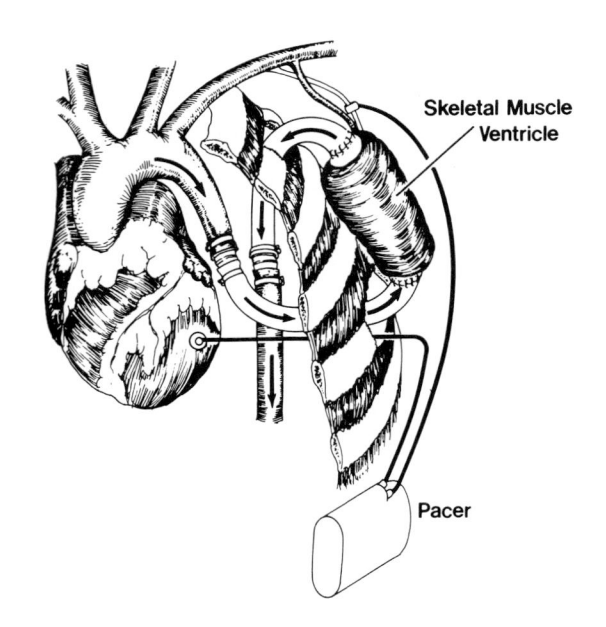

Fig. 85 Skeletal muscle tube ventricle (SMTV) interposed into the descending aorta for use as a diastolic arterial counterpulsator. Pacemaker stimulating electrode is connected to the thoracodorsal nerve and the sensing electrode to the left ventricle.

sisted cardiac cycle (SMTV contraction). The forward blood flow was 29%, 40%, and 63% greater during the assisted cardiac cycle than during the unassisted normal cycle at 25, 43, and 85 Hz, respectively. Arterial pressure tracings obtained from the same dog after 14 days of continuous pumping at these burst frequencies are shown in Figure 87.

These SMTVs functioned in circulation for up to 11 weeks. In all animals, the SMTV was functioning well up until termination. The two longest survivors, 5 weeks and 11 weeks respectively, both died due to complications of renal failure. Autopsy demonstrated multiple renal and splenic infarcts, without evidence of cerebrovascular or coronary thromboembolic disease. Despite these complications, this study demonstrated for the first time that skeletal muscle could perform significant circulatory assistance for several weeks.

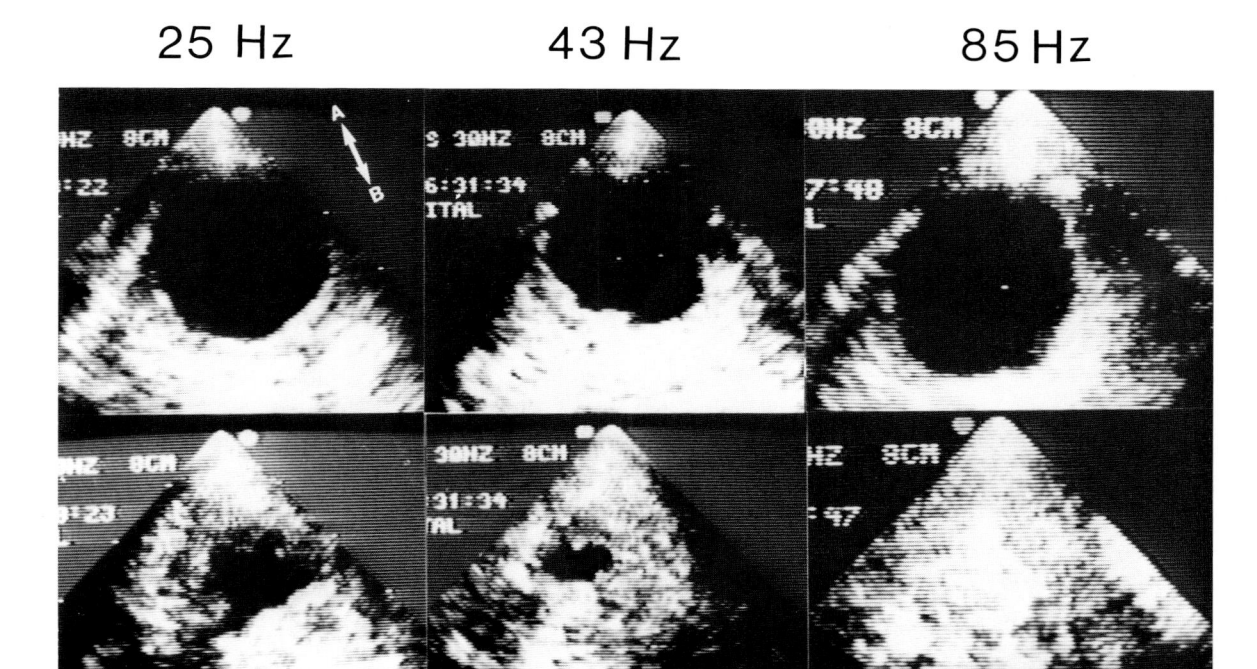

Fig. 86 Two-dimensional echocardiogram, short axis view, of midpoint of SMTV obtained from one dog on postoperative day 12. Top row illustrates the cross-sectional area at enddiastole. Bottom row illustrates the cross-sectional area during contraction. Increasing the burst frequency(25 Hz, 43 Hz, 85 Hz) leads to increasing ejection fraction.

Right Ventricular Replacement

Our previous mock circulation studies have used a preload of 40 mmHg chronically (1,2). Similarly, SMTVs functioning as aortic counterpulsators have a high preload - equal to aortic diastolic pressure. Using mathematical modelling techniques described below, we redesigned SMVs for potential performance as right ventricular replacements, with preloads of only 10 to 20 mmHg. These SMVs (unpublished data) were able to exceed right ventricular power output at low preloads for up to several weeks. Macoviak et al have used preconditioned SMTVs to pump blood for hours in the right-sided circulation (62). In a pilot experiment, we constructed an SMV acutely, and using valved Gortex conduits, anastomosed this device to the right atrial appendage (inflow), and to the proximal pulmonary artery (outflow). Right ventricular outflow was excluded, using an umbilical tape placed around the pulmonary artery proximal to the entrance of the SMV conduit. Right ventricular inflow was excluded using a 30 cc Foley catheter balloon, placed through the right atrium, and pulled retrograde against the tricuspid valve. The results are summarized in Figure 88.

Mechanics of Skeletal Muscle; Modelling and Design

Despite the constraints of muscle orientation, neural innervation, and blood supply, a substantial degree of freedom exists in the specification of the ventricle geometry for SMVs constructed from a single latissimus dorsi muscle. As illustrated in Figure 83, SMVs can be constructed as cylinders,

2. Artificial Heart

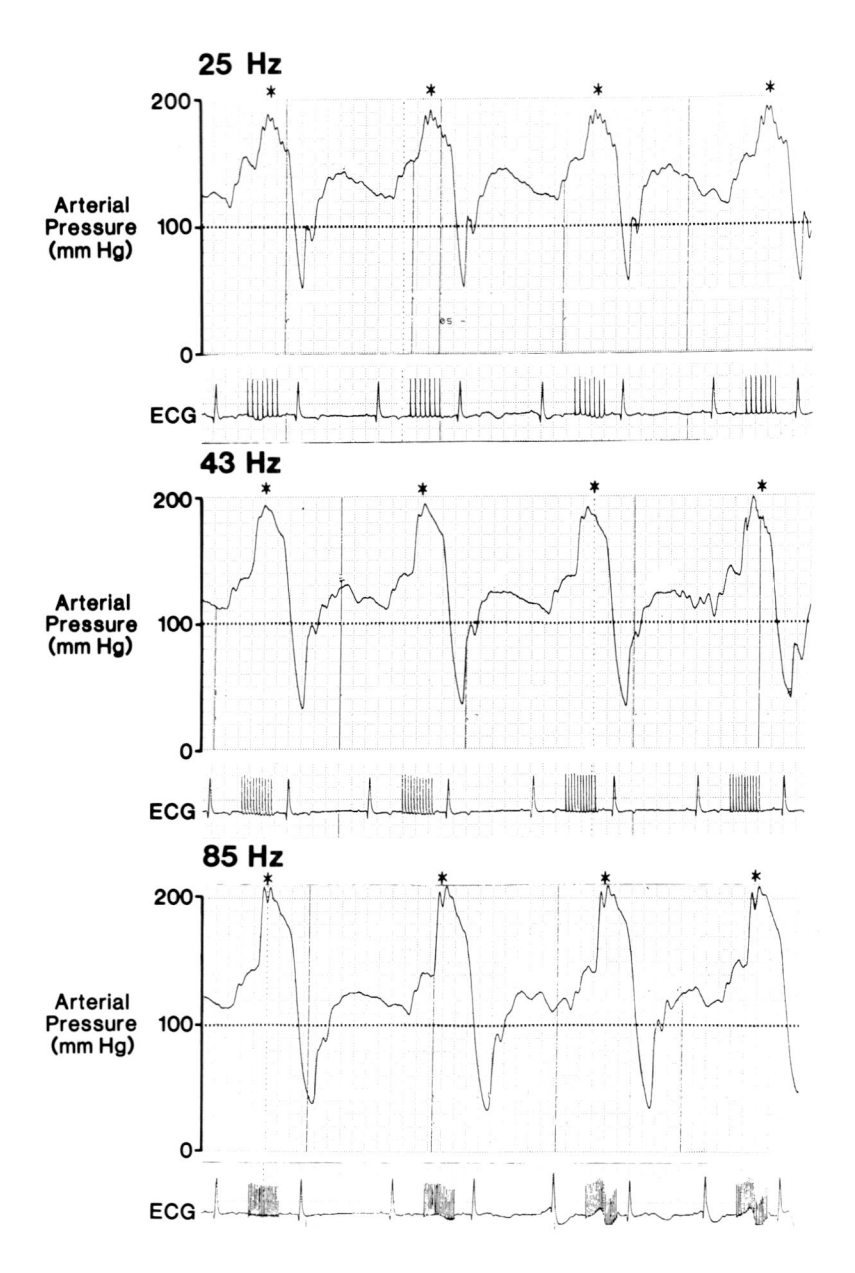

Fig. 87 Distal aortic pressure and electrocardiogram tracings in the same dog as in Figure 6 on postoperative day 14 at burst frequencies of 25 Hz, 43 Hz and 85 Hz. Diastolic augmentation of 130 mmHg occurs at 85 Hz burst frequency. (*) indicates diastolic augmentation. Note corresponding superimposed burst pattern on electrocardiogram.

cones, ellipses or spheres of a variety of sizes, depending on the number of muscle wraps employed, and depending on the geometry of the mandrel around which the muscle is wrapped. Optimal ventricle design varies as a function of the preload and afterload at which the ventricle will be expected to function. Ventricles designed to function as aortic counterpulsators, left atrial-to-systemic left ventricular assist devices, and right ventricular replacements are likely to have different optimal geometries. We present here the first attempt to develop a detailed theoretical model of the SMV based on the principles of large deformation elasticity theory. Using an alternative ap-

2. Artificial Heart

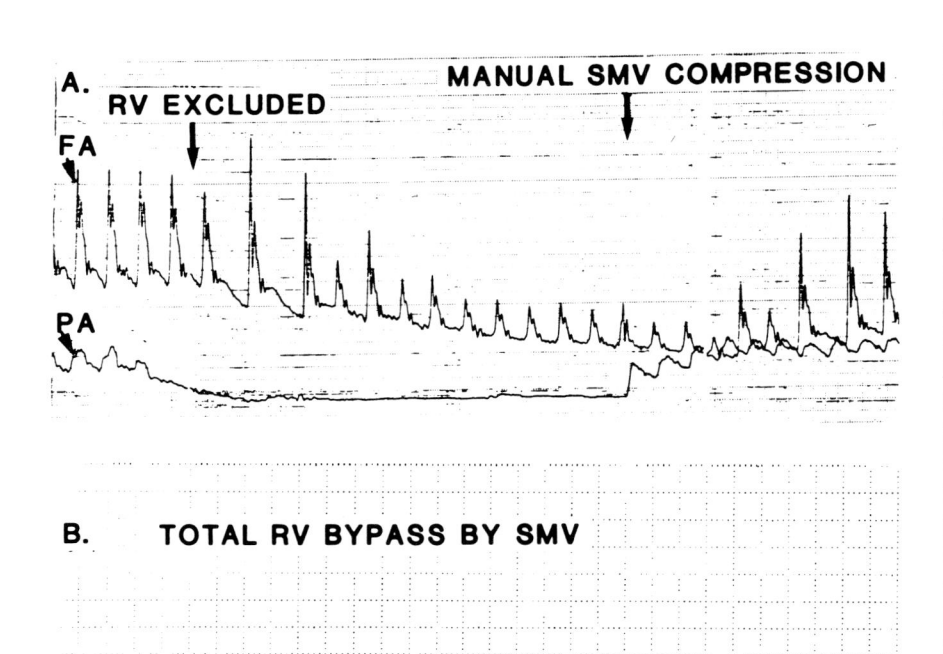

Fig. 88
Right ventricular (RV) bypass with skeletal muscle ventricle (SMV). FA = femoral artery, PA = pulmonary artery. Panel A illustrates RV exclusion and corresponding fall in arterial pressure. Arterial pressure is restored by manual compression of the SMV. Panel B illustrates maintenance of arterial pressure using the SMV for total bypass of the right ventricle (25 Hz burst frequency, contraction rate = 54/min).

proach, Khalafalla has also applied quantitative methods to SMV design (63).

We model the SMV here as a thick-walled axisymmetric structure. The fiber orientation is assumed to be concentric, and therefore the strain in the meridional direction is ignored. The material is assumed to be homogeneous and incompressible. Based on our observations of cineangiograms of pumping SMVs, the assumption that meridional strain is negligible is a reasonable first approximation. The model is similar to the thick-walled axisymmetric model derived by Janz et al (64) for the left ventricle. The model derived here allows calculation of pressure as a function of the elastic parameters U_p, and K_p (passive stress), and U_s (active stress), for a given volume. The wall volume V_w and the resting volume V_o (volume at zero pressure in diastole) must be known. V_o is estimated by the volume of the mandrel used to construct the SMV. By constructing SMVs of known V_w, V_o, and experimentally measuring isovolumetric passive and active pressure-volume curves, the coefficients U_p, U_s, and K_p are estimated using a curve-fitting routine.

The diastolic pressure (P_d) and systolic pressure (P_s) are calculated as follows (see Appendix). The notation used here is similar to that of Bogen et al (65).

2. Artificial Heart

$$P_d = -\int_{a'}^{b'} \frac{U_p(\lambda^{-K_p} - \lambda^{K_p})d\lambda}{\lambda(1-\lambda^2)} \quad (1)$$

$$P_s = -\int_{\lambda_c a''}^{b''} \frac{U_s(\lambda^{-2} - \lambda^2)d\lambda}{\lambda(1-\lambda^2)} + P_d \quad (2)$$

where

$$b' = \sqrt{\frac{V + V_w}{V_0 + V_w}} \quad (3)$$

$$a' = \sqrt{\frac{V}{V_0}} \quad (4)$$

$$b'' = \sqrt{\frac{V + V_w}{\lambda_c^{-2} V_0 + V_w}} \quad (5)$$

tracted sarcomere length, and is typically ~ 1.18 for cardiac muscle (66,67). Volume is $V_0/(\lambda_c)^2$. λ is the extension or deformed length/resting length in the circumferential direction. V_0 is the diastolic resting volume. The ventricular wall volume V_w is measured for each SMV. The resting volume V_0 is approximated by the volume of the mandrel used to construct the SMV.

The parameters U_p, K_p (passive); and U_s, λ_c (active) completely describe the mechanical properties of the SMV using this model. Given these parameters, and the values for V_0 and V_w, equations (1-5) allow calculation of theoretical isovolumetric pressure-volume curves in systole and diastole. Using the equation (A7, Appendix) the model can also be used to calculate stress throughout the thickness of the SMV wall. Note that though explicitly derived for a thick-walled cylinder (see Appendix) these equations are valid for an arbitrarily shaped axisymmetric ventricle with negligible meridional strain.

The parameters U_p, K_p, U_s, and λ_c were estimated using a curve fitting procedure as described above. Experimental systolic and diastolic isovolumetric pressure-volume curves were measured in three dogs with conical SMVs after 1-3 weeks of continuous electrical stimulation at 25 Hz burst frequency. In all three cases, there was an excellent fit between the theoretical and experimental isovolumetric pressure-volume curves. The mean estimated values of the parameters were $K_p = 21.2$, $\lambda_c = 1.25$, $U_s = 370$ mmHg, and a reliable estimate of U_p could not be obtained. Of note, Janz and Waldron found the estimated value of U_p to be unreliable using a thick-walled spherical model, applied to the human left ventricle (68). The value of K_p estimated here is somewhat higher than estimated here is somewhat higher than the values estimated previously for cardiac muscle. Janz and Waldron (68) and Rabinowitz (69), using a similar approach, found $K_p = 14.9$ for the human left ventricle and $K_p = 16$ for the canine left ventricle, respectively. In rabbit papillary muscle, Mirsky et al (70) found $K_p = 18$. The value of U_s for the SMV is also higher than the value of 151.9 mmHg estimated by Bogen et al (65) for the human left ventricle.

Given these parameters, we investigated the effect of altering the resting volume of the SMV on SMV stroke volume. Figure 89 demonstrates the SMV output for an SMV constructed from a latissimus dorsi muscle with a mass of 100 gm - typical for a 15 kg dog. In addition, an afterload of 80 mmHg and a preload of 20 mmHg are assumed. Values of $K_p = 25.4$, $\lambda_c = 1.35$, $U_s = 410$ mmHg, and $U_p = 7.7$ mmHg obtained from one dog are used in these calculations. The SMV output is calculated assuming a contraction rate of 54 beats per minute. A clear maximum in the predicted SMV output is demonstrated for an SMV constructed using a mandrel with a volume of approximately 50 ml. The theoretical SMV output for this SMV, 850 ml/min, is more than twice the 400 ml/min output, of an SMV constructed from a 17 ml mandrel. Since our previous studies have generally employed a mandrel size of 17 ml (1,2), it is likely that optimization of SMV design may result in a doubling of SMV stroke work. These results suggest that the SMV is somewhat less compliant than the left ventricles in diastole, but that its ability to generate pressure in systole is several fold greater than an equal mass of left ventricular muscle.

In summary, a great deal of progress has been made in the application of skeletal muscle to assist the circulation. Major and formidable obstacles such as muscle fatigue and ischemia have been largely overcome. SMVs have been useful in circulation as diastolic counterpulsators for up to 11 weeks. A quantitative approach to the design of skeletal muscle ventricles using the principles of solid mechanics and mathematical modelling is likely to lead to substantial improvements in mechanical pumping efficiency. There are still some questions, however, that need to be answered before we can determine if SMVs will become clinically useful. How long can the SMVs function effectively as blood pumps? What methods will be best for coupling SMVs with the systemic and pulmonary circulation? Perhaps we can avoid the thrombo-embolic complications of blood-surface interactions that have plagued the artificial heart. Since skeletal muscle has such an abundant blood supply, it is likely that a layer of endothelial cells would find its surface a friendly and desirable environment.

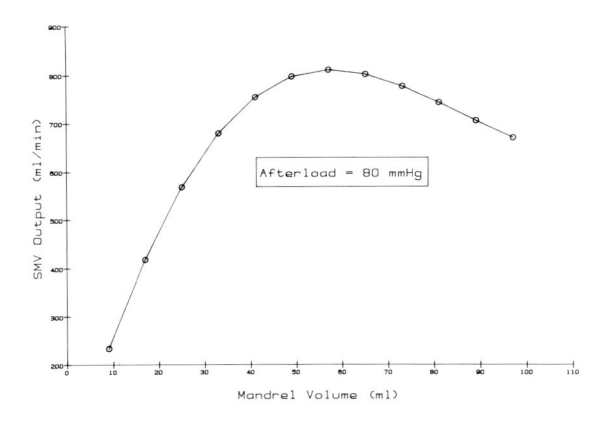

Fig. 89 Theoretical SMV output for a conical SMV, as a function of the resting volume (mandrel volume) for an SMV constructed from a 100 gram latissimus dorsi muscle. SMV output = stroke volume x 54 contractions per minute.

2. Artificial Heart

Appendix

Derivation of the Thick-Walled Cylindrical Model of the SMV

The equation of equilibrium for a thick-walled cylinder is expressed as

$$\frac{d\sigma_r}{dr} + \frac{(\sigma_r - \sigma_\theta)}{r} = 0 \tag{A1}$$

where σ_r is the radially directed stress and σ_θ is the circumferential stress. Integration of this equation results in an expression for σ_r:

$$\sigma_r(r) = -\int_a^r (\sigma_r - \sigma_\theta)\left(\frac{d\xi}{\xi}\right) + \sigma_r(a) \tag{A2}$$

The pressure gradient across the wall is equal to the difference in radial stresses

$$\Delta P = P_{in} - P_{out} = \sigma_r(b) - \sigma_r(a)$$

$$\Delta P - \int_a^b (\sigma_r - \sigma_\theta)\left(\frac{d\xi}{\xi}\right) \tag{A3}$$

where a is the inner radius and b is the outer radius of the cylinder. Let λ_θ be the extension in the radial direction and λ_θ the extension (length/undeformed length) in the circumferential direction. Incompressibility implies $\lambda_r \lambda_\theta = 1$ (no meridional strain) and if r is defined as the deformed radial coordinate and r_0 defined as the undeformed radial coordinate, then

$$\lambda_r = \frac{dr}{dr_0} \quad \text{and} \quad \lambda_\theta = \frac{r}{r_0}$$

Using this change of variables in equation (A3) the following expression for ΔP is derived:

$$\Delta P = -\int_{a'}^{b'} \frac{(\sigma_r - \sigma_\theta)d\lambda}{\lambda(1 - \lambda^2)} \tag{A4}$$

where

$$a' = \sqrt{\frac{V}{V_0}} \tag{A5}$$

and

$$b' = \sqrt{\frac{V + V_w}{V_0 + V_w}} \tag{A6}$$

2. Artificial Heart

V_0 is the undeformed volume in diastole and V_w is the wall volume. If a strain energy function of the form assumed by Ogden (71) is assumed, then

$$\sigma_r - \sigma_\theta = U_p\left(\lambda^{-K_p} - \lambda^{K_p}\right) \tag{A7}$$

If K_p and U_p are elastic constants describing mechanical properties of SMV muscle in diastole.

$$P_d = -\int_{a'}^{b'} \frac{U_p(\lambda^{-K_p} - \lambda^{K_p})d\lambda}{\lambda(1-\lambda^2)} \tag{A8}$$

$$P_s = -\int_{a'\lambda_c}^{b''} \frac{U_s(\lambda^{-2} - \lambda^2)d\lambda}{\lambda(1-\lambda^2)} + P_d \tag{A9}$$

$$\text{active} \qquad\qquad \text{passive}$$

where λ_c is the the ratio of the rest length of muscle fibers in diastole to the rest length in systole.

$$b'' = \sqrt{\frac{V + V_w}{\lambda_c^{-2}V_0 + V_w}} \tag{A10}$$

This result is equivalent to specifying $\lambda_c^{-2}V_0$ as the resting volume in systole. Note that the systolic pressure is the sum of active and passive components. U_s and K_s are the elastic constants describing SMV muscle in systole.

Finally, the value $K_s = 2$ is assumed. This is equivalent to assuming that the stress-strain relationship is linear, see Ogden (71), for active stress generation in the region of interest as has been shown for papillary muscle and over a physiological range of extensions (66). Therefore

$$P_s = -\int_{a'\lambda_c}^{b''} \frac{U_s(\lambda^{-K_s} - \lambda^{K_s})d\lambda}{\lambda(1-\lambda^2)} + P_d \tag{A11}$$

The SMV is completely characterized by knowledge of V_w, V_0, U_s, U_p, K_p and λ_c.

2. Artificial Heart

References

1. Acker MA, Hammond RL, Mannion JD, Salmons S, Stephenson LW. An autologous biologic pump motor. J Thorac Cardiovasc Surg 92, 733, 1986.

2. Acker MA, Hammond RL, Mannion JD, Salmons S, Stephenson LW. Skeletal muscle as a potential power source for a cardiovascular pump: assessment in vivo. Science 236, 324, 1987.

3. Acker MA, Anderson WA, Hammond RL, Chin AJ, Buchanan JW, Morse CC, Kelly AM, Stephenson LW. Skeletal muscle ventricles in circulation: one to eleven weeks experience. J Thorac Cardiovasc Surg 94, 163, 1987.

4. Mannion JD, Hammond RL, Stephenson LW. Canine latissimus dorsi hydraulic pouches. Potential for left ventricular assistance. J Thorac Cardiovasc Surg 91, 534, 1986.

5. Mannion JD, Velchik MA, Acker M, Hammond R, Staum M, Duckett S, Stephenson LW. Transmural blood flow of multilayered latissimus dorsi skeletal muscle ventricles during circulatory assistance. Trans Am Soc Artif Intern Organs 32, 454, 1986.

6. Mannion JD, Acker MA, Hammond RL, Stephenson LW. Four-hour circulatory assistance with canine skeletal muscle ventricles. Surg Forum 37, 211, 1986.

7. Mannion JD, Acker MA, Hammond RL, Faltemeyer W, Duckett S, Stephenson LW. Power output of skeletal muscle ventricles in circulation: short term studies. Circulation 76, 155, 1987.

8. Leriche R, Fontaine R. Essai experimental de traitement de certains infarctus du myocarde et de l'aneuvrisme du cœur par une greffe de muscle strie. bull Soc Nat Chir 59, 229, 1933.

9. Beck CS. A new blood supply to the heart by operation. Surg Gynec & Obstet 61, 407, 1935.

10. Petrovsky BV. The use of the diaphragm grafts for plastic operations in thoracic surgery. J Thorac Cardiovasc Surg 41, 348, 1961.

11. Petrovsky BV. Surgical treatment of cardiac aneurysms. J Cardiovasc Surg 2, 87, 1966.

12. Sola OM, Dillard DH, Ivey TD, Haneda K, Itoh T, Thomas R. Autotransplantation of skeletal muscle into myocardium. Circulation 71, 341, 1985.

13. Kantrowitz A, McKinnon W. The experimental use of the diaphragm as an auxiliary myocardium. Surg Forum 9, 266, 1959.

14. Kusaba E, Schraut W, Sawatani S, Jaron D, Freed P, Kantrowitz A. A diaphragmatic graft for augmenting left ventricular function: a feasibility study. Trans Am Soc Artif Intern Organs 19, 251, 1973.

15. Termet H, Chalencon JL, Estour E, Gaillard P, Favre JP. Transplantation sur le myocarde d'un muscle strie excite par pacemaker. Ann Chir Thor Cardio 5, 260, 1966.

16. Dewar ML, Drinkwater DC, Wittnich C, Chiu RCJ. Synchronously stimulated skeletal muscle graft for myocardial repair. J Thorac Cardiovasc Surg 87, 325, 1984.

17. Nakamura K, Glenn WWL. Graft of the diaphragm as a functioning substitute for the myocardium. J Surg Res 4, 435, 1964.

18. Shepherd MP. Diaphragmatic muscle and cardiac surgery. Ann R Coll Surg Engl 45, 212, 1969.

19. Hume WI. Construction of a functioning accessory myocardium. Trans Southern Surg Assoc 79, 200, 1968.

20. Macoviak JA, Stephenson LW, Spielman S, Greenspan A, Likoff M, St. John-Sutton M, Riechek N, Rashkind WJ, Edmunds LH Jr. Electrophysiological and mechanical characteristics of diaphragmatic autograft used to enlarge the right ventricle. Surg Forum 31, 270, 1980.

21. Macoviak JA, Stephenson LW, Spielman S, Greenspan A, Likoff M, St. John-Sutton M, Riechek N, Rashkind WJ, Edmunds LH Jr. replacement of ventricular myocardium with a diaphragmatic skeletal muscle: acute studies. J Thorac Cardiovasc Surg 81, 519, 1981.

22. Macoviak JA, Stephenson LW, Alavi A, Kelly AM, Edmunds LH Jr. Effects of electrical stimulation on diaphragmatic muscle used to enlarge the right ventricle. Surgery 90, 271, 1981.

23. Macoviak JA, Stephenson LW, Kelly A, Likoff M, Reichek N, Edmunds LH Jr. Partial replacement of the right ventricle with a synchronously contracting diastolic counter-pulsators skeletal muscle autograft. Proceedings of III Meeting of the International Society for Artificial Organs 5 (Suppl), 550, 1981.

24. Carpentier A, Chachques JC. Myocardial substitute with a stimulated skeletal muscle: first successful clinical case. Lancet 1, 1267, 1985.

25. Magovern GJ, Park SB, Magovern GJ Jr, Benckart DH, Tullis G, Rozar E, Kao R, Chrislieb I. Latissimus dorsi as a functioning synchronously paced muscle component in the repair of a left ventricular aneurysm. Ann Thorac Surg 41, 116, 1986.

26. Anderson WA, Andersen JS, Acker MA, Hammond RL, Chin AJ, Douglas PS, Salmons S, Stephenson LW. Skeletal muscle applied to the heart: a word of caution. Circulation (submitted November 1987).

27. Kusserow BK, Clapp JF. A small ventricle-type pump for prolonged perfusions: construction and initial study including attempts to power a pump biologically with skeletal muscle. Trans Amer Soc Intern Organs 8, 74, 1964.

28. Juffe A, Ricoy JR, Marquez J, Castillo-Olivares JL, Figuera D. Cardialization: a new source of energy for circulatory assistance. Vasc Surg 12, 10, 1978.

29. Vachon BR, Kunor H, Zingg W. Mechanical properties of diaphragm muscles in dogs. Med Biol Eng 13, 252, 1975.

30. Spotnitz HM, Merker C, Malm JR. Applied physiology of the canine rectus abdominis. Trans Amer Soc Artif Intern Organs 20, 747, 1974.

31. Adams R, Schwartz A. Comparative mechanisms for contraction of cardiac and skeletal muscle. Chest 78, 123, 1980.

32. Chiu RCJ, Walsh GL, Dewar ML, De Simon JH, Khalafalla AS. Implantable extra-aortic balloon assist powered by transformed fatigue-resistant skeletal muscle. J Thorac Cardiovasc Surg 94, 694, 1987.

33. Chachques J, Grandjean P, Vasseur B, Hero M, Perier P, Bourgeois I, Fardeau M. Myocardial assistance. In: Nose Y, Kjellstrand C, Ivanovich P. Progress in Artificial Organs. Cleveland, Ohio: ISAO Press, 409, 1985.

2. Artificial Heart

34. Mannion JD, Velchik M, Alavi A, Stephenson LW. Blood flow in conditioned and unconditioned latissimus dorsi muscle (Abstract). Second Vienna Muscle Symposium, p. 28, 1985.

35. Glenn W, Phelps M. Diaphragm pacing by electrical stimulation of the phrenic nerve. Neurosurgery 17, 974, 1985.

36. Ciesielski TE, Fukuda Y, Glenn W, Gorfien J, Jeffery K, Hogan JF. Response of the diaphragm muscle to electrical stimulation of the phrenic nerve. J Neurosurg 58, 92, 1983.

37. Kim JH, Manuelidis EE, Glenn W, Fukuda Y, Cole DS, Hogan JF. Light and electron microscopic studies of phrenic nerves after long-term electrical stimulation. J Neurosurg 58, 84, 1983.

38. Acker MA, Mannion JD, Brown WE, Salmons S, Henriksson J, Bitto T, Gale DR, Hammond R, Stephenson LW. Canine diaphragm muscle after one year of continuous electrical stimulation: its potential as a myocardial substitute. J Appl Physiol 62, 1264, 1987.

39. Acker MA, Clark BJ, Subramanian H, McCully K, Hammond B, Salmons S, Chance B, Stephenson LW. In vivo P-NMR spectroscopy of electrically conditioned skeletal muscle. Circulation 74(Suppl), 415, 1986.

40. Acker MA, Anderson WA, Hammond RL, Di Meo F, McCullum J, Staum M, Velchik M, Brown WE, Gale D, Salmons S, Stephenson LW. Oxygen consumption of fatigue-resistant muscle. J Thorac Cardiovasc Surg 94, 702, 1987.

41. Armenti FR, Bitto T, Macoviak JA, Kelly AM, Chase CT, Hoffman BK, Rubinstein NA, St. John-Sutton M, Edmunds LH Jr, Stephenson LW. Transformation of skeletal muscle for cardiac replacement. Surgical Forum 35, 258, 1984.

42. Bitto T, Hammond R, Macoviak JA, Rashkind WJ, Edmunds LH Jr, Stephenson LW. Pectoralis and rectus abdominus muscle for potential correction of congenital heart defects. Pediatric Cardiology, Proceedings of the Second World Congress of Pediatric Cardiology. New York, Springer-Verlag, p. 609, 1986.

43. Bitto T, Mannion J, Hammond R, Cox J, Yamashita J, Duckett SW, Salmons S, Stephenson LW. Preparation for fatigue-resistant diaphragmatic muscle grafts for myocardial replacement. In: Nose Y, Kjellstrand C, Ivanovich P. Progress in Artificial Organs, Cleveland, Ohio: ISAO Press, 441, 1985.

44. Frey M, Thoma H, Gruber H, Stohr H, Huber L, Havel M, Steiner E. The chronically stimulated muscle as an energy source for artificial organs: Preliminary results of a basic study in sheep. Eur Surg Res 16, 232, 1984.

45. Hoffman BK, Gambke B, Stephenson LW, Rubinstein NA. Myosin transitions in chronic stimulation do not involve embryonic isozymes. Muscle Nerve 8, 796, 1985.

46. Macoviak JA, Stephenson LW, Armenti F, Kelly AM, Alavi A, Mackler T, Cox J, Palatianos GM, Edmunds LH Jr. Electrical conditioning of in situ skeletal muscle for replacement of myocardium. J Surg Res 32, 429, 1982.

47. Mannion JD, Bitto T, Hammond R, Rubinstein N, Stephenson LW. Histochemical fatigue characteristics of conditioned canine latissimus dorsi muscle. Circ Res 58, 298, 1986.

48. Mannion JD, Acker MA, Hammond RL, Stephenson LW, Khalafalla A, Henriksson J, Salmons S. Chronic burst stimulation of canine latissimus dorsi muscle: a further step towards the use of skeletal muscle for cardiac augmentation. Proceedings, PADOVA Muscle Symposium, 1986 (in press).

49. *Pette DL. Activity-induced fast to slow transitions in mammalian muscle. Med Sci Sports Exerc 16, 517, 1984.*

50. *Pette DL, Vrbova G. Neural control of phenotype expression in mammalian muscle fibers. Muscle Nerve 8, 676, 1985.*

51. *Pette D, Muller W, Leisner E, Vrbova G. Time dependent effects on contractile properties, fibre population, myosin light chains and enzymes of energy metabolism in intermittently and continuously stimulated fast twitch muscles of the rabbit. Pfluegers Arch 364, 103, 1976.*

52. *Salmons S, Vrbova G. The influence of activity on some contractile characteristics of mammalian fast and slow muscles. J Physiol (London) 210, 535, 1969.*

53. *Salmons S, Henriksson J. The adaptive response of skeletal muscle to increased use. Muscle Nerve 4, 94, 1981.*

54. *Buller JC, Eccles JC, Eccles RM. Differentiation of fast and slow muscles in the cat hind limb. J Physiol 150, 399, 1960.*

55. *Henry CG, Lowry OH. Quantitative histochemistry of canine cardiac Purkinje fibers. Am J Physiol 245, H824, 1983.*

56. *Eisenberg BR, Salmons S. The reorganization of subcellular structure in muscle undergoing fast-to-slow type transformation. Cell Tissue Res 220, 449, 1981.*

57. *Crow MT, Kushmerick MJ. Myosin light chain phosphorylation is associated with a decrease in the energy cost for contraction in fast twitch mouse muscle. J Biol Chem 257, 2121, 1982.*

58. *Wendt IR, Gibbs CL. Energy production of mammalian fast- and slow-twitch muscles during development. Am J Physiol 226, 642, 1974.*

59. *Von Recum A, Stulc JP, Hamada O, Baba H, Kantrowitz A. Long-term stimulation of a diaphragm muscle pouch. J Surg Res 23, 422, 1977.*

60. *Stevens L, Brown J. Can non-cardiac muscle provide useful cardiac assistance? Am Surg 52, 423, 1986.*

61. *Neilson IR, Brister SJ, Khalafalla AS, Chiu RCJ: Left ventricular assistance in dogs using a skeletal muscle powered device for diastolic augmentation. J Heart Transplant 4, 343, 1985.*

62. *Macoviak JA, Stinson EB, Starkey TD, Hansen DE, Cahill PD, Miller DC, Shumway NE: Myoventriculoplasty and neoventricles myograft cardiac augmentation to establish pulmonary blood flow: preliminary observations and feasibility studies. J Thorac Cardiovasc Surg 93, 212, 1987.*

63. *Khalafalla AS: Muscle mass and design requirement for cardiac assist systems. in: Chiu RC (ed), Biomechanical Cardiac Assist - Cardiomyoplasty and Muscle Powered Devices. Futura Publishing, pp 151, 1986.*

64. *Janz RF, Kubert BR, Mirsky I, Korecky B, Taichman GC. The effect of age on passive elastic stiffness of rat heart muscle. Biophys J 16, 281, 1976.*

65. *Bogen DK, Rabinowitz SA, Needleman A, McMahon TA, Abelmann WH. An analysis of the mechanical disadvantage of myocardial infarction in the canine left ventricle. Circ Res 47, 728, 1980.*

2. Artificial Heart

66. Grimm AF, Katele KV, Kubota R, Whitehorn WV. Relation of sarcomere length and muscle length in resting myocardium. Am J Physiol 218, 1412, 1970.

67. Spotnitz HM, Sonnenblick EH, Spiro D. Relation of ultrastructure to function in the intact heart: Sarcomere structure relative to pressure-volume curves of intact left ventricles of dogs. Circ Res 18, 49, 1966.

68. Janz RF, Waldron RJ. Predicted effect of chronic apical aneurysms on the passive stiffness of the human left ventricle. Circ Res 42, 255, 1978.

69. Rabinowitz SA. Myocardial mechanics: constitutive properties and pumping performance of the infarcted ventricle (Ph D thesis). Cambridge, Mass., Harvard University, 1978.

70. Mirsky I, Janz RF, Kubert BR, Korecky B, Taichman GC. Passive elastic wall stiffness of the ventricle: a comparison between linear theory and large deformation theory. Bull Math Biol 38, 239, 1976.

71. Ogden RW. Large deformation isotropic elasticity - on the correlation of theory and experiment for incompressible rubber-like solids. Proc R Soc Lond A326, 565, 1972.

2.6. An Electromagnetic Actuator Using Recently Developed Rare Earth Permanent Magnets

MV Koroly[1], N Ida[2], LR Roemer[2]

[1] Department of Vascular Research,
Akron City Hospital, Akron, Ohio, USA, and
Applied Biotechnologies, Inc, Akron, Ohio, USA

[2] Department of Electrical Engineering,
University of Akron, Akron, Ohio, USA

Abstract

Total artificial heart programs throughout the world can be categorized on the basis of their method of actuation. Current programs include pneumatic technology, hydraulic hybrids of pneumatic technology, and electro-mechanical hearts with motors, gears, and cams. The purpose of this study was to investigate an alternative type of actuator which operates efficiently without external drive lines, gears, or motors.

An electromagnetic voice coil type actuator was constructed using state-of-the-art Neodymium-Iron-Boron (Nd FeB) permanent magnets. The actuator is attached to a diaphragm and positioned between two chambers which alternate, filling and discharging fluid in a reciprocal fashion. The current inside the coil is reversed as the actuator moves from side to side. By varying the amount of current in the coil, the attracting force (and therefore the intraventricular pressure) can be controlled.

In its non-optimized form, the voice coil actuator was capable of delivering near physiologic pressures while using about 20 Watts in a continuous duty cycle. The model weighed 900 grams (including all external fittings, etc). The pump is 95 mm high and 80 mm in diameter.

The feasibility of this type of actuator was proven. The pump uses a minimum of moving parts and promises to be very efficient. Optimization of the voice coil actuator on mock circulation loops (currently in progress) using shaped pulses and a shortened duty cycle, allow for a variety of physiologic pressures with a minimum of power consumption.

Introduction

A new generation of permanent magnets is available today that is very different from those available only a few years ago. Not only are new materials being used, but the properties of these new magnets are improving steadily. Rare earth magnets are used today al-

2. Artificial Heart

most exclusively for applications where performance is critical.

The Permanent Magnets properties consist of:

1. High Coercive Force
   - difficult to demagnetize improved stability in external magnetic fields

2. High Remnant Flux
   - the maximum flux density available

3. High Energy Product
   - product of the flux density and coercive force
   - measure of the energy stored in the magnet

4. Linearity of the Demagnetization curve
   - allows simpler calculation of the magnetic field and shape of the magnet

5. Stability
   - improved stability to temperature variations

The Neodymium-Iron-Boron (NdFeB) magnets seem to be ideal as far as overall properties are concerned. It was not possible to design such a device in the past because the necessary materials were not available.

Methods and Materials

The actuator proposed here consists of two permanent magnets connected such that their fields oppose each other, and a coil (one or more) is positioned between the REPM. The operation of the actuator relies on the fact that, be-

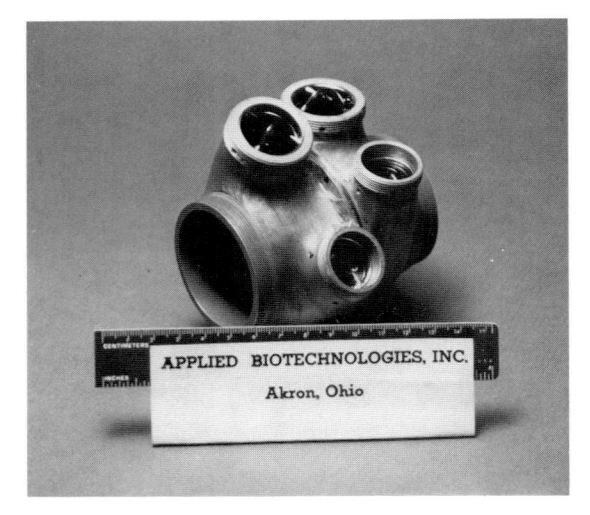

Fig. 90

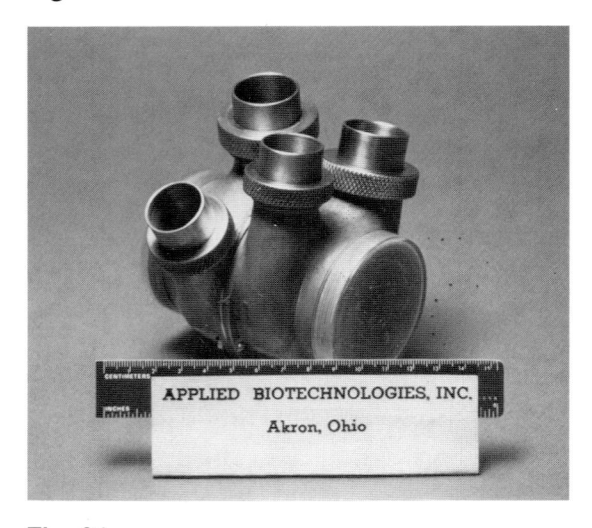

Fig. 91

cause of the opposing fields of the two magnets, the coil is attracted by one magnet and repelled by the other. This dual force contributes significantly to the overall efficiency of the device.

The control of the mechanism is very simple. In essence, reversing the current in the coil will change the direction of movement of the coil, while modulation of the current will affect the pressure directly.

The controller itself is essentially a low power microprocessor with some power transistors to handle the current through the coils. This allows both con-

2. Artificial Heart

trol and programmability of the actuator to match the need of the device.

A prototype actuator has been built (Figure 90 and 91) consisting of two permanent magnets, 50mm in diameter and 19 mm thick. The two magnets are separated by 51 mm and the coil is 15 mm thick. The stroke volume is 105 cc. Neither the coil nor the permanent magnets are optimal.

Results

To measure the efficiency of the prototype pump, the input and output of the pump were measured. The measurements presented here were made at a pressure differential (between inlet and outlet) of about 25cm.

At lower rates the efficiency is lower than for higher rates, primarily because the power is on longer, while pumping does not occur. Also, this is a continuous duty cycle (Table 29).

Discussion

The results clearly demonstrate feasibility of this approach to actuation. Although voice coil actuators generally have a lower efficiency than most electromagnetic devices, the use of high intensity permanent magnets makes such an actuator feasible. Considerable improvements in efficiency can be expected through extensive optimization of the various parts of the actuator.

A finite element computer code will be used to optimize the interaction of the electromagnet (coil) and the permanent magnets. Greater opportunity for optimization exists at this stage.

Optimization of the pump housing will also receive extensive attention. In general, the wider and flatter the housing, the narrower the air gap between the magnets and therefore the larger the force available.

Software development and controller design represent a third area for potential improvement. It is anticipated that a CMOS (Complementary Metal Oxide Semiconductor) microprocessor device will be incorporated for low power consumption, reliability, and immunity to external noise.

Efficiency Measurements
At 0.26 Ampere (6.5 Watts)
a. 50 beats/min, efficiency = 9,86%
b. 75 beats/min, efficiency = 8,85%
At 0.4 Ampere (15 Watts)
a. 50 beats/min, efficiency = 6,43%
b. 75 beats/min, efficiency = 8,85%

Table 29

The actuator described here should prove to be of significant advantage over existing devices, primarily because of its reliance on all-electric operation without the need for complex mechanical devices or impractical pneumatic lines.

2.7. Blood Platelets during Experimental and Clinical Total Artificial Heart Replacement

MR Mueller, A Wohlfahrt, A Lee, P Zilla, R Fasol, E Wolner

Department of Surgery 2 and Ludwig Boltzman Institute, University of Vienna, Austria.

The occurrence of thromboembolism during the use of the total artificial heart (TAH) as a bridge for transplantation is one of the major problems (1). Unfortunately, these complications appear more frequently during clinical application than in experimental use in calves. In 1986, for instance, Levinson and coworkers reported a 64% thromboembolic complication rate with the use of the Jarvik 7 TAH (1).

These primarily platelet-related events are likely to be due to both the contact of blood with the artificial surfaces of the pump, and the unphysiological high shear forces of blood cells. Until now, however, it is not clear whether the surface contact or the shear stress is mainly responsible for the initiation of these thromboembolic events.

On the one hand it has been suggested that contact with artificial surfaces would lead to platelet destruction, loss of membrane integrity (2), and leakage of granular contents, together with an impaired platelet reactivity to various stimulants. On the other hand, high shear forces were shown to result in platelet activation, shape change, and aggregate formation (3,4,5,6,7).

Although one is aware of the effects of extracorporeal circulation (ECC) on haemostasis (8,9,10,12,13) very little is known about the subsequent platelet alterations during the clinical application of the TAH. To gain a better insight into this topic, we initially observed platelets of the calf during 10 experimental applications of the "Ellipsoid Heart". The subsequent comparison of experimental and clinical data should lead to greater knowledge about the situation in man.

The total artificial heart device used in this study was a pneumatically driven membrane pump of the ellipsoid type. It consists of two separate polyurethane ventricles, each with a volume of 120 ml and an inflow and outflow Bjork-Shiley valve.

Platelet and haemolysis parameter were determined over a period of up to 26 days.

We measured platelet function by impedance aggregometry (whole blood aggregometer), using different dosages of collagen for induction of platelet aggregation. Radioimmunoassays were applied to investigate the release of the platelet granular contents beta-thromboglobulin (β-TG) and platelet factor 4 (PF4) as well as of the cyclo-oxygenase product thromboxane A_2 (TXA_2) by measuring its stable metabolite thromboxane B_2 (TXB_2). Apart from platelet

2. Artificial Heart

release products, surface morphology of circulating platelets was quantitatively determined (2,9,13,14,15).

Blood samples were taken one day before operation to determine basal values. Further samples were taken at the beginning of the operation, at the onset of CPBP, and after 15, 30, 60 and 120 minutes of bypass. The same pattern was used after implantation of the artificial heart. During the further follow-up, blood samples were taken after 4 hours and then every 24 hours.

In our bovine experiments a significant reduction of platelet function was found immediately after the onset of CPBP. During bypass the platelet reactivity to collagen remained very low. Four hours after the end of CPB, at the onset of TAH perfusion, platelet function began to increase to a first peak until the end of day 1. After a period of relatively unaltered platelet function, a second peak was reached at the 7th and 8th day (Figure 92).

However, the measurement of bovine cyclo-oxygenase activity showed an even more rapid recovery: thromboxane B2 levels showed a peak of 120 ng/ml after the end of bypass, but rapidly decreased to normal values within the first 24 hours of perfusion with the artificial heart (Figure 93).

In analogy to our bovine experiments, those patients who did not receive any antiplatelet agents or thrombocyte substitutes, showed a similar course of platelet function, although bovine platelets were generally found to be much less sensitive to collagen stimulation than human ones (Figure 94).

Figure 95 shows the response of the platelets of one patient to aggregometry, using 4 different dosages of collagen. To stress the trends more clearly, the results are also shown as relative data in Figure 96. In this patient, the significantly reduced response to all dosages on day 6 was due to a two day period of haemofiltration.

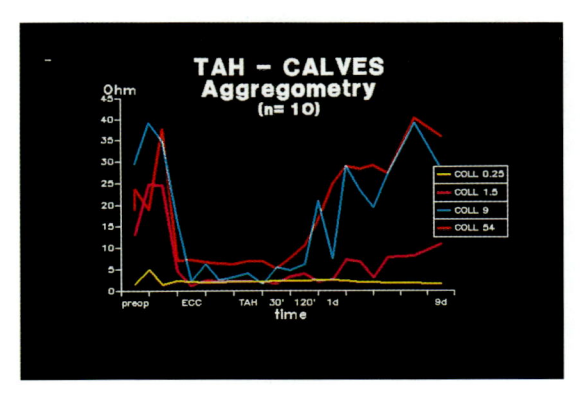

Fig. 92 Whole blood aggregometry, using increasing dosages of collagen. Note the drastic decrease of platelet function at the end of extracorporeal circulation. A marked recovery of platelet reactivity to pre-operative values can be seen between days 1 and 8 after total artificial heart (TAH) replacement, when a high concentration of collagen was used. The threshold dosis of 1.5 µg collagen/ml still reveals a continual, slightly diminished aggregability.

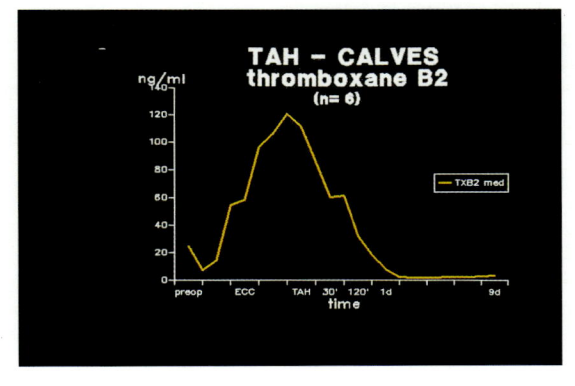

Fig. 93 Mean values of thromboxane B$_2$ (TXB$_2$) in plasma. A successive increase towards the end of extracorporeal circulation is followed by a sharp decrease. Plasma levels below the pre-operative value are reached on day 1.

2. Artificial Heart

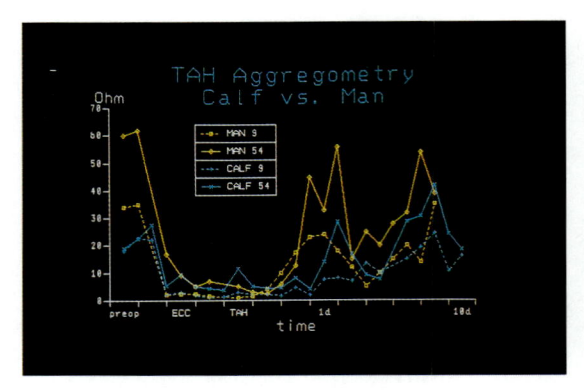

Fig. 94 Comparison of platelet function in man and calves. Platelet reactivity to high dose (9 µg/ml) and very high dose (54 µg/ml) collagen-stimulation is displayed over a 10 day period. In both species the recovery of aggregability shows 2 peaks - one on day 1 and a second on day 8. It is obvious that the sensitivity of human platelets is distinctly higher than that of bovine platelets.

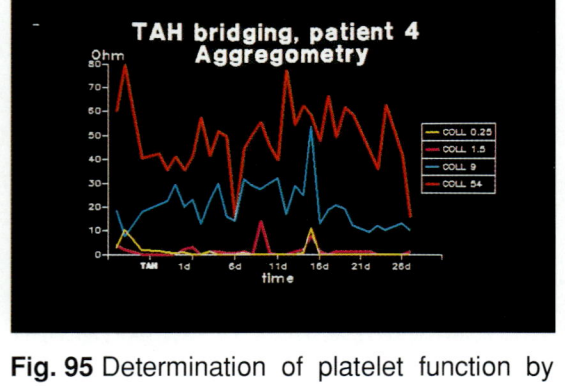

Fig. 95 Determination of platelet function by whole blood aggregometry in one of the patients after TAH replacement. The recovery of platelet function until day 16 with a subsequent loss of aggregability is best shown when 9 µg/ml collagen are added.

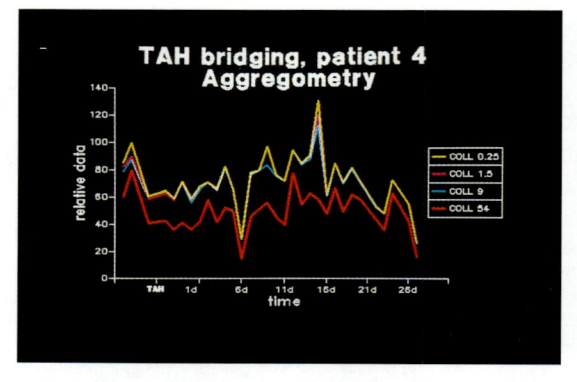

Fig. 96 Relative aggregability of platelets of the same patient as in Fig 95. When the results are compared to the pre-operative values, it is evident in all 4 dosages of collagen that platelet sensitivity on day 16 is even higher than pre-operatively.

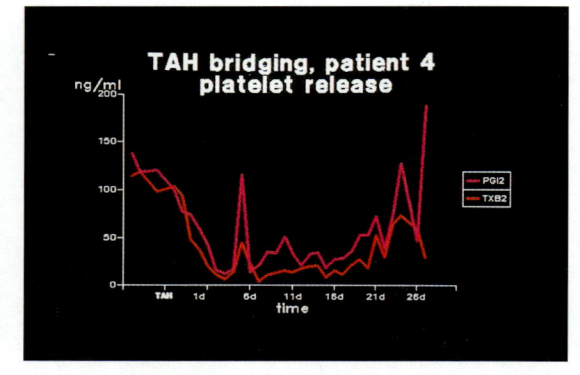

Fig. 97 The measurement of the antagonistic endoperoxide products prostacyclin (PGI_2) and thromboxane A_2 (TXA_2) via their stable metabolites (PG-6 keto F, alpha and TXB_2) reveal a similar time course; both decrease at a time when platelet function recovers (Fig 95 and 96) and subsequently increase when platelet function decreases. Note the peak on day 6, indicating haemofiltration caused by platelet activation.

In the same patient, the comparison of the levels of TXB_2 and of the PGI_2 metabolite prostaglandin 6-keto-F-alpha (Figure 97) with the platelet specific proteins βTG and PF4 (Figure 98) showed a rapid decrease of all substances within 24 hours after cardiopulmonary bypass (CPBP). The levels of βTG took longer to decrease, due to a longer half life of this alpha granule compound. Only on day 6, at the time of haemofiltration, did alpha-granular platelet release products, as well as endoperoxide products show, an impressive increase in levels. When we compare the overall time course of platelet release products with the percentage of morphologically activated platelets (Figure 99) we found a close correlation, again with the distinct platelet activation during the 2 days of haemofiltration. Moreover, when we compared haemolysis parameters like free Hb with alpha-granular release products and TXB_2 (Figure 100), it became obvious that the two groups of substances had similar time changes of their levels. Therefore, elevated plasma levels of platelet release products were apparently caused by both platelet activation and platelet lysis. In order to reduce platelet activation, we used aspirin as an antiplatelet agent in our third patient. The success of this concept was proved by the interpretation of the morphology of circulating platelets, which is probably the most sensitive method to determine platelet activation (14,15).

Figure 101 demonstrates the relative distribution of circulating activated and unactivated platelets in this patient. At the onset of TAH perfusion we found 90% unactivated and 10% activated platelets. This pattern changed after 32 hours, when the percentage of activated and unactivated platelets was similar. After administration of 2g acetyl salicylic acid (ASA) per day, the percentage returned to about 80% unactivated and 20% activated platelets. After withdrawal of this medication, the distribution returned to the situation prior to the treatment with acetyl salicylic acid. During the whole period of observation, primarily early forms of platelet activation were found. Only between 16 and 32 hours of TAH replacement, a small percentage of platelets was found to be in "late shape-change".

These ASA specific findings were similar in the bovine experiments and in the human application. However, "late shape change" morphology was found only in the clinical case.

In summary, our observations indicate similar changes of platelet function during experimental bovine and clinical human TAH replacement. This could be of future interest, since this would make it easier to establish mean values for clinical use.

However, we found, that hemolysis closely parallels platelet release reaction as well as the percentage of "shape change" platelets during the initial phase of the clinical use of the TAH. This means that platelets are not only highly activated but also damaged. We believe that it should be beneficial to lower the plasma levels of platelet specific release products in order to prevent other functional intact thrombocytes from being co-activated. Our findings in SEM during aspirin medication are a hint in this direction.

2. Artificial Heart

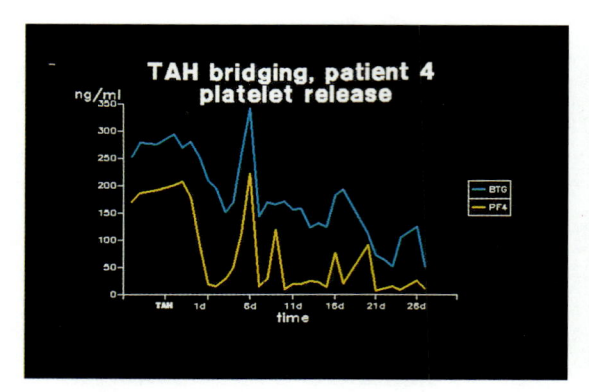

Fig. 98 Time-course of plasma levels of platelet factor 4 (PF4) and beta-thrombogobuline (βTG) over 4 weeks in the same patient; in contrast to cyclo-oxygenase activity (Fig 97) and platelet aggregability (Fig 95,96), alpha granular release shows a different pattern; after the same peak levels on day 6, platelet release successively decreases over the following 3 weeks.

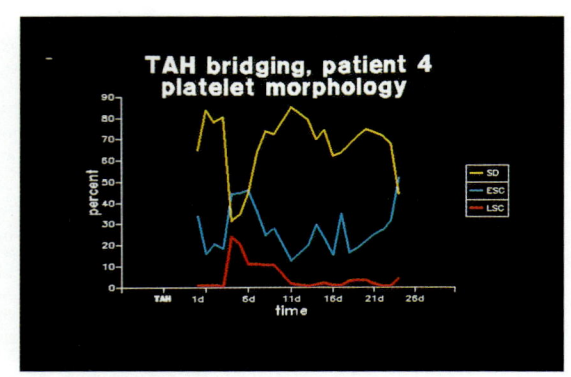

Fig. 99 Qualitative analysis of surface morphological changes in circulating platelets. The time course of activation is similar to that indicated by alpha-granular release products (Fig 98): Unactivated, smooth discoid platelets (SD) drastically decrease in number before day 6 (Haemofiltration). At the same time, the percentage of "early" (ESC) and "late shape changed" platelets (LSC) increase with the duration of TAH pumping. The decreasing number of unactivated smooth discoid platelets (SD) indicates that the percentage of activated platelets actually increases.

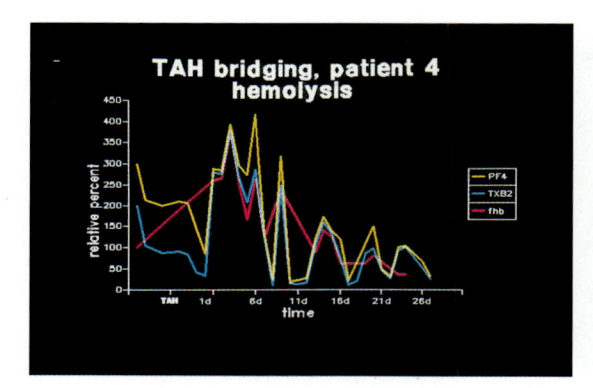

Fig. 100 Comparison of the platelet activation parameters thromboxane B_2 (TXB_2) and platelet factor 4 (PF4) with the lysis parameter free haemoglobin (fHb). The similar time course of the three substances indicates that platelet lysis seems to be partially responsible for the increase of activation parameters.

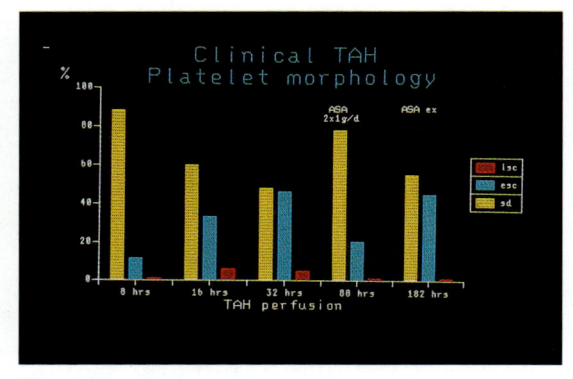

Fig. 101 Influence of acetyl salicylic acid (ASA) therapy on the surface morphological appearance of circulating platelets: after 32 hours of TAH pumping, a higher percentage of platelets is morphologically activated (ESC and LSC) than unactivated (SD). After the onset of ASA therapy, more than 80% of circulating platelets have regained the smooth, discoid appearance of the unactivated stage (SD), while only 20% remain in "early shape change" (ESC), which is typical for the earliest phase of platelet activation. Shortly after ASA therapy was stopped, platelets return to their pre-therapeutic stage of activation.

2. Artificial Heart

References

1. Levinson MM, Smith RG, Cork RC, Gallo J, Emery RW, Icenogle TB, Ott RA, Burns GL, Copeland JG. Thromboembolic complications of the Jarvik-7 total artificial heart: case report. Art Organs 10, 236, 1986.

2. Fasol R, Zilla P, Fischlein T, Deutsch M. Surface morphology of circulating platelets: a suggested parameter for the monitoring of endothelial seeded grafts. J Cardiovasc Surg 1988, in press.

3. Wurzinger LJ, Schmid-Schönbein H. Species differences in platelet aggregation and the influence of citrate and heparin anticoagulation thereon. J Am Soc Art Int Organs 4, 149, 1981.

4. Jen CJ, McIntire LV. Characteristics of shear-induced aggregation in whole blood. J Lab Clin Med 115, 1984.

5. Hardwick RA, Gritsman HN, Stromberg RR, Friedmann LI. The biochemical mechanism of shear-induced platelet aggregation. Trans Am Soc Artif Intern Organs 29, 448, 1983.

6. Dostal M, Vasku J, Sotolova O, Urbanek E, Cerny J, Gregor Z, Sladek T, Hanzelka P, Urbanek P, Pavlicek V. Effects of the total artificial heart on the blood components and plasma free hemoglobin level. Scripta Medica 53, 3, 1980.

7. Hung TC, Hochmuth RM, Joist JH, Sutera SP. Shear-induced aggregation and lysis of platelets. Trans Amer Soc Artif Int Organs 22, 285, 1976.

8. Zilla P, Fasol R, Deutsch M, von Oppell U, Knöbl P, Vukovich T, Laufer G, Wollenek G, Hammerle A, Müller MM. Whole blood aggregometry and platelet adenine nucleotides during cardiac surgery. Scand J Thoracic Cardiovasc Surg 22, 165, 1988.

9. Zilla P, Fasol R, Hammerle A, Yildiz S, Kadletz M, Laufer G, Wollenek G, Seitelberger R, Deutsch M. Scanning electron microscopy of circulating platelets reveals new aspects of platelet alteration during cardiopulmonary bypass operations. J Tex Heart Inst 14, 13, 1987.

10. De Jong JC, Smit Sibinga CT, Wildevuur CR. Platelet behaviour in extracorporal circulation. Transfusion 19, 72, 1979.

11. Knöbl PN, Zilla P, Fasol R, Muller MM, Vukovich TC. The protein C system in patients undergoing cardiopulmonary bypass. J Thorac Cardiovasc Surg 94, 600, 1987.

12. Van den Dungen JJ, Karliczek G, Brenken U, Homan van der Heide JN, Wildevuur CR. Clinical study of blood trauma during perfusion with membrane and bubble oxygenators. J Thorac Cardiovasc Surg 83, 108, 1982.

13. Zilla P, Fasol R, Groscurth P. Blood platelets in cardiopulmonary bypass surgery: recovery occurs after initial stimulation rather than continual activation. J Thorac Cardiovasc Surg 1988 (in press).

14. Zilla P, Groscurth P, Rhyner K, von Felten A. Surface morphology of human platelets during in vitro aggregation. Scand J Hematol 33, 440, 1984.

15. Zilla P, Groscurth P, Varga G, Fischlein T, Fasol R. PGI_2 and PGE_1 induce morphological alterations in human platelets similar to those of the initial phase of activation. Exp Hematology 15, 741, 1987.

3. Endothelial Cell Lining

3.1. Introduction: Endothelialization of Cardiovascular Prostheses

R Fasol, P Zilla, B Reichart

*Department of Cardio-Thoracic Surgery,
Groote Schuur Hospital,
University of Cape Town, South Africa*

Vascular surgery started in 1879 with experiments in vascular anastomoses by Eck. The first human vascular replacement with a vein graft for a popliteal aneurysm was reported by Goyannes in 1906. Experiments to explore the possibility of vascular replacement using synthetic materials were carried out by Carrel and Guthrie during the first part of this century.

In the trial-and-error process by which vascular grafts were developed, only one of the many functions of the artery was initially recognised - that of a mechanical conduit. Little was known about the biology of the arterial wall, but this was not thought to be of much importance in the development of vascular prostheses.

With the increasing recognition of the failure of current small-diameter synthetic vascular prostheses, it became apparent that further study was necessary in at least three areas:

Firstly, renewed efforts to develop a better synthetic polymer,
secondly, the pharmacological modification of the surface of the graft by heparin bonding, by the administration of antiplatelet agents or by the administration of a thromboxane A2 synthetase inhibitor
thirdly, an improved interface response between the circulating blood and the vascular graft - possibly a completely endothelial-lined graft.

Over the last ten years the attitude of at least a minority of cardiovascular surgeons has changed with regard to the importance of cell-biological efforts to overcome the high failure rate of cardiovascular implants. These surgeons now believe that future research should be directed towards the creation of an endothelium on cardiovascular prostheses.

With regard to this growing awareness of the various endothelial cell functions which distinguish an endothelialized from a non-endothelialized cardiovascular prosthesis, we provided selected basic information on endothelial cell functions in the first part of the relevant chapter of this book.

Theodor Vukovich (University of Vienna, Austria) gives a survey on the role of endothelial cells in the coagulation system, emphasizing the recently discovered protein C/protein S system. To understand the mechanisms and sensitivity of endothelial cell reactivity, Una Ryan (University of Miami, Florida) explains how endothelial cells, with their numerous receptors, translate a signal into a response. Another basic

3. Endothelial Cell Lining

scientific contribution emphasizes that endothelial cells are not only targets of immune response, but also express properties that may be directly involved in immune functions; this was previously believed to be restricted to bone marrow cells. This article by Peter Libby (Tufts University, Boston) is probably the most convincing demonstration of the challenge for cardiovascular surgeons to get a deeper understanding of endothelial cells, since it is of equal importance for both those involved in transplantation and those involved in surface endothelialization.

As mentioned above, the main reason for the failure of synthetic vascular grafts is lack of complete endothelialization. Two possible solutions - the *in vitro* endothelialization via cell culture techniques on the one hand, and the stimulation of the natural endothelial cell ingrowth onto the synthetic surface on the other - are both dependent on potential initiators of endothelial cell proliferation. Thomas Maciag (American Red Cross, Maryland) describes such a group of 'initiators' which belongs to a family of polypeptides which are commonly known as 'heparin-binding growth factors'.

Historically, the onset of a dramatic increase of basic knowledge of endothelial cell functions with Jaffe's first endothelial cell culture was relatively soon followed by the first approach of cardiovascular surgeons to utilize this information. These developments of endothelial cell research in cardiovascular surgery during the last 10 years are reviewed by Allan Callow (Tufts University, Boston) together with a critical analysis of the pitfalls and the most recent trends.

Two approaches to endothelialize cardiovascular prostheses are single-staged techniques, which use either freshly harvested endothelial cells from a major vessel like the saphenous vein - a process known as 'endothelial cell seeding' - or freshly harvested microvascular endothelial cells from fat tissue - known as 'endothelial cell sodding'. A third approach is *in vitro* endothelialization. In the following chapter, two contributions deal directly with 'seeding', one with 'sodding' and three with *in vitro* lining. Bernhard Bourke (University of New South Wales, Sidney) describes, for the first time, an additional systemic effect of 'seeding' after intravenous application of autologous endothelial cells, and Per Oertenwall (University of Gothenborg, Sweden) reports on his experience with 36 'seeded' vascular grafts in humans. Results of initial human trials with 'sodding' - the younger of the two techniques - are presented by Steven Schmidt (Akron, Ohio).

Since a better cell yield is desirable for all three approaches, James Stanley's (University of Michigan, Ann Arbor) experience with improved harvest efficiencies by using the enzyme Dispase instead of Collagenase is a most important contribution.

A further basic field of research which is important for both 'seeding' and 'sodding' on the one hand, and *in vitro* endothelialization on the other, is the surface modification of cardiovascular prostheses to improve endothelial cell adherence and shear stress resistance. In order to find an ideal substrate for the precoating of synthetic surfaces, Richard Kempczinski (University of Cincinatti, Ohio) compares the commonly used fibronectin precoating of PTFE grafts with a matrix-coating, which resembles natural, endothelial-cell-derived extracellular matrix in its composition. In a different approach, Jan Kaehler, from our group, correlates the primary adherence of endothelial cells with their attachment area on various collagenous matrices, on glycoproteins, and on fibrin glue. Bruce Jarrell's group (Jefferson University, Philadelphia) goes one step further and determines the shear stress resistance of endothelial cells on different precoating substrates.

Since *in vitro* endothelialization has the disadvantage that a period of time is needed for the cultivation of autologous endothelial cells, reports on successful homologous seeding encouraged our own group to implant into baboons, *in vitro* endothelialized, small-diameter PTFE grafts lined with blood-group identical, pooled, homologous endothelial cells. W Müller-Glausner (University of Zurich, Switzerland) added to his interesting results with *in vitro* endothelialization the aspect of graft compliance by introducing a novel, compliant polyurethane graft. The last contribution from our group demonstrates that the application of graft endothelialization is not necessarily limited to vascular prostheses. We summarize in this article, our research efforts, extending over five years, to endothelialize the inner surface of artificial hearts. Our hope is that these cardiac prostheses may regain their attractiveness for long-term implantation, provided endothelialization drastically reduces their thromboembolic risk.

3. Endothelial Cell Lining

3.2. Basics of Enthothelial Cell Lining

3.2.1. Anticoagulant Properties of Vascular Endothelium

TC Vukovich, PN Knöbl

*Department of Medical Physiology,
University of Vienna,
Vienna, Austria*

The term "endothelium" for the description of the luminal surface of blood vessels was created in the nineteenth century by the Swiss anatomist Wilhelm His. Originally, endothelium had been considered to be a rather passive barrier between the vascular wall and the enclosed blood. Until a few years ago, little was known about the role of endothelial cells in haemostasis. Although the antithrombotic properties of the endothelial cells were evident from the observation that blood platelets adhere to injured areas of vascular endothelium but not to healthy endothelium, the mechanisms of endothelial-cell-related antithrombotic properties remained unclear.

However, since the development of methods for the isolation and culture of endothelial cells by EA Jaffe in 1973 (1), enormous progress in elucidating the haemostatic functions of endothelial cells has been made. A variety of mechanisms have been discovered by which vascular endothelium actively contributes to the maintenance of the blood fluidity and the preventions of hemorrhage by controlling the whole haemostatic system, comprising blood coagulation, platelet function, and fibrinolysis. For this reason, the haemostatic properties of vascular endothelial cells should not be considered in isolation but rather in common with the haemostatic mechanisms of the enclosed blood.

Although the present article focuses on the anticoagulant properties of endothelial cells, it should be noted that endothelial cells also possess significant procoagulant, fribinolytic, antifribinolytic, and platelet-aggregatory properties, manifested by the generation of tissue thromboplastin, coagulation factor V, tissue-type plasminogen activator, plasminogen activator inhibitor, platelet activating factor, and von Willebrand factor. Figure 102 summarizes these endothelial-cell-related functions.

Active and Passive Thromboresistance Mediated by Endothelial Cells

General Considerations
Under physiological conditions endothelial cells maintain the fluidity of blood by passive and active mechanisms. The passive thromboresistance

3. Endothelial Cell Lining

```
ANTITHROMBOTIC                          ANTIHEMORRHAGIC
 PROPERTIES                               PROPERTIES
```

ANTITHROMBOTIC	ANTIHEMORRHAGIC
INHIBITION OF COAGULATION Glycosaminoglycans Thrombomodulin (Protein C System) Protein S	**COAGULATION** Tissue Factor Factor V
FIBRINOLYSIS Tissue Type Plasminogen Activator	**INHIBITION OF FIBRINOLYSIS** Plasminogen Activator Inhibitor – 1

ENDOTHELIAL CELL

PLATELET	
ANTIAGGREGATION Prostacyclin	**AGGREGATION** Platelet Activating Factor von Willebrand Factor Thromboxane

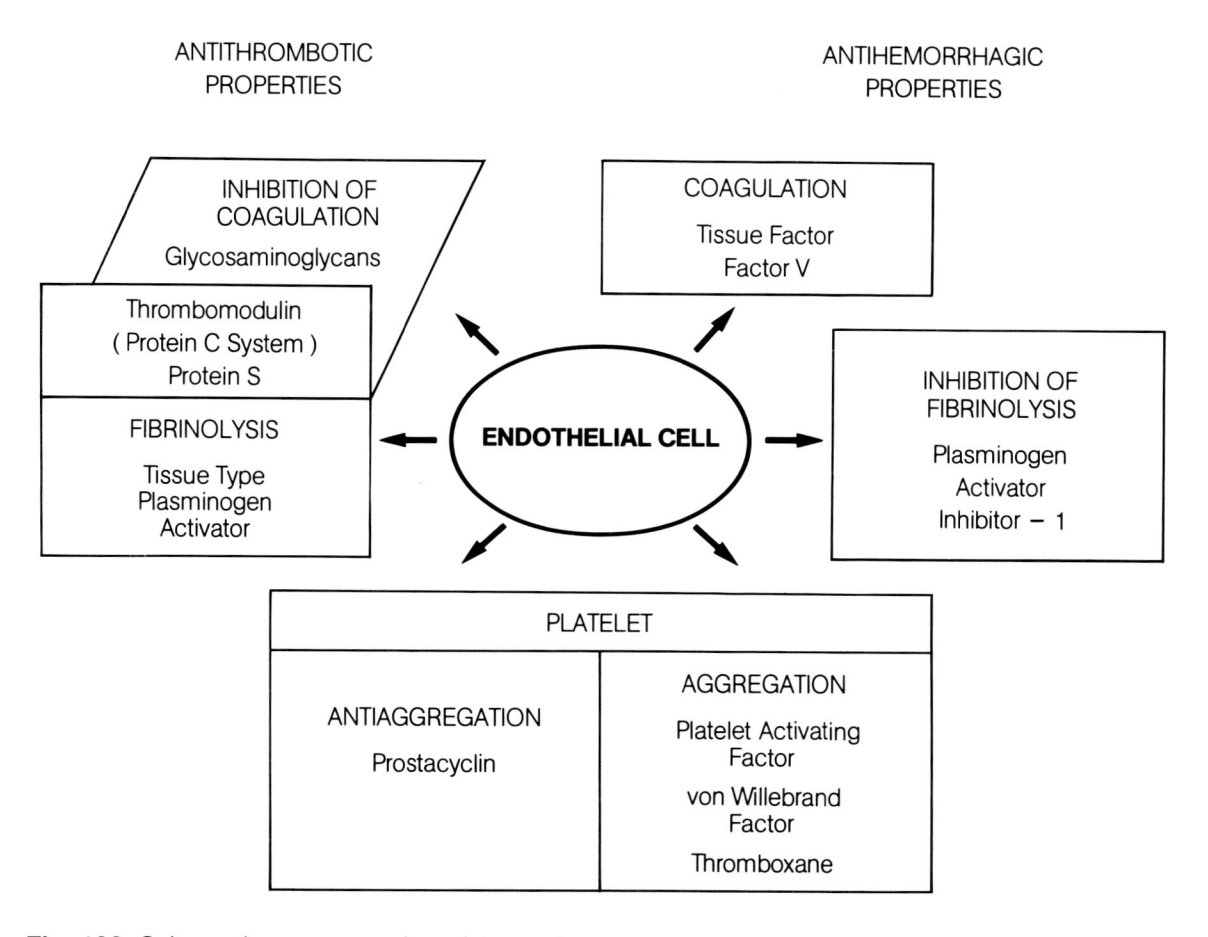

Fig. 102 Schematic representation of the endothelial-cell-mediated haemostatic mechanisms.

of the endothelium is based on a "barrier effect" which separates the haemostatic components of the blood from the thrombophilic subendothelial tissue. When the haemostatic system is not activated, the various coagulation factors circulate in plasma as inactive precursors and platelets exist in an "unstimulated" form. Contact with subendothelial tissue, however, leads to activation of the coagulation cascade and adhesion of blood platelets and leucocytes (2). The active thromboresistance of the endothelium is based on a variety of quite different effects such as generation of thrombomodulin, a component of the protein C-system with anticoagulatory and profibrinolytic activity, production of heparin sulphate, which increases the anticoagulant activity of antithrombin III, induction of fibrinolysis through generation of tissue-type plasminogen activator, and synthesis and release of inhibitors of platelet aggregation.

Thrombomodulin and the Protein C-System

Physiological Consideration

The protein C-system consists of protein C (3) and protein S (4), two vitamin K-dependent plasma proteins, and of thrombomodulin (5), an insoluble protein synthesized in endothelial cells and expressed on the luminal surface of the vascular wall. Thrombomodulin is a receptor for thrombin; it removes this fibrin-producing and platelet-activating enzyme from the circulation by complex

3. Endothelial Cell Lining

formation. Furthermore, thrombomodulin changes the substrate specificity of thrombin from fibrinogen to protein C (6).

The thrombin-thrombomodulin complex converts protein C from its zymogenic form to the enzyme form, protein Ca (5). In the presence of protein S, which is a cofactor of protein Ca, synthesized in liver and endothelial cells (7), protein Ca exerts potent anticoagulatory activity by inactivation of coagulation factors V and VIII (8). Furthermore, once protein C has been activated by the thrombin-thrombomodulin complex on the endothelial cell surface, it acts with its cofactor protein S to promote fibrinolysis. Endothelial cells produce the fibrinolysis inducing enzyme tissue type plasminogen activator and also its main antagonist, the "fast-acting" plasminogen activator inhibitor (9). Under physiological conditions endothelial cells release an excess of the inhibitor over the plasminogen activator and therefore no "free" activity of tissue type plasminogen activator can be detected in the blood plasma (10). In the presence of activated protein C, however, the balance between the plasminogen activator and its inhibitor is shifted towards the fribinolytic enzyme, since activated protein C degrades proteolytically the "fast acting" inhibitor of tissue type plasminogen activator (11,12). Figure 103 illustrates the activation and functions of protein C.

Optimal conditions for reactions between thrombomodulin, located on the endothelial cell and the plasma proteins thrombin and protein C must presumably occur in the microcirculation. The closest contact between the components of the protein C-system takes place within the capillaries, since, in these vessels, the blood flow velocity is

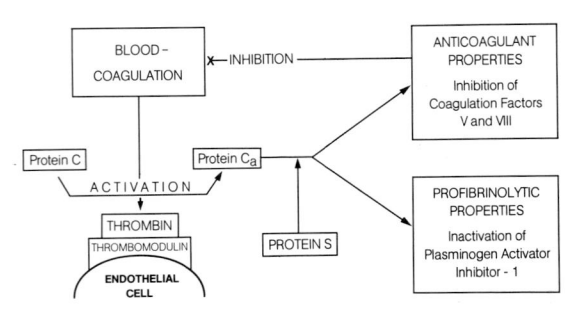

Fig. 103 Schematic illustration of the activation and functions of protein C.

slow and the ratio between the endothelial surface bearing thrombomodulin and the volume of blood contained in these vessels is much higher than in arteries and veins. Since activated protein C is rapidly inactivated in the circulation through a specific protein C inhibitor (13) one may conclude that the highest protein C-related anticoagulant potential is located in capillaries and venules. Figure 104 illustrates the quantitative differences of thrombin-initiated haemostatic mechanisms in macro- and micro-vessels.

Clinical Significance of the Protein C-system

Acquired and congenital deficiency states of protein C or protein S have been reported to result in a thrombophilic state. At present little is known about thrombomodulin deficiency states, since there is no simple method available for detecting the expression of thrombomodulin on the vascular endothelium.

The homozygous (complete) form of congenital protein C-deficiency results in severe thromboembolic complications, which are most commonly seen in the early postnatal period (14,15,16, for review 17). Only two patients have been reported to present after this period, at an age of 1 (18) and 18 years (19). Without substitution therapy

3. Endothelial Cell Lining

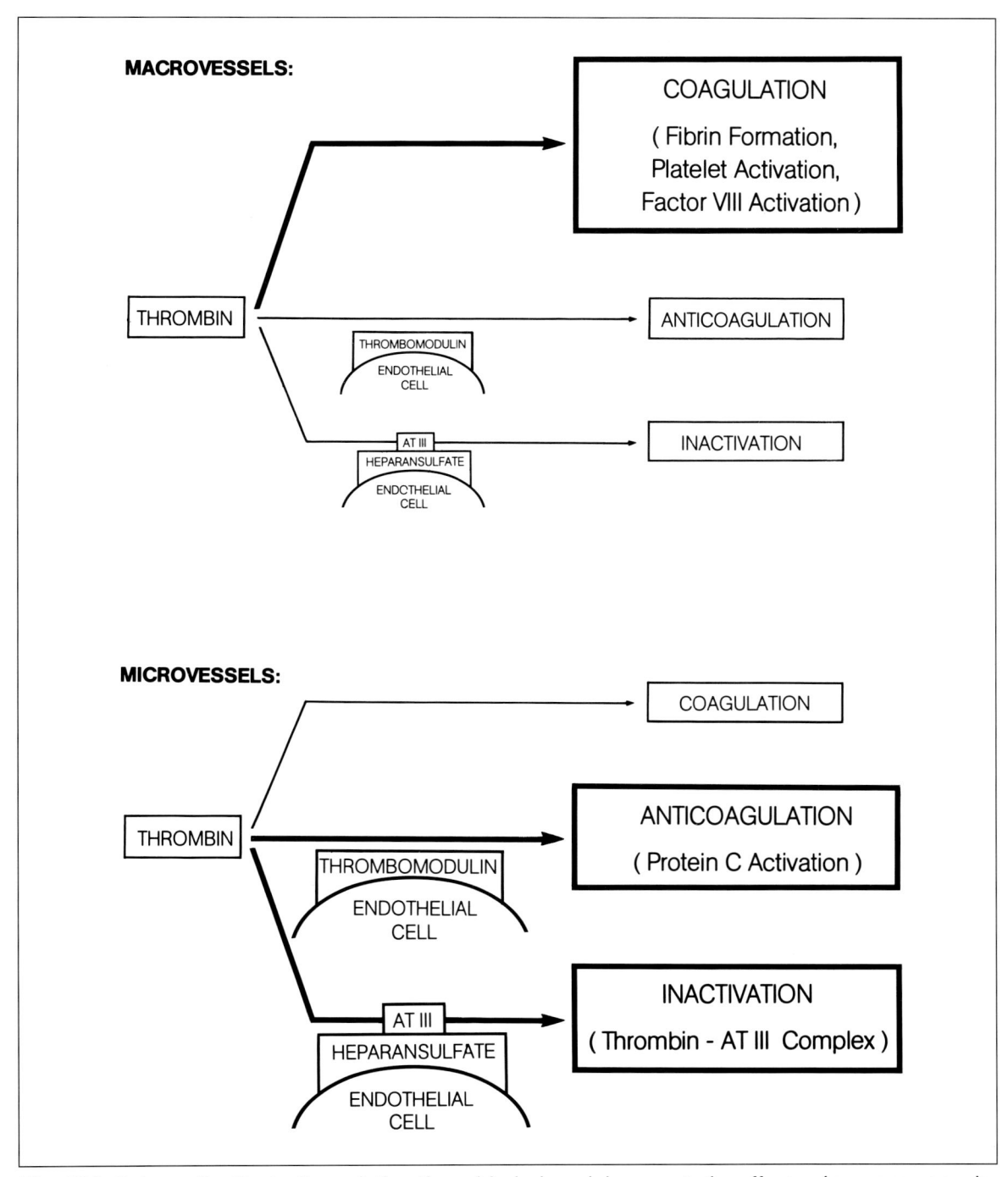

Fig. 104 Schematic illustration of the thrombin-induced haemostatic effects. In macrovessels, thrombin induces predominantly coagulation, in microvessels, where the contact to endothelial cells is closer, anticoagulation.

using fresh frozen plasma, factor IX concentrate (16), or protein C concentrate (18), the infants develop skin ecchymoses, intracerebral haemorrhages, and purpura fulminans - which is a syndrome of dermal microvascular thrombosis - and subsequent haemorrhagic skin necrosis.

The heterozygous form of protein C-deficiency manifests itself most commonly between adolescence and the age of 30 years, and leads to recurrent

221

3. Endothelial Cell Lining

thromboembolic events as superficial thrombophlebitis, deep venous thrombosis, and pulmonary embolism (20). The thrombophilia can be controlled by reducing procoagulant activity with oral anticoagulation. However, when oral anticoagulant therapy is initiated, an additional risk for the development of thromboembolic events is incurred. coumarin drugs suppress both the vitamin K-dependent coagulation factors and the anticoagulant proteins C and S. Since the plasma level of protein C declines at the beginning of coumarin therapy more rapidly than most vitamin K-dependent coagulation factors because of its short half life of about 8 hours (21), the balance between anti- and procoagulant potential shifts paradoxically in favour of procoagulant activity. During this initial period of oral anticoagulation, the patients may develop coumarin-induced skin necrosis caused by thrombotic obliteration of skin venules. Substitution therapy using protein C concentrates at the start of coumarin therapy can prevent skin necrosis in patients with heterozygous protein C-deficiency (22). Subsequently, in the phase of stable oral anticoagulation, the decrease in vitamin K-dependent coagulation factors overcomes the decrease in protein C and protein S.

The clinical picture of congenital protein S deficiency is very similar to that of protein C deficiency. Up to now no homozygous (complete) protein S deficiency has been described; the heterozygous deficiency state has been reported to be associated with recurrent thromboembolic events (23,24).

Besides coumarin therapy, acquired protein C deficiency states have been described in a variety of clinical conditions resulting in activation of the coagulation system. Examples include: disseminated intravascular coagulation, acute respiratory distress syndrome, and the postoperative period (25,26). Since protein C and protein S are synthesized in the liver, hepatic dysfunction results in a decrease in plasma levels of both proteins. However, this form of protein C and protein S deficiency is also associated with a reduced hepatic synthesis of several coagulation factors. The decrease in both anti- and procoagulant proteins tends to cause a haemophilic rather than a thrombophilic state. Furthermore, reduced plasma levels of protein C and protein S without reduction of coagulation factors, have been found in diabetic patients and have been linked to the high thromboembolic risk associated with diabetes mellitus (27,28).

Recently, we investigated the protein C-system in patients undergoing cardiopulmonary bypass surgery (29). Although all patients investigated were anticoagulated with heparin, a progressive increase in plasma levels of crosslinked fibrin degradation products and thrombin-antithrombin III complexes (30) was found, which indicates a marked activation of the coagulation system during extracorporeal circulation. Protein C levels were found to decrease significantly in the late phase of extracorporeal circulation, probably as a result of its activation and subsequent clearance from the circulation. Protein S levels were found to increase significantly soon after onset of extracorporeal circulation. This effect might be due to an enhanced release of protein S from thrombin-stimulated endothelial cells or platelets. A pronounced release of elastase from blood granulocytes into the plasma during extracorporeal circulation has recently been described by others (31). In a subsequent study we found evidence of a consumption of several plasmatic protease inhibitors, such as alpha-1-antitrypsin, the primary plasma inhibitor of elastase and antithrombin III, a secondary elastase inhibitor (30). These findings may well be attributed to the release of elastase from granulocytes. Once plasmatic protease inhibitors have been consumed, the protein C-system may conceivably be the only means of preventing intravascular coagulation.

The above-mentioned syndrome of purpura fulminans appears not only in patients with congenital protein C deficiency but also in association with septicemia. In the course of a recent outbreak of Neisseria meningitis infection in California, patients with purpura fulminans were found to have severely reduced plasma levels of protein C and protein S (32). Furthermore, in vitro experiments showed endotoxin-induced suppression of the expression of thrombomodulin on endothelial cells (33). The results of both reports strongly support the view that septicemia associated purpura fulminans is due to a combined reduction of the anticoagulant activity of the protein C-system.

Therapeutical Potential of the Protein C-System

Besides the obvious therapeutic potential for concentrates of purified protein C and/or protein S in congenital protein C or protein S deficiency states (18,22), other evidence indicates that these concentrates may be useful in a variety of clinical conditions. Fibrinolytic therapy using tissue plasminogen activator for thrombolysis may be improved by combined administration with protein C and protein S; activated protein C and protein S would depress additional thrombus formation whilst it also enhances fibrinolysis by degrading the inhibitor of plasminogen activator. The therapeutic potential of protein C in endotoxin-induced shock has recently been investigated. In baboons it has been demonstrated that the coagulopathic, hepatotoxic and lethal effects of LD_{100} concentrations of intravenously applied Escherichia coli can be prevented by simultaneous infusion of activated protein C. Further experiments of an antibody directed against protein C reduces the concentration of Escherichia coli required to elicit a lethal response by at least tenfold (34). The first pharmacological data about intravenously applied thrombomodulin have been published fairly recently. Detergent solubilized purified rabbit thrombomodulin was injected into rabbits, resulting in a significant and surprisingly long prolongation of the partial thromboplastin clotting time (35).

Heparin Sulphate Proteoglycans and Antithrombin III

Physiological Considerations

Antithrombin III is a member of the serpins, a family of plasma proteins with protease inhibitory capacity. In the same way as its relatives (plasminogen activator inhibitor, antiplasmin, alpha-1-antitrypsin, and antichymotrypsin), antithrombin III forms equimolar complexes with its target proteases which are then rapidly cleared from the circulation. In contrast to several of its relatives, antithrombin III alone has only a weak inhibitory activity. However, antithrombin III forms a complex with heparin, resulting in an approximately 10 000-fold increase in the inhibitory efficacy of antithrombin III (36,37). The main target of the heparin-antithrombin III complex is thrombin; secondary targets are activated coagulation factor X and other serine proteases of the intrinsic coagulation system.

Heparin was first prepared in 1916 by McLean (38) from the liver. For a long time, mast cells have been thought to be the sole site of heparin synthesis (39). In 1973 Damus and co-workers postulated that the thromboresistance of the vascular endothelium might be partly due to the presence of heparin-like substances on the luminal surface (40). In recent investigations, heparin sulphate was extracted from animal micro- and macro-vessels and purified by fractionation on immobilized antithrombin III. These fractions strongly potentiated the inhibitory capacity of antithrombin III against thrombin and activated coagulation factor X (41). Endothelial cells were identified as the site of generation of heparin sulphate by using cloned endothelial cells. Endothelial cells cultured from macro-vascular tissue were found to express about 1×10^{-3} USP units of heparin-like activity per 10^6 cells, whereas the activity expressed by cells cultured from micro-vascular endothelium was roughly 3 times higher (42).

The biological significances of heparin sulphate on the luminal vessel wall surface has been investigated in animal models. Perfusion of the vascular tree of the rat hindlimb with a solution containing thrombin and antithrombin III resulted in a twenty-fold acceleration in the rate of complex formation between thrombin and antithrombin III, when compared with in vitro mixtures. Although the eluted perfusion solution was free of any detectable heparin-like substances that might accelerate thrombin-antithrombin III complexation, the phenomenon of acceleration was clearly related to endothelium-linked heparin-like substances, since it was absent when the rat limb was perfused with a heparin-degrading enzyme (43, for review 44).

The inactivation mechanisms of thrombin by heparin sulphate on the endothelial cell surface is graphically shown in Figure 105. Because of the low blood flow velocity in capillaries and the high ratio between the endothelial surface bearing heparin sulphate, and the volume of blood enclosed, the optimal reaction conditions for thrombin

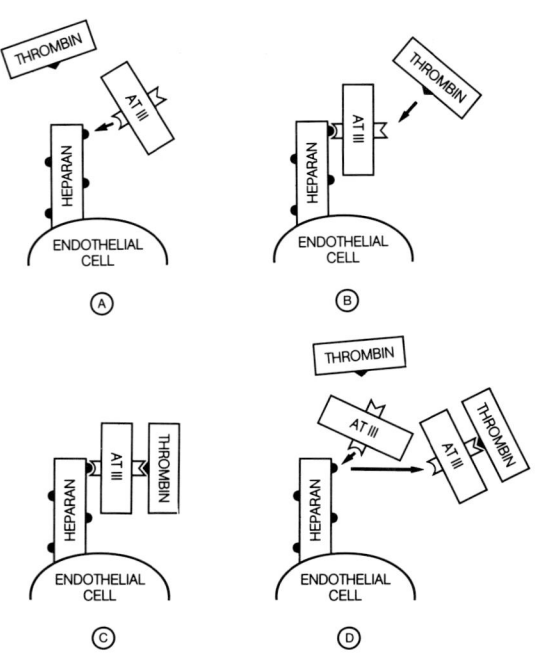

Fig. 105 Reaction steps on the luminal surface of endothelial cells, leading to inactivation of thrombin by antithrombin III (AT III).

and antithrombin III must presumably exist in micro-vessels (see Figure 104).

Clinical Significance of the Heparin-Antithrombin III System

Congenital and acquired antithrombin III deficiency states have been described by several investigators (45,46).

Patients heterozygous for antithrombin III-deficiency who demonstrate about 50% of normal antithrombin III activity, have a high risk of developing deep vein thrombosis and pulmonary embolism. The homozygous condition has never been reported, indicating that a complete antithrombin III deficiency is not compatible with intra-uterine life.

Acquired deficiency states have been found in patients with hepatic dysfunction, resulting in reduced hepatic synthesis (47), in patients with nephrotic syndrome resulting in urinary loss of the protein (48), and in a variety of clinical conditions associated with intravascular activation of the coagulation system, such as septicemia (49), major surgery (50), and eclampsia (51). In patients with nephrotic syndrome, it has been reported, that a reduction of plasma antithrombin III activity to only 75% of normal, leads to thromboembolic events in 60 out of 100 patients (48).

In conditions with intravascular coagulation, the decrease in antithrombin III is a result of consumption of the inhibitor as is evident from the simultaneous appearance of thrombin-antithrombin III complexes in the circulation (30,51). The appearance of cross-linked fibrin degradation products in plasma indicates that in cases of marked intravascular activation of the coagulation system (as found in patients suffering from eclampsia (51), or during extracorporeal circulation (30)) the antithrombin III and protein C-related natural anticoagulant potency is not sufficient to prevent intravascular fibrin generation. This view is also supported by the well-documented improvement of the clinical situation in patients with intravascular coagulation following enhancement of the antithrombin III-related anticoagulant potency by intravenous application of therapeutical concentrates of antithrombin III (52,53, for review 54).

Acknowledgements

The most valuable suggestions in preparation of the manuscript by Judy M Stephenson, MD are thankfully acknowledged. This article was supported by Schwab & Co Vienna, Austria.

3. Endothelial Cell Lining

References

1. Jaffe EA, Nachman RL, Becker CG, Minick CR. Culture of human endothelial cells derived from human umbilical cord veins. J Clin Invest 52, 2745, 1973.

2. Simionescu M, Simionescu N. Functions of the endothelial cell surface. Ann Rev Physiol 48, 279, 1986.

3. Stenflo J. A new vitamin K-dependent protein. J Biol Chem 251, 355, 1976.

4. Walker FJ. Regulation of activated protein C by a new protein: a possible function for bovine protein S. J Biol Chem 255, 5521, 1980.

5. Esmon NL, Owen WG, Esmon CT. Isolation of a membrane-bound cofactor for thrombin-catalyzed activation of protein C. J Biol Chem 257, 859, 1982.

6. Esmon CT. Regulation of protein C activation by components of the endothelial cell surface. In Vascular Endothelium in Haemostasis Thrombosis, Gimbrone MA Ed. New York: Churchill Livingstone; pp 99-119, 1986.

7. Flair DS, Marlar RA, Levin EG. Human endothelial cells synthesize protein S. Blood, 67, 1168, 1986.

8. Walker FJ, Sexton PW, Esmon CT. The inhibition of blood coagulation by activated protein C through the selective inactivation of activated factor V. Biochim Biophys Acta 571, 333, 1979.

9. Levin EG. Latent tissue plasminogen activator produced by human endothelial cells in culture: evidence of an enzyme-inhibitor complex. Proc Natl Acad Sci USA 80, 6804, 1983.

10. Korninger C, Wagner O, Binder BR. Tissue plasminogen activator inhibitor in human plasma: development of a functional assay system and demonstration of a correlating Mr 50.000 antiactivator. J Lab Clin Med 105, 718, 1985.

11. Van Hinsbergh VWM, Bertina RM, van Wijngaarden A, van Tilburg NH, Emeis JJ, Haverkate F. Activated protein C decreases plasminogen activator inhibitor activity in endothelial cell conditioned medium. Blood, 65, 444, 1985.

12. De Fouw NJ, Haverkate F, Bertina RM, Koopman J, van Wijngaarden A, van Hinsbergh VWM. The cofactor role of protein S in acceleration of whole blood clot lysis by activated protein C in vitro. Blood 67, 1189, 1986.

13. Suzuki K, Nishioka J, Hashimoto S. Protein C inhibitor: purification from human plasma and characterization. J Biol Chem 258, 163, 1983.

14. Griffin JH, Evatt B, Zimmerman TS, Kleis AJ, Wideman C. Deficiency of protein C in congenital thrombotic disease. J Clin Invest 68, 1370, 1981.

15. Marciniak E, Wilson HD, Marlar RA. Neonatal purpura fulminans: a genetic disorder related to the absence of protein C in blood. Blood 65, 15, 1985.

16. Sills RH, Marlar RA, Montgomery RR, Deshpande GN, Humbert JR. Severe homozygous protein C deficiency. J Pediatr 105, 409, 1984.

17. Clouse LH, Comp PC. The regulation of hemostasis. N Engl J Med 314, 1298, 1986.

18. Vukovich TH, Weil J, Auberger K, Engelmann H, Knöbl P, Hadorn HB. Replacement therapy of a severe homozygous protein C deficiency state using a concentrate of human protein C and S. Brit J Haematol 70, 435, 1988.

19. Manabe S, Matsuda M. Homozygous protein C deficiency combined with heterozygous dysplasminogenemia found in a 21-year-old thrombophilic male. Thromb Res 39, 333, 1985.

20. Broekmans AW, Veltkamp JJ, Bertina RM. Congenital protein C deficiency and venous thromboembolism. A study in three Dutch families. N Engl J Med 309, 340, 1983.

21. Riess H, Binsack T, Hiller E. Protein C antigen in prothrombin complex concentrates: content, recovery and half life. Blut 50, 303, 1985.

22. Riess H, Riewald M, Wagner M, Reinhardt B, Vukovich TH, Hiller E. Protein C concentrate and coumarin necrosis: a case report. Blut, 53, 182, 1986.

23. Schwarz HP, Fischer M, Hopmeier P, Batard MA, Griffin JH. Plasma protein S deficiency in familial thrombotic disease. Blood, 64 1297, 1984.

24. Comp PC, Esmon CT. Recurrent venous thromboembolism in patients with a partial deficiency of protein S. N Engl J Med 311, 1525, 1984.

25. Griffin JM, Mosher DF, Zimmermann TS, Kleiss AJ. Protein C an antithrombotic protein, is reduced in hospitalized patients with intravascular coagulation. Blood 60, 261, 1982.

26. Manucci PM, Vigano S. Deficiencies of protein C, an inhibitor of blood coagulation. Lancet 2, 463, 1982.

27. Vukovich TC, Schernthaner G. Decreased protein C levels in patients with insulin-dependent type I diabetes mellitus. Diabetes 35, 617, 1986.

28. Schwarz HP, Schernthaner G, Griffin JH. Decreased plasma levels of protein S in well-controlled type I diabetes mellitus. Thromb Haemostas 57, 240, 1987.

29. Knöbl PN, Zilla P, Fasol MD, Müller MM, Vukovich TC. The protein C system in patients undergoing cardiopulmonary bypass. J Thorac Cardiovasc Surg 94, 600, 1987.

30. Vukovich TC, Knöbl PN, Havel MP, Andert RC, Müller MM. Elastase inhibitory capacity, antithrombin III, and antiplasmin levels in patients undergoing cardiopulmonary bypass. Manuscript in preparation.

31. Havel MP, Graninger W, Moritz A, Griesmacher A, Priess P, Müller MM, Wolner E. Release of granulozyte elastase during cardiopulmonary bypass. J Europ Soc Artificial Organs 4, Suppl 2, 210, 1986.

32. Powars DR, Rogers ZR, Patch MJ, McGehee WG. Francis RB. Purpura fulminans in meningococcemia: association with acquired deficiencies of proteins C and S. N Engl J Med 317, 571, 1987.

33. Moore KL, Andreoli SP, Esmon NL, Esmon CT, Bang NU. Endotoxin enhances tissue factor and suppresses thrombomodulin expression of human vascular endothelium in vitro. J Clin Invest 79, 124, 1987.

34. Taylor FB, Chang A, Esmon CT, D'Angelo A, Vigano-D'Angelo S, Blick KE. Protein C prevents the coagulopathic and lethal effects of Escherichia coli infusion in the baboon. J Clin Inves 79, 918, 1987.

35. Ehrlich HJ, Bang NU, Esmon CT. In vivo behaviour of detergent solubilized purified rabbit thrombomodulin injected into rabbits. Thromb Haemostas 58, 320, 1987.

36. Rosenberg RD, Damus PS. The purification and mechanism of action of human antithrombin-heparin cofactor. J Biol Chem 248, 6490, 1973.

3. Endothelial Cell Lining

37. Jordan RE, Oosta GM, Gardner WT, Rosenberg RD. The kinetics of haemostatic enzyme-antithrombin III interactions in the presence of low molecular weight heparin. J Biol Chem 255, 10081, 1980.

38. McLean J, The thromboplastic action of cephalin. Am J Physiol 41, 250, 1916.

39. Pepsy J, Edwards AM (Editors). The mast cells. Kent, England Pitman Medical p. 842, 1979.

40. Damus PS, Hick M, Rosenberg RD. Anticoagulant action of heparin. Nature 246, 355, 1973.

41. Marcum JA, Rosenberg RD. Anticoagulantly active heparin-like molecules from vascular tissue. Biochem 23, 1730, 1984.

42. Marcum JA, Rosenberg RD. Heparin-like molecules with anticoagulant activity are synthesized by cultured endothelial cells. Biochem Biophys Res Commun 126, 365, 1985.

43. Marcus JA, McKenney JB, Rosenberg RD. Acceleration of thrombin-antithrombin complex formation in rat hindquarters via heparin-like molecules bound to the endothelium. J Clin Invest 74, 341, 1984.

44. Marcum JA, Reilly CF, Rosenberg RD. The role of specific forms of heparin sulphate in regulating blood vessel wall function. In: Progress in Haemostasis and Thrombosis (editor Coller BS); Grune & Stratton, Orlando. 8, 185, 1986.

45. Egeberg O. Inherited antithrombin deficiency causing thrombophilia. Thromb Diath Haemorrh 13, 516, 1965.

46. Sas G, Petö I, Banghegyi D, Domjan G, Blasko G. Heterogeneity of the classical antithrombin III deficiency. Thromb Haemostas 43, 133, 1980.

47. Thaler E. Pathogenese und klinische Bedeutung des erworbenen Antithrombin III Mangels in der inneren Medizin. Wien Klin Wschr 93, 563, 1981.

48. Kaufmann RH, Veltkamp JJ, Tilburg NH, van Es LA. Aquired antithrombin III deficiency and thrombosis in nephrotic syndrome. Am J Med 65, 607, 1978.

49. Thaler E. Disseminerte intravasculäre Gerinnung: Antithrombin III und Heparin. Folia Haematol, 104, 740, 1977.

50. Stamatikis JD, Lawrence D, Kakker VV. Surgery, venous thrombosis and anti Xa. Brit J Surg 64, 709, 1977.

51. Kobayashi T, Terao T. Preeclamsia as chronic disseminated intravascular coagulation. Study of two parameters: thrombin-antithrombin III complexes and D-dimers. Gynecol Obst Invest 24, 170, 1987.

52. Hellgren M, Javelin L, Hägnevik K, Blombäck M. Antithrombin III concentrate as adjuvant in DIC treatment. A pilot study in 9 severely ill patients. Thromb Res 35, 459, 1984.

53. Blauhut B, Kramer H, Vinazzer H, Bergmann H. Substitution of antithrombin III in DIC: a randomized study. Thromb Res 39, 81, 1985.

54. Vinazzer H. Clinical use of antithrombin III concentrates. Vox Sang 53, 193, 1987.

3.2.2. Heparin-Binding Growth Factors

T Maciag

*Laboratory of Molecular Biology,
Jerome H Holland Laboratory for the Biomedical Sciences,
American Red Cross,
Rockville, Maryland, USA*

Introduction

Angiogenesis is the formation of new blood vessels *in vivo*. During this process, quiescent vessel wall-derived cells are activated by hormonal-like agents which induce cellular migration, proliferation, and differentiation *in situ*. Because the migration of the endothelial cell is the presumed initiator of the dynamics of neovascularization, biological agents, which modulate endothelial cell function, may contribute significantly to the phenomena of angiogenesis *in situ*. Likewise, an orchestrated series of integrated events, involving the hormonal modulation of the pericyte, fibroblast, macrophage, and smooth muscle cell, occur in tandem during the cascade with angiogenesis. Indeed, biological agents, which affect the dynamics of these cell types *in vitro* can also modulate the process of neovascularization *in vivo*. Thus, the variety of cell types involved in the process of angiogenesis *in situ* may account for the structural variety of biochemical angiogenics (1,2,3). However, consideration of these angiogenic effectors as potential initiators of human endothelial cell proliferation reduces this variation in structure to a family of polypeptides collectively known as the heparin-binding growth factors (4,5,6,7).

The Heparin-Binding Growth Factors

Two polypeptide mitogens have been characterized as potent stimulators of human endothelial cell proliferation in vitro and initiators of angiogenesis in vivo (8,9). Fibroblast growth factor (FGF) and endothelial cell growth factor (ECGF) represent two brain-derived growth factors which have been purified based upon their avid affinity for immobilized heparin (10,11). Prior to structural characterization, the two polypeptide mitogens could be identified as distinct activities by their different isoelectric points and affinity for heparin. These differences are highlighted by the nomenclature which describes the acidic polypeptide as heparin-binding growth factor-I (HBGF-I) and the basic polypeptide as heparin-binding growth factor-II (HBGF-II) (13). Table 30 lists the nomenclature previously used to describe the polypeptides. Both growth factors possess a similar range of biological targets (Table 31) with the exception that HBGF-I, unlike HBGF-II, cannot stimulate human melanocyte proliferation in vitro (12). Table 31 summarizes the physical, chemical, and biological properties of both polypeptides.

Although distinguishable by isoelectric points and heparin affinity, the abil-

3. Endothelial Cell Lining

Previous Nomenclature for the Heparin-Binding Growth Factors

HBGF-I

Acidic-fibroblast growth factor
Endothelial cell growth factor, (alpha,beta)
Astroglial growth factor-I
Prostate endothelial cell growth factor (prostatropin)
Anionic-hypothalamus growth factor
Eye-derived growth factor-II
Retina-derived growth factor
Brain-derived growth factor-I

HBGF-II

Basic-fibroblast growth factor
Astroglial growth factor-II
Cationic-hypothalamus growth factor
Eye-derived growth factor-I
Brain-derived growth factor-II

Table 30

ity of heparin to potentiate the biological activity of the acidic polypeptide, is a property not shared by HBGF-II (14). Further, radioreceptor and immunological methods have been employed to study the ability of heparin to stabilize the biological activity of HBGF-I (14), presumably by conformational stability. Likewise, heparin blankets the acidic polypeptide and creates a situation where HBGF-I is refractory to proteolytic modification by trypsin and plasmin. Although heparin does not potentiate the biological activity of HBGF-II, heparin does induce conformational stability in both HBGF-I and HBGF-II (14). Table 31 summarizes the similarity and distinguishing characteristics of the interaction between HBGF I and HBGF-II, and heparin.

The Structural Properties of the Heparin-Binding Growth Factors

The structures of HBGF-I and HBGF-II have been deduced by traditional protein chemistry methods (4,5,6,7) and cDNA cloning (16,17).

Both growth factor classes are single chain polypeptides containing a methionine residue within a single disulfide loop.

Although the structures of HBGF-I and HBGF-II are distinct, the polypeptides demonstrate a high degree (55%) of sequence similarity to each other. This similarity is most apparent in the COOH terminal end of the polypeptides. Although a number of different forms of both polypeptides have been characterized, all variations within the structures of HBGF-I and HBGF-II are modifications of the growth factors in the NH_2-terminal domain in both classes (5,7). The isolation of biologically active NH_2-terminal-truncated forms of both HBGF-I and HBGF-II suggest that the NH_2-terminal domain of both polypeptide classes do not contain structural information relevant to the biological activity of polypeptides as functional mitogens in vitro. Whether the non-homologous sequences associated with the NH_2-terminus of HBGF-I and HBGF-II, contain structural information relevant to other biological activities, is presently unclear.

Properties of the Heparin-Binding Fibroblast Growth Factors

	HBGF-I	HBGF-II
Heparin Elution (NaCl)	1.0M	>2.0M
Structural Similarity	55%	55%
Structural Similarity to int-2	33%	45%
Structural Similarity to hst/ks	34%	48%
Isoelectric Point	4.6	> 9.0
M_r/Amino Acid Residues	155	> 155
Signal Peptide Sequence	None	None
Blocked Amino Terminus	Yes	ND
Biological Activities:		
Endothelial Cells	+	+
Fibroblasts	+	+
Smooth Muscle Cells	+	+
Myoblasts	ND	+
Kerantinocytes	+	ND
Melanocytes	-	+
Neurite Extension	+	+
Potentiation by Heparin (Biological Activity)	Yes	No
Protection by Heparin (Denaturation, Proteases)	Yes	Yes
Competitive Receptor Binding Between Ligands	+(30-40%)	+(ND)
M_r Receptor (Cross-Linking)	≅150,000	≅150,000
Receptor-Associated Tyrosine Kinase Activity	Yes	ND
Stimulates Angiogenesis *In Vivo*	Yes	Yes

Table 31

The genes encoding both the acidic and basic polypeptides have been isolated and the deduced amino acid sequences agree with the polypeptide structures obtained by protein chemistry methods (15,16). Comparison of the human and bovine sequences for HBGF-I suggest that the HBGF-I gene is conserved among mammals. Although the upstream sequence encoding the open-reading frame for HBGF-II has not presently been deduced, it is thought that this domain in HBGF-II, like HBGF-I, will not contain a signal peptide sequence (15,16). This observation suggests that biosynthetic HBGF-I and HBGF-II are not secreted by cells in the traditional endocrine manner. This is consistent with the apparent absence of HBGF-I from biological fluids such as plasma (14). Although the biological reason for the absence of a signal peptide sequence in the structures of HBGF-I and HBGF-II is not known, the inability to secrete the polypeptides may reflect a degree of conservation by nature which restricts the potent biological properties of these polypeptides in situ. Likewise, the absence of a signal peptide sequence also suggests that cell death, in the form of necrosis, and/or ischemia, may play an important role in the release of these wide-spectrum biological mitogens.

The genes encoding HBGF-I and HBGF-II have been localized to different chromosomes (15). Interestingly, HBGF-I residues on human chromosome 5q31.3-33.2, a very rich hormone receptor region which includes the platelet-derived growth factor receptor and the receptor for colony-stimulating factor-1, the c-fms proto-oncogene. The significance of this observation is presently not known.

Structural Sequence Similarities between the Heparin-Binding Growth Factors and other Growth Factors and Oncogenes

HBGF-I and HBGF-II share sequence similarities with the growth factor family of interleukins (IL). HBGF-I contains a 16% structural similarity with IL-1 alpha and a 20% homology with IL-1 beta (6). Likewise, HBGF-II contains a 14% sequence similarity with IL-1 alpha and a 20% structural homology with IL-1 beta. Interestingly, the interleukens do not contain a consensus signal peptide sequence, a property which is shared by HBGF-I and HBGF-II. These homologies suggest that the interleukins and heparin-binding growth factors may have arisen from a single primordial gene which diverged into two polypeptide families (16). However, the interleukins do not share the biological attributes associated with the heparin-binding growth factors.

Recently, two new oncogenes have been discovered and their polypeptide sequences deduced from their nucleotide sequences. The oncogene, hst/ks, was independently isolated from a human stomach tumor (17) and a human Kaposi sarcoma (18). In addition, the oncogene, int-2, was isolated from a mouse mammary carcinoma (19). Interestingly, both oncogenes contain amino acid sequences which are homologous with HBGF-I and HBGF-II. The oncogenes, hst/ks and int-2, contain approximately a 45% and 33% structural similarity with HBGF-II and HBGF-I respectively. The presence of a potential disulfide loop containing a single methonine residue is conserved in the structures of both hst/ks and int-2. This property is consistent with the design of HBGF-I and HBGF-II. Further, the most significant sequence homologies between the two oncogenes and the heparin-binding growth factors occur in the COOH-terminal domain of the polypeptides. In contrast to the precursor structures of HBGF-I and HBGF-II, both hst/ks and int-2 possess precursor forms containing NH_2-terminal hydrophobic sequences which may serve as a signal peptide. Thus, unlike HBGF-I and HBGF-II, int-2 and hst/ks are most likely secreted in the traditional endocrine manner. Whether the hst/ks and int-2 polypeptides can bind heparin, compete for HBGF-I and HBGF-II receptor occupancy, or exert an angiogenic or mitogenic response, is presently unknown. However, the existence of these oncogenes serves to highlight the anticipated complexity of angiogenesis and the possible function of putative growth factor-helper genes during this process *in vivo*.

Sites of Synthesis for the Heparin-Binding Growth Factors

Although both polypeptides were initially isolated from bovine brain, the absence of these polypeptides in plasma and serum suggests that they do not utilize the circulatory system as a carrier to biological sites of need. Studies designed to evaluate the role of plasma-derived cells as potential carriers of the heparin-binding growth factors have suggested that the mRNA transcript for HBGF-I is not expressed in these cells. In contrast, the mRNA transcript for HBGF-II has been found to be present in the macrophage/monocyte, suggesting that HBGF-II, but not HBGF-I, may be carried to angiogenic sites (20). Within the vessel wall, vascular human smooth muscle cells, but not human endothelial cells, express the HBGF-I mRNA transcript and a HBGF-I-like polypeptide (21). Further, it is also known that human endothelial cells express the PDGF-B chain, a potent smooth muscle cell mitogen (21). Surprisingly, the heparin-binding growth factors are also potent mitogens for vascular smooth muscle cells in vitro (21). These data suggest that a potential paracrine situation may be established between the vascular smooth muscle and endothelial cells in which both cell types may contribute to the potential proliferative ability of their neighbor. This could also serve to mediate or amplify the role of the macrophage and platelet in vascular injury. Such a model would require cell death as an important component, since HBGF-I and HBGF-II do not possess signal peptide sequences for polypeptide secretion.

The ability of the vascular smooth muscle cell to synthesize the HBGF-I mRNA transcript may explain the induction of angiogenesis which accompanies atherogenesis *in vivo*. The recruitment of the endothelial cell from the vasa vasorum may indeed be the responsibility of the heparin-binding growth factors. Likewise, angiogenesis, which accompanies the growth of solid tumors *in vivo*, may also involve the expression of the heparin-binding growth factors. However, in situations where the angiogenic growth factors are released from cellular constraints, it is likely that only a small amount reached the appropriate paracrine receptor, while most remains adsorbed to the extracellular matrix (26), perhaps complexed with the heparin sulfate proteoglycan. Such mechanisms stress the importance of the extracellular matrix as a potential modulator of heparin-binding growth factor function in physiology and pathology and further demonstrate the potential biochemical complexity of angiogenesis *in situ*.

The Receptor(s) for the Heparin-Binding Growth Factors

High affinity receptors for HBGF-I and HBGF-II are present on the surface of endothelial cells. Ligand-binding assays from HBGF-I have established that the HBGF-I receptor is rapidly down-regulated by receptor occupancy; an event which is a prerequisite for the initiation of DNA synthesis (14). These properties suggest that the receptor system(s) for the heparin-binding growth factors will most likely be similar to the receptors for other polypeptide mitogens (22). Table 31 lists the properties of the receptors for HBGF-I and HBGF-II. Although it is presently unclear whether two independent receptors exist for HBGF-I and HBGF-II, covalent ligand: receptor cross-linking strategies with both ligands have yielded at least two receptor candidates for both ligands with molecular weights (M_r) of approximately M_r 170,000 and M_r 150,000 (23,24). Whether these putative receptor candidates represent a covalent modification of a common precursor or two distinct receptor systems is presently not known. However, both receptor species appear to be phosphorylated by a tyrosine kinase activity which is activated by ligand occupancy of the receptor (25). Further studies promise to define the structure of the receptor(s) for this polypeptide growth factor family; information which is critical to our understanding the function of these polypeptides *in situ*.

Addendum: This subject has been recently reviewed in depths in: Burgess WH, Maciag T. Annual review of biochemistry, 1989.

3. Endothelial Cell Lining

References

1. *Folkman J. Science (Wash, DC), 235, 442, 1987.*
2. *Maciag T. Prog Hemost Thromb 7, 167, 1984.*
3. *Folkman J and Klagsbrun M. Science (Wash, DC), 235, 442, 1987.*
4. *Harper JW et al. Biochemistry 25, 4097, 1986.*
5. *Esch F et al. Proc Natl Acad Sci USA 82, 6507, 1985.*
6. *Thomas KA et al. Proc Natl Acad Sci USA 82, 6409, 1985.*
7. *Burgess WH et al. Proc Natl Acad Sci USA 83, 7216, 1986.*
8. *Thomas KA Gimenez-Gallego G. Trends in Biochem Sci 11, 81, 1986.*
9. *Hayek A et al. Biochem Biophys Res Comm 147, 876, 1987.*
10. *Shing T et al. Science (Wash, DC), 223, 1296, 1984.*
11. *Maciag T et al. Science (Wash, DC), 225, 932, 1984.*
12. *Halaban T et al. In Vitro Cell. Dev Biol 23, 47, 1987.*
13. *Lobb RR et al. Analyt Biochem 154, 1, 1986.*
14. *Schreiber AB et al. Proc Natl Acad Sci. USA 82, 6138, 1985.*
15. *Jaye M et al. Science (Wash, DC), 233, 541, 1986.*
16. *Abraham JA et al. Science (Wash, DC), 233, 345, 1986.*
17. *Taira M et al. Proc Natl Acad Sci USA 24, 2980, 1987.*
18. *DelliBovi P et al. Cell 50, 729, 1987.*
19. *Dickson C et al. Cell 37, 529, 1984.*
20. *Baird A, Ling N. Biochem Biophys Res Comm 142, 428, 1987.*
21. *Winkles JA et al. Proc Natl Acad Sci USA 84, 7124, 1987.*
22. *James R, Bradshaw RA. Ann Rev Biochem 53, 259, 1984.*
23. *Friesel R et al. J Biol Chem 261, 7581, 1986.*
24. *Neufeld G, Gospodarowicz D. J Biol Chem 261, 13860, 1985.*
25. *Huang SS, Huang JS. J Biol Chem 260, 9568, 1986.*
26. *Vlodavsky L et al. Proc Natl Acad Sci USA 84, 2292, 1987.*

3. Endothelial Cell Lining

3.2.3. Active Responses and Signal Transduction in Endothelial Cells

US Ryan

*University of Miami, School of Medicine,
Miami, Florida, USA*

Abstract

Endothelial cells form the natural blood interface and it is now well recognized that physical or chemical treatment of artificial biomaterials to render them blood compatible frequently reproduces only one or a few of the properties of the natural endothelial lining. Since pannus ingrowth into implanted prostheses in humans is not extensive, many investigators have attempted to improve the situation by seeding with endothelial cells, their derivatives or products. However, endothelialization is not an inert treatment that can be applied to a surface, it consists of a monolayer of highly metabolically active, responsive cells that react to blood-borne and tissue-derived stimuli in ways that change the hemostatic and immunologic profile of the blood-vessel interface. We now know that, in addition to their barrier properties, endothelial cells can regulate the quality of blood by selective metabolism of circulating bioactive substances. In addition, endothelial cells possess a wide variety of receptors, engagement of which leads to an equally wide variety of endothelial cell responses. However, the mechanisms by which the endothelial cell translates the signal into the response are not well known. We have studied signal transduction in endothelial cells focusing particularly on the role of calcium. We have studied the response to vasodilator agonists that cause release of endothelial derived relaxing factors (EDRF), responses to platelet activating factor and responses to phagocytosis of bacteria. We have applied a variety of techniques, including the use of fluorescent indicators INDO-1 and FURA-2, to measure intracellular calcium concentration, $[Ca^{2+}]_i$, measurement of Ca^{2+} fluxes using ^{45}Ca loaded endothelial cells, and patch-clamp techniques to measure ionic currents in the endothelial cell membrane. We have shown that:

- agonist action is controlled by intracellular free calcium levels, $[Ca^{2+}]_i$,
- agonists may exert their actions on endothelial cells via activation of phosphoinositide turnover,
- Ca^{2+} entry through receptor-operated ion channels contributes to excitation-secretion coupling in endothelial cells,
- a negative feedback mechanism that blocks receptor-mediated increase in intracellular calcium is triggered as a result of activation of protein kinase C.

Thus, endothelial cells seeded into vascular prostheses cannot be assumed to be metabolically stable. Their functions and dysfunctions are controlled by highly sensitive mechanisms similar to stimulus-response coupling systems in a wide variety of excitable and reactive cell types.

Introduction

Techniques for culture of endothelial cells are now at a stage where reproducible long-term, large-scale cultures can be obtained routinely (1-4). Furthermore, there are now a number of techniques that allow seeding of endothelial cells from a variety of sources onto vascular prostheses (5, see also chapters by Callow, Kempczinski, Risberg, Schmidt, Stanley). Thus the question is no longer: Is vascular seeding possible, but rather: Is vascular seeding desirable? It still remains true that the normal blood vessel lining, composed of a single layer of endothelial cells, is the only surface known over which blood flows for a lifetime. The endothelium that appears extremely thin in cross section (Figure 106) is remarkably durable and the turnover of individual cells is very low. However, it is a mistake to regard the endothelium simply as an inert lining layer endowed with non-thrombogenic and passive permeability properties.

Endothelial cells possess a wide range of active metabolic functions (6,7) and are capable of responding to a plethora of blood-borne and tissue-derived molecules. Endothelial responses to such stimuli include the synthesis and release of a number of bioactive molecules that affect neighboring cells and target organs at a distance. Interactions between endothelial cells and other molecules, cell-types or particulates together constitute the overall

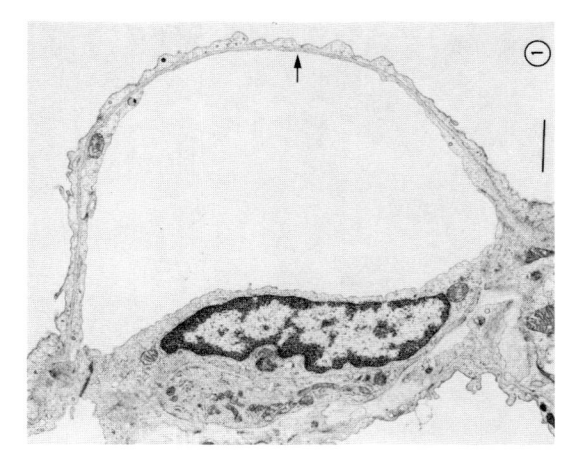

Fig. 106 Transmission electron micrograph of blood-free rat pulmonary capillary illustrating the extreme thinness of the endothelial cells which, at the gas exchanging surface, is barely thicker than its two cell membranes (arrow). Bar = 0.5 μm.

functional significance of the endothelial layer. In this chapter, the active responses of endothelial cells to some of these stimuli are described and the mechanisms whereby endothelial cells transduce the signal into the response are considered. The aim is to improve understanding of the cellular and molecular biology of the endothelial cell and the conditions under which endothelial seeding of vascular prostheses can be used to the best advantage.

Techniques for Endothelial Cell Culture and Seeding

Despite earlier scattered reports, the culture of endothelial cells as a routine procedure dates from the early 1970s, when endothelial cultures from umbilical vein (8,9) and pulmonary artery (10) were established. The isolation techniques used proteolytic enzymes, usually trypsin or collagenase, to remove the cells and trypsin/EDTA mixtures for passaging. Since proteolytic enzymes remove endothelial surface enzymes,

3. Endothelial Cell Lining

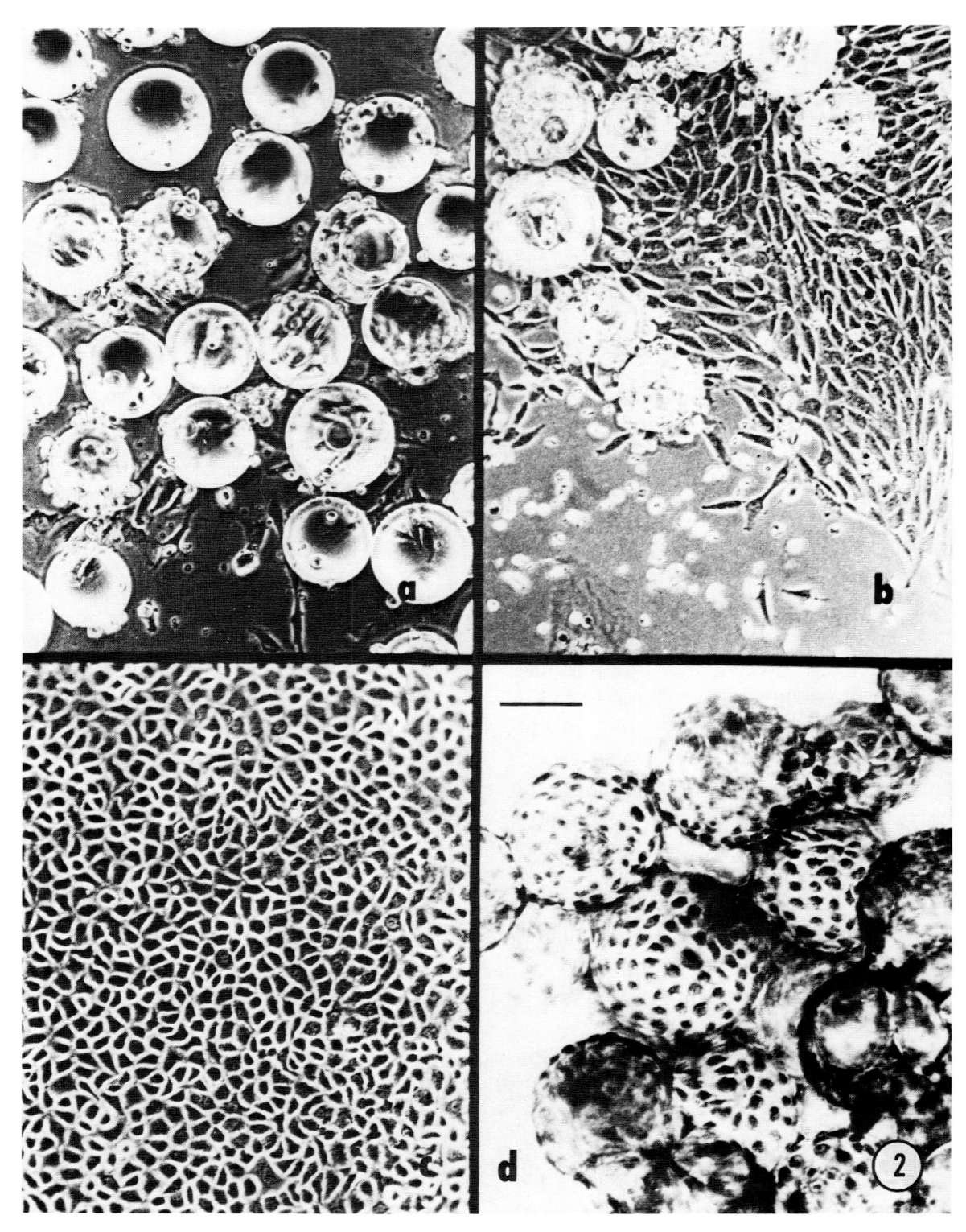

Fig. 107 As shown in the sequence: Figs a-d, endothelial cells isolated on microcarriers **(a)** can be introduced into flasks **(b)**, allowed to form stationary monolayer cultures **(c)**, and then seeded back onto microcarriers for scale-up in roller bottles **(d)**. Bar = 100 μm; from referenc14.

receptors and some extracellular matrix molecules, techniques have been developed more recently for the non-enzymatic isolation and long-term culture of endothelial cells. Endothelial cells can be removed from large vessels mechanically by scraping with a scalpel (12) and subcultured either on microcarriers (13) or with a rubber policeman. Isolation of microvascular endothelial cells can be accomplished using microcarriers of 40-70 microns, the approximate diameter of the vessels from which the desired endothelial cells are collected (Figure 107). Endothelial cells can be collected from both the arterial and venous microcirculation of the lungs, and potentially from any organ, by this method (14-16). Once in monolayer culture, the cells can be subcultured on microcarriers (2,13) or with a rubber policeman, as for large vessel endothelium.

Endothelial cells in culture from a variety of sources can be used for seeding vascular grafts. A number of procedures result in good coverage of the graft surface in vitro and confluence can be achieved within two weeks. Nevertheless the problems associated with seeding vascular grafts relate more to detachment of the endothelial cell layer in vivo or during surgical manipulations, and to the need to use autologous endothelium or else to find alternative means for avoiding immunological problems.

Gortex grafts can be seeded successfully if a preclotting step is included (Figure 108) while Corvita polyurethane grafts that have a gelatin impregnated surface can be seeded directly (Figure 109). Thus, the potential for endothelial seeding in the operating room exists and some attachment of endothelial cells within 15 mins is seen even though confluence itself cannot be achieved under these conditions.

Metabolic Activities of Endothelial Cells

Endothelial cells are now known to be capable of metabolizing a wide variety of circulating vasoactive substrates including peptides, adenine nucleotides, prostaglandins and amines (6, 7,17). Thus, angiotensin converting enzyme situated on the luminal surface of endothelial cells (10,11), is capable of degrading bradykinin and of converting angiotensin I to angiotensin II (17). Endothelium is also able to degrade the adenine nucleotides by means of ectoenzymes (18-20) and to take up adenosine (20,21) formed in the process or derived from other sources. Endothelial cells are capable of uptake of prostaglandins but probably transport them to extravascular sites for processing. Endothelial cells in culture metabolize leucotrienes (22). Vasoactive amines such as norepinephrine and 5-HT undergo endothelial uptake and intracellular metabolism by monoamine oxidase (23).

In addition endothelial cells possess carboxypeptidase N, an enzyme important in the processing of the anaphylatoxins (24). They also possess carbonic anhydrase which indicates that endothelial cells can play a role in facilitating the release of CO_2 from vessels and in regulating the pH of blood (25). A number of xenobiotic substances are also metabolized by endothelial cells (26). The disposition of some of the enzymes involved in the metabolic functions described above are illustrated in Figure 110.

All in all, the ability of endothelial cells to process (activate, inactivate or other-

3. Endothelial Cell Lining

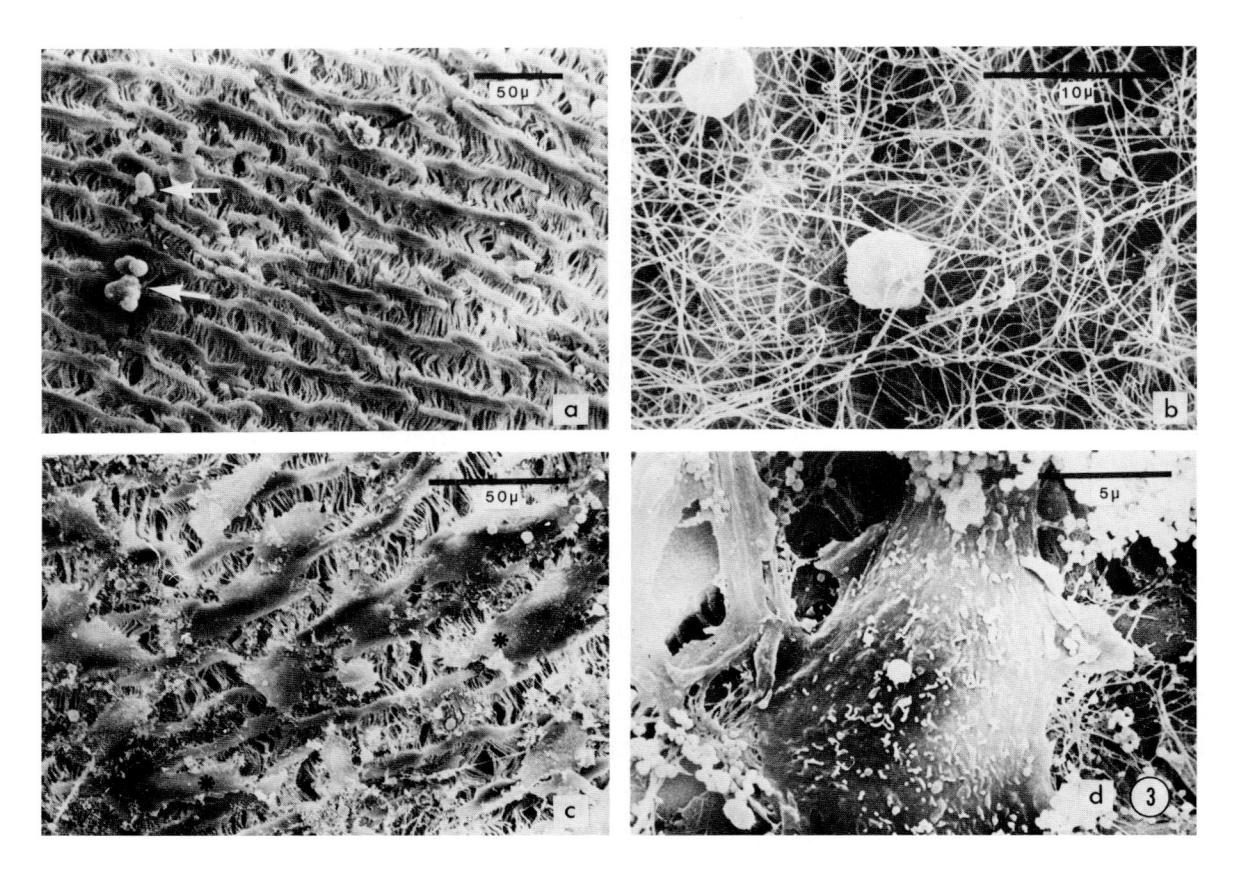

Fig. 108 **a)** Endothelial cells (arrows) seeded onto untreated Gore-tex graft, no attachment or spreading. **b)** Gore-tex surface preclotted and washed. **c)** Gore-tex surface, preclotted, seeded with endothelial cells (*). **d)** High power of endothelial cell on pretreated graft (5).

wise remove) circulating vasoactive substances constitutes an important physiological function of endothelium. It will be important to ensure that the endothelium that colonizes or is seeded onto vascular grafts is not compromised in this respect.

Responses of Endothelial Cells to Blood-Borne Stimuli

In addition to being able to process blood-borne vasoactive substances, endothelial cells are also able to react to them. For example, substances such as bradykinin, thrombin and ATP are metabolized by endothelial cells but also interact with endothelial cells to cause release of prostacyclin PGI_2 (27), platelet activating factor (PAF) (28) and endothelium dependent relaxing factor (EDRF) (29). However the mechanisms of signal transduction involved in the release of these active products are not well known. It has been postulated that increased intracellular free calcium concentration could trigger the release of these substances. Increase in intracellular calcium, $[Ca^{2+}]\sim_i$, can be the result of increased influx from extracellular sources, release from intracellular stores, or a combination of both processes.

The studies described here were designed to elucidate the relationship between release of active products derived from endothelial cells and agonist induced calcium movements.

3. Endothelial Cell Lining

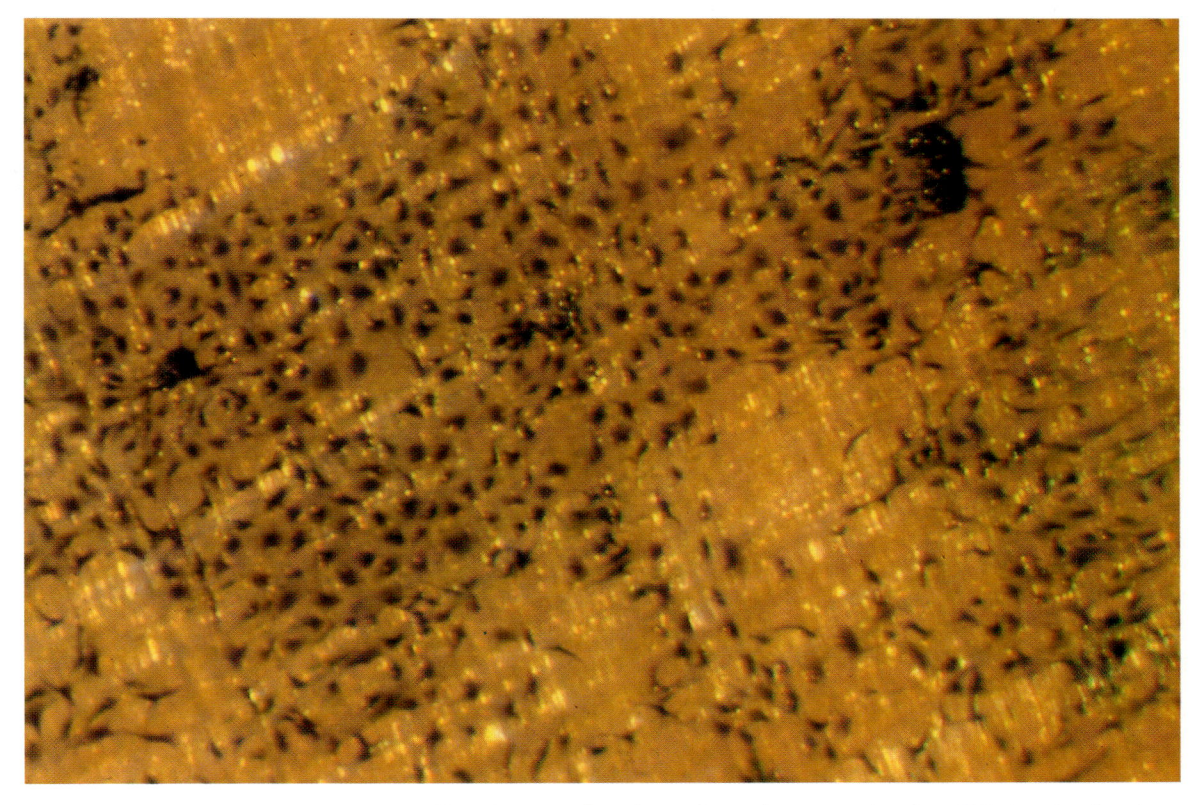

Fig. 109 Endothelial cells seeded directly onto Corvita polyurethane graft, after 68h incubation in a roller-bottle incubator. Bar = 100 µm.

Release of EDRF

Endothelial cells in vivo engage in close structural and functional interactions with smooth muscle cells. Myoendothelial junctions occur in a variety of vessels, and are abundant in small pulmonary arteries (30). Their function is not known. They may be involved in mechanical interactions, ionic interactions or could conceivably act as specific conduits for chemical messengers.

Functional interactions between endothelial cells and smooth muscle have been demonstrated involving the release of endothelium dependent vasodilators (29,31) and contracting substances (32). Clearly, interactions between endothelium and smooth muscle are not germane to the situation in artificial grafts. However, endothelium dependent relaxing factor(s) also act on platelets to reduce aggregation, a situation critical to graft survival (Figure 111).

Release of EDRF was assayed on both smooth muscle and platelets and the effect of various agonists on the release of EDRF from cultured bovine pulmonary artery endothelial cells was investigated. Thrombin, ATP, bradykinin and calcium ionophore A23187 each caused relaxation of a precontracted de-endothelialized rabbit aortic strip when added to a column of endothelial cells on microcarriers mounted above the assay tissue (33). None of these agonists had any relaxing action if added directly to the assay strip, bypassing the endothelial cell column (33).

Release of EDRF can occur in response to bradykinin or ATP in the absence of extracellular calcium (EGTA, 2

3. Endothelial Cell Lining

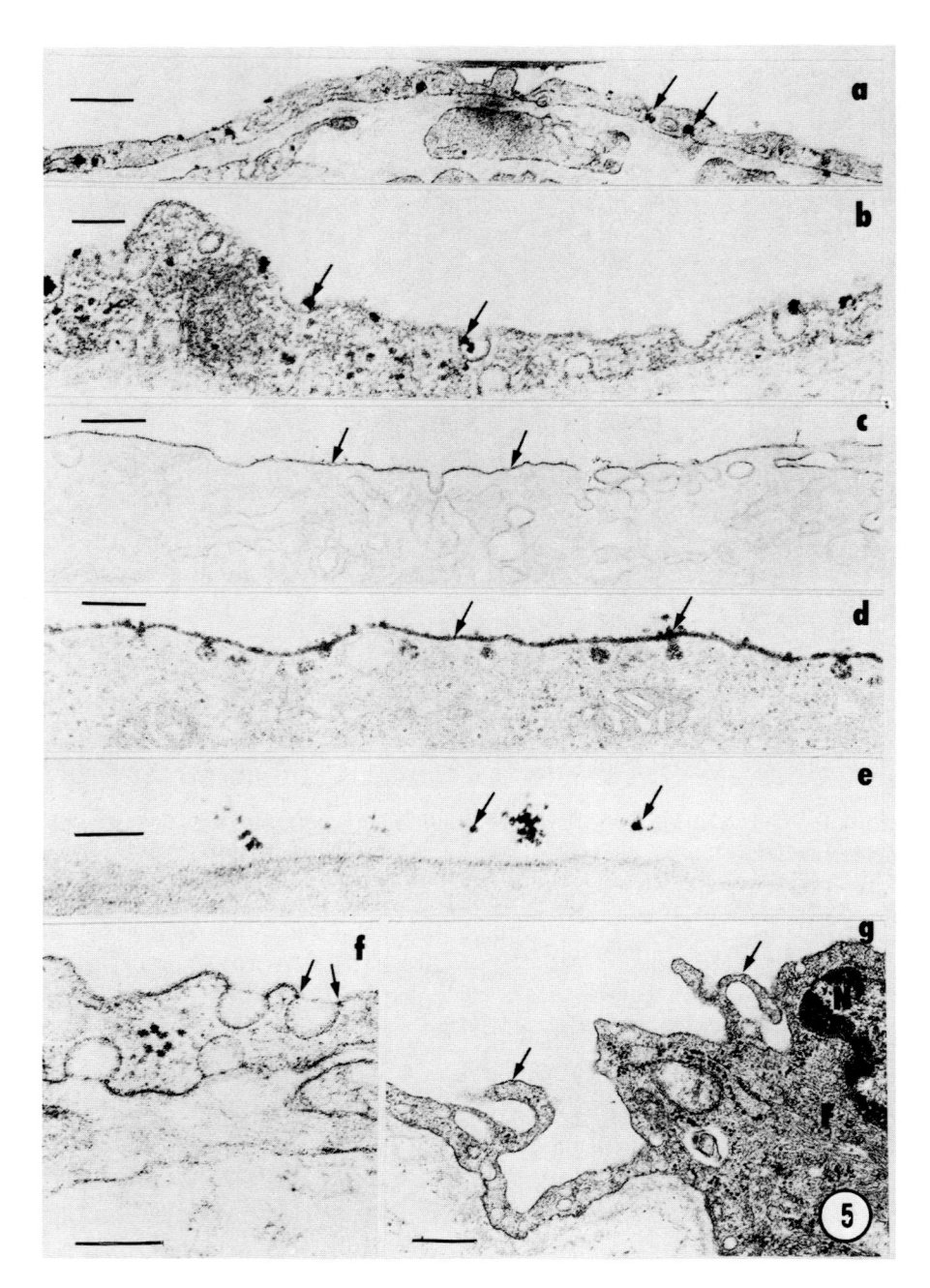

Fig. 110 Enzymes of the endothelial plasma membrane and associated caveolae. **a)** Cytochemical localization of ATPase indicating sites of ATPase activity specifically localized in caveolae (arrows). Bar = 0.2 μm. **b)** Cytochemical localization showing sites of 5'-=nucleotidase activity localized on caveolae (and in incipient caveolae) facing the vascular lumen (arrows). Bar = 0.1μm. **c)** Immunocytochemical localization of ACE one a pulmonary endothelial cell in culture. The electron-dense reaction product indicating sites of immunoreactive ACE (arrows) is localized along the plasma membrane, including caveolae. Bar = 0.2 μm. **d)** Immuno-cytochemical localization of carboxypeptidase N (CPN) on the plasma membrane and associated caveolae (arrows). Bar = 0.2 μm. **e)** Immunocytochemical localization of carbonic anhydrase. Sites of reactivity (arrows) are localized on the plasma membrane; the ferritin tag is restricted by a layer approximately 100 over A thick. Bar = 0.05 μm. **f)** Part of a capillary endothelial cell showing caveolae and diaphragms composed of a single lamella. Dense knobs at junctions of diaphragm with caveola membrane and plasma membrane (arrows) may represent a skeletal rim or ring of beads, which could help to maintain patency of the stoma and integrity of the diaphragm. Bar = 0.1 μm. **g)** Portion of an endothelial cell with its nucleus (N). Fibrillar strands (F) are present in the subnuclear cytoplasm. Endothelial projections (arrows) occur both on the main body of the cell and on the tenuous peripheral pertions. Bar = 10 μm. From reference 42.

3. Endothelial Cell Lining

Endothelium Dependent Inhibition of Platelet Aggregation

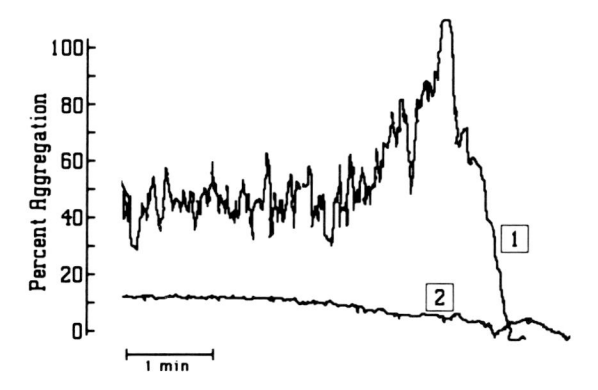

[1] Media, thrombin (0.5 U/ml),PRP
[2] Endothelial cells, thrombin (0.5 U/ml),PRP

Fig. 111 Thrombin added directly to human platelet-rich plasma results in a rapid increase in aggregation, the same concentration of thrombin added to a column of endothelial cells mounted immediately above the platelets causes release of a substance that inhibits platelet aggregation. From: Vargas-Cuba, RD and Ryan, US. Unpublished.

mM) but only one response and a reduced response is seen. A subsequent challenge does not produce a response until calcium is reintroduced into the extracellular solution (33). This suggests that intercellular calcium may be sufficient for a single diminished release of EDRF but that replenishment from extracellular sources is required for a repeated or sustained response.

EDRF also exerts effects on platelets. Figure 111 shows the anti-aggregatory actions of thrombin-stimulated release of EDRF from endothelial cells. Therefore, the presence of an intact, healthy endothelial layer should contribute to maintaining vessel patency through release of EDRF, while in the absence of endothelium, opportunities for thrombus formation could proceed unchecked.

Role of Calcium

In order to test whether [Ca^{2+}]$_i$ is altered in response to vasodilators that stimulate release of EDRF, endothelial cells were grown on the inner surface on quartz or plastic cuvettes, loaded with the fluorescent intracellular calcium indicators INDO-1 or FURA-2 and examined by the multiwavelength (34) or two wavelength methods (35). [Ca^{2+}]$_i$ was elevated in response to a wide variety of agonists such as bradykinin, thrombin, histamine, ATP, PAF and the calcium ionophore A23187 (Figure 112), although some differences in responsiveness were noted in endothelial cells from different species or different vascular beds.

Calcium fluxes and calcium content were investigated using endothelial cells loaded with ^{45}Ca (33). Bradykinin

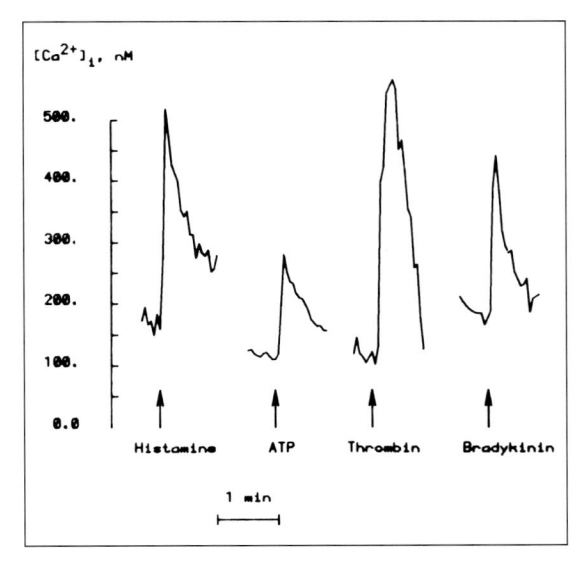

Fig. 112 The influence of histamine (100 μM), thrombin (1 U/ml), ATP (200 μM) or bradykinin (10 μg/ml) on [Ca^{2+}]$_i$ in endothelial cells. The cells were incubated in a Medium 199 with a 2 mM additional exogenous Ca^{2+} at 37C. From reference 34.

3. Endothelial Cell Lining

and thrombin caused an increase in the calcium content of endothelial cells. Thus, both the results obtained using fluorescent indicators and those using ^{45}Ca-loaded cells indicate that engagement of receptors for substances that trigger release of EDRF from endothelial cells leads to elevation of $[Ca^{2+}]_i$.

Since transient elevation of cytosolic free calcium levels can be achieved by release from intracellular stores such as the endoplasmic reticulum or by influx from extracellular sources, it was necessary to investigate the source of the observed increase.

Evidence for release from intracellular calcium stores can be obtained from more than one line of evidence. Studies using FURA-2 (35) have shown that in the presence of extracellular calcium the resting level of $[Ca^{2+}]_i$ in pulmonary artery endothelial cells was 100-200 nM. $[Ca^{2+}]_i$ increased in response to bradykinin (5 uM), ATP (20 uM) and to a lesser extent thrombin (1.5 U/ml). Bradykinin and ATP elevated $[Ca^{2+}]_i$ both in the presence and absence of extracellular Ca^{2+}_i. Our data indicate that in the presence of extracellular calcium the kinetics of agonist-induced increase of $[Ca^{2+}]_i$ consisted of two components. Fast elevation and decrease of $[Ca^{2+}]_i$ represent mobilization of intracellular Ca^{2+} and its reuptake. The second slower phase is apparently due to entry of extracellular calcium ion. In order to separate these components, the agonist-induced increase in $[Ca^{2+}]_i$ was first measured in the absence of extracellular Ca^{2+}. After $[Ca^{2+}]_i$ reached its peak level and returned to baseline, extracellular Ca^{2+} was added and the second response to the agonists was seen. $[Ca^{2+}]_i$ increased in 20-30 sec and then slowly returned to the basal state (35).

Agonists such as platelet activating factor (PAF), a substance likely to be released in vessels occluded by platelet plugs, cause an increased polyphosphoinositide turnover in endothelial cells (6). In response to PAF, inositol phosphate (IP), inositol bisphosphate (IP$_2$) and inositol 1,4,5-triphosphate (IP$_3$) are increased approximately threefold (Figure 113). IP$_3$ can act to release calcium from intracellular stores, suggesting an involvement of this source in the calcium elevation seen in response to PAF. A further consequence of receptor-mediated hydrolysis of inositol phospholipids is diacylglycerol-induced activation of proteinkinase C. The response of endothelial cells to PAF appears to involve activation of protein kinase C (36). Treatment of endothelial cells with PMA (phorbol myristate acetate), an activator of protein kinase C, inhibits the PAF induced increase in IP, IP$_2$ and IP$_3$ (36) and inhibits the increase in $[Ca^{2+}]_i$ in response to agonist action (34). Thus a negative feedback mechanism involving activation of protein kinase C appears to play a role in endothelial responses to some agonists (36).

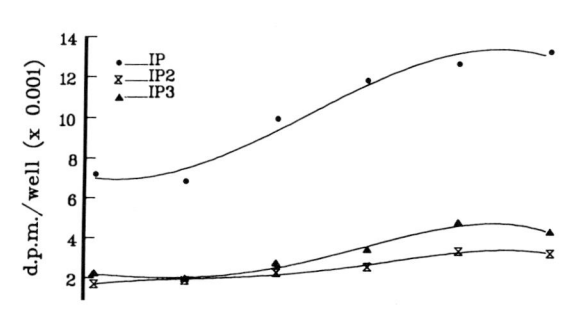

Fig. 113 Dose-response curves from PAF-stimulated release of inositol phosphates by bovine pulmonary artery endothelial cells. From reference 36.

3. Endothelial Cell Lining

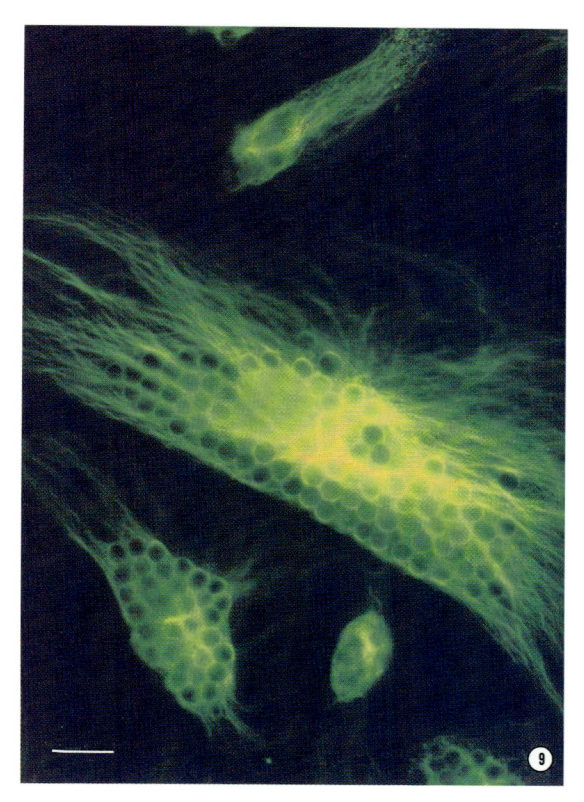

Fig. 114 Fluorescence localization of endothelial cytoskeletal filaments during ingestion of 5-10 beads using monoclonal antibodies to vimentin (kindly supplied by Dr Marina Glukhova, Cardiology Institute, Moscow, USSR). Bar = 20 μm. From reference 39.

Receptor mediated entry of extracellular calcium was measured using patch clamp recording techniques that have been reviewed in more detail elsewhere (33,37). Briefly, endothelial cells appear to respond to agonists such as bradykinin and thrombin via activation of a cation selective channel (33). In addition, endothelial cells possess a histamine-induced current associated with activation of calcium-dependent ionic channels. Stimulation of endothelial cells with PAF causes a marked outward current dependent on the presence of Ca^{2+} in the external solution (38). Thus, endothelial cells possess a variety of ionic currents in their membranes and entry of extracellular calcium is clearly an important component of the transient increases in cytosolic calcium measured in response to agonists.

Endothelial Responses to Bacteria

Occlusion of vascular grafts is not solely the result of thrombus formation and coagulapathies but may involve bacterial infection. Likewise, endothelial responses are not limited to release of EDRF, PGI_2 and PAF and are not elicited only by soluble mediators and agonists. Although one does not normally think of endothelial cells as phagcytic, they are capable of binding and ingesting a variety of particulates (Figures 114) including bacteria (Figures 115 and 116). Phagocytosis results in a number of dramatic responses. Endothelial cells that have ingested bacteria respond by unmasking Fc receptors, releasing toxic oxygen radicals such as superoxide anion (O_2), and by behavioral "activation" responses including increased migration, division and further phagocytosis (39, 40).

The release of superoxide anion may cause bactericidal action depending on the strain, size of inoculum and time of incubation (41) but in any event release of active oxygen species from endothelial cells is of great significance in vascular pathology. Oxygen radicals are a cause of severe vascular damage, in, for example, ischemia-reperfusion injury and in inflammatory reactions. It is now clear that endothelial cells may not simply be the target of oxygen radicals released from neutrophils but may also suffer from attack of neighboring endothelial cells. Phagocytosis of bacteria (e.g. the Remutant of S. minnesota) causes a substan-

245

3. Endothelial Cell Lining

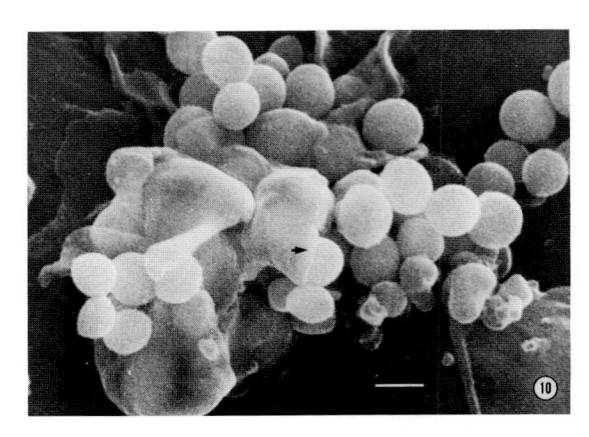

Fig. 115 Scanning electron micrograph showing binding (15 mins) of Staphylococcus aureus to the surface of a pulmonary endothelial cell and engulfment by membrane flaps (arrow). Bar = 1μm. From reference 39.

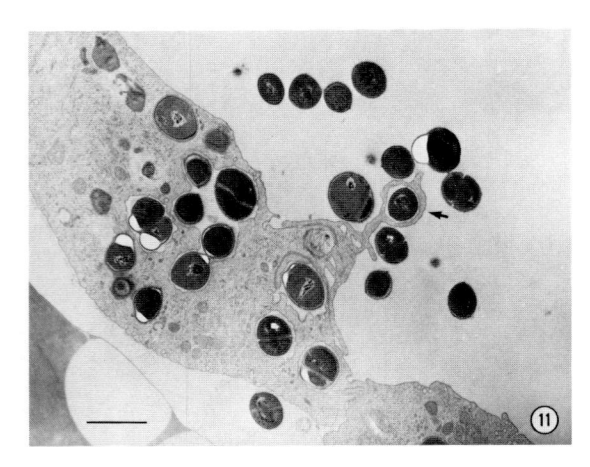

Fig. 116 Transmission electron micrograph showing engulfment of Staphylococcus aureus by membrane extensions (arrow) and internalization within a pulmonary endothelial cell. Bar = 1μm. From reference 39.

tial release of O_2 from endothelial cells (40).

Since the calcium ionophore A23187 and PMA cause a much greater release of O_2 from endothelial cells than the sum of either substance acting alone the release of O_2 from endothelial cells appears to be controlled by calcium and proteinkinase C, perhaps acting synergistically (40,41).

Discussion

It is clear that the presence or absence of the endothelial layer makes a profound difference to the functioning of the normal vascular wall. Endothelial derived substances such as EDRF and PGI_2 act both as vasodilators and as anti-aggregatory substances, thus their agonist-stimulated release in the presence of endothelium tends towards maintaining patency and flow. However, the very agonists that cause release of EDRF, acting directly on smooth muscle in the absence of endothelial, tend to vasoconstrict thus leading to vasospasm, with thrombus formation on subendothelial layers. Clearly, the presence or absence of endothelium is likely to be equally important for maintaining patency of vascular grafts.

Release of substances such as PAF and superoxide anion from endothelium cells would tend to cause vascular damage and platelet aggregation. It is interesting that endothelium is both a source and a target of action of each of these substances.

We now know that endothelium can receive a variety of signals that lead to a multiplicity of effector actions. It is clear that calcium plays an important role in stimulus-response coupling and that activation of protein kinase C is involved in some receptor mediated responses. Thus endothelium possesses many of the signal transduction mechanisms common to excitable and secretory cells in general. The very conservatism of signal transduction mechanisms may indicate that endothelium can become activated by a large number of commonly occurring stimuli. The challenge will be to understand the steps leading from specific stimuli to specific responses and to understand the total response of endothelium to signals likely to pertain after implantation of vascular prostheses, which, if inappropriately expressed, could signal pathophysiological rather than physiological outcomes.

Acknowledgements

Supported by grants from the National Institutes of Health (HL 21568, HL 33064) and from the Council of Tobacco Research (814).

References

1. Ryan US, Maxwell G. Isolation, culture and subculture of bovine pulmonary artery endothelial cells: mechanical methods. J Tissue Cult Methods 10, 3, 1986.

2. Ryan US, Maxwell G. Microcarrier cultures of endothelial cells. J Tissue Cult Methods 10, 7, 1986.

3. Ryan US. Culture of pulmonary endothelial cells on microcarrier beads. In Biology of the Endothelial Cell (ed EA Jaffe), Marthinus Nijhoff, The Netherlands, Chapter 4, p. 34, 1984.

4. Ryan US. Isolation and culture of pulmonary endothelial cells. Environmental Health Perspectives 56, 103, 1984.

5. Ryan US, Olazabal B. Endothelial seeding of filters, grafts and tubes. J Tissue Cult Methods 10, 61, 1986.

6. Ryan US. Metabolic activity of pulmonary endothelium: Modulation of structure and function. Ann Rev Physiol 48, 263, 1986.

7. Ryan US. Pulmonary endothelium: a dynamic interface. Clin Invest Med 9, 124, 1986.

8. Jaffe EA, Nachman RL, Becker CG, Minick CR. Culture of human endothelial cells derived from umbilical veins. J Clin Invest 52, 2745 1973a.

9. Gimbrone MA, Cotran RS, Folkman J. Human vascular endothelial cells in culture: growth and DNA synthesis. J Cell Biol 60, 673, 1974.

10. Ryan US, Ryan JW and Chiu AT. Kininase II (angiotensin-converting enzyme) and endothelial cells in culture. Adv Exp Med Biol 70, 217, 1976.

11. Ryan, US, Ryan, JW, Whitaker, C and Chiu, A: Localization of angiotensin converting enzyme (kininase II). II. Immunocyto-chemistry and immunofluorescence. Tissue & Cell 8, 125, 1976.

12. Ryan US, Clements E, Habliston D, Ryan JW. Isolation and culture of pulmonary artery endothelial cells. Tissue & Cell 10, 535, 1978.

13. Ryan US, Mortara M, Whitaker C. Methods for microcarrier culture of bovine pulmonary artery endothelial cells avoiding the use of enzymes. Tissue & Cell 12, 619, 1980.

14. Ryan US, White L, Lopez M, Ryan JW. Use of microcarriers to isolate and culture pulmonary microvascular endothelium. Tissue & Cell 14, 597, 1982.

15. Ryan US, Ryan JW. Inflammatory mediators, contraction and endothelial cells. In: Progress in Microcirculation Research, II (eds. FC Courtice, DG Garlick and MA Perry), Sydney: Committee in Postgraduate Medical Education, University of New South Wales, p. 424, 1984.

3. Endothelial Cell Lining

16. Ryan US, White L. Microvascular endothelium, isolation with microcarriers: Arterial, venous. J Tissue Cult Methods 10, 9, 1986.

17. Ryan US. Processing of angiotensin and other peptides by the lungs. In Handbook of Physiology - The Respiratory System 1 (eds AP Fishman and AB Fisher), Amer Physiol Soc, Bethesda, MD, Chapter 10, p. 351, 1985.

18. Smith, U, Ryan JW. Pniocytotic vesicles of the pulmonary endothelial cell. Chest 59, 12s, 1971.

19. Ryan JW, Smith U. Metabolism of adenosine-5'-monophosphate during circulation through the lungs. Trans Assoc Am Physcns 84, 297, 1971.

20. Crutchley DJ, Ryan US, Ryan JW. Effects of aspirin and dipyridamole on the degradation of adenosine diphosphate by cultured cells derived from bovine pulmonary artery. J Clin Invest 66, 29, 1980.

21. Pearson JD, Hallewell PG. Adenosine transport and ectonucleotidase activity in pulmonary and aortic endothelial cells. In: Carrier-mediated transport of solutes from blood to tissue, pp. 213, Yudilevich, DL and Mann, GE (eds) Longman, New York, 1985.

22. Johnson AR, Revtyak GE, Ibe PO, Campbell WB. Endothelial cells metabolize but do not synthesize leukotrienes. Prog Clin Biol Res 199, 185, 1985.

23. Gillis CN, Pitt BR. The fate of circulating amines within the pulmonary circulation. Ann Rev Physiol 44, 269, 1982.

24. Ryan US, Ryan JW. Endothelial cells and inflammation. In: Clinics in Laboratory Medicine (ed. PA Ward), WB Saunders Publishing Company, Volume 3, p. 577, 1983.

25. Ryan US, Whitney PL, Ryan JW. Localization of carbonic anhydrase on pulmonary artery endothelial cells in culture. J Appl Physiol 53, 914, 1982.

26. Ryan US, Grantham CJ. Metabolism of endogenous and xenobiotic substances by pulmonary vascular endothelial cells. Pharmocology & Therapeutics, in press, 1989.

27. Crutchley DJ, Ryan JW, Ryan US, Fisher GH. Bradykinin-induced release of prostacyclin and thromboxanes from bovine pulmonary artery endothelial cells. Studies with lower homologs and calcium antagonists. Biochem Biophys Acta 751, 99, 1983.

28. McIntyre TM, Zimmerman GA, Satoh K, Prescott SM. Cultured endothelial cells synthesize both platelet-activating factor and prostacyclin in response to histamine, bradykinin and adenosine triphosphate. J Clin Invest 76, 271, 1985.

29. Furchgott RF. Role of endothelium in the responses of vascular smooth muscle to drugs. Ann Rev Pharmacol Toxicol 24, 175, 1984.

30. Ryan US, Ryan JW. Vital and functional activities of endothelial cells. In: Pathobiology of the Endothelial Cell (eds. HL Nossel and HJ Vogel), Academic Press, NY, p. 455, 1982.

31. Johns A, Khalil RA, Ryan US, van Breemen C. Endothelium-Derived Relaxing Factor. In: Endothelial Cells. (ed. US Ryan) CRC Press, Boca Raton, Florida, in press, 1987.

32. Rubanyi GM. Endothelium-derived vasoconstrictor factors. In: Endothelial Cells. (ed US Ryan) Chapter 32, CRC Press, Boca Raton, Florida, 1988.

33. Johns A, Lategan TW, Lodge NJ, Ryan US, van Breemen C, Adams DJ. Calcium entry through receptor-operated channels in bovine pulmonary artery endothelial cells. Tissue & Cell 19, 1, 1987.

3. Endothelial Cell Lining

34. Ryan US, Avdonin PV, Pozin E Ya, Popov EG, Danilov SM, Tkachuck VA. Influence of vasoactive agents on cytoplasmic free calcium concentration in INDO-1 loaded vascular endothelial cells. J Appl Physiol 65, 2221,1988.

35. Avdonin PV, Hayes BA, Pozin EY, Popov EG, Gavrilov IY, Tkahuk VA, Ryan US. Dual-phase response of bovine pulmonary artery endothelial ccells to the agonists inreasing free cytoplasmic calcium concentration. Tissue & Cell, 21, 1989.

36. Grigorian GY, Ryan US. Platelet-activating factor effects on bovine pulmonary artery endothelial cells. Circulation Research 61, 389, 1987.

37. Bregestovski PD, Ryan US. Voltage-gated and receptor mediated ionic currents in the membrane of endothelial cells. J Molec Cell Cardiol 21, Suppl, 1989.

38. Ryan US, Grigorian GY, Avdonin PV, Bregestovski P. Platelet-activating factor effects on endothelial cells. In: New Trends in Lipid Mediators Res 1., 144, Karger, Basel, 1988.

39. Ryan US. Endothelial cell activation responses. In: Pulmonary Endothelium in Health and Disease. (ed US Ryan), Marcel Dekker, Inc, NY 32, 3, 1987.

40. Ryan US. Phagocytic properties in endothelial cells. In: Endothelial Cells, rd III (ed. US Ryan), CRC Press, Boca Raton, Florida, Chapter 31, p. 50, 1988.

41. Ryan US, Vann JM. Cultured endothelial cells as probes for in vivo biology. Alternative Methods in Toxicology, Vol 6, 49, 1988.

42. Ryan US, Ryan JW. Cell biology of pulmonary endothelium. Circulation 70, III-46, 1984.

3.2.4. Immune Functions of Vascular Wall Cells

P Libby, SJC Warner, L Birinyi

*Departments of Medicine (Cardiology) and Surgery,
Tufts University and New England Medical Center,
Boston, Massachusetts, USA.*

Introduction

In the traditional view, regulatory or effector roles in the immune response were thought to be limited to leukocytes such as T-cells, B-cells, or monocyte/macrophages. These were the only cells considered capable of presenting antigens or secreting molecules that regulate the immune response. This view regarded the parenchymal cells of most organs (including blood vessels) solely as targets of immune responses generated and regulated by cells derived from the bone marrow. Results from a number of laboratories over the last several years have broadened this classical view in important ways. It now appears that a surprising variety of cell types share several of the functions previously believed restricted to leukocytes. In particular, vascular endothelium and smooth muscle cells of the blood vessel wall can express functions that may contribute to local inflammation, injury, and immune responses. These findings have a number of important implications in the pathogenesis of certain vascular diseases, and suggests a novel view of the role of blood vessel cells in the pathogenesis of allograft rejection. Since host immune cells first encounter recipient cells in the blood vessel, these newly appreciated immune functions of vascular wall cells have considerable interest in the context of transplantation biology.

Cellular Immunology Oversimplified

Appreciation of the rôles of vascular wall cells in the local immune response requires review of some of the elementary concepts of cellular immunology related to recognition and elimination of foreign cells. This discussion is necessarily drastically oversimplified, but describes the elements necessary to understand the newly recognized immune functions of vascular cells. The basic principles involved in these processes are actually quite straightforward. However, the three-dimensional networks and the combination of stimulatory and inhibitory regulatory loops render understanding of the immune response formidable for non-specialists (including surgeons and cardiologists). An additional major obstacle for non-immunologists to understanding immunology is the arcane and abbreviation-laden language that has evolved to describe these phenomena. We provide a listing of some frequently encountered terms (Table 32), with the proviso that this decoding and our explanations are incomplete. Rather than

Immune Functions of Vascular Wall Cells: Some Relevant Abbreviations and Explanations

T-cell	Thymus-derived lymphocyte
T_H	Helper-induced subset of T-cells (bear CD4 or T4 antigen)
T_{CTL}	Cytolytic or killer T-cell
Ti	Receptor for antigen on the surface of T-cells ("T-cell receptor")
HLA	Human Leukocyte Antigens
MHC	Major Histocompatibility Complex
Class I	HLA found on most nucleated cells most of the time (HLA-A,B,C)
Class II	HLA (HLA-DR, DQ, DP etc) found on antigen-presenting cells
Ia	Synonym for class II antigen, Immune response associated
IL	Interleukin - a family of biologically active mediators associated with leukocytes
IL-1	Interleukin-1, T-cell co-activator, endogenous pyrogen (two isoforms α and β)
IL-2	a T-cell growth factor
CD	Cell Determinant - a family of serologically defined surface molecules
CD 2	Found on T-cell surface, helps binding to interacting cells via LFA-3
CD 3	Transmembrane signalling component or T-cell antigen receptor complex
CD 4	Class II binding molecule on helper T-cell (synonym T4)
CD 8	Found on suppressor and killer T-cell surface (synonym T8)
LFA	Leukocyte function antigen - a family of surface proteins involved in adhesion
LFA-1	Found on lymphocytes (cognate ligand ICAM-1)
LFA-3	Receptor on peripheral cells for T-cell surface protein CD 2
CAM	Families of Cellular Adhesion Molecules associated with cell surfaces
ICAM-1	Receptor for LFA-1 found on many cell types involved in intercellular adhesion
ELAM-1	Endothelial-Leukocyte Adhesion Molecule
TNF	Tumor necrosis factor
TNF-α	form of TNF secreted by monocyte/macrophages
TNF-β	lymphotoxin, form of TNF secreted by lymphocytes

Table 32

citations to primary research papers in the immunological literature, we felt it would be more useful to provide references to recent review articles intended for generalists.

The peripheral blood of the mature immunocompetent individual contains several distinct functional classes of thymus-derived lymphocytes (T-cells). In the context of transplantation, the most important subclasses of T-cells are the helper T-cells (T_H) and cytolytic T-cells (T_{CTL} or CTL,) also known as "killer" T-cells (Nossal, 1987; Bach, 1987). The surface of T_H cells contains a serologically defined molecule known as CD4 (cell determinant 4, also known as T4). The surface of CTL generally exhibits the distinct marker CD8 or T8 also delineated by specific antibodies. The property of T-cells to recognize specific antigens is due to the presence of another complex of surface molecule known as the T-cell receptor for an-

3. Endothelial Cell Lining

tigen, often abbreviated "T-cell receptor" or Ti by immunologists (Royer and Reinhertz, 1987; Marrack and Kappler, 1987). The details of mechanisms that generate diversity of the T-cell receptors are well beyond the scope of this paper. In brief, each of the major polypeptide chains of the mature T-cell receptor varies in structure because it is the product of a gene remodelled during ontogeny of this specific family of T-cells by reassortment of various pieces of DNA in the genome. These rearrangements lead to numerous different possible combinations of structures, a process that resembles the generation of antibody diversity.

The peripheral blood contains T-cells of only a few functional repertoires, but many millions of individual potential antigenic specificities (due to Ti heterogeneity) within each functional subclass. Under usual circumstances these T-cells are at rest; they neither divide at a rapid rate, nor secrete factors that signal T-cell proliferation (e.g. interleukins or tumor necrosis factor) or that stimulate the expression of histocompatibility antigens (gamma interferon, lymphotoxin). The resting cytolytic T-cells are not "armed for warfare" by being primed to release the cytotoxic contents of their granules. The ability of the cellular immune system to respond to a foreign invader, be it a virus or an organ transplanted from an unrelated donor, requires both quantitative and qualitative changes in the resting state of the T-cell (Nossal, 1987).

The T-cells in the peripheral blood continuously sample their environment by cell-cell interactions. A variety of intercellular adhesion ligand-receptor pairs (e.g. LFA-1/ICAM-1) probably promote frequent physical interactions between leukocytes (homotypic interactions) or between leukocytes and endothelial cells in blood vessels and lymphoid organs (heterotypic interactions) (Table 33) (Springer, 1985). In the basal uninfected and untransplanted state these collisions and adhesive encounters between cells are transitory and of little consequence, since neither these T_H or the CTL receptors will re-

---

Cell Surface Molecules Involved in Intercellular Adhesion and ImmunRecognition:
Cognate Ligand/Receptor Pairs

Cell Type	Ligand/Receptor Pair		Cell Type
Lymphocytes	LFA-1	ICAM-1	Peripheral cells
Peripheral cells	LFA-3	CD2	T-cells
Macrophages	Mac-1	C3bi	Complement protein

The ligand or receptor is expressed on the surface of the cell type joined by dashed lines. Non-covalent interactions between ligand/receptor pairs are indicated by dotted lines.

Table 33

3. Endothelial Cell Lining

cognize any specific antigenic stimulus due to deletion of self-reactive clones during T-cell ontogeny in the individual (Nossal, 1987; Bach, 1987).

When these cells encounter tissue from an unrelated donor, the situation is altogether different. The cellular immune system distinguishes self and non-self on the basis of antigens on the surface of cells, products of genes of the major histocompatibility complex (MHC) (Benacerraf, 1981; Bach, 1987). The two types of MHC antigens in man consist of class I (HLA-A,B, and C; expressed on most nucleated cells) or class II (HLA-DR, DQ, DP, etc, usually expressed on lymphoid tissue). Helper T-cells only recognize foreign (allogenic) tissue as being non-self if their surface contains foreign MHC antigens. Since cells of a transplanted organ can bear foreign class II determinants, the interaction of the recipient's helper cells with the donor tissue may no longer be casual. Most encounters between the recipient helper cell and the donor organ will still fail to activate the T_H since the T-cell antigen receptor will not be engaged. However, a minority of the helper T-cells will contain a T-cell receptor complementary to and bind with high affinity to the specific foreign histocompatibility antigens of the donor. This crucial recognition event "activates" the engaged helper T-cell to secrete a number of mediators including interleukin-2 (IL-2), a well characterized T-cell growth factor, and to express receptors for this molecule on its surface (Figure 118) (Dinarello and Mier, 1987). After engagement with its specific antigen this helper T-cell will propagate, expanding this particular clone. In addition, the activated T-helper cell will secrete a form of interferon (gamma interferon or immune in-

THE AFFERENT LIMB OF CELLULAR IMMUNITY:
Antigen Presenting Cell (APC) and recognition by Helper T-cells (T_H)

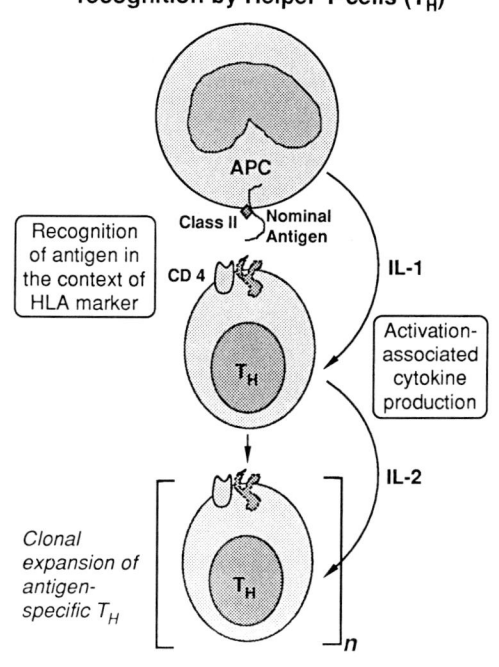

Fig. 117 Helper T-cell recognition of antigen and proliferation. Foreign antigens are processed by the antigen presenting cell (APC) by partial degradation and de-naturation. The antigen presenting cell inserts the processed or "normal" antigen into the surface membrane in direct physical contact with the class II histocompatibility molecule. The helper T-cell with an antigen receptor T_i com- plementary to this particular combination of nominal antigen and class II will recognize this complex and form a "fit" that will activate the T-cell. Interleukin-1 (IL-1) secreted by the antigen presenting cell amplifies the T-cell response during the activation process, a property known as co-stimulation. The IL-1 may be inserted into the membrane of the presenting cell as well as secreted. The activated T-cell will begin to produce interleukin-2 (IL-2) and express receptors for this growth factor. This autocrine growth stimulation will result in proliferation of the clone of T-cells specific for this particular antigen. The above scenario applies to the recognition by helper T-cells of foreign antigens other than MHC products. In the case of allogeneic tissue it is the foreign histocompatibility antigen itself that is recognized by the helper T-cell and is sufficient to activate and cause expansion of the allospecific clone.

253

3. Endothelial Cell Lining

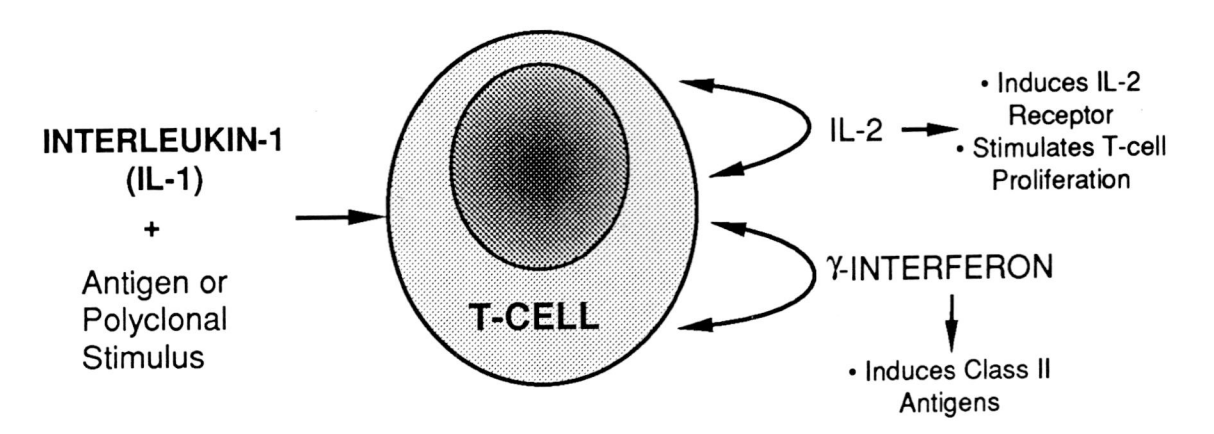

Fig. 118 A schematic view of T cell activation
This diagram presents a more detailed view of the rôle of cytokines in T-cell activation. Interleukin-1 complements the triggering stimulus of antigen, foreign MHC, or polyclonal activators such as plant lectins. The T-cell reacting to these ligands makes a response to IL-2 as described in the legend to Figure 117. In addition, the activated T-cell secretes gamma-interferon. This immune form of interferon acts to induce class II antigens on a number of cell types, including endothelial cells and smooth muscle cells. The amplification of the activating stimulus may strengthen the local cellular immune response.

terferon, abbreviated IFN-γ that can, in turn, increase the expression of class II histocompatibility antigens on nearby cells (Figure 118).

Meanwhile, the CTL precursors also continuously sample their environment (Figure 3). Again, only a tiny minority of the CTL will bear a T-cell receptor specific for the donor histocompatibility antigens. The CTL which bear CD 8 recognize class I determinants. When a "fit" occurs, the killer T-cell then displays its own "activation program", including the expression of IL-2 receptors and the ability to release cytotoxic substances that can lead to the death of the cell it has embraced. In many cases the CTL will not produce IL-2 even when activated by contact with specific antigen. Thus, expansion of this clone of killer T-cells usually depends on the "help" of IL-2 released locally by activated helper T-cells. In this manner, the generation of the cellular immune response requires close co-operation between antigen-presenting or foreign cells, and at least two classes of T-lymphocytes (the CTL and T_H). When these cells encounter specific antigens that they recognize as foreign, their activation causes quantitative (clonal expansion) (Figure 117) and qualitative changes including lymphokine secretion by T_H (Figures 117 and 118), and target-specific killing by CTL (Figure 119).

Helper T-cells usually encounter foreign antigens other than MHC products on the surface of an "antigen presenting cell". In the case of infectious agents such as viruses, the macrophage will engulf an infected cell, partially degrade macromolecules, such as viral glycoproteins, and "present" the partially degraded and denatured or "processed" nominal antigen on its surface in intimate association with class II MHC product (Unanue and Allen, 1987). The mechanism of generation of an individual's own T-cell population in the thymus early in life accounts for the commitment of T-cells to recognize foreign antigens in the context of MHC. The thymus does not have "samples" of

3. Endothelial Cell Lining

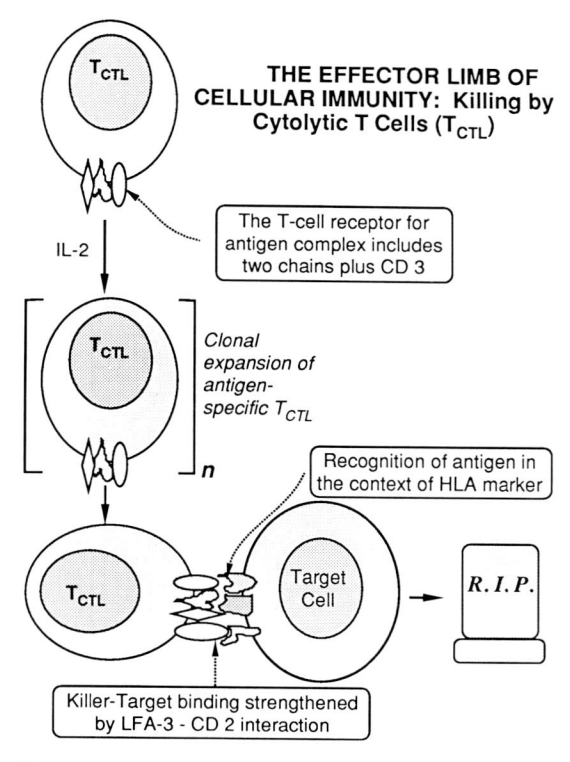

Fig. 119 Killing of target cells by cytolytic T-cells (T_{CTL})

The cytolytic T-cells containing receptors specific for specific antigen proliferate in response to IL-2 secreted by helper T-cells in the vicinity of the local immune reaction. The interaction between the activated killer cell and the target is increased by the LFA-3 - CD2 interaction as diagramed. Cytolytic T-cells that bear CD8 determinants recognize class I antigenes on target cells. It is now apparent that killer T-cells can also bear CD4 determinants. In this case the killer cell recognized class II antigens. After close approximation due to specific Ti mediated and non-specific interaction, the cytotoxic cell releases the toxic components of its granules that kill the target cell.

Figure labels: THE EFFECTOR LIMB OF CELLULAR IMMUNITY: Killing by Cytolytic T Cells (T_{CTL}); The T-cell receptor for antigen complex includes two chains plus CD 3; Clonal expansion of antigen-specific T_{CTL}; Recognition of antigen in the context of HLA marker; Target Cell; R.I.P.; Killer-Target binding strengthened by LFA-3 - CD 2 interaction

all of the infectious agents to which an individual may have to mount a response during life. Instead, the intrathymic developmental process uses cell surface markers that are available (i.e. self MHC product) as templates to select permitted clones of T-cells. Clones that recognize self precisely and with high affinity must be "forbidden" to avoid autoreactivity. Rather, the selected T-cell clones fit the templates (self MHC) imperfectly i.e. with low affinity (Benacerraf, 1985). This strategy proves successful because foreign antigens encountered during later life are presented as processed fragments in conjunction with self MHC products, and thus resemble self closely yet imprecisely. Non-MHC antigens (e.g. a viral protein) must be perceived together with self MHC product in order to mimic modified self MHC.

There is a crucial distinction between the recognition of grafted foreign tissue (that bears non-self MHC antigens) and other types of antigens. An individual's own T-cells can recognize foreign MHC products on the surface of allografted cells without processing or presentation by a specialized cell. This mechanism contrasts sharply with non-MHC foreign antigens that are recognized exclusively in the context of self MHC product. Because of the homology in structures of the highly polymorphic but related HLA proteins, an individual's T-cells perceive foreign histocompatibility antigens as altered self without modification or juxtaposition with another molecule. In the case of the allograft then, expression of foreign class II histocompatibility antigens by donor cells suffices to trigger the host T_H and CTL. The limitations that histocompatibility barriers impose on organ grafting, while a nuisance in modern clinical transplantation, result from these primordial protective mechanisms. From a teleologic point of view, the polymorphism and complexity of the MHC recognition system must confer a selective advantage through enhanced resistance to infection (Benacerraf, 1981 and 1985).

3. Endothelial Cell Lining

The mononuclear phagocyte that has processed this antigen generally expresses its own program of effector functions. In the context of antigen presentation, another important contribution of the accessory cell (classically the mononuclear phagocyte) is the ability to produce the peptide hormone interleukin-1 (IL-1) (Dinarello and Mier, 1987; Oppenheim, 1985). Interleukin-1 has a myriad of effects on immunocompetent and other cells as well (Dinarello et al, 1986). Most importantly in the context of the immune response, IL-1 sensitizes T helper cells, resulting in amplified responses to low concentrations of specific antigen, or (as commonly used in the laboratory) polyclonal activators derived from plant sources such as the lectins phytohemagglutinin (PHA) or poke weed mitogen (Rosenwasser and Dinarello, 1981). Interleukin-1 is not only secreted by mononuclear phagocytes, but may remain associated with the cell membrane (Unanue and Allen, 1987). In this strategic location IL-1 maintains its functional capacity for participating in helper cell activation in conjunction with nominal antigen and class II molecules on the presenting cell surface.

Expression of Class II Histocompatibility Antigens and Antigen Presentation by Vascular Wall Cells

The ability to express class II determinants and thus to present antigen in the appropriate context for recognition by antigen-specific helper T-cells has traditionally been considered a unique property of highly specialized antigen presenting cells such as monocyte/macrophages or dendritic cells of the skin. One theory of allograft rejection even postulated that "passenger" leucocytes or dendritic cells introduced inadvertently with implantation of the grafted organ engendered the host immune response to transplanted organ (Pober et al, 1986a). We now realize that the capacity to present antigens is less restricted than previously appreciated. A wide variety of cells not derived from bone marrow can display class II histocompatibility antigens on their surface (Wong and Schrader, 1985). In particular, the ability of vascular endothelial cells to express class II determinants and act as antigen presenting cells may have particular relevance to the rejection of allografts (Pober et al, 1986). The endothelial lining of the blood vessel of transplanted organs forms the crucial interface between host leukocytes and donor cells. The host immune system first encounters foreign tissue on the luminal surface of the graft's vascular endothelium, the first potential target of host effector cells (e.g. macrophages or CTL).

Under usual circumstances in vitro and probably in vivo the vascular endothelium does not express class II histocompatibility antigens. However, when exposed to immune interferon (but no other cytokine yet examined) these cells transcribe genes for class II molecules and express these determinants on their surface (Pober et al., 1982 and 1983a; Collins et al, 1984a; Wagner et al, 1985a; Groenewegen et al, 1985). Work from a number of laboratories indicates that endothelial cells that bear these class II or Ia determinants can present antigen to helper T-cells (Pober et al, 1983b; Collins et al, 1984b; Geppert and Lipsky, 1985; Wagner et al., 1984 and 1985 a and b).

Once activated, T-cells localized in the vicinity of the foreign endothelial cells can elaborate gamma interferon which can induce class II antigen expression by endothelium and amplify the local immune response.

Smooth muscle cells comprise the bulk of the cell mass in arteries and veins and also exhibit inducible expression of class II histocompatibility antigens (Pober et al, 1986a; Warner and Libby, unpublished observations). As in the case of endothelium, smooth muscle cells under usual circumstances do not appear to express these molecules. In response to gamma interferon, smooth muscle cells accumulate messenger RNA that encodes class II determinants and express these molecules on their surface (Warner and Libby, unpublished observations). Immunohistochemical studies have verified that these cells are capable of expressing HLA-DR antigens in vivo in human vascular lesions (Jonasson et al, 1985 and 1986; Hansson et al, 1986).

Thus, vascular smooth muscle cells may also present antigen and participate in amplification of alloreactivity under circumstances in which they would contact helper T-cells. Smooth muscle cells may also participate in autoimmune responses in the absence of allogeneic tissue. Lymphocytes sensitized to syngeneic smooth muscle cells grown from brain microvessels in vitro can produce a granulomatous vasculitis when injected into an H-2 identical mouse (i.e., one with identical major histocompatibility determinants) (Hart et al, 1985 and 1987). This syngeneic sensitization may be due to the ability of smooth muscle cells to express the class II antigens. Whether this phenomenon observed in mice applies to the human situation or is involved in certain types of autoimmune disease is not yet certain.

Vessel Wall Cells as Sources of Immunoregulatory Cytokines

Another type of important function previously considered exclusively a property of bone marrow-derived cells is the ability to produce immunoregulatory cytokines such as IL-1. As described above, IL-1 is a potent activator of T_H that dramatically lowers the threshold for activation of these cells to antigen-specific or polyclonal stimuli. Until recently, mononuclear phagocytes were considered the sole important source of IL-1. Activated monocytes express two distinct genes that encode protein products (IL-1 α and β) which differ substantially in amino acid sequence and physical properties but exhibit indistinguishable biological activities. Over the last few years, several groups found thymocyte-activating activity that resembled IL-1 in supernatants of cultured human endothelial cells (Windt and Rosenwasser, 1984; Wagner et al, 1985b; Stern et al, 1985; Miossec et al, 1986). We found that these cells do not secrete IL-1 under basal conditions in vitro. However, mediators such as Gram negative bacterial endotoxin, tumor necrosis factor, or IL-1 itself, strongly stimulate IL-1 gene expression in human endothelial cells (Libby et al, 1986a; Warner et al, 1987b).

These stimuli cause both accumulation of IL-1 messenger RNA and secretion of thymocyte co-stimulation activity neutralizable by selective anti-IL-1 antibodies. Furthermore, human vascular endothelial cells can localize functionally intact IL-1 on their surface membranes as originally described in the case of mononuclear phagocytes (Kurt-Jones et al, 1987). It is little wonder that endothelial cells are particularly effective stimulators of allogeneic responses since they exhibit both inducible class

II antigen and IL-1 activity on their surfaces where these molecules may interact with T helper cells. In this regard, it is noteworthy that gamma interferon, the same stimulus which induces class II expression on the endothelial surface, also increases the level of an intercellular adhesion molecule denoted ICAM-1 (Rothlein et al, 1986; Dustin et al, 1986; Pober et al, 1986b). This molecule provides a receptor for a particular leukocyte function antigen (LFA-1) molecule on the surface of leucocytes including T helper cells thought to be important in the initial adhesive reactions between lymphocytes and endothelium (Haskard et al, 1986; Mentzer et al, 1986; Pohlman et al, 1986).

To our initial surprise, we recently found that vascular smooth muscle cells are an even more robust source of IL-1 than are endothelial cells (Libby et al, 1986b). The smooth muscle cells by far outnumber endothelial cells in the walls of macrovessels. Stimuli such as bacterial endotoxin, tumor necrosis factor, or IL-1 itself, induce IL-1 gene expression in smooth muscle cells much more rapidly and in greater amounts than in endothelial cells from the same source (Libby et al, 1987; Warner et al, 1987a). The ability of smooth muscle cells to transcribe IL-1 genes corresponds to the synthesis and secretion of biologically active IL-1 as judged by the ability to participate in thymocyte stimulation. Thus, both major cell types of the blood vessel wall, endothelium and smooth muscle, can secrete this important immunostimulatory molecule in an inducible manner. Under some circumstances, human smooth muscle cells can transcribe a gene for the cytokine tumor necrosis factor (TNF), and secrete biologically and immunoreactive TNF (Libby et al, 1987; Warner and Libby, unpublished observations).

In addition to allograft rejection, these newly recognized immune functions of vascular wall cells have important implications for a variety of vascular diseases such as vasculitis or atherosclerosis. For example, IL-1 produced locally by vessel wall cells could act in an autocrine or paracrine manner to change the usually anticoagulant and antithrombotic luminal endothelium to a procoagulant and thrombogenic surface at sites of local immune responses, infection, inflammation, or injury (Bevilacqua et al, 1984, 1985, 1986a and b, and 1987; Nachman et al, 1986). Both IL-1 and TNF sensitize human endothelial cells to lysis by antibodies found in the serum of patients with Kawasaki syndrome, a disease characterized by a pan-vasculitis with a predilection for involvement of the coronary arteries (Leung et al, 1986). Tumor necrosis factor also stimulates angiogenesis, and could thus contribute to the neovascularization of atherosclerotic lesions which may predispose to haemorrhage into complicated plaques (Leibovich et al, 1987). An additional effect of TNF related to vascular immune function is its ability to increase expression of class I MHC antigens on endothelial cells (Collins et al, 1986).

The Role of Endothelium in Lymphocytes Recirculation

Under usual circumstances in vivo, lymphocytes are not activated but circulate between the vascular space and lymphoid organs constantly sampling their environment. Far from random, this recirculation of lymphocytes is highly targeted and in part controlled by endothelial-dependent mechanisms (Rosen et al, 1985; Jalkanen et al,

1986a; Gallatin et al, 1986). Peripheral lymph nodes contain venules lined with endothelial cells that have a cuboidal rather than the typical squamous morphology found in larger vessels. The specialized cells are called "high" venular endothelial cells because of this distinct appearance. In vitro experiments demonstrated that various subclasses of lymphocytes exhibited differential affinity for adherence to high endothelial venules in different locales. For example, venules in Peyer's patches attract one lymphocyte population while peripheral extra-intestinal lymph nodes attract another. It is now clear that the selectivity of endothelium in these various beds is due to specific membrane molecules defined by monoclonal antibodies (Siegelman et al, 1986; Jalkanen et al, 1986b). Gamma interferon increases the surface expression of at least one of these lymphocyte receptors (Duijvestijn et al, 1986). The rôle of endothelial cells in directing lymphocyte recirculation provides another example of active participation of vascular cells in the immune response as well as regulation by cytokines of immune-related functions of endothelium.

The Role of Endothelium in Delayed-Type Hypersensitivity and other Local Immune or Inflammatory Responses

Infiltration of tissues by leukocytes is a classical hallmark of local inflammatory and immune responses. From the foregoing discussion it should be apparent that the recruitment of leukocytes in this context probably depends on endothelial-dependent mechanisms. Under basal conditions, vascular endothelium, as well as a variety of other cells (e.g. fibroblasts), expresses the intercellular adhesion molecule ICAM-1 that binds to the leukocyte membrane protein LFA-1 alluded to above (Rothlein et al., 1986; Dustin et al, 1985). LFA-1 belongs to a class of widely distributed molecules that mediate cellular interactions with other cells or substrata known as the integrin superfamily (Springer, 1985; Ruoslahti and Pierschbacher, 1987; Hynes, 1987). These basally-expressed adhesion mechanisms may be important in leukocyte margination on the vessel wall as well as in the routine encounters between lymphocytes and endothelium during immune surveillance.

At sites of arterial injury, inflammation, or immune responses, more selective mechanisms of leukocyte - endothelial adherence probably help to recruit specific populations of leukocytes. As mentioned above, gamma interferon increases ICAM-1 expression on endothelial cells in vitro. In addition, endothelial cells can exhibit specific leukocyte adhesion properties in response to other cytokines such as IL-1 or tumor necrosis factor (TNF). Exposure of human endothelial cells to IL-1 or TNF increases the adhesion of all classes of leukocytes tested, including granulocytes, monocytes, and T and B lymphocytes (Bevilacqua et al, 1985; Haskard et al, 1986; Mentzer et al, 1986; Pohlman et al, 1986; Cavender et al, 1986; Schleimer and Rutledge; 1986). IL-1-treated endothelial monolayers show increased adhesion, even for cells of the HL-60 promyelocytic leukemia line, which do not express LFA-1 determinants and thus do not depend on ICAM-1 for intercellular adhesion (Bevilacqua et al, 1985).

Studies with monoclonal antibodies raised against IL-1-treated human endothelial cells have revealed an endothelial surface molecule induced by IL-1 or TNF that mediates leukocyte binding in vitro (Pober et al, 1986b; Bevilacqua et al, 1987). In contrast to the LFA-1/ICAM-1 system, the endothelial leukocyte adhesion molecule defined by these antibodies (denoted ELAM-1) is found only on cytokine-activated endothelial cells and not on other cell types tested. This example illustrates an endothelial-specific leukocyte adhesion mechanism induced by inflammatory mediators in vitro. Important recent observations have established the in vitro significance of ELAM-1. Normal human tissues do not contain ELAM-1 when examined by immunohistochemical techniques. By contrast, in human delayed-type hypersensitivity reactions, post-capillary venules express this antigen in temporal and spatial proximity to the leukocyte infiltration (Cotran et al, 1986). The venular endothelial cells in the skin of patients undergoing lymphokine-activated killer cell (LAK) therapy also express ELAM-1 (Cotran et al, 1987). These observations suggest an important role of endothelial-dependent leucocyte adhesion mechanism in the recruitment of leukocytes to sites of immune and inflammatory reactions in vivo.

Implications for Atherogenesis

The application of modern immunohistochemical techniques has recently added a new dimension to the morphologic analysis of human atherosclerosis. Study of human atheromata with selective monoclonal antibodies confirmed the presence of vascular smooth muscle cells and macrophages, long suspected on the basis of routine morphology and animal experimentation. A surprising finding emanating from the work of Lena Jonasson in Göran Hansson's laboratory and of Gown, Tsukada, and Ross in Seattle was that T-lymphocytes comprise an important component of the cellular composition of advanced human atheromata (Jonasson et al, 1985, 1986; Gown et al, 1986). These lesions also contain smooth muscle cells which bear class II determinants in the vicinity of these T-cells (Jonasson et al, 1985; Hansson et al, 1986). These morphologic findings provide evidence that the T-cells in human atheromata are activated and secrete gamma interferon, the only known stimulus to class II expression in vascular cells. It is not yet known how T-cells might play a primary or secondary role in the pathogenesis of human arteriosclerosis.

The ability of mononuclear phagocytes and vascular endothelial and smooth muscle cells to produce IL-1 suggests a possible scenario for T-cell involvement in atherogenesis. If the monocyte-derived foam cells in early atheromata, or in the necrotic core of complicated human lesions, or the intimal smooth muscle cells secrete IL-1, they will beget more IL-1 due to the phenomenon of IL-1-induced IL-1 gene expression (Warner et al, 1987a and b; Dinarello et al, 1987). The human atheroma is a potential source of large amounts of IL-1 activity. This cytokine can recruit T-cells by inducing leukocyte adhesion molecules on the endothelial surface and by acting as a direct chemoattractant for T lymphocytes (Hunninghake et al, 1987). Interleukin-1 not only calls forth T-cells, but lowers their threshold for activation (Rosenwasser and Dinarello, 1981; Oppenheim, 1985; Dinarello and Mier,

1987). Activated T-cells in turn produce gamma interferon which can induce class II antigens on both smooth muscle cells and endothelial cells in the region of the lesion.

A missing link in this schema is the antigenic or other stimulus for T-cell activation in concert with IL-1, which by itself does not activate T-cells. A putative candidate for this activating stimulus could be class II molecules on the surface of smooth muscle cells themselves. As explained above, exposure of murine lymphocytes to syngeneic smooth muscle cells in culture somehow confers autoreactivity (Hart et al, 1985 and 1987). A more likely prospect is that the initial nidus of inflammation in the nascent lesion leads to non-specific immune reactions. In the developing human atheroma, such nonspecific activation of immune functions of the vascular wall cells such as IL-1 release could cause secondary involvement of lymphocytes or mononuclear phagocytes that would perpetuate and amplify the local inflammatory response. Although there is no reason to expect that antigen-specific immune responses play a primary rôle in the usual form of human atherosclerosis, in one special type of atherosclerosis, that associated with cardiac allografts, an antigen-specific immune response may well be of primary and central pathogenic significance (see below).

Implications of the Immune Functions of Vascular Wall Cells for Organ Transplantation in Man

The recognition that vascular endothelium can express class II histocompatibility determinants and present antigen bears obvious relevance to the problem of allograft rejection. As noted above, host lymphocytes first encounter the grafted organ via the endothelial lining of the vasculature (Pober et al, 1986a). Furthermore, effector cells such as macrophages or cytotoxic T-cells must traverse the endothelium to gain access to the underlying parenchymal cells. The recognition that cells of the graft blood vessel wall can exhibit all of the immune functions necessary to engender an allo-specific immune response obviates the need to invoke the transfer of "passenger" leukocytes with the engrafted organ (Pober et al., 1986a). Since endothelial and smooth muscle cells both exhibit inducible class II antigen and IL-1 gene expression, it is unlikely that any procedure that involves the transfer of viable vascular wall cells from unrelated donors will bypass the immune response and permit grafting across major histocompatibility barriers. This prediction has important implications for the selection of the source of endothelial cells used for seeding of cardiovascular prostheses. In addition, similar cautions apply to the application of homografting or the construction of artificial blood vessels from donor cells in vitro.

Although both endothelial and smooth muscle cells can express class II antigens and secrete IL-1, the endothelial cells appear to stimulate allogenic responses more readily than smooth muscle cells from the same donor (Pober et al, 1986a). Human fibroblasts also appear less immunogenic than endothelial cells (Geppert and Lipsky, 1985). This disparity could result from a differential ability of these two cell types to express membrane IL-1, but this point is still under investigation (Pober et al, 1986a; Kurt-Jones et al, 1987). None-

3. Endothelial Cell Lining

theless, this observation may explain why, in recent experiments performed on rats, deendothelialized aortic allografts resisted rejection much more than did vessels with intact endothelium (Galumbeck et al, 1987).

With the advent of cyclosporine therapy, cardiac allografting, first performed in Cape Town 20 years ago, has now become a nearly routine procedure in many centers around the world. In the post-cyclosporin era of cardiac transplantation arteriosclerosis of the arteries of the engrafted heart has emerged as a major limitation to the long-term success of this procedure. These lesions can differ substantially from ordinary coronary atherosclerosis in man. The lesions of graft-associated arteriosclerosis tend to be concentric and diffuse rather than eccentric and focal as in the usual form of spontaneous coronary atherosclerosis (Figure 120). Accumulation of lipids is also much less prominent in the lesions in transplanted coronary arteries. Furthermore, the graft-associated lesions are commonly associated with leukocytic infiltration of the exuberantly hyperplastic intima. The graft-associated arteriosclerosis may be quite rapidly progressive and commonly occurs in patients whose own hearts had normal coronary arteries and patients who lack other risk factors for atherosclerosis. A primary immune mechanism may well be of etiologic significance in this transplant-associated form of proliferative arterial disease.

The infiltration with leucocytes and ongoing immune stimulation initiated by the foreign histocompatibility antigens could initiate and perpetuate this process. Recent findings from our laboratory could help to explain the hyperplastic nature of this proliferative lesion. We found that exposure of

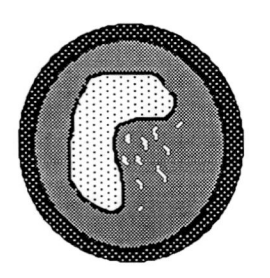

Typical Atherosclerosis
- eccentric lesion
- lipid deposits
- focal distribution

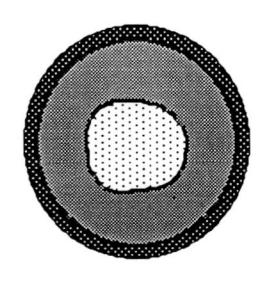

Graft Arteriosclerosis
- concentric lesion
- little or no lipid
- diffuse narrowing

Fig. 120 Comparison of the lesions of typical atherosclerosis and allograft-associated coronary arteriosclerosis
Left hand panel: In the usual form of human atherosclerosis, the lesions are typically most severe in particular locations within the epicardial coronary artery. The diagram of a cross section through such a stenotic area depicts the eccentric nature of the lesion, which leaves a crescent-shaped and narrowed lumen. The necrotic core of the lesion usually contains fatty deposits, represented by the white areas in the diagram.
Right hand panel: The coronary arteries of hearts transplanted from unrelated donors can develop a distinct form of arteriosclerosis characterized by exuberant smooth muscle hyperplasia in addition to leukocytic infiltration. These lesions tend to involve the entire epicardial coronary vessel and produce a more diffuse lesion than does the usual form of human atherosclerosis. The coronary arteriograms in such cases show diffuse narrowing without discrete stenoses. These lesions typically are more concentric than the usual atherosclerotic lesion and in some cases contain little or no lipid accumulation.

cultured human vascular smooth muscle cells to IL-1 for several days furnished a strong mitogenic stimulus (Libby et al., 1988). Under certain conditions IL-1 was as potent a smooth muscle mitogen as platelet-derived growth factor (PDGF), the prototypical activator of smooth muscle growth. The IL-1-induced smooth muscle cell proliferation appeared not to be secondary to endogenous production of PDGF due to IL-1, as determined by studies with selective antisera. Furthermore, IL-1 caused expression of the growth-related c-*fos* proto-oncogene with rapid kinetics, identical to those observed with PDGF, another indication that IL-1's mitogenic action is independent of other growth fators. It is very likely that IL-1 would be secreted locally at the site of vascular immune reactions in allografted tissues. These considerations suggest that IL-1 may provide one important mitogenic stimulus for the exuberant hyperplasia of smooth muscle cells. This abnormal proliferation of smooth muscle cells characterizes coronary arteriosclerosis in allografted hearts, an important remaining obstacle to the long-term success of this procedure.

Conclusions

Results from many laboratories over the last few years have considerably broadened our comprehension of the range of cell types that can participate actively in the generation of immune responses. The "classical" view of cellular immunologists accorded a monopoly to bone marrow-derived leucocytes as immunocompetent cells. This view is no longer tenable. A number of "peripheral" cells previously thought of simply as targets for the immune response may play a major role in localized immune responses, including those in the blood vessel wall. In general, antigen-specific recognition events do indeed appear to be restricted to lymphocytes in accord with the classical view. However, many functions previously thought to be limited to mononuclear phagocytes such as class II histocompatibility antigen expression, antigen processing and presentation, and elaboration of potent immunoregulatory molecules such as IL-1, are shared by vascular wall cells, notably vascular endothelium and smooth muscle cells.

The foregoing conclusion emphasizes the potential in vivo significance of these findings in the pathogenesis of vascular diseases and rejection of transplanted organs. In general, the bone marrow derived cells or "professional immunocytes" function more efficiently in this regard than their peripheral tissue counterparts. What value might accrue to the organism from maintenance of these specialized immune functions in the peripheral non-lymphoid tissues of multicellular organisms? We propose that the ability to localize elements of the immune response to a specific focal area can serve not only to amplify or intensify the local reaction, but might also limit its unnecessary and potentially deleterious propagation. Dissemination of immune responses (such as those produced by a grafted organ) throughout the vasculature and lymphoid system could prove dangerous to the host. Such diffuse immune activation may account for the generalized and severe pathology associated with lymphokine-activated killer cell therapy in man. This syndrome includes widespread vascular changes, including capillary leak that produces anasarca and pulmonary edema, as well as systemic alterations such as fever and obtundation. The ability of endothelium to recruit antigen-specific T-cells or other potent effectors of the inflammatory response to specific foci may tend to limit these responses to the area where they are needed and avoid such undesirable effects of a generalized immune response. Activation of helper T-cells and cytolysis by killer T-cells clearly require intimate cell-cell contact. Non-antigen-specific effects of cytokines such as modulation of histocompatibility antigen expression or co-activation of thymocytes by IL-1 might best be restricted to the particular site of injury or inflammation. These considerations indicate how the ability of vascular wall cells to express these non-antigen-specific immune functions may provide a benefit to the host.

Acknowledgements

We thank Drs Jordan S Pober, Charles A Dinarello, Göran Hansson, and Baruj Benacerraf for enlightening discussions regarding the application of immunology to vascular diseases. Drs Sheldon M Wolff and Alan D Callow have provided both intellectual and material support for our experimental work over the years. We are grateful to Drs Richard J Cleveland, Douglas Payne, Thomas F O'Donnell, William C Mackey, and other members of the Department of Surgery at our institution for their co-operation in obtaining specimens of human vascular tissue for our investigations. Ms Joan L Leonard provided excellent secretarial and administrative assistance for the preparation of this manuscript. Maria W Janicka, Cindy B Galin, Gary B Friedman, and Nathan H Margolis contributed technical expertise to the studies performed in our laboratory. This work is supported by grants from the US National Institutes of Health; National Heart, Lung and Blood Institute, Grants HL34636 to PL and HL36898 to Drs Callow and Libby. PL is an Established Investigator of the American Heart Association and SJCW is the Howard B Sprague Fellow of the American Heart Association, Massachusetts Affiliate for 1987-1988.

References

1. Bach FH, Sachs DH. Current Concepts: Immunology. Transplantation immunology. N England J Med 317, 489, 1987.

2. Benacerraf B. Role of MHC gene products in immune regulation. Science 212, 1229, 1981.

3. Benacerraf B. Significance and biological function of class II MHC molecules. Am J Pathol 120, 333, 1985.

4. Bevilacqua MP, Pober JS, Majeau GR, Cotran RS, Gimbrone MA Jr. Interleukin-1 (IL-1) induces biosynthesis and cell surface expression of procoagulant activity in human vascular endothelial cells. J Exp Med 160, 618, 1984.

4. Bevilacqua MP, Pober JS, Majeau GR, Cotran RS, Gimbrone MA Jr. Interleukin -1 acts on cultured human vascular endothelium to increase the adhesion of polymorphonuclear leukocytes, monocytes and related leukocyte cell linies. J Clin Invest 76, 2003, 1985.

5. Bevilacqua MP, Pober JS, Majeau GR, Fiers W, Cotran RS, Gimbrone MA Jr. Recombinant tumor necrosis factor induces procoagulant activity in cultured human vascular endothelium: characterization and comparison with the actions of interleukin-1. Proc Natl Acad Sci USA 83, 4533, 1986a.

6. Bevilacqua MP, Schleef R, Gimbrone MA Jr, Loskutoff DJ. Regulation of the fribinolytic system of cultured human vascular endothelium by interleukin-1. J Clin Invest 78, 587, 1986b.

7. Bevilacqua MP, Pober JS, Mendrick DL, Cotran S, Gimbrone MA Jr. Identification of an inducible endothelial-leukocyte adhesion molecule. Proc Natl Acad Sci USA (in press).

8. Cavender DE, Haskard DO, Joseph B, Ziff M. Interleukin-1 increases the binding of human B and T lymphocytes to endothelial cell monolayers J Immunol 136, 203, 1986.

9. Collins T, Korman AJ, Wake CT, Boss JM, Kappes DJ, Fiers W, Ault KA, Gimbrone MA Jr, Strominger JL, Pober JS. Immune interferon activates multiple class II major histocompatibility complex genes and the associated invariant chain gene in human endothelial cells and dermal fibroblasts. Proc Natl Acad Sci USA 81, 4917, 1984.

10. Collins T, Krensky AM, Clayberger C, Fiers W, Gimbrone MA Jr, Burakoff SJ, Pober JS. Human cytolytic T lymphocyte interactions with vascular endothelium and fibroblasts: role of effector and target cell molecules. J Immunol 133, 1878, 1984.

11. Collins T, Lapierre LA, Fiers W, Strominger JL, Pober JS. Recombinant human tumor necrosis factor increases MRNA levels and surface expression of HLA-A, B antigens in vascular endothelial cells and dermal fibroblasts in vitro. Proc Natl Acad Sci USA 83, 446, 1986.

12. Cotran RS, Gimbrone MA Jr, Bevilacqua MP, Mendrick DL, Pober JS. Induction and detection of a human endothelial activation antigen in vivo. J Exp Med 164, 661, 1986.

13. Cotran RS, Pober JS, Gimbrone MA Jr, Springer TA, Wiebke EA, Gaspari AA, Rosenber SA, Lotze MT. Endothelial activation during interleukin-2 (IL-2) immunotherapy: a possible mechanisms for the vascular leak syndrome. J Immunol (in press).

14. Dinarello CA, Ikejima T, Warner SJC, Orencole SF, Lonnemann G, Cannon JG, Libby P. Interleukin-1 in rabbits in vivo and in human mononuclear cells in vitro. J Immunol 139, 1902, 1987

3. Endothelial Cell Lining

15. Dinarello CA, Cannon JG, Mier JW, Bernheim HA, LoPreste G, Lynn DL, Love RN, Webb AC, Auron PE, Reuben RC, Rich AR, Wolff SM, Putney SD. Multiple biological activities of human recombinant interleukin-1. J Clin.Invest 77, 1734, 1986.

16. Dinarello CA, Mier JW. Lymphokines. N Engl J Med 317, 940, 1987.

17. Duijvestijn AM, Schreiber AB, Butcher EC. Interferon- regulates an antigen specific for endothelial cells involved in lymphocyte traffic. Proc Natl Acad Sci USA 83, 9114, 1986.

18. Dustin ML, Rothlein R, Bhan AK, Dinarello CA, Springer TA. Induction by IL-1 and interferon-gamma: tissue distribution, biochemistry, and function of a natural adherence molecule (ICAM-1). J Immunol 137, 245, 1986.

19. Gallatin M, St John TP, Siegelman M, Reichert R, Butcher EC, Weissman IL. Lymphocyte homing receptors. Cell 44, 673, 1986.

20. Galumbeck M, Hagen PO, Seabar A and Urbaniak J. Inhibition of vascular allograft rejection by removal of the endothelium. Circulation 76, IV-55, 1987.

21. Geppert TD, Lipsky PE. Antigen presentation by interferon--treated endothelial cells and fibroblasts: differential ability to function as antigen-presenting cells despite comparable Ia expression. J Immunol 135, 3750, 1985.

22. Gown AM, Tsukada T, Ross R. Human atherosclerosis II. Immunocytochemical analysis of the cellular composition of human atherosclerotic lesions. Am J Pathol 125, 191, 1986.

23. Groenewegen G, Buurman WA, van der Linden CJ. Lymphokine dependence of in vivo expression of MHC class II antigens by endothelium. Nature 316, 361, 1985.

24. Hansson GK, Jonasson L, Holm J, Claesson-Welsh L. Class II MHC antigen expression in the atherosclerotic plaque: smooth muscle cells express HLA-DR, HLA-DQ and the invariant gamma chain. Clin Exp Immunol 64, 261, 1986.

25. Hart MN, Tassell SK, Sadewasser KL, Schelper RL and Moore S A. Autoimmune vasculitis resulting from in vitro immunization of lymphocytes to smooth muscle. Am J Pathol, 119, 448, 1985.

26. Hart MN, Waldschmidt MM, Hanley-Hyde JM, Moore SA, Kemp JD, Schelper RL. Brain microvascular smooth muscle expresses class II antigens. J Immunol 138, 2960, 1987.

27. Haskard D, Cavender D, Beatty P, Springer T, Ziff M. T lymphocyte adhesion to endothelial cells: mechanisms demonstrated by anti-LFA-1 monoclonal antibodies. J Immunol 137, 2901, 1986.

28. Hunninghake GW, Glazier AJ, Monick MM, Dinarello CA. Interleukin-1 is a chemotactic factor for human T-lymphocytes. Am Rev Respir Dis 135, 66, 1987.

29. Hynes RO. Integrins: a family of cell surface receptors. Cell 48, 549, 1987.

30. Jalkanen S, Reichert RA, Gallatin WM, Bargatze RF, Weissman IL, Butcher EC. Homing receptors and the control of lymphocyte migration. Immunol Rev 91, 39, 1986a.

31. Jalkanen ST, Bargatzem RF, Herron LR, Butcher EC. A lymphoid cell surface glycoprotein involved in endothelial cell recognition and lymphocyte homing in man. Eur J Immunol 16, 1195, 1986b.

32. Jonasson L, Holm J, Skalli O, Gabbiani G, Hansson GK. Expression of class II transplantation antigen on vascular smooth muscle cells in human atherosclerosis. J Clin Invest 76, 125, 1985.

33. Jonasson L, Holm J, Skalli O, Bondjers G, Hansson GK. Regional accumulations of T-cells, macrophages, and smooth muscle cells in the human atherosclerotic plaque. Atherosclerosis 6, 131, 1986.

34. Kurt-Jones EA, Fiers W, Pober JS. Membrane interleukin-1 induction on human endothelial cells and dermal fibroblasts. J Immunol 139, 2317, 1987.

35. Leibovich SJ, Polverini PJ, Shepard HM, Wiseman DM, Shively V, Nuseir N. Macrophage-induced angiogenesis is mediated by tumour necrosis factor-. Nature 329, 630, 1987.

36. Leung DY, Geha RS, Newburger JW, Burns J C, Fiers W, Lapierre L A, Pober JS. Two monokines, interleukin-1 and tumor necrosis factor, render cultured vascular endothelial cells susceptible to lysis by antibodies circulating during Kawasaki syndrome. J Exp Med 164, 1958, 1986.

37. Libby P, Ordovas JM, Auger KR, Robbins AH, Birinyi LK, Dinarello CA. Endotoxin and tumor necrosis factor induce interleukin-1 beta gene expression in adult human vascular endothelial cells. Am J Pathol 124, 179, 1986a.

38. Libby P, Ordovas JM, Birinyi LK, Kruger KR, Dinarello CA. Inducible interleukin-1 expression in human vascular smooth muscle cells. J Clin Invest 78, 1432, 1986b.

39. Libby P, Warner SJC, Galin CB. Human vascular smooth muscle can transcribe the tumor necrosis factor/cachectin gene and respond to this inflammatory mediator. Clinical Research 35, 297A, 1987.

40. Libby P, Warner SJC, Friedman GB. Interleukin-1: a mitogen for human vascular smooth muscle cells that induces the release of growth-inhibitory prostanoids. J Clin Invest (in press).

41. Marrack P and Kappler J. The T-cell receptor. Science 238, 1073, 1987.

42. Mentzer SJ, Burakoff SJ, Faller DV. Adhesion of T-lymphocytes to human endothelial cells is regulated by the LFA-1 membrane molecule. J Cell Physiol 126, 285, 1986.

43. Miossec P, Cavender D and Ziff M. Production of interleukin-1 by human endothelial cells. J Immunol, 136, 2486, 1986.

44. Nachman RL, Hajjar KA, Silverstein RL and Dinarello CA. Interleukin-1 induces endothelial cell synthesis of plasinogen activator inhibitor. J Exp Med, 163, 1595, 1986.

45. Nossal GJV. Current Concepts: Immunology. The basic components of the immune system. N Engl J Med, 316, 1320, 1987.

46. Oppenheim JJ. Antigen nonspecific lymphokines: an overview. Methods in Enzymology 166, 357, 1985.

47. Pober JS, Gimbrone MA Jr. Expression of Ia-like antigens by human vascular endothelial cells is inducible in vitro: demonstration by mononuclear antibody binding and immunoprecipitation. Proc Natl Acad Sci USA 79, 6641, 1982.

48. Pober JS, Gimbrone MA Jr, Cotran RS, Reiss CS, Burakoff SJ, Fiers W, Ault K A. Ia expression by vascular endothelium is inducible by activated T-cells and by human interferon. J Exp Med 157, 1339, 1983a.

49. Pober JS, Collins T, Gimbrone MA Jr, Cotran RS, Gitlin JD, Fiers W, Clayberger C, Krensky AM, Burakoff SJ, Reiss CS. Lymphocytes recognize human vascular endothelial and dermal fibroblast Ia antigens induced by recombinant immune interferon. Nature 305, 726, 1983b.

3. Endothelial Cell Lining

50. Pober JS, Collins T, Gimbrone MA Jr, Libby P, Reiss CS. Inducible expression of class II major histocompatibility complex antigens and the immunogenicity of vascular endothelium. Transplantation 41, 141, 1986a.

51. Pober JS, Gimbrone MA Jr, Lapierre L A, Mendrick DL, Fiers W, Rothlein R, Springer TA. Overlapping patterns of activation of human endothelial cells by interleukin-1, tumor necrosis factor and immune interferon. J Immunol 137, 1893, 1986b.

52. Pober JS, Bevilacqua MP, Mendrick DF, Lapierre L A, Fiers W, Gimbrone MA Jr. Two distinct monokines interleukin-1 and tumor necrosis factor, each independently induce biosynthesis and transient expression of the same antigen of the surface of cultured human vascular endothelial cells. J Immunol 136, 1680, 1986c.

53. Pohlman TH, Stanness KA, Beatty PG, Ochs HD, Harlan JM. An endothelial cell surface factor(s) induced in vitro by lipopolysaccharide, interleukin-1, and tumor necrosis factor-alpha increases neutrophil adherence by a CDw 18-dependent mechanism. J Immunol 136, 4548, 1986.

54. Rosen SD, Singer MS, Yednock TA, Stoolman LM. Involvement of sialic acid on endothelial cells in organ-specific lymphocyte recirculation. Science 228, 1005, 1985.

55. Rosenwasser LJ, Dinarello CA. Ability of human leukocyte pyrogen to enhance phytohemagglutinin-induced murine thymocyte proliferation. Cell Immunol 63, 134, 1981.

56. Rothlein R, Dustin ML, Marlin SD, Springer TA. A human intercellular adhesion molecule (ICAM-1) distinct from LFA-1. J Immunol 137, 1270, 1986.

57. Royer HD, Reinhertz EL. T-lymphocytes: Ontogeny, function and relevance to clinical disorders. N Engl J Med 317, 1136, 1987.

58. Ruoslahti E, Pierschbacher MD. New perspectives in cell adhesion: RGD and integrins. Science 238, 491, 1987.

59. Schleimer RP, Rutledge BK. Cultured human vascular endothelial cells acquire adhesiveness for neutrophils after stimulation with interleukin-1, endotoxin and tumor-promoting phorbol diesters. J Immunol 136, 649, 1986.

60. Siegelman M, Bond M W, Gallatin WM, St John T, Smith HT, Fried VA, Weissman IL. Cell surface molecule associated with lymphocyte homing is a ubiquitinated branched-chain glycoprotein. Science 231, 823, 1986.

61. Springer TA. The LFA-1, Mac-1 glycoprotein family and its deficiency in an inherited disease. Federation Proc 44, 2660, 1985.

62. Stern DM, Bank I, Nawroth PP, Cassimeris J, Kisiel W, Fenton JW II, Dinarello CL, Chess DI, Jaffe EA. Self-regulation of procoagulant events on the endothelial cell surface. J Exp Med 162, 1223, 1985.

63. Unanue ER, Allen PM. The basis for the immunoregulatory role of macrophages and other accessory cells. Science 236, 551, 1987.

64. Wagner CR, Vetto RM, Burger DR. The mechanisms of antigen presentation by endothelial cells. Immunobiology 168, 453, 1984.

65. Wagner CR, Vetto RM, Burger DR. Subcultured human endothelial cells can function independently as fully competent antigen-presenting cells. Hum Immunol 13, 33, 1985a.

66. Wagner CR, Vetto RM, Burger DR. Expression of I-region-associated antigen (Ia) and interleukin-1 by subcultured human endothelial cells. Cell Immunol 93, 91, 1985.

3. Endothelial Cell Lining

67. Warner SJC, Auger KR, Libby P. Human interleukin-1 induces interleukin-1 gene expression in human vascular smooth muscle cells. J Exp Med 165, 1316, 1987a.

68. Warner SJC, Auger KR, Libby P. Interleukin-1 induces interleukin-1.-II. Recombinant human interleukin-1 induces interleukin-1 production by adult human vascular endothelial cells. J Immunol 139, 1911, 1987b.

69. Windt MR, Rosenwasser LJ. Human vascular endothelial cells produce interleukin-1. Lymphokine Res 315, 641, 1984.

70. Wong GHW, Schrader JW. Regulation of H-2, Ia, TL, and Qa antigen expression by interferon. Lymphokines 11, 47, 1985.

3. Endothelial Cell Lining

3.3. Ten Years of Endothelial Cell Seeding

3.3.1. The Tissue Culture Arterial Graft

AD Callow
New England Medical Center,
Boston, Massachusetts, USA

An intensive investigative effort has been underway in many laboratories throughout the world during the last ten years in an attempt to overcome the problem of the high failure rate of synthetic bypass grafts with an internal diameter of 4 mm or less. These prostheses anastomosed to the vessels of the distal calf display patency rates of 15-20% in less than three years from insertion (1). In the aortoiliac and femoropopliteal positions, patency rates at ten years are approximately 100% and 50% respectively. (2) Below the inguinal ligament, the reversed and in situ saphenous, yield a patency rate of approximately 65 to 70% at eight years, compared to Dacron grafts in the same position of only 10% (2). For expanded polytetrafluoroethylene grafts below the knee, the three year patency rate is approximately 25% and the denatured human umbilical vein is only slightly better (3,4).

From the first use, bypass grafts, as well as the arteries they were intended to replace, were regarded as simple mechanical conduits. Appreciation of the biological complexity of the arterial wall, and its response to the foreign body that was the graft, awaited the discoveries of cell biologists during the 1970s and 80s.

In the experimental animal model, an endothelial or endothelial-like lining develops on the wall of the synthetic graft. It was incorrectly assumed that this also occurred in the human. There is no conclusive evidence that this is so. Moreover, there is a paucity of evidence, other than simple morphologic observations that a true intima is indeed regenerated in the dog or other animal models (5). In the human, except for a perianastomotic zone of endothelial cells of approximately 1-2 cm, and which are assumed to originate from endothelial cells of the adjacent host artery, a completely lined endothelial graft has not been realized. Rather, an inner capsule of a largely acellular, proteinaceous nature gradually accumulates. When unchecked, this perianastomotic neointimal fibroplasia slowly increases, resulting in flow reduction and secondary retrograde thrombosis of the graft. The realization that the superior performance of the saphenous vein might be due to the endothelial lining of the vein, coupled with recently available technology for harvesting human vascular endothelial cells, led to the introduction of seeding techniques by Herring and his associates in 1978 (6). Vascular endothelial cells from many species - the dog, sheep, baboon and human - can now be successfully seeded (7,8,9).

Early attempts of seeding endothelial cells on polymer surfaces were not uniformly successful nor reproducible. Mere attachment to the surface did not guarantee cell growth. Spreading to confluence did not preclude substantial cell loss in a dynamic flow environment. Substrates such as fibronectin, fibrin, laminin, and a variety of types of collagen, as well as simple autologous clot were utilized to encourage attachment and replication of the endothelial cell. Occasional success with simple endothelial lined prosthetics in current use have been reported from the laboratory. Whittemore and associates (10) seeded Dacron grafts coated with Type I bovine collagen with venous endothelial cells and implanted them in the femoral position in the dog. Unseeded contralateral grafts served as the control. Explanted after one month, the seeded grafts demonstrated an 86% patency rate in contrast to only 14% of the unseeded controls. This is too short a period of observation for neointimal hyperplasia to develop.

Questions also arise concerning functional integrity of the attached cells, especially since the report by Gimbone of endothelial cell phenotype modulation (11).

Many highly specialized functions of the endothelial cell have been identified

Paralleling the increase in information about the endothelial cell is a similar expansion of knowledge of the smooth muscle cell. There is a growing

Partial Listing of Endothelial Cell Products and Activities

Luminal Surface

Procoagulant
    Tissue factor
    vWf
Enzymes
    ACE I & II
    Nucleotidases
    Histamine
    Bradykinin

Inducible immune functions
    Class II HLA determinants
    Interleukin-I production
Anticoagulant
    Prostacyclin
    Thrombomodulin
    t-PA
    Heparin-like molecules

Abluminal Surface

Biosynthesis of extracellular matrix
    Collagens
    Fibronectin
    Laminin
    Glycosaminoglycans
Growth Stimulators
    C-sis product
    Interleukin-I

Elaboration of vasodilators
    Prostacyclin
    'Endothelial-dependent
    relaxation factor'

Growth Inhibitors
    Heparin-like molecules

Table 34 (12)

3. Endothelial Cell Lining

awareness of the importance of other components of the arterial wall, such as basement membrane, extracellular matrix, and the participation of innumerable "wayfarers" in the blood, proteins, platelets and white cells, to name a few.

It has yet to be demonstrated that the endothelial cell in the abnormal environment of the synthetic surface continues to function as it does in its differentiated state, that is, to express those functions such as control of thrombosis and smooth muscle cell growth which the cell does in its normal environment of the intact arterial wall. Indeed, there is increasing information from the laboratory that the reverse is true (13).

An additional area of concern is the failure of clinical trials to demonstrate convincingly that long-term patency rates are improved by allegedly successful endothelial cell coverage of the prosthetic graft (6). Lack of standardization of harvesting and seeding techniques, lack of precision in intermediate and late evaluation of the seeded surface, variations in the size of the cell innoculum as well as amount of surface coverage at the time of implantation of the graft, and the difficulty of evaluating continuing function of the endothelial cell, make interpretation of these trials difficult and uncertain.

Anastomotic neointimal fibroplasia is probably the most frequent cause of late failure of synthetic grafts. With the identification and purification of platelet derived growth factor for vascular smooth muscle cells by Ross, et al (14,15) and the observation that injury and denudation of the endothelial layer were followed by platelet adhesion, aggregation and release of smooth muscle cell mitogen from the alpha granule, the platelet was assumed to play a prominent role in the development of the hyperplastic response. Control of platelet adhesion and aggregation might, it was reasoned, inhibit not only thrombus formation, the chief cause of early failure, but late failure secondary to smooth muscle cell proliferation as well.

Results of studies of platelet deposition and activation on endothelialized Dacron and ePTFE grafts are inconsistent. In our studies, no difference in platelet accumulation was noted between the seeded and the unseeded grafts at the end of 24 hours, utilizing baboon cells grown to confluence and implanted in the carotid position. (7, 8,16). Other studies have shown reduction in platelet deposition from the earliest observations (17,18). A reduction in neointimal fibroplastic hyperplasia in both ePTFE grafts and coronary artery vein bypass grafts has been shown when antiplatelet drugs have been administered (19,20,21,22).

Administration of aspirin plus dipyridamole has been shown to improve patency of human coronary bypass grafts at 12 months after operation (23, 24). Moreover, thrombocytopenia inhibits intimal fibromuscular hyperplasia after aortic intimal injury (25). The flaw in these and other studies has been a lack of distinction between failure due to platelet initiated thrombosis and failure secondary to anastomotic hyperplasia. Late failure due to downstream progression of occlusive disease must also be included.

In the canine model, neointimal fibroplasia at the anastomoses of Dacron grafts demonstrated progression as long as 60 days after implantation, despite formation of a confluent layer of endothelial cells and despite no evidence of platelet adhesion (26). Burkel and associates (27) and Sharefkin and associates (17) have demonstrated that endothelial cell seeded Dacron grafts with confluent linings show continuing late hyperplasia of the smooth muscle cell beneath the confluent lining, even in the absence of evidence of graft/platelet interactivity. Doses of aspirin and dipyridamole large enough to reduce platelet aggregation by 90% failed to decrease neointimal fibroplasia after injury of the rabbit aortic intima (28). Furthermore, administration of aspirin prior to surgery in doses large enough to result in 99% inhibition of platelet aggregation in the canine model, failed to prevent or even reduce neointimal fibromuscular hyperplasia at a sham carotid endarterectomy site (29). Finally, no improvement in patency rates of human femoral popliteal bypass grafts followed over a two year period was noted with administration of aspirin and dipyridamole (18).

As early as 1977, Clowes and Karnovsky (30) suggested that although antiplatelet agents may assist in the prevention of thrombosis of the graft, the concept that platelet derived growth factor from platelets alone was the sole cause of neointimal fibroplasia deserved more careful study. Utilizing 4 mm ePTFE arterial bypass grafts in the baboon, endothelium and smooth muscle cells from the cut ends of the adjacent host artery established a new intima. These endothelial cells migrated together along the luminal surface of the graft at approximately 0.2 mm/day. Both endothelial and smooth muscle cell types proliferated in association with the growing edge. An important observation was that both endothelial cells and smooth muscle cells located discretely over the anastomoses continued to proliferate despite complete endothelial coverage. Thus, the platelet theory for the formation of neointimal hyperplasia was further weakened. Neointimal hyperplasia occurs in areas covered by endothelium to which platelets apparently cannot adhere and, despite administration of antiplatelet agents in generous doses in the clinical area, neointimal fibromuscular hyperplasia is not prevented.

From these observations, the hypothesis arose that intermediate and late perianastomotic cellular stenosis might be due to chronic endothelial injury and turnover accompanied by continuing SMC proliferation and intimal thickening. Strandness summarized this information in his overview of peripheral vascular disease research: "lesions tend to form where endothelium is preserved or restored and not where it is absent" (31).

Numerous observations have confirmed the expression of a platelet derived growth factor-like protein by cultured endothelial cells. (32,33). By 1984 it was reported that there were multiple growth factors of the cultured endothelial cell, stimulative to connective tissue cells (34). Collins and associates demonstrated that the cultured human endothelial cell expressed platelet derived growth factor B chain (35) as well as the A chain (36). Somewhat earlier, Castellot et al had demonstrated that these same cultured cells produce a heparin-like inhibitor of smooth muscle cell growth (37,38). Inasmuch as endothelial cells, therefore, can produce smooth muscle cell mitogens, it must be surmised that, in the normal state, EC's are in a quiescent or nonproliferating phase releasing little if any smooth muscle cell mitogen. Probably as a consequence of unnatural stimuli, a phenotype change occurs which not only may result in expression

3. Endothelial Cell Lining

of procoagulant functions, but also the release of smooth muscle cell mitogens.

There are a host of additional endothelial cell functions, some of which are the expression of the normal endothelial cell, and others of the transposed or seeded cell. The normal cell can be thought of as quiescent and differentiated, whereas the abnormal cell is in a more active phase and has been described as dedifferentiated. In all likelihood the same statements can be made concerning the smooth muscle cell, e.g. in its normal resting state within the arterial wall, it expresses a number of functions acting singly or in concert on the micro-domain of the arterial wall. Grown in culture or seeded on an abnormal substrate or injured in some other way (such as resting on a bioresorbable or non-resorbable polymer), the smooth muscle cell, too, may undergo phenotype modulation. In this secretory phase, the SMC may express functions quite distinct from those when in its normal quiescent and contractile phase.

It has become increasingly clear that the construction of a tissue culture arterial graft is enormously complex. Thus, a second generation biological graft is needed - as great as quantum leap beyond the simple endothelial cell seeded synthetic graft as that concept is beyond the raw or unseeded prosthesis. Studies are underway in several laboratories directed to coculture and inoculation of smooth muscle as well as endothelial cells, and in one instance, of fibroblasts as well. The inoculated "scaffolds" consist of materials, some of which are biodegradable or bioresorbable; others are not. Still others are of biologic or natural origin. Various blends of synthetic materials are under study.

Biodegradation has been described as a breakdown process resulting in loss of tensile strength and other mechanical properties of the material, with the resulting development of fragmentation debris. These particles are recognized as foreign bodies by the host. The tissue compatibility of the original material in its intact state on implantation may not be the same for its degradation products. The initial material on implantation may be biologically inert. Its fragmentation products may not be. Bioresorbtion is the process by which the host not only biodegrades the implant but, in addition, eliminates the resulting products through several largely enzymatic mechanisms.

As early as 1962, Wesolowski and others mixed collagen and Dacron in an effort to develop a bioresorbable arterial prosthesis (39,40,41,42). In 1972 prostheses made of Dacron and poly DL lactic acid were reported (42). In 1978, Vicryl - polyglactin 910 - a copolymer consisting of 90% polyglycolic acid and 10% poly L-lactic acid was produced in a tubular configuration with the intent that it would be totally bioresorbable (43). In most of these instances, aneurysmal dilatation is a major obstacle. This is well demonstrated by the performance of tubular configurations made of 100% polyglycolic acid (Dexon) (44).

Using prostheses made of various blends of polymers or other suitable materials with "suitable porosity", compliance and biodegradability to serve as scaffolds for cellular invasion of inoculated cells, arterial "walls" have been grown in the laboratory and implanted in an animal model. Further growth has been observed in vivo.

Van der Lei and associates reported, in 1985, fabrication of a small diameter

3. Endothelial Cell Lining

microporous, compliant and bioresorbable prosthesis made of a mixture of polyurethane and poly L-lactic acid in a mixture 95/5% respectively. This mixture was satisfactory for optimal regeneration of the newly formed arterial wall leading to replacement of the prosthesis. Prosthesis compliance was thought to correlate with enhancement of regeneration of the new arterial wall (45,46,47,48,49,40). Van der Lei noted a predominantly longitudinal arrangement of the smooth muscle cells in the neomedia. This observation needs confirmation and interpretation because of the correlation between cyclic stretching and the synthesis of extracellular matrix components noted by Glagov et al (51). Further, the formation of elastic laminae appears to correlate to the pulsatile stimulation of smooth muscle cells of the neointima (46,47). If the orientation of neointimal smooth muscle cells is controlled by the tension to which they are subjected (52) and if cells become arranged predominantly in circular fashion with circumferential expansion of the prosthesis (52), circular orientation may be of crucial importance for the performance of the "regenerated" artery.

Greisler and associates (53) reported a substantially thicker internal capsule on polyglycolic acid prostheses as compared to that forming on Dacron prostheses in current use. The thickness appeared to vary with the amount of PLLA incorporated in the base bioresorbable polyurethane prosthesis (49, 50). Possibly as a consequence of latic dehydrogenase and hydrolysis of PLLA, increase in lactic dehydrogenase activity has been observed with these bioresorbable materials. Increase of fibroblast activation also occurs (54,55,565). During the bioresorbtion process, de-polymerization of the synthetics may result in the development of a macrophage derived growth factor which, in turn, results in increased fibroblast proliferation (57,58). The consequent proliferation of fibroblasts and the production of collagen as well as other limitations, suggests that these materials may be unacceptable (59).

In addition to applying vascular endothelial and smooth muscle cells, Weinberger and Bell have also added fibroblasts. (60) Wildevuur and associates (48) have utilized the concept of coculture of endothelial and vascular smooth muscle cells on collagen tubes. Endothelial like and smooth muscle like cells have been demonstrated within these "regenerated" arterial walls. What has not been demonstrated is the functional state of the cells growing on these materials. Is this smooth muscle in a contractile or a "synthetic" phase? Is this endothelial cell in a differential quiescent phase and capable of expressing normal functions? Lastly, the presence of a basement membrane has not been convincingly demonstrated.

Small diameter grafts may have improved patency if they possess compliance comparable to that of the natural vessel as well as a mature smooth muscle substrate upon which can be established a stable and nonthrombogenic neoendothelial layer. Galletti, et al have chosen as their goal a fully resorbable graft tested in the dog (59). As with most polyurethane based prostheses, these underwent aneurysmal dilatation in a matter of a few weeks to months.

Barrett and his group demonstrated expression of the sis-gene by endothelial cells in culture and in vivo in 1984 (61) showing that PDGF gene sequences are not only expressed by en-

3. Endothelial Cell Lining

dothelium but also in the proliferative vascular lesions. Analysis of plaques from the carotid artery removed at surgery revealed 5 to 10 times more PDGF B chain transcription signal than did the normal carotid artery, although the cell type producing the transcript has not been identified as to endothelial, smooth muscle, or macrophage origin (62).

The inescapable conclusion from these and other data suggests that the endothelial cell can exist in two phenotypic states: the normal state in the normal environment of the normal artery. In this differentiated state the cell is quiescent as indicated by thymidine labeling index of less than 0.01%. The cell expresses the normal antithrombogenic functions and, presumably through production of heparin like molecules (63), inhibits or suppresses smooth muscle cell proliferation. The abnormal, de-differentiated cell is in a highly active state as demonstrated by a high mitotic index (64), production of smooth muscle cell mitogens (65), irregular cytoskeleton patterns (66), and uncoupling of the boundary junctions (67). The physiologic dilemma is illustrated by the need on one hand to have an active proliferating endothelial cell which can replicate to complete coverage of the prosthesis, yet not stimulate increased and potentially harmful activity by other elements of the cellular and humoral orchestra such as the macrophage, platelet, and the smooth muscle cell. Can the proliferating ultimately confluent endothelial cell layer be persuaded to enter a quiescent phase, cease expression of undesirable functions, and resume its expression of those functions characteristic of the normal differentiated cell?

A number of possible solutions come to mind. It may be possible to prepare a basement membrane or membrane-like material which will support and sustain the endothelial cell growth until it reaches confluence, and then permit it to return to a quiescent state. At this time, it may then suppress smooth muscle cell proliferation and subsequent development of a hyperplastic lesion. Is it possible to develop a biomaterial that allows only endothelial cell growth but by its own characteristics, either intrinsic or applied, may suppress the production of growth factor or render it ineffective? A number of possibilities come to mind. Each requires expenditure of time, energy and thought. Unravelling the mysteries of the endothelial cell, of the accompanying smooth muscle cell, and of the many factors operating on both, seems possible in the light of discoveries of the past decade (31,68,69,70,71,72).

3. Endothelial Cell Lining

References

1. Sauvage LR, Berger K, Wood SJ et al. Grafts for the 80s (The Bob Hope International Heart Research Institute, Seattle 1981).

2. Darling RC, Linton RR. Durability of femoropopliteal reconstructions. Am J Surg 123, 472, 1972.

3. Gupta SK, Veitch FJ. Three year experience with expanded polytetrafluoroethylene arterial grafts for limb salvage. Am J Surg 140, 214, 1980.

4. Bergan JJ, Veitch FJ, Bernhard VM et al. Randomization of autogenous vein and polytetrafluoroethylene grafts in femorodistal reconstruction. Surgery 92, 921; 1982.

5. Sauvage L, Berger K, Wood S, et al. Interspecies healing of porous arterial prostheses. Arch Surg 109, 698, 1974.

6. Herring M, Gardner A, Glover J. A single-staged technique for seeding vascular grafts with autogenous endothelium. Surgery 84, 498, 1978.

7. Shepard AD, Eldrup-Jorgensen J, Keough EM, Foxall TF, Ramberg K, Connolly RJ, Mackey WC, Gavris V, Auger KR, Libby P, O'Donnell TF, Callow AD. Endothelial cell seeding of small-caliber synthetic grafts in the baboon. Surgery 99, 318, 1986.

8. Callow AD, Foxall TF, Shepard AD, Mackey WC, Ramberg KL et al. Endothelial cell seeded small caliber artery grafts; preliminary results in baboons (Abstract). Circulation 70, II/164, 1986.

9. Foxall TL, Auger KR, Callow AD, Libby P. Adult human endothelial cell coverage of small-caliber Dacron and polytetrafluoroethylene vascular prostheses in vitro. J Surg Res 41, 158-172, 1986.

10. Shindo S, Takagi A, Whittemore AD. Improved patency of collagen-impregnated grafts after in vitro autogenous endothelial cell seeding. J Vasc Surg 6, 3254, 1987.

11. Gimbrone MA. Vascular endothelium in hemostasis and thrombosis. Edinburgh, Churchill Livingston 1986.

12. Callow AD. The "tissue culture" arterial graft. How soon? In Greenhalgh, Jamieson, Nicolaides (eds). Vascular Surgery Issues in Current Practice. London, Grune & Stratton, pp 211, 1986.

13. Libby P, Birinyi LK, Callow AD. Functions of endothelial cells relating to seeding of vascular prostheses: the unanswered questions. In: Herring M, Glover JL (eds): Endothelial Seeding in Vascular Surgery. Orlando, Grune & Stratton, pp 17, 1987.

14. Ross R, Glomset J, Kariya B, Harker L. A platelet-dependent serum factor that stimulates the proliferation of arterial smooth muscle cells in vitro. Proc Nat Acad Sci USA 71, 1207, 1971.

15. Ross R, Raines EW, Bowen-Pope DF. The biology of platelet-derived growth factor. Cell 46, 155, 1986.

16. Shepard AD, Connolly RJ, Callow AD, Ramberg K, Foxall TL, Libby P, Keough EM, O'Donnell TF. Endothelial cell seeding of small-caliber synthetic vascular prostheses in the primate: sequential indium-III platelet studies. ACS Surg Forum 35, 432, 1984.

17. Sharefkin JB, Latker C, Smith M, Clagett GP, Gruess D, Rich NM. Early normalization of platelet survival by endothelial seeding of Dacron arterial prostheses in dogs. Surgery 92, 385, 1982.

3. Endothelial Cell Lining

18. Kohler TR, Kaufman JL, Kacoyanis GP, Clowes AW, Donaldson C, Kelly E, Skillman J, Whittemore AD, Couch NP, Mannick JA, Salzman EW. Effect of aspirin and dipyridamole on the patency of femoral artery bypass grafts. Surgery 96, 462, 1984.

19. Oblath RS, Buckley FO, Green RM, Schwartz SI, DeWeese JA. Prevention of platelet aggregation and adherence to prosthetic vascular grafts by aspirin and dipyridamole. Surgery 84, 37, 1984.

20. Hagen PO, Wang ZG, Mikat EM, Hackel DB. Antiplatelet therapy reduces aortic intimal hyperplasia distal to small diameter vascular prostheses (PTFE) in nonhuman primates. Ann Surg 195, 328, 1982.

21. Metke MP, Lie JT, Fuster V, Josa M, Kaye M. Reduction of intimal thickening in canine coronary bypass vein grafts with dipyridamole and aspirin. Am J Cardiol 43, 1144, 1979.

22. McCann RL, Hagen PO, Fuchs JCA. Aspirin and dipyridamole decrease intimal hyperplasia in experimental vein grafts. Ann Surg 191, 238, 1980.

23. Lorenz RL, Weber M, Kotzuk J, Thiesen K, Schacky CV, Meister W, Reichardt B, Weber PC. Improved aortocoronary bypass patency by low dose aspirin (100 mg daily). Lancet 9, 1261, 1984.

24. Brown BG, Cukingnan RA, DeRouen T, Goede LV, Wong M, Fee HJ, Roth JA, Carey JS. Improved graft patency in patients treated with platelet-inhibiting therapy after coronary bypass surgery. Circulation 72, 138, 1985.

25. Friedman RJ, Stemerman MB, Wenz et al. The effect of thrombocytopenia on experimental arteriosclerotic lesion formation in rabbits. Smooth muscle proliferation and re-endothelialization. J Clin Invest 60, 1191, 1977.

26. LoGerfo FW, Quist WC, Nowak MD, Crawshaw HM, Haudenschild CC. Downstream anastomotic hyperplasia. A mechanism of failure in Dacron arterial grafts. Ann Surg 197, 479, 1983.

27. Burkel WE, Ford JW, Vinter DW, Kahn RH, Graham LM, Stanley JC. Fate of knitted Dacron velour vascular grafts seeded with enzymatically derived autologous canine endothelium. Trans Am Soc Artif Internal Organs 28, 127, 1982.

28. Radic ZS, O'Malley MK, Mikat EM, Makhoul RG, McCann RL, Cole CW, Hagen PO. The role of aspirin and dipyridamole on vascular DNA synthesis and intimal hyperplasia following deendothelialization. J Surg Res 41, 84, 1986.

29. Bush HL, Jakubowski JA, Sentissi JM, Curl GR, Hayes JA, Deykin D. Neointimal hyperplasia occurring after carotid endarterectomy in a canine model: effect of endothelial cell seeding versus perioperative aspirin. J Vasc Surg 5, 118, 1987.

30. Clowes AW, Karnovsky MJ. Failure of certain antiplatelet drugs to affect myointimal thickening following arterial endothelial injury in the rat. Lab Invest 36, 452, 1977.

31. Strandness DE. An overview of research in peripheral vascular disease. J Vasc Surg 5, 636, 1987.

32. Gajdusek C, DiCorleto P, Ross R, Schwartz SM. An endothelial cell-derived growth factor. J Cell Biol 85, 467, 1980.

33. DiCorleto PE, Bowen-Pope DF. Cultured endothelial cells produce a platelet-derived growth factor-like protein. Proc Nat Acad Sci USA 80, 1919, 1983.

3. Endothelial Cell Lining

34. DiCorleto PE. Cultured endothelial cells produce multiple growth factors for connective tissue cells. Exp Cell Res 153, 167, 1984.

35. Collins T, Ginsburg D, Boss JM, Orkin SH, Pober JS. Cultured human endothelial cells express platelet derived growth factor B chain: cDNA cloning and structural analysis. Nature 316, 748, 1985.

36. Collins T, Gimbrone MA Jr, Hammachaer A, Betsholtz C, Westermark B, Heldin CH. Culture human endothelial cells express platelet-derived growth factor A chain. Am J Path 127, 7, 1987.

37. Castellot JJ, Addonizio ML, Rosenberg R, Karnovsky MJ. Cultured endothelial cells produce a heparinlike inhibitor of smooth muscle cell growth. J Cell Biol 90, 372, 1981.

38. Castellot JJ, Favreau JV, Karnovsky MJ, Rosenberg RD. Inhibition of vascular smooth muscle cell growth by endothelial cells-derived heparin: possible role of platelet endoglycosidase. J Biol Chem 257, 11256, 1982.

39. Wesolowski SA, Fries CC, Liebig WJ, Sawyer PN, Deterling RA. The synthetic vascular graft: new concepts, new materials. Arch Surg 84, 56, 1962.

40. Wesolowski SA, Fries CC, Domingo RT, Liebig WJ, Sawyer PN. The compound prosthetic vascular graft: a pathologic survey. Surgery 53, 19, 1963.

41. Cronenwett JL, Zelenock GB. Alternative small diameter arterial graft. In Stanley JC, Burkel WE, Lindenauer SM, Bartlett RH, Turcotte JG (eds). Biologic and Synthetic Vascular Prostheses. New York, Grune & Stratton, pp 595, 1982.

42. Rudeman RJ, Hegyeli AF, Hattler BG, Leonard F. A partially biodegradable vascular prosthesis. Trans Am Soc Artif Intern Organs 18, 30, 1972.

43. White RA, Hirose FM, Sproat RW, Lawrence RS, Nelson RJ. Histopathologic observations after short-term implantations of two porous elastomers in dogs. Biomaterials 2, 171, 1981.

44. Goglewski S, Pennings AJ. Biodegradable materials of polyactides, porous biomedical materials based on mixtures of polyactides and polyurethanes. Makromol Chem, Rapid Commun 3, 839, 1982.

45. Van der Lei B, Wildevuur CRH, Nieuwenhuis P. Compliance and biodegradation of vascular grafts stimulate the regeneration of elastic laminae in neoarterial tissue: an experimental study in rats. Surgery 99, 45, 1986.

46. Van der Lei B, Wildevuur CRH, Nieuwenhuis P. Mechanical stimulation of smooth muscle cells by arterial pulsation. An important stimulus for the formation of elastic lamina in arterial tissue. Cell Biology International Reports. 9, 2, 1984.

47. Van der Lei B, Wildevuur CRH, Nieuwenhuis P, Blaauw EH, Dijk F, Hulstaert CE, Molenaar I. Regeneration of the arterial wall in microporous, compliant, biodegradable vascular grafts after implantation into the rat abdominal aorta. Cell Tissue Res 242, 569, 1985.

48. Wildevuur CRH, van der Lei B. Smooth muscle cell seeding enhances the regeneration of a new arterial wall. Life Support Systems 4, 109, 1986.

49. Lommen E, Gogolewski S, Pennings AJ, Wildevuur CRH, Nieuwenhuis P. Development of a neo-artery induced by a biodegradable polymeric vascular prosthesis. Trans Am Soc Artif Inter Organs 29, 255, 1983.

50. Van der Lei B, Bartels HL, Nieuwenhuis P, Wildevuur CRH. Microporous, compliant, biodegradable vascular grafts for the regeneration of the arterial wall in rat abdominal aorta. Surgery 98, 955, 1985.

3. Endothelial Cell Lining

51. Leung DYM, Glagov S, Mathews MB. Cyclic stretching stimulates synthesis of matrix components by arterial smooth muscle cells in vitro. Science 191, 475, 1976.

52. Noishiki Y. Pattern of arrangement of smooth muscle cells in neointimae of synthetic vascular prostheses. J Thor Cardiovasc Surg 75, 894, 1978.

53. Greisler HP, Kim DU, Price JB, Voorhees AB. Arterial regenerative activity after prosthetic implantation. Arch Surg 120, 315, 1985.

54. Slathouse TN, Matlaga BF. Tissue regeneration associated with lactide containing implants. Trans Soc Biomat 10, 272, 1984.

55. Revis NW, Cameron AJV. The relationship between fibrosis and lactate dehydrogenase isoenzymes in the experimental hypertrophic heart of rabbits. Cardiovascular Research. 12, 348, 1987.

56. Hunt TK, Connolly WB, Aronson SB, Goldstein P. Anaerobic metabolism and wound healing: an hypothesis for the initiation and cessation of collagen synthesis in wounds. Am J Surg 135, 328, 1978.

57. Leibovich SJ, Ross R. A macrophage-dependent factor that stimulates the proliferation of fibroblasts in vitro. Amer J Path 84, 501, 1976.

58. Bitterman PB, Rennard SI, Hunninghake GW, Crystal RG. Human alveolar macrophage growth factor for fibroblasts. J Clin Invest 70, 806, 1982.

59. Galletti PM, Aebischer P, Sasken HF, Goddard M, Chiu TH. Experience with fully bioresorbable aortic grafts in the dog. Surgery 1987 (in press)

60. Weinberg CB, Bell E. A blood vessel model constructed from collagen and cultured vascular cells. Science 231, 397, 1986.

61. Barrett, TB, Gajdusek CM, Schwartz SM, McDougall JK, Benditt EP. Expression of the sis gene by endothelial cells in culture and in vivo. Proc Nat Acad Sci USA 81, 6772, 1984.

62. Barrett TB, Benditt EP. Sis (platelet-derived growth factor B chain) gene transcript levels are elevated in human atherosclerotic lesions compared to normal artery. Proc Nat Acad Sci USA 84, 1099, 1987.

63. Majack RA, Clowes AW. Inhibition of vascular smooth muscle cell migration by heparin-like glycosaminoglycans. J Cellular Physiol 118, 253, 1984.

64. Goldsmith JC, McCormick JJ, Yen A. Endothelial cell cycle kinetics: changes in culture and correlation with endothelial properties. Lab Invest 51, 643, 1984.

65. Jaye M, McConathy E, Drohan W, Tong B, Duel T, Maciag T. Modulation of the sis gene transcript during endothelial cell differentiation in vitro. Science 228, 882, 1985.

66. Dethlefsen SM, Butterfield CE, Ausprunk DH. Structural changes induced in capillary endothelial cells by growth factors: altered distribution of cytoskeletal elements and organelles in cells spreading in the presence of tumor conditioned medium and hypothalamus-derived growth factor. Tissue & Cell 18, 827, 1986.

67. Zimmerman M, McGeachie J. Quantitation of the relationship between aortic endothelial intracellular cleft morphology and permeability to albumin. Atherosclerosis 59, 277, 1986.

68. Folkman J, Klagsbrun M. Angiogenic factors. Science 235, 442, 1987.

69. Baird A, Ling N. Fibroblast growth factors are present in the extracellular matrix produced by endothelial cells in vitro: implications for a role of heparinase-like enzymes in the neovascular response. Biochem Biophy Res Comm 142, 428, 1987.

70. Gospodarowicz D, Cheng J. Heparin protects basic and acidic FGF from inactivation. J Cellular Physiol 128, 475, 1986.

71. Vlodavsky I, Folkman J, Sullivan R, Fridman R, Ishai-Michaeli R, Sasse J, Klagsbrun M. Endothelial cell derived basic fibroblast growth factor: synthesis and deposition into sunendothelial extracellular matrix. Proc Nat Acad Sci 84, 2292, 1987.

72. Malone JM, Brendel K, Duhamel RC, Reinert R. Detergent-extracted small-diameter vascular prostheses. J Vasc Surg 1, 181, 1984.

3.4. Endothelial Cell Seeding and Sodding

3.4.1 Technique and Experience with Clinical Endothelial Cell Seeding

P Örtenwall [1], H Wadenvik [2], J Kutti [2], B Risberg [1]

[1] Departments of Surgery and [2] Medicine, Östra Sjukhuset,
University of Göteborg, Sweden

Implantation of vascular artificial devices has been followed by thrombotic complications. Systemic anticoagulation using heparin or dicumarol preparations has been the conventional mode of dealing with this problem. Reduction of platelet reactivity using antiplatelet drugs, such as acetylsalicylic acid, has also been used. An ideal vascular surface should preferably have inherent antithrombotic properties.

In vitro culture of endothelial cells has permitted detailed studies of the antithrombotic endothelial surface. It used to be thought that endothelium had only anticoagulant activity, but, more recently, it has been demonstrated that, when properly stimulated, the endothelial cells can express procoagulant activity as well. Fortunately for the progress of seeding techniques the procoagulant activities of endothelium were not identified until after initiation of animal and clinical experiments.

Endothelial Anticoagulant Activities

Vascular endothelium produces factors involved in the process of coagulation and fibrinolysis.

Prostacyclin

Prostacyclin (PGI_2) is a dominant endothelial product in the arachidonic acid cascade. Its main actions are vasodilation and prevention of platelet aggregation. It has a half-life of only a few minutes and its effects are mediated by stimulated adenylate cyclase and elevated levels of cyclic AMP (1). Factors involved in the haemostatic process can modulate synthesis of PGI_2. Thrombin stimulates PGI_2 production (2). Of interest is that substances involved in the immunesystems, such as interferon and interleukin 1, stimulates PGI_2 synthesis (3,4) indicating important pathways between the immunesystem and endothelial cells.

Plasminogen Activator

Tissue plasminogen activators (t-PA) are endothelial products (5,6,7). t-PA cleaves plasminogen inducing formation of plasmin. t-PA is probably continuously produced and released from the endothelial cells. Regulation of t-PA release is closely related to the haemostatic system as well as to the

3. Endothelial Cell Lining

immunesystem. t-PA effects can be modulated by thrombin, protein C, platelet activating factor, and interleukin 1 (8,9,10,11,12). The cleavage of plasminogen by t-PA is greatly enhanced by the presence of fibrin ensuring a localized activation on the fibrin clot (13).

Neutralization of thrombin can be achieved through many routes. Surface bound antithrombin III effectively neutralizes thrombin, especially in the presence of heparin or heparin-like glucosaminoglucanes on the endothelial cell surface (14). Antithrombin III as well as glucosaminoglycanes are produced by endothelial cells (15). Thrombomodulin is an endothelial surface receptor or thrombin (8). When thrombin is bound to thrombomodulin, protein C, a vitamin K depending inhibitor of the coagulation cascade, is activated. The anticoagulant activity is mediated by inhibition of activated coagulation factor V and VIII (16, 17).

Endothelial Procoagulant Activities

Endothelial cells synthesize several coagulation factors and can bind enzymes, co-factors, and substrates to its surface. The cells can produce the von Willebrand factor (18), factor V (19) and also tissue factor (20). The endothelial cells have surface receptors for coagulation factors (21). The whole series of reactions in the coagulation cascade, including factor X activation and formation of prothrombinase complexes, leading to thrombin formation, can occur on the surface of the endothelial cell (22). Normally this thrombin formation is modulated by the mechanisms described above, such as neutralization bt antithrombin III, glucosaminoglucanes, and protein C activation. If this balance is out of tune, coagulation is initiated with aggregation and activation of platelets, resulting in formation of a clot. During quiescent and normal conditions the anticoagulant activities dominate but when the endothelial cells are stimulated (= perturbated) e.g. by endotoxin, pro-coagulation is initiated (22).

Plasminogen activator inhibitor (PAI) is the dominant inhibitor of the fibrinolytic system. It is produced in endothelial cell as a main product of endothelial protein synthesis (23,24). The inhibitor is present in plasma in concentrations high enough to effectively neutralize free t-PA. Many recent studies indicate that clinically apparent changes in fibrinolytic activity are regulated by shifts in inhibitor levels (25,26,27,28).

Seeding Technique

In the late seventies animal experiments on endothelial cell seeding (29) were initiated and also the first clinical trial started (30).

For in vivo seeding, two approaches are available: a one-stage or a two-stage procedure.

In the one-stage procedure freshly harvested vascular endothelial cells (VEC) are immediately seeded onto the vascular graft. The cells are either enzymatically or mechanically harvested. A cell suspension in culture medium is achieved that subsequently is inoculated into the prosthesis. This procedure is fairly easy to perform and sterility problems are easily overcome.

As a rule the operative procedure is not prolonged since isolation of the cell suspension does not take more than 45-60 minutes. The number of cells available for seeding using this approach is limited. Using human venous EC a number of $4.4 \times 10^2 - 3.1 \times 10^3$

3. Endothelial Cell Lining

cells/cm^2 graft has been reported (31, 32). Taking into account that probably the majority of these cells are flushed away once flow is instituted, only a limited number of cells are adherent after 24 hours of flow. In animal experiments Rosenman et al (33) found that only approximately 4% of harvested cells were adherent after 72 hours. Refinement in techniques of harvesting and enhancing adherence to the prosthesis could improve the number of cells initially available for replication on the graft. However, with this technique the maximal number of cells available is limited by the number of cells in the donor vein. For practical reasons only a short vein segment will be available for harvest. Using this technique immediate coverage of the whole vascular surface is not possible. Notwithstanding that human endothelial cells have a high reproductive capacity in vivo (34) it has been calculated that confluence would require a period of months (35). Thus, with the one-stage approach, using a donor vein, an effective antithrombotic surface cannot be anticipated in the immediate postoperative period.

To overcome this problem, researchers have turned into other sources of endothelial cells. Microvessels have been used as sources for endothelial cells. EC from fat microvessels can be isolated by enzymatic techniques. Such cells have been used for experimental seeding (36,37). With this approach a large number of cells can be achieved that rapidly form a monolayer on the graft (38) (= "sodding").

Another approach towards high yield of EC could be the use of homogolous endothelial cells. Unfortunately endothelial cells express antigens and to prevent rejection of transplanted cells, immunosuppression will be necessary (39, 40).

Peritoneal mesothelial cells have fibrinolytic properties and have been tried in seeding of grafts (41).

So far, only adult venous EC have been used in clinical seeding. The future potential of other EC sources, described above, has to be explored further.

Two-stage procedure. Using this approach, harvested EC are multiplied in a culture laboratory before inoculation. When a large number of cells has been achieved, they can be used for intraoperative seeding (42). Still another approach is inoculation of these cultured cells in vitro onto a prosthetic graft where they are allowed to grow to confluence. Such a totally endothelialized graft can then be implanted into the patient (43). This approach is theoretically appealing, but sterility problems may be difficult to overcome.

Clinical Endothelial Cell Seeding

The vast majority of knowledge in endothelial cell seeding stems from animal experiments. Dogs, sheep, pigs and baboons have been used (44,45, 46,47,48). Species differences, however, make extrapolations to the clinical situation hazardous (49). In animal experiments documentation of endothelialization is easily accomplished by biopsies from the experimental vessel. Endothelial cells can then be identified both morphologically and functionally. In the clinical setting, this is impossible, and demonstration of endothelialization has to be indirect. Estimation of patency or external detection of radiolabelled platelet deposition on the vascular graft have been used.

The first clinical study was initiated by Herring et al in 1978 (50). Seeded and non-seeded Dacron grafts in the femoropoliteal position were compared. Endothelial cells were harvested by mechanical scraping. There was no statistically significant difference in patency between the two groups when followed for 7 years. The detrimental effect of smoking was noticed. The mechanical harvesting used in that study was probably not optimal.

In another recent report, mechanical harvesting of venous endothelial cells was also used (51). Thirteen patients with predominantly femoropoliteal reconstructions had a seeded PTFE graft implanted. When compared to 20 control patients with unseeded grafts, the cumulative patency at 9 months was slightly in favour of the seeding procedure, although not statistically significant. The patients were also monitored at intervals postoperatively with external scanning of III-Indium labelled platelets. At 3 months, deposition of platelets was less on seeded than on unseeded grafts, but statistical significance was not reached. The PTFE grafts in this study were prewetted with absolute alcohol to render them more susceptible to the cell suspension. The inoculation was made with pressure to force the cells into the interstices of the graft.

Three clinical trials have been carried out using enzymatic harvesting of EC. Herring et al demonstrated (52,53) a patency that was, to a statistically significant degree, better in 39 patients with seeded grafts than in 15 patients with unseeded grafts at 24 months (84.6% compared with 44.5% respectively). This difference was even more remarkable in smokers where non-seeded grafts did significantly worse than seeded grafts (p<0.005). In this study patency alone was used as end point. To the individual patient the question of open or occluded reconstruction is of extreme interest. However, patency is influenced by so many factors that it is very difficult to relate differences in patency to only one factor e.g. seeding. At the present stage we need better methods for evaluation of endothelial attachment and coverage to improve efficacy of the seeding technique. The electronmicroscopical observation by the Indianapolis group of an endothelial lining in a seeded PTFE graft is extremely interesting (54).

Enzymatic harvesting was also used in the study by Zilla et al (32). Eighteen patients with either femoropopliteal or femorocrural PTFE prostheses were studied. Nine patients were seeded and 9 served as controls. EC were harvested from external jugular veins and the grafts were pretreated with fibrin. The number of cells seeded per cm^2 of graft was 3.1×10^3. The patients were followed postoperatively with double-isotope platelet and erythrocyte scanning and simultaneous measurement of several platelet parameters. No significant difference in platelet deposition on the grafts was found. Levels of 2 alpha-granulae factors, platelet factor 4 and beta-thromboglobulin, were significantly reduced in the seeded patients. Platelet function as measured by aggregometry was improved in seeded patients after 3 months. From that study it was likely that islands of EC were growing on the grafts but that no complete endothelialization was reached.

Compiled data from published studies on clinical seeding are presented in Table 35.

Clinical Seeding: The Göteborg Experience

The first clinical seeding experiments started in 1984. The experience until

3. Endothelial Cell Lining

Author	Region	Donor vein	Harvest	Cells /cm^2	Graft/Pre treatment	Post treatment	Evaluation	Patients	Results
Herring et al 1984	FEM-POP	Sub-cutaneous	Mechanical	-	Dacron Blood	-	Patency	19 seeded 17 non-seeded	NS
Herring et al 1987	Fem-pop	Ext.jug	Enzyme	-	PTFE	-	Patency	39 seeded 15 non-seeded	$p<0.05$ $p<0.005$ (smokers)
Walker et al 1987	Fem-pop	Saphenous	mechanical	-	PTFE ABS, alcohol	Dicumarol	Patency platelet scan	13 seeded 20 non-seeded	NS
Zilla et al 1987	Fem-pop Fem-dist	Ext-Jug	Enzyme	3.1×10^3	PTFE Fibrin	ASA Dipyridamol	Platelet function and scan	9 seeded 9 non-seeded	$p<0.05$ (function NS (scan)
Risberg et al	Bifurcation	Saphenous	Enzyme	2.2×10^3	Dacron Blood	-	Platelet scan	22	$p<0.02$
Present Series	Fem-pop	Saphenous	Enzyme	3.2×10^3	PTFE Blood	Dicumarol	Platelet scan	14 Each patient his own control	$p<0.02$

Table 35 Compiled data from studies on clinical seeding.

now includes 22 patients with seeded aortic bifurcation grafts (knitted Dacron) and 14 with seeded femoropopliteal or femorofemoral PTFE grafts. Of the 22 patients with bifurcation grafts 12 were operated on because of infrarenal abdominal aortic aneurysm and 10 because of aortoiliac occlusive disease. The patients with peripheral reconstructions were operated on due to critical ischemia or disabling claudication using criteria as defined by Rutherford et al (55).

Endothelial cell harvesting. A small part of the greater saphenous vein in the ankle was excised. The vein was handled with non-traumatic technique and a cell suspension was prepared using a 0.1% collagenase solution as previously described (46). The cell pellet was resuspended in culture medium. Samples were taken for cell counting and for demonstration of cell viability (plating efficiency).

Surgical procedure. Surgery started with excision of the vein. The cell suspension was prepared during the preparative surgery. Since the cell preparation did not take more than 45-60 minutes the surgical procedure was not (or only slightly) prolonged. In patients having an aortic bifurcated graft, a random graft limb was seeded with endothelial cells and the other limb was sham-seeded with culture medium. The resuspended cells were mixed with an equal volume of blood and inoculated in two steps, 5 minutes apart, into the limb to be seeded. Just before completion of the distal anastomosis, clamps were removed and the graft limb was flushed with arterial blood. Patients with bifurcation grafts had no anticoagulant or antiplatelet therapy postoperatively.

Patients with peripheral reconstruction. (13 patients with bypasses between iliac/femoral and politeal arteries and 1 patient with a femorofemoral

3. Endothelial Cell Lining

crossover). The great saphenous vein was used as donor vein, except in one case where the external jugular vein was used. Surgery started by preparing the vein as described above. The cells were resuspended in culture medium. Before implantation the PTFE graft was cut into an appropriate length. It was filled and "precoated" with blood under pressure for 10 minutes before implantation. The graft was rinsed free of blood clots with heparin/saline solution. Random half of the graft was seeded with endothelial cells. The other half was sham-seeded with culture medium. The cells were allowed to settle for 10 minutes after which the graft was rotated by 180° and another 10 minutes incubation was accomplished.

Platelet scanning. Graft-platelet interactions were studied using 111-indium labelled autologous platelets and a thrombogenicity index (TI) was calculated as described previously (46). Patients were scanned 24, 48, 72, and 96 hours after reinfusion of radiolabelled platelets. Patients with aortic bifurcation grafts were studied with this technique 1, 4, and 12 months after surgery. Patients with peripheral reconstructions were studied 1 and 4 months postoperatively.

Statistical Analysis

Statistical analyses were performed using paired and unpaired Student's t-test for comparison of thrombogenicity index at different imaging times. Data are presented as mean ± SEM if not otherwise stated.

Results

The seeding procedure did not appear to cause any complications.

The number of cells seeded per cm^2 of the graft was $2.2-3.2 \times 10^3$. Plating efficiency was 62-66%. Endothelial cells were identified by morphology and factor VIII related antigen. The admixture of other cells types in these cultures was less than 5%.

Platelet Scanning

1. Dacron grafts

One month postoperatively there was a significant reduction in TI. At all imaging times, 24, 48, 72, and 96 hours, there was a significant difference between seeded and control grafts in favour of the seeded graft limbs ($p<0.01$).

Four months postoperatively, the thrombogenicity of the whole graft was lower than it had been 1 month postoperatively. TI in both seeded and control limbs was significantly reduced at this time compared to values at 1 month postoperatively. However, the difference between the seeded and unseeded limbs was still statistically significant ($p<0.02$).

Twelve months postoperatively 15 patients have been examined. The overall thrombogenicity index in the prosthesis was at a similar level as at 4 months. The difference between seeded and unseeded limbs persisted ($p<0.01$).

2. PTFE grafts

In patients with distal reconstruction the TI in the seeded half of the PTFE graft was compared to the non-seeded control half of the graft. The seeded portions of the grafts had significantly lower TI ($p<0.02$).

Details are presented in Table 36.

3. Endothelial Cell Lining

	Seeded Graft	Control Graft	
Day 2	1.05 ± 0.20	1.63 ± 0.29	p < 0.002
Day 3	1.76 ± 0.27	2.28 ± 0.30	p < 0.02
Day 4	1.60 ± 0.27	2.36 ± 0.41	p < 0.007

Table 36 Thrombogenicity index (TI) from 14 patients with seeded femoropopliteal or femorofemoral PTFE grafts. TI from platelet scans 2, 3 and 4 days after infusion of 111 Indium labelled autologous platelets 1 month postoperatively. Seeded portions of the graft are compared to non-seeded control portions within the same patients.

Present Status of Clinical Endothelial Cell Seeding

The procedure is theoretically appealing and it is commonly felt that there is a great potential in this field.

Clinical experiments with endothelial cell seeding have been conducted in a few centres as presented above. Clinical studies have either been started or are being planned in other centres. Clinical data presented so far have not been conclusively informative on the benefit of the concept. The studies presented differ in many various aspects.

Differences in harvesting techniques may give a highly various number of cells available for seeding. Zilla et al (32) reported almost 10 times more harvested cells from the external jugular vein than Risberg et al (31) from a similar area of distal saphenous veins. Not only the number of cells may differ but also the viability. Collagenase has been utilized in most studies for harvesting and various batches of collagenase may differ in cytotoxicity and harvesting efficiency. Mechanical scraping of endothelial cells is considered to be less efficient and seems to carry a higher degree of contamination from other cells (53).

The best means of attaching the inoculum to the prosthetic surface is unknown. Dacron and PTFE differ in their retention of EC. Animal experiments documented that Dacron prostheses were superior to PTFE for retention of EC 24 hours after restoration of blood flow (56). In contrast Herring et al (57) found PTFE grafts to endothelialize more rapidly than Dacron. The configuration of Dacron fabric is probably important as documented in a study by Herring et al (58). The structure of the PTFE graft usually does not permit tissue in-growth. However, a more porous PTFE prosthesis allows ingrowth and apparently endothelializes faster following seeding compared to the regular PTFE graft (59). Regular PTFE grafts have 30 microns internodular distance. The porous graft with 60 microns internodular distance was found to permit rapid capillary ingrowth and endothelialize completely in the baboon (59,60,61,62). The different materials, Dacron or PTFE, may differ in the way they activate the complement system. Shepard et al (63) demonstrated that Dacron stimulated this complement cascade more than PTFE. Complement activation could lead to adherence of leukocytes to the graft surface. Accumulation of leukocytes and their

3. Endothelial Cell Lining

activation is potentially harmful to the inoculated endothelial cells. In a canine model it was found that retention of seeded endothelial cells after restoration of blood flow was much better in leukopenic animals than in animals with normal leukocyte count (64).

Attachment of endothelial cells furthermore depends on the pre-coating of the graft. Generally it has been found that pre-coating with fibronectin is beneficial for attachment and retention of endothelial cells on the graft surface (65,66,67,68,69). Coating with plasma may also improve EC attachment (70). Various proteins in the extra cellular matrix can also enhance the attachment (62,71). Laminin can enhance adherence and retention of EC on grafts (69,72). Collagen has been used alone or in combination with other proteins (69,73,74). Both experimentally and clinically PTFE grafts have been coated with a fibronectin containing fibrin glue to create an artificial matrix (32,73). The presence of smooth muscle cells on the surface may also improve endothelialization of grafts (75). In clinical studies pre-coating with autologous blood have been utilized (31,50,52). The wide variability in pre-coating of grafts indicates that the surface ideal for endothelialization has yet to be determined.

Another problem when different studies are compared is the multiple ways by which the procedure is evaluated. In experimental animals, biopsies from seeded vessels are easily obtained, whereas this is impossible in the clinical setting except in extreme situations (54). So far no direct methods can be used. Patency is a too rough end-point. The other methods used, platelet scanning and measurement of platelet release products in plasma, can also not be considered as ideal. When comparing studies it is of course critical that the means of evaluation are precise and directly related to the presence of a nonthrombogenetic endothelial lining.

The postoperative treatment of the patients with drugs interfering in the haemostatic process may also affect the outcome and make interpretation of different studies difficult. In the clinical studies reported, patients were either not treated, or treated with antiplatelet drugs or dicumarol (Table 1).

The problems related above are obvious when comparing different studies. However, they may be relevant also in the individual study where different patients are compared. Most of these drawbacks can be eliminated when the patient serves as his own control.

The concept of endothelial cell seeding as a means of reducing thrombogenicity in vascular grafts has been confirmed in animal experiments. Based on this, more clinical studies are needed. The studies on patients presented until now indicate that seeding can reduce the thrombogenicity of implanted vascular grafts. Whether this will improve the patency rate and the clinical outcome for these patients still has to be determined.

Acknowledgements

This work was supported by grants from the Medical Faculty, University of Göteborg, the Swedish Medical Society, the Medical Society of Göteborg, and the Swedish National Association against Heart and Chest Diseases.

3. Endothelial Cell Lining

References

1. Gorman RR, Bunting S, Miller OV. Modulation of human platelet adenylate cyclase by prostacyclin (PGX). Prostaglandins 13, 377, 1977.

2. Weksler BB, Ley CW, Jaffe EA. Stimulation of endothelial cells prostacyclin production by thrombin, trypsin and the inophore A23187. J Clin Invest 62, 923, 1978.

3. Eldor A, Fridman R, Vlodavsky I, Hy-Am E, Fukz Z, Planet A. Interferon enhances prostacyclin production by cultured vascular endothelial cells. J Clin Invest 73, 251.

4. Rossi V, Brevario F, Ghezzi P, Dejana E, Mantovani A. Prostacyclin synthesis induced in vascular cells by Interleukin I. Science 229, 174, 1985.

5. Todd AS. The histological localization of fibrolysin activator. J Path Bact 78, 281, 1959.

6. Levin E, Loskutoff DJ. Comparative studies of the fibrinolytic activity of cultured vascular cells. Thromb Res 15, 869, 1979.

7. Risberg B. Fibrinolysis in the lung. Acta Chir Scand suppl 458, 1975.

8. Esmon CT, Owen WG. Identification of en endothelial cell cofactor for thrombin catalyzed activation of protein C. Proc Natl Acad Sci USA 78, 2249, 1981.

9. Loskutoff DJ. Effect of thrombin on the fibrinolytic activity of cultured bovine endothelial cells. J Clin Invest 64, 329, 1979.

10. Levin EG, Loskutoff DJ. Regulation of plasminogen activator production by cultured endothelial cells. Ann NY Acad Sci 401, 184, 1982.

11. Emeis JJ, Kluft C. PAF-acether induced release of tissue-type plasminogen activator in vessel walls. Blood 66, 86, 1985.

12. Emeis JJ, Koistra T. Interleukin I and lipopolysaccarid A induces an inhibitor of tissue-plasminogen activator in vivo and in cultured endothelial cells. J Exp Med 163, 1260, 1986.

13. Holyaerts M, Rijken DC, Lijnen HR, Collen D. Kinetics of the activation of plasminogen by human tissue plasminogen activator. Role of fibrin. J Biol Chem 257, 2912, 1982.

14. Marcum JA, McKenney JB, Rosenberg RD. The acceleration of thrombin-antithrombin complex formation in rat hindquarters via naturally occurring heparin-like molecules bound to the endothelium. J Clin Invest 74, 341, 1984.

15. Marcum JA, Rosenberg RD. Heparin-like molecules with anticoagulant activity are synthesized by cultured endothelial cells. Biochem Biophys Res Com 126, 365, 1985.

16. Stenflo J. A new vitamin K-dependent protein: purification from bovine plasma and preliminary characterization. J Biol Chem 251, 355, 1976.

17. Walker FJ, Sexton PW, Esmon CT. The inhibition of blood coagulation by activated protein C through the selective inactivation of activated factor V. Biochim Biophys Acta 571, 333, 1979.

18. Jaffe EA, Hoyer LW, Nachman RL. Synthesis of antihaemophilic factor antigen in cultured human endothelial cells. J Clin Invest 52, 2757, 1973.

19. Cerveny T, Fass D, Mann. Synthesis co-factor V by cultured bovine endothelial cells. Blood 63, 1456, 1984.

3. Endothelial Cell Lining

20. Lyberg T, Galdal KS, Evensen SA, Prydz H. Cellular cooperation in endothelial thromboplastin synthesis. Br J Haematol 53, 85, 1983.

21. Stern DM, Drillings M, Nossel HL, Hurlet-Jensen A, La Gamma K, Owen J. Binding of factors IX and IXa to cultured vascular endothelial cells. Proc Natl Acad Sci (USA) 80, 4119, 1983.

22. Nawroth PP, Stern DM. Endothelial cells as active participants in procoagulant reactions. In: "Vascular endothelium in hemostasis and thrombosis". Gimbrone MA, (ed). Edinburgh, Churchill Livingstone, pp 14, 1986.

23. Sprengers ED, Kluft C. Plasminogen activator inhibitors. Blood 69, 381, 1987.

24. Risberg B, Hansson GK, Eriksson E, Wiman. Immunohistochemical localization of plasminogen activator inhibitor (PAI) in tissue. Thromb Haemostas 58, 446, 1987.

25. Hesel W, Kluft C. Advance in clinical fibrinolysis. Clin Haematol 15, 443, 1986.

26. Hamsten A, Wiman B, DeFaire U, Blombäck M. Increased plasma levels of a rapid inhibitor of tissue plasminogen activator in young survivors of myocardial infarction. N Engl J Med 313, 1557, 1985.

27. D'Angelo A, Kluft C, Verheijen JH, Rijken DC, Mozzi E, Mannucci PM. Fibrinolytic shutdown after surgery: impairment of the balance between tissue-type plasminogen activator and its specific inhibitor. Eur J Clin Invest 15, 308, 1985.

28. Juhan-Vague I, Moerman B, DeCock F, Aillaud F, Collen D. Plasma levels of a specific inhibitor of tissue-type plasminogen activator (and urikinase) in normal and pathological conditions. Thromb Res 33, 523, 1984.

29. Graham LM, Burkel WE, Ford JW, Vinter DW, Kahn RH, Stanley IC. Immediate seeding of enzymatically derived endothelium on Dacron vascular grafts: early experimental studies with autogenous canine cells. Arch Surg 115, 1289, 1980.

30. Herring MB, Gardner AL, Glover J. A single staged technique for seeding vascular grafts with autogenous endothelium. Surgery 84 (4), 498, 1978.

31. Risberg B, Örtenwall P, Wadenvik H, Kutti J. Endothelial cell seeding: experience and first clinical results in Göteborg. In "Endothelialization of vascular grafts". Zilla P, Fasol P, Deutsch M (eds). Karger, Basel. pp 225, 1987.

32. Zilla P, Fasol R, Deutsch M, Fischlein T, Minar E, Hammerle A, Krupicke O, Kadletz M. Endothelial cell seeding by polytetrafluoroethylene vascular grafts in humans: a preliminary report. J Vasc Surg 6, 535, 1987.

33. Rosenman JE, Kempczinski RF, Pearce WH, Silberstein EB. Kinetics of endothelial cell seeding. J Vasc Surg 2, 778, 1985.

34. Watkins MT, Sharefkin JB, Zajtchuk R, Maciag TM, D'Amore PA, Ryan US, van Wart H, Rich NM. Adult human saphenous vein endothelial cells. Assessment of their reproductive capacity for use in endothelial seeding of vascular prostheses. J Surg Res 36, 588, 1984.

35. Schima H, Tsangaris S, Zilla P, Fasol R, Kadletz M. Simulation of pulsatile wall shear stress in peripheral arteries by means of a mock circulation. In "Endothelialization of vascular grafts". Zilla P, Fasol R, Deutsch M. (eds). Karger, Basel, pp 189, 1987.

36. Jarrel BE, Williams SK, Stokes G, Hubbard FA, Carabasi RA, Koolpe E, Greener D, Pratt K, Moritz MJ, Radomski J, Speicher L. Use of freshly isolated capillary endothelial cells for the immediate establishment of a monolayer on a vascular graft at surgery. Surgery 100, 392, 1986.

3. Endothelial Cell Lining

37. Williams SK, Jarrel BE, Rose DG. Isolation of human fat-derived microvessel endothelial cells for use in vascular graft endothelialization. In: "Endothelialization of vascular grafts". Zilla P, Fasol R, Deutsch M. (eds). Karger, Basel, pp 211, 1987.

38. Jarrel BE, Williams SK, Carabasi RA, Hubbard FA. Immediate vascular grafts monolayers using microvessel endothelial cells. In: "Endothelial seeding in vascular surgery". Herring M, Glover JL, (eds). Grune and Stratton Inc Orlando Fl. pp 37, 1987.

39. Cerilli J, Brasile L, Galouzis T et al. The vascular endothelial cell antigen system. Transplantation 39, 286, 1985.

40. Eskin SG, Navarro LT, Zamora JL, Ives CL, Anderson JM, Weilbaecher DG, Gao ZR, Noon GP. Preliminary studies on autologous versus homologous endothelial seeding of arteriovenous grafts. In: "Endothelial seeding in vascular surgery". Herring M, Glover JL, (eds). Grune and Stratton Inc, Orlando Fl. pp 155, 1987.

41. Clarke JMF, Pittilo RM, Nicholson LJ, Woolf N, Marston A. Seeding Dacron arterial prostheses with peritoneal mesothelial cell: a preliminary morphological study. Br J Surg 71, 492, 1984.

42. Burkel WE, Ford JW, Vinter DW, Kahn RH, Graham LM, Stanley JC. Endothelial seeding of enzymatically derived and cultured cells on prosthetic grafts. In: Biologic and synthetic vascular prostheses. Stanley JC, (ed). pp 631. Grune & Stratton, New York, 1982.

43. McCall E, Povey J, Dumonde DC. The culture of vascular endothelial cells to confluence on microporous membranes. Thromb Res 24, 417, 1981.

44. Stanley JC, Burkel WE, Ford JW, Vinter DW, Kahn RH, Whitehouse WM, Graham L. Enhanced patency of small-diameter externally supported Dacron iliofemoral grafts seeded with endothelial cells. Surgery 92, 994, 1982.

45. Clagett GP, Burkel WE, Sharefkin JB, Ford JW, Hufnagel H, Vinter DW, Kahn RH, Graham LM, Stanley JC. Antithrombotic character of canine endothelial cell-seeded arterial prostheses. Surgical Forum 33, 471, 1982.

46. Örtenwall P, Wadenvik H, Kutti J, Risberg B. Reduction in deposition of Indium-III labelled platelets after autologous endothelial seeding of Dacron aortic bifurcation grafts in humans: a preliminary report. J Vasc Surg 6, 17, 1987.

47. Hollier LH, Fowl RJ, Pennell RC, Heck CF, Winter KAH, Fass DN, Kaye MP. Are seeded endothelial cells the origin of neointima on prosthetic vascular grafts? J Vasc Surg 3, 65, 1986.

48. Shepard AD, Eldrup-Jorgensen J, Keough EM, Foxall TF, Ramberg K, Connelly RJ, Mackey WC, Gavris V, Auger KR, Libby P, O'Donnell TF, Callow AD. Endothelial cell seeding of small-caliber synthetic grafts in the baboon. Surgery 99, 318, 1986.

49. Örtenwall P, Bylock A, Kjellström T, Risberg B. Seeding of ePTFE carotid interposition grafts in sheep and dogs: species dependent results. Surgery 103, 199, 1988.

50. Herring MB, Gardner AL, Glover JL. Seeding of human arterial prostheses with mechanically derived endothelium. The detrimental effects of smoking. J Vasc Surg 1, 279, 1984.

51. Walker MG, Thomson GJL, Shaw JW. Endothelial cell seeded versus non-seeded ePTFE grafts in patients with severe peripheral vascular disease. In: "Endothelialization of vascular grafts". Zilla P, Fasol R, Deutsch M. (eds). Karger, Basel, pp 245, 1987.

52. Herring MB, Compton RS, LeGrand DR, Gardner AL, Madison DL, Glover JL. Endothelial seeding of polytetrafluoroethylene popliteal bypasses. A preliminary report. J Vasc Surg 6, 114, 1987.

3. Endothelial Cell Lining

53. Herring MB, Compton RS, Gardner AL, LeGrand DR. Clinical experiences with endothelial seeding in Indianapolis. In: "Endothelialization of vascular grafts". Zilla P, Fasol R, Deutsch M (eds). Karger, Basal, p. 218, 1987.

54. Herring MB, Baughman S, Glover J. Endothelium develops on seeded human arterial prosthesis, a brief clinical report. J Vasc Surg 2, 727, 1985.

55. Rutherford RB, Flanigan DP, Gupta SK, Johnston KW, Karmody A, Wittermore AD, Baker D, Ernst CB. Suggested standards for reports dealing with lower extremely ischemia. J Vasc Surg 4, 80, 1986.

56. Schmidt SP, Hunter TJ, Hirko M, Belden TA, Evancho M, Sharp WV, Donovan DL. Small diameter vascular prostheses. Two designs of PTFE and endothelial cell seeded and non-seeded Dacron. J Vasc Surg 2, 292, 1985.

57. Herring MB, Baugham S, Glover JL, Kesler K, Jesseph J, Campbell J, Dilley R, Evan A, Gardner A. Endothelial seeding of Dacron and polytetrafluoroethylene grafts. The cellular events of healing. Surgery 96, 745, 1984.

58. Herring MB, Gardner A, Glover JL. Seeding endothelium into canine arterial prostheses. The effects of grafts design. Arch Surg 114, 679, 1979.

59. Kempczinski RF, Rosenman JE, Pearce WH, Roedersheimer LR, Berlatzky Y, Ramalanjaona G. Endothelial cell seeding of a new PTFE vascular prostheses. J Vasc Surg 2, 424, 1985.

60. Clowes AW, Gown AM, Hanson SR, Reidy MA. Mechanisms of arterial graft failure. I. Role of cellular proliferation in early healing of PTFE prostheses. Am J Path 118, 43, 1985.

61. Clowes AW, Kirkman TR, Reidy MA. Mechanisms of arterial graft healing: rapid transmural capillary ingrowth provides a source of intimal endothelium and smooth muscle in porus PTFE prosthesis. Am J Path 123, 220, 1986.

62. Thompson RW, D'Amore PA. Growth control of cultured endothelial cells. In: "Endothelialization of vascular grafts" Zilla P, Fasol R, Deutsch M (eds). Karger, Basal. p. 100, 1987.

63. Shepard AD, Gelfand JA, Callow AD, O'Donnell TF. Complement activation by synthetic vascular prosthesis. J Vasc Surg 1, 829, 1984.

64. Emerick S, Herring MB, Arnold M et al. Leukocyte depletion enhances cultured endothelial retention on vascular prosthesis. J Vasc Surg 1987 (in press).

65. Kessler KA, Herring MB, Arnold MP, Glover JL, Hee-myung Park, Helmig MN, Bendick PJ. Enhanced strength of endothelial attachment of polyester elastomer and polytetra-fluoroethylene graft surfaces with fibronectin substrate. J Vasc Surg 3, 58, 1986.

66. Ramalanjaona G, Kempczinski RF, Rosenman JE, Douville EC, Silberstein EB. The effect of fibronectin coating on endothelial cell kinetics on polytetrafluoroethylene grafts. J Vasc Surg 3, 264, 1986.

67. Seeger JM, Klingman N. Improved endothelial cell seeding with cultured cells and fibronectincoated grafts. J Surg Res 38, 641, 1985.

68. Sentissi JM, Ramberg K, O'Donnell Jr. TF, Connolly RJ, Callow AD. The effect of flow on vascular endothelial cells grown in tissue culture on polytetrafluoroethylene grafts. Surgery 99, 337, 1986.

69. Köveker GB, Graham LM, Burkel WE, Sell R, Magill T, Stanley JC. ePTFE grafts in an AV shunt model. In: "Endothelialization of vascular grafts". Zilla P, Fasol R, Deutsch M, (eds). Karger, Basal, p. 177, 1987.

3. Endothelial Cell Lining

70. Williams SK, Jarrell BE, Friend L, Radomski JS, Carabasi RA, Koolpe E, Mueller SN, Thornton SC, Marinucci T, Levine E. Adult human endothelial cell compatibility with prosthetic graft material. J Surg Res 38, 618, 1985.

71. Macarak EJ, Howard PS. Adhesion of endothelial cells to extracellular matrix proteins. J Cell Physiol 116, 76, 1983.

72. Schnittler HJ, Franke RP, Fuhrman R, Petermeyer M, Jung F, Mittelmayer C, Drenckhahn D. Influence of various substrates on the action filament system of cultured human vascular endothelial cells exposed to fluid shear stress. In: "Endothelialization of vascular grafts". Zilla P, Fasol R, Deutsch M, (eds). Karger, Basal, p. 183, 1987.

73. Zilla P, Fasol R, Preiss P, Kadletz M, Deutsch M, Schima H, Tsangaris S, Groscuth P. Use of fibrin glue as a substrate for in vitro endothelialization of PTFE vascular grafts. Surgery (in press).

74. Baker KS, Williams SK, Jarrell BE, Koolpe EA, Levine E. Endothelialization of human collagen surfaces with human adult endothelial cells. Am J Surg 150, 197, 1985.

75. Van Oene GH, Yue X, van der Lei B, Schakenraad JM, Kuit JH, Feijen J, Wildevuur CRH. Smooth muscle cell seeding enhances neo-endothelialization. In: "Endothelialization of vascular grafts". Zilla P, Fasol R, Deutsch M, (eds). Karger, Basal, p. 160, 1987.

3.4.2. Endothelial Cell Seeding of Synthetic Vascular Grafts - Evidence for a Systemic Effect on Early Patency

BM Bourke, TS Reeve, M Appleberg

The Department of Surgery, University of Sydney and the Department of Vascular Surgery, The Royal North Shore Hospital, Sydney, Australia

Abstract

In an attempt to study the effects of endothelial seeding in an animal which is prone to intimal hyperplasia and thrombosis, 60 carotid interposition grafts were performed in sheep using 10 cm lengths of 4 mm diameter thin-walled polytetrafluoroethylene. Each animal received one experimental and one control graft. Experimental grafts were either seeded with endothelial cells suspended in culture medium, (n = 10), or sham seeded with medium alone, (n = 20), before insertion. Of the 20 animals receiving sham seeded grafts, 9 were injected with freshly harvested endothelial cells into the systemic circulation. Scanning and transmission electron microscopy confirmed the presence of 'endothelial like' cells (ELC) lining the luminal surfaces of patent seeded grafts (PSG). Patent control grafts (PCG) did not exhibit such a cellular lining except for those regions immediately adjacent to the anastomoses. Autologous indium-111-oxine labelled platelet studies showed that PSG's were less thrombogenic than PCG's which showed excessive luminal thrombus. Radioactivity counts from the central regions were significantly reduced by the seeding process (p = 0.03). There was no significant early (2 weeks) patency difference between experimental and control grafts in the 'seeded group'. Control grafts in animals receiving endothelial cells (either via a seeded graft or via injection) showed significantly higher patency rates than control grafts in animals not receiving cells (p = 0.04 - Fisher's exact probability). The overall graft (experimental and control) patency in animals receiving injected cells was significantly greater than in those animals not receiving cells (p = 0.03 - Fisher's exact probability).

These results suggest that freshly harvested endothelial cells may trigger a systemic effect which is advantageous to early graft patency.

Introduction

Autogenous vein lined with normal endothelium is a more successful small diameter arterial substitute than any of the currently available synthetic or biografts. The two main causes of graft failure are thrombogenicity of the graft luminal surface and anastomotic nar-

3. Endothelial Cell Lining

rowing caused by intimal hyperplasia. As endothelium is the most non-thrombogenic surface known, lining a synthetic graft with functional endothelium should theoretically reduce the graft's thrombogenicity. In addition, by lessening the platelet vessel wall interaction endothelialization may decrease intimal hyperplasia (by reducing the release of platelet derived vascular smooth muscle growth factor). Previous studies have demonstrated that, when seeding techniques are employed, experimental arterial grafts more rapidly endothelialize than control grafts (1,2,3,4,5,6,7,8).

Other workers have shown that these grafts are less thrombogenic than control grafts (9,10,11). Despite these encouraging findings, at least one recent study has demonstrated the very low attachment efficiency of directly seeded endothelial cells on PTFE grafts (12).

This report is a study of endothelial cell seeding of 4 mm PTFE in sheep, an animal which appears to thrombose grafts readily and to be prone to intimal hyperplasia (13).

Material and Methods

Study Design

Figure 121 illustrates the experimental design and the three groups into which the animals were randomly divided.

Group I consisted of 20 grafts inserted into 10 animals. Experimental grafts were directly seeded with en-

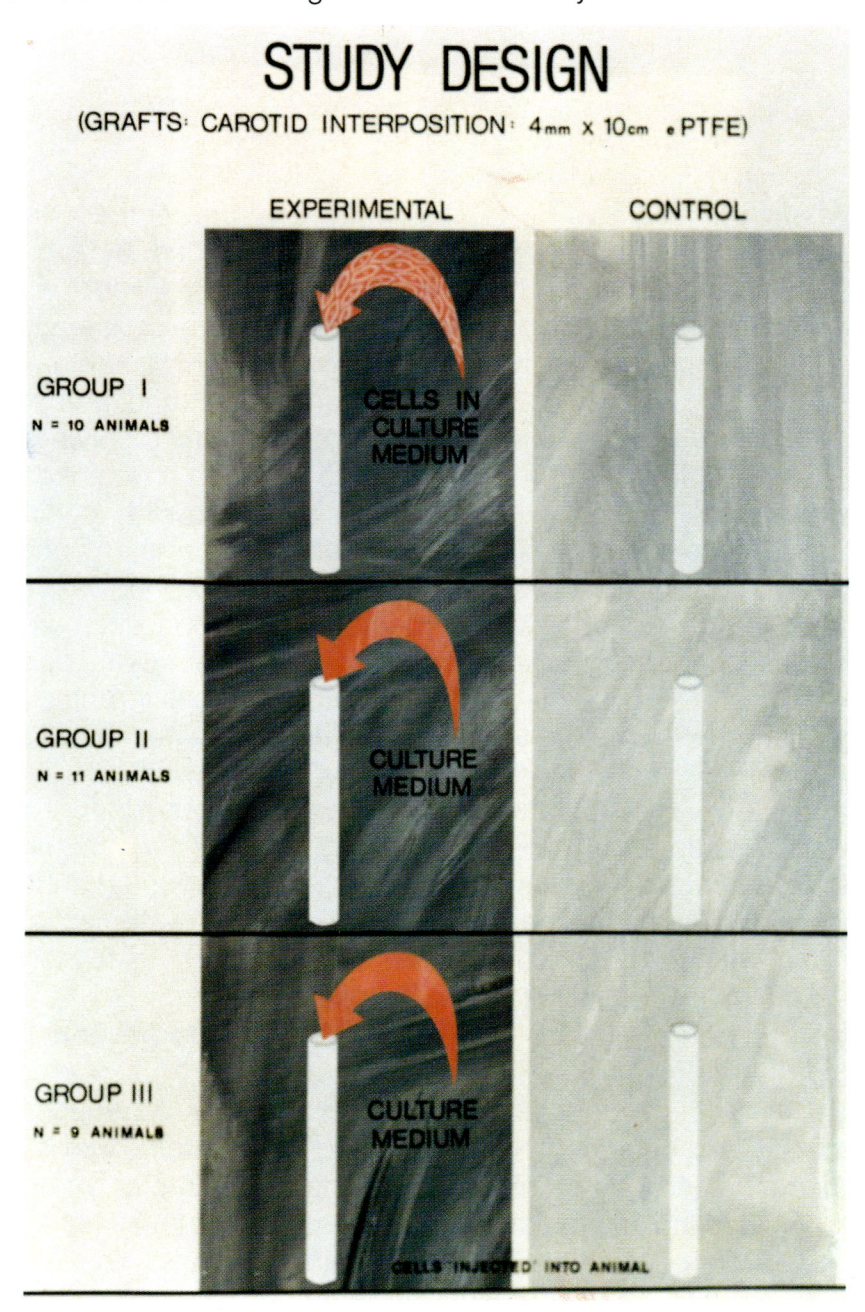

Fig. 121 Study Design (See Text).

dothelial cells suspended in culture medium.

Group II consisted of 22 grafts in 11 animals; experimental grafts being sham seeded with culture medium alone.

Group III consisted of 18 grafts in 9 animals. Experimental grafts were sham seeded but these animals were injected with endothelial cells into the systemic circulation.

Animals

Grafts were inserted into 30 healthy 12 to 18 month old Border Leicester female sheep weighing 35 to 40 kg. This animal has a long neck and constant jugular veins making it an ideal model for such a study. Animals were housed in individual pens and accustomed to their surroundings for approximately one week before use. Permission for the use of the animals was gained from the Animal Ethics Review Committee of the Royal North Shore Hospital and School of Life Sciences, NSW Institute of Technology, Sydney, Australia. Animals were handled according to the principles set out in the publication, "Code of Practice for the Care and Use of Animals in Research in Australia" NH and MRC/CSIRO 1982. Experimentation was stopped as soon as statistical requirements were fulfilled.

Sheep were given oral aspirin 900 mg twice daily commencing 48 hours prior to surgery and continuing for the first 7 post-operative days. They were also given 5 000 units of sodium heparin subcutaneously twice daily for the first post-operative week. Each animal received one million units of intramuscular penicillin with the induction of anaesthesia and this was repeated 8 and 16 hours following surgery.

Cell Harvest

Our method of cell harvest has been previously reported (14). Sheep were anaesthetized with intravenous pentobarbitone, (30 mg/kg), and a jugular vein was exposed through a longitudinal cervical incision. Care was taken to ligate the many fine tributaries of the vein to prevent subsequent leakage. The vein segment was placed in phosphate buffered saline (PBS), pH 7.4, at room temperature. Cannulation was performed by inserting portex vinyl tubing (4 mm bore) (Boots, Australia) into the distal end of the vein and ligating it over the tubing with a silk ligature. A three-way plastic stopcock (AHS, Australia) was then inserted into the portex tubing. The proximal end of the vein was cannulated with another three-way plastic stopcock and similarly ligated with a silk ligature.

The vein was then flushed from proximal to distal with 40 mls of PBS to remove red cells and then an appropriate volume of collagenase solution (465 units per ml) (Worthington, Type II, Cooper Biomedical, USA), previously warmed to 37°C, was instilled into the vein such that it became slightly dilated just beyond its in vivo natural calibre. Both three-way stopcocks were then closed and the preparation was placed into a kidney dish containing PBS and held at 37°C. The enzyme was left to act for 30 minutes. The enzyme solution was allowed to run into a 50 ml plastic centrifuge tube (Corning) and the vein was flushed with a further 30 mls of PBS while simultaneously gently massaging the external surface of the vein with the fingers.

The enzyme-PBS mixture was centrifuged at 400 x g for ten minutes to generate a pellet containing endothelial cells and some red cells. The resulting endothelial cell pellet was resuspended in 1.25 mls of Dulbecco's Modified Eagle Medium (DME) (Gibco Labs NY).

Graft Insertion

Through the same incision used for removal of the jugular vein the ipsilateral carotid artery was displayed. The contra-lateral carotid artery was exposed through a separate longitudinal incision. Arteries were then randomly chosen to receive either a control or experimental graft. Four millimeter diameter, thin-walled polytetrafluoroethylene (PTFE) (WL Gore & Assoc, Flagstaff, Arizona) was used as the graft material.

Control grafts were inserted according to the manufacturer's instructions. Experimental grafts were initially filled with autologous unheparinized blood and squeezed so that the blood appeared through the interstices of the graft (5). After a 10 minute period the contents of the graft were allowed to escape and the graft filled with either fresh culture medium containing the suspended endothelial cells, in the case of the seeded grafts, or with fresh medium alone, in the case of sham seeded grafts. The graft was allowed to lie on one side for ten minutes and then on the reverse side for ten minutes prior to implantation.

After systemic heparinization (sodium heparin 5 000 units), the carotid artery was clamped at both ends and a 10 cm length of artery removed. Using standard vascular surgical techniques and with the aid of 2.5 loupe magnification a 10 cm length of PTFE was then inserted as an interposition graft using end-to-end anastomoses, (8 x interrupted 7/0 Prolene sutures at each end). The culture medium was retained within the experimental grafts during their insertion with the use of small arterial clamps and was allowed to escape from the graft just prior to the restoration of arterial flow within the carotid system. The total time during which the culture medium was in contact with the luminal surface of experimental grafts was approximately fifty minutes.

Cell Injection

In those animals allocated for injection, endothelial cells were harvested in the same fashion as described and the endothelial cell pellet was resuspended in 1.25 mls of Dulbecco's Modified Eagle Medium (DME) (Gibco Labs, New York). This suspension was gently mixed with 5 mls of freshly drawn autologous blood and then drawn into a plastic syringe and injected into a jugular vein through a 19 French gauge plastic cannula. The cells were injected between the completion of the first graft insertion and the commencement of the second graft insertion.

Autologous Indium-Platelet Methods

We have previously reported on the use of this substance as a platelet label in the sheep model (15). In a sterile fashion, sixty mls of whole blood were drawn into a plastic syringe through a 19 gauge needle. Two lots of thirty mls were then added each to 3 mls of citrate in separate plastic centrifuge tubes, (Corning). The two tubes were centrifuged in a bench centrifuge (Clements) at 400 x g for 10 minutes to generate platelet rich plasma (C-PRP). Using a disposable plastic transfer pipette, (Samco, San Fernando, CA, USA), and avoiding excessive foaming, 1 ml of C-

PRP was retained for aggregation studies and 10 mls were added to a round-bottomed plastic tube, (Corning) to which 2 mls of acid citrate previously had been added. The contents were mixed by inverting the tube three times and centrifuged at 1000 x g for 10 minutes to generate a platelet pellet and acid citrated platelet poor plasma (AC-PPP). The latter was decanted and retained, and the pellet was washed with modified Tyrode's Solution (MTS) (16), warmed to 37°C. The washing procedure was as described by Hawker et al (17). The pellet was then resuspended in 3 mls of MTS at 37°C again using a sterile disposable plastic transfer pipette (as above).

Indium-111-oxine, (approx. 500 µCi), was then carefully drawn up using a 1 ml insulin syringe, gently mixed with the platelet suspensions and allowed to stand in a water bath for 10 minutes at 37°C. The suspension was then made to 10 mls by adding 7 mls of AC-PPP. The tube containing the labelled platelet suspension and the original 2 citrated centrifuge tubes were centrifuged at 1000 x g for 10 minutes. This produced a labelled platelet pellet with supernatent (10 mls) and citrated platelet poor plasma (C-PPP). 0.5 ml of the radioactive supernatent was taken for radioactive counts. The remainder of the supernatent was removed and the labelled platelets were resuspended in C-PPP (the suspension being made up to 10 mls). 1 ml of C-PPP was also retained for aggregation studies. 0.5 ml of the labelled platelet suspension was retained for radioactivity counts and 1 ml for aggregation studies. The remainder of the labelled platelet suspension was re-injected into the animal. All steps were performed using strict sterile techniques.

Graft Removal

Graft removal was performed under general anaesthesia and systemic heparinization. The proximal and distal carotid arteries were exposed and the carotid systems were flushed with PBS to remove red cells. The grafts were then perfusion-fixed with glutaraldehyde 2.5% in 0.1 M cacodylate buffer, PH 7.4. These precautions ensured that red blood cells were not artefactually fixed to the surface of the grafts and also ensured optimal preparation for subsequent histological evaluation. After removal, the grafts were placed into a dissecting tray containing glutaraldehyde fixative, opened longitudinally and if patent, a colour photograph was taken. The grafts were then divided into four segments, the two central segments each of 3 cm length and the proximal and distal segments each of 2 cm length (with a small segment of attached parent artery).

Radioactivity Studies

Each graft was placed into a bottle of fixative and its radioactivity measured in an autogamma scintillation spectrometer (Packard). Gamma images were also obtained from selected animals prior to graft removal.

Electron Microscopic (EM) Studies

Representative samples of the removed grafts were submitted for scanning, (SEM), and transmission, (TEM), electron microscopy. The specimens were fixed in 2.5% glutaraldehyde in 0.1 M sodium cacodylate buffer, pH 7.4, for 60 minutes. Specimens were then rewashed in cacodylate buffer, pH 7.4, with two changes for a total of 5 minutes. They were then dehydrated in 40% ethanol for 15 minutes and 60% ethanol for 15 minutes and block

3. Endothelial Cell Lining

stained with 2% uranyl acetate in 80% ethanol for 60 minutes. They were further dehydrated in 95% ethanol for 15 minutes and 100% ethanol for 15 minutes (the latter step being repeated a further 2 times). Specimens were then infiltrated with a propylene oxide (100%) twice (5 minutes each) and then with propylene oxide: Spurr's epoxy resin - 1:1 for 30 minutes and 1:3 for 30 minutes. This was followed by infiltration with Spurr's epoxy resin (100%) for at least 60 minutes. The specimens were embedded in Spurr's resin for at least 8 hours in an embedding oven at 70°C. Thin sections were stained with uranyl acetate and lead citrate and viewed with a transmission electron microscope (Joel JEM 100S Japan).

The following description applies to the methods employed by the pathologists at WL Gore and Associates. SEM was utilized to perform the endothelial-like cell (ELC) coverage estimates from the glutaraldehyde fixed specimens (i.e. half the peri-anastomotic two 2 cm segments and the proximal middle 3 cm segment), (Figure 122). Estimates were calculated from data obtained by linear transect methods.

Briefly, low magnification SEM micrographs were taken over the entire length of the luminal surface of each graft specimen. Longitudinally-orientated line transects were constructed over each micrograph. Along each transect, the length intersecting ELC covered areas

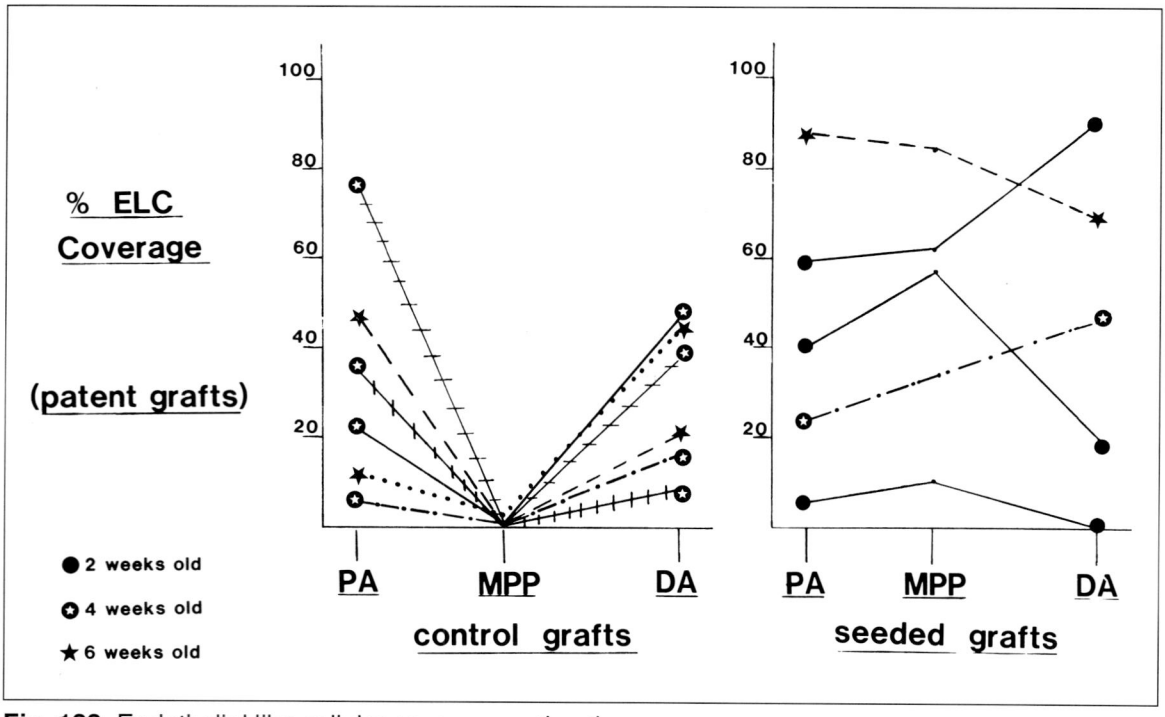

Fig. 122 Endothelial like cellular coverage estimation
(As Assessed by Scanning Electron Microscopy).
PA = Proximal Anastomotic Segment (i.e. the first 2 cm of graft split longitudinally into two equal parts one of which being examined by SEM).
MPP = Proximal Middle Segment (i.e. the next 3 cm segment of graft beyond PA).
DA = Distal Anastomotic Segment (i.e. the last 2 cm of graft split longitudinally into two equal parts one of which being examined by SEM).

3. Endothelial Cell Lining

was measured as a ratio of the total transect length. At sufficient SEM accelerating voltages ELC covered regions usually contrasted against uncovered regions. Higher magnification was used to confirm ELC morphology in the covered regions. Areas of scattered ELC mixed with blood clot were not counted.

Statistical Methods
Difference in graft patency was assessed by Fisher's exact probability test and differences in radioactivity counts and ELC coverage were assessed by the non-parametric Mann-Whitney U test (18).

Results

Graft Patency

A summary of graft patency at removal is shown in Table 137.

Although there was no significant patency difference between experimental and control grafts in directly seeded animals, the overall patency in this group was significantly better than in those animals not receiving cells ($p = 0.01$ - Fisher's exact probability). Interestingly the graft patency in animals receiving cells via systemic injection was significantly better than in those animals not receiving cells ($p = 0.03$ - Fisher's exact probability). The overall patency for control grafts was significantly better in those animals receiving endothelial cells at a site remote from their insertion (Groups I & III) than in those animals not receiving cells ($p = 0.04$ - Fisher's exact probability).

Radioactivity Studies

These studies were only performed in Group I animals. In only two animals in which these studies were performed were both control and experimental grafts patent at removal. In each case radioactivity counts were greater in the control grafts (by a factor of 14 in one case and a factor of 73 in the other case).

Graft Patency at Removal

	Experimental	Control	
Group I "Seeded"	5	6	Patent
N = 20	5	4	Occluded
Group II "Sham-seeded"	1	2	Patent
N = 22	10	9	Occluded
Group III "Sham-seeded" (and injected)	3	6	Patent
N = 18	6	3	Occluded

Overall graft patency: Group I vs Group II: P = 0.01
Overall graft patency: Group III vs Group II: P = 0.03
Control graft patency: Groups I + III vs Group II: P = 0.04
(Fisher's Exact Probability)

Table 37

3. Endothelial Cell Lining

Analyses of the distribution of radioactivity along the grafts were performed in 8 of the 11 patent conduits. The percentage of total graft radioactivity per cm was significantly higher from the 'middle segments' of control grafts compared to their 'peri-anastomotic segments' (p = 0.03). In seeded grafts the opposite applied, there being significantly less radioactivity in the central regions compared to the ends (p = 0.04), (Figure 123).

Luminal Thrombus

Inspection of 35 mm colour transparencies showed a striking increase in luminal thrombus on PCG's compared to PSG's. Thrombus formation was maximal in the central regions of the control grafts.

A direct comparison could only be made in the two animals in which both grafts remained patent. Clot-free surface approximated 70% in the two seeded grafts compared to 20% in the two control grafts.

Electron Microscopic Studies
(i) Studies from this institution:
SEM revealed that PSG's exhibited substantial 'endothelial like' cellular coverage and this lining was distributed throughout the length of the graft. Apart from limited in-growth of endothelium at the anastomoses (maximum 6-10 mm) PCG's did not exhibit cellular coverage at all (Figure 124). Patent sham seeded grafts (Groups II & III) were similar to PCG's showing endothelial coverage only adjacent to the anastomoses.

TEM showed that endothelial like cells covering seeded grafts had characteristics of 'true' endothelial cells, including flat bi-polar configuration with plasmalemnal vesicles at both cell surfaces interdigitating cell

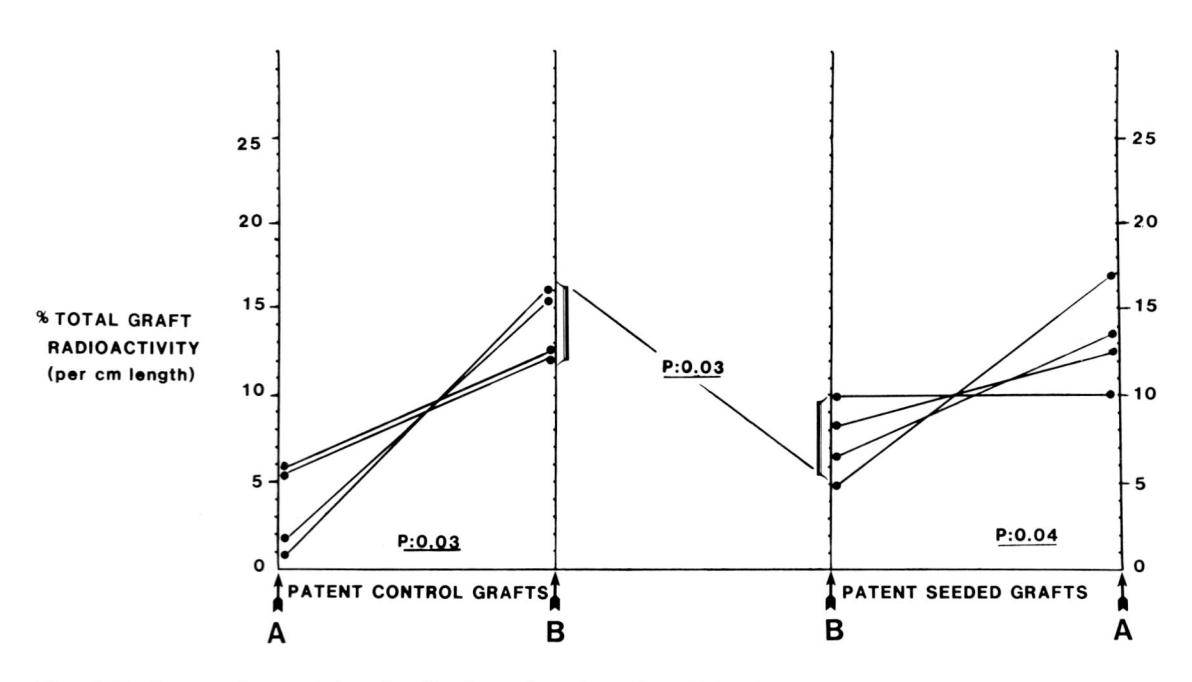

Fig. 123 Comparison of the distribution of graft radioactivity (after removal) in autologous indium-III-oxine platelet labelled sheep. The seeded grafts are significantly less thrombogenic in their centres.   A: Anastomotic regions,   B: Central regions.

3. Endothelial Cell Lining

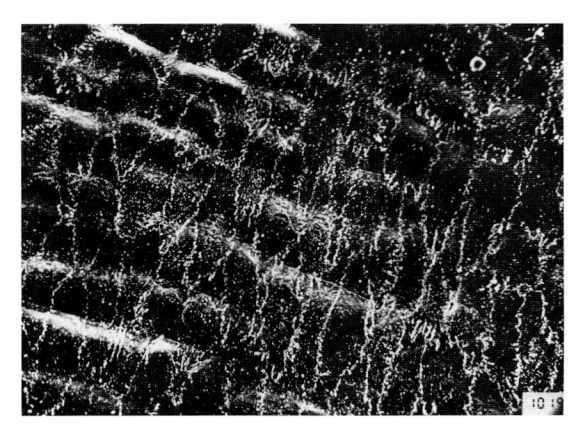

Fig. 124 Endothelial like cells lining the luminal surface of a seeded graft. This example was taken from the middle segment of a seeded graft and such an appearance was not seen in control or sham seeded grafts. Note the underlying pattern of the PTFE structure.
SEM: Original magnification x 1050.

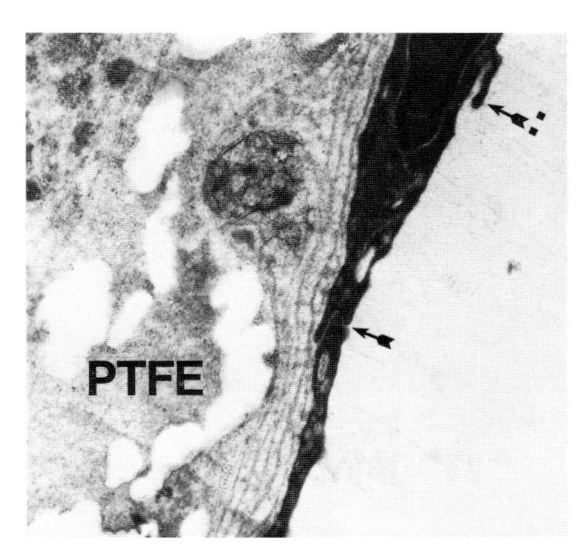

Fig. 125 Endothelial like cells forming a monolayer over the luminal surface of the middle segment of a seeded graft. (6 weeks post insertion). Note the bipolar nature of the cells and the multiple basement laminae lying directly on the polytetrafluoroethylene (PTFE). The 'arrow' indicates an interdigitating intercellular junction; another arrow indicates an endothelial projection, both features of true endothelial cells. TEM: Original Magnification x 38 000.

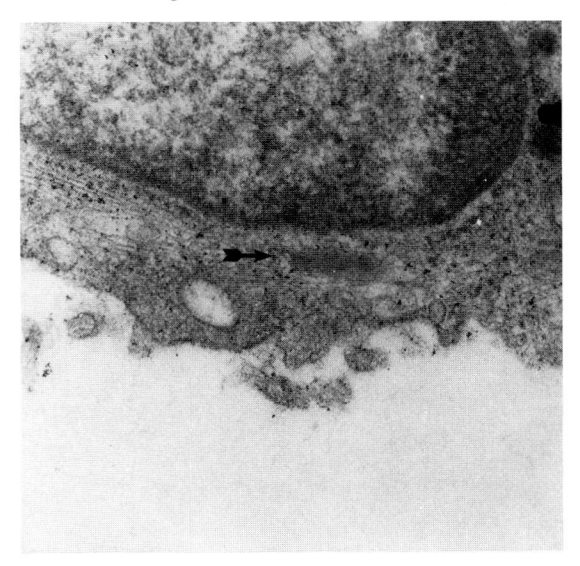

Fig. 126 High power micrograph of a lining cell from the middle segment of a seeded graft. The structure indicated by the arrow measures 0.4 μm (left to right) and appears to be surrounded by its own membrane - a possible Weibel-Palade body. TEM: Original magnification x 45 000.

borders, multiple basement laminae, and possibly Weibel-Palade bodies (Figures 125 and 126) (21).

(ii) Studies from WL Gore & Assoc:
The results of the estimated ELC coverage obtained from the SEM studies of the glutaraldehyde fixed specimens are shown in Figure 122. Table 38 shows the comparison between the coverage on the mid-proximal 3 cm segments of the patent control and seeded grafts. There was a highly significant increase in ELC coverage over the seeded grafts (P= 0.008).

Discussion

Although there are many studies demonstrating beneficial effects for endothelial cell seeding synthetic vascular prostheses in animal models (1-11,19), the value of seeding artificial conduits in humans is yet to be determined. Interpretation of seeding studies is difficult because of the variations in

3. Endothelial Cell Lining

% Endothelial-Like Cell Coverage - Patent Grafts
(proximal middle 3 cm)

Seeded	Control	Duration
57.1	(occluded)	2 weeks
62.7	(occluded)	2 weeks
9.6	(occluded)	2 weeks
(occluded)	0.0	4 weeks
(occluded)	0.0	4 weeks
(occluded)	0.0	4 weeks
34.4	0.0	4 weeks
84.9	0.0	6 weeks
(occluded)	1.0	6 weeks

P = 0.008 (Mann Whitney U Test)

Table 38

methodology, graft designs, graft lengths and duration of implantation, and because of doubts about the efficacy of attachment of seeded cells (12). Further confusion arises due to the existence of interspecies variation and the unknown ability of the particular animal under consideration to "autoendothelialize a graft". Man has virtually no ability to endothelialize a synthetic conduit of the length and diameter used in vascular reconstrutive procedures. The canine model has often been chosen in seeding studies because dogs are also thought to have limited ability to line grafts with autogenous endothelium (20). Despite this, some studies have shown that dogs endothelialize grafts in certain situations (21,22).

Other investigators have found that sheep are prone to intimal hyperplasia and graft thrombosis and occlude arterial synthetic conduits more readily than dogs (13). The length of 4 mm PTFE used (10 cm) was well above the 'maximum critical length' beyond which there is little chance of prolonged graft patency without anticoagulation (7,23). Therefore, in this study, a high rate of graft occlusion would be expected.

Most other endothelial cell seeding studies performed with both arterial and venous synthetic replacements have failed to demonstrate a beneficial effect on early (2-3 weeks post-insertion) patency rate of seeded grafts. The results in this paper are consistent with these studies (references 2-21, 24). These reports have, however, shown that seeded grafts which remain patent develop an endothelial cell lining and that control grafts, apart from limited endothelial cell coverage near the anastomoses, do not. One exception was the study by Plate et al (21), which did not show any difference in endothelialization between seeded and sham seeded grafts. It is of interest that this study was performed in the venous system of dogs using relatively wide diameter PTFE (8 mm). Their method of seeding PTFE differed from that described in this study and from that described by others (5,7).

By using autologous 111-indium labelled platelet methods, other workers have shown that seeding reduces platelet-vessel wall interactions (9,10,11). In this study, direct comparison of graft radioactivity could only be made in the two animals in which both the seeded and control graft remained patent. In both cases there was a striking reduction in the thrombogenicity of the seeded graft. When all patent grafts were considered seeded, grafts were significantly less radioactive in their centres compared to contral grafts. It appears, therefore, that a successfully seeded graft is less thrombogenic and that seeding tends to reduce thrombus formation in the central regions of the graft. Consistent with this suggestion was the finding of maximal macroscopic thrombus in the central regions of control grafts.

Previous studies have shown improved patency in seeded grafts after cessation of antithrombotic agents (4,11,25).

Another study (19), demonstrated an early patency rate for control grafts in seeded animals which was better than would be expected from the predictions of Herring et al (23). In the same report the patency rate in unseeded animals was consistent with these predictions. Although the present study did not consider long term patency, distinct advantages for PSG's (endothelial like cellular lining, increased clot-free surface, decreased thrombogenicity) suggests that their long-term patency may be better than PCG's.

The high occlusion rate of grafts in sham seeded animals is consistent with the predictions of Herring et al (23), especially in sheep (13). This occlusion rate is, however, higher than that reported by Hunter and Carson (13) who also used 10 cm lengths of 4 mm PTFE in sheep. Possible explanations include different graft insertion (single 10 cm crossover graft compared to bilateral 10 cm interposition grafts), different breeds of sheep (Columbian type compared to Border Leicester) and different size of animal (40-55 kg compared to 30-40 kg) (23). These authors demonstrated Thromboxane A2 production (TXA2) by the sheep carotid artery following surgery and an alteration in the ratio of prostacyclin to TXA2, with dominance of TXA2. They postulate that vessel wall trauma during surgery, clamping and graft insertion may be among the factors causing this alteration. If this were true, the insertion of two grafts into one animal would be expected to be more detrimental to overall graft patency than the insertion of two grafts into separate animals.

This study differs from other seeding studies in small diameter (4 mm or less) arterial prostheses in that control grafts were not sham seeded but inserted according to the manufacturer's instructions whereas sham seeded grafts were inserted into separate animals along with their own control. The difference between the patency rate in these two groups of animals was significant in spite of there being no apparent patency advantage for seeded grafts compared to their own controls. All grafts were removed at 2 weeks from "sham seeded animals" whereas most grafts were removed from "seeded animals" at longer time intervals, thus serving to emphasize the remarkable difference in overall patency between the two groups. The significant difference in patency between group II & III and between the controls of groups I &

3. Endothelial Cell Lining

III combined and the controls of group II, is evidence that a systemic effect is operative to favour patency for grafts inserted at a site remote from the introduction of endothelial cells.

A possible explanation is that a proportion of seeded cells detach, circulate and either bind 'pro-occluding' factors or are activated to release factors which favour graft patency. The currently employed cell harvest methods are injurious to many endothelial cells (14) and it is also possible that such cells release factors favouring graft patency. Endothelial cells are known to produce prostacyclin (26) plasminogen activator (27) to bind thrombin (28) to interact with heparin (29) and to possess other antiplatelet aggregating functions (28).

Circulating endothelial cells conceivably could be activated to perform these functions when coming into contact with a foreign surface. Endothelial cells also produce a factor which inhibits smooth muscle cell growth (30) and this may be relevant to intimal hyperplasia. Kempczinski et al (12) have shown that less than 5% of harvested endothelial cells remain attached to PTFE grafts 24 hours after seeding. There can be no doubt that many endothelial cells are released into circulation. This "circulating factor" theory could explain the results of other studies which have attributed the early equality of seeded and control graft patency to the use of anti-platelet agents in the perioperative period.

According to this theory any cells which remained attached to the seeded graft would proliferate, provided the graft remained patent, and may assist to maintain graft patency while control grafts would tend to occlude as the "circulating factor" dissipated. Consistent with this proposal was the remarkable difference in ELC coverage of the mid portions of the patent seeded grafts compared to that of the mid-portions of the patent control grafts. One could also speculate that the few cells which do remain attached to directly seeded grafts are stimulated to proliferate by the "circulating factor". (Figure 127).

This theory would explain the excellent histological results of many workers involved in endothelial cell seeding in the face of probable low seeding efficiency.

Acknowledgements

The authors wish to thank Mr P Jamieson of the Electronmicroscopy Unit,

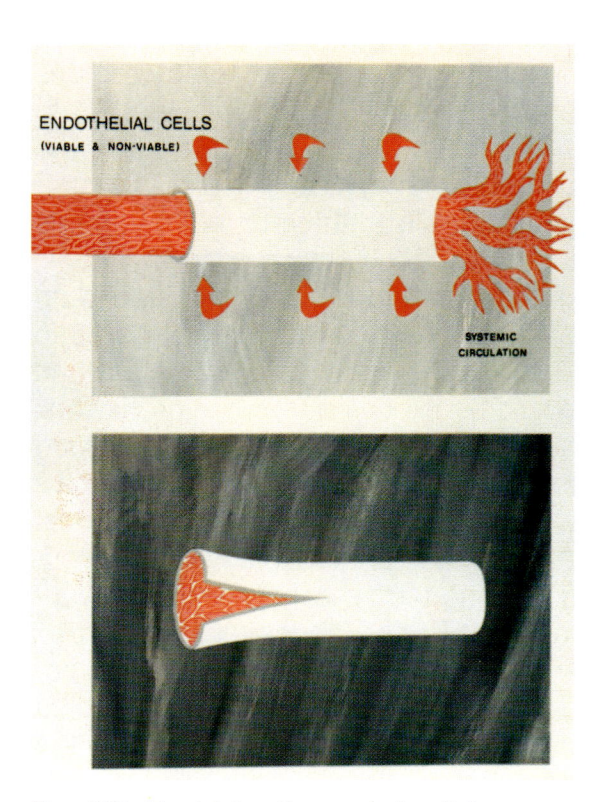

Fig. 127 Most "directly seeded cells" escape into the circulation (12). Do these cells have feedback effects on the graft maintaining patency and stimulating attached cells to proliferate?

NSW Institute of Technology, Gore Hill, and Mr R Kearns of the Wellcome Experimental Laboratory, The Royal North Shore Hospital, for their excellent technical assistance. We are also grateful to the departments of Nuclear Medicine, Haematology, and Endocrinology, The Royal North Shore Hospital for their assistance.

I would also like to thank my wife who typed this paper and who has supported me throughout.

Polytetrafluoroethylene vascular grafts were a generous gift from WL Gore and Associates (Flagstaff, Arizona, USA). We also thank the pathologists at WL Gore (Arizona) for their contribution to the histological evaluation of the grafts.

This work was supported in part by the Ethel and Olive Hewitt Medical Research Scholarship awarded by the Postgraduate Medical Committee, University of Sydney.

3. Endothelial Cell Lining

References

1. Herring M, Gardner A, Glover J. A single-staged technique for seeding vascular grafts autogenous endothelium. Surgery 84, 498, 1978.

2. Graham LM, Burkel WE, Ford JW, Vinter DW, Kahn RH, Stanley JC. Seeding of enzymatically derived endothelium in Dacron vascular grafts. Early experimental studies with autologous Canine cells. Arch Surg 115,1289, 1980.

3. Graham LM, Vinter DW, Ford JW, Kahn RH, Burkel WE, Stanley JC. Endothelial cell seeding of prosthetic vascular grafts. Early experimental studies with cultured autologous Canine endothelium. Arch Surg 115, 929, 1980.

4. Stanley JC, Burkel WE, Ford JW, Vinter DW, Kahn RH, Whitehours WM, Graham LM. Enhanced patent of small-diameter externally supported Dacron iliofemoral grafts seeded with endothelial cells. Surgery 92, 994, 1982.

5. Herring M, Baugham S, Glover J, Kesler K, Jesseph J, Campbell J, Dilley R, Evan A, Gardner A. Endothelial seeding of dacron and polytetrafluoroethylene grafts: the cellular events of healing. Surgery 96,745, 1984.

6. Graham LM, Burkel WE, Ford JW, Vinter DW, Kahn RH, Stanley JC. Expanded Polytetrafluoroethylene vascular prostheses seeded with enzymatically derived and cultured canine endothelial cells. Surgery 91, 550, 1982.

7. Kempczinski RF, Rosenman JE, Pearce WH, Roedersheimer LR, Berlatzky Y, Ramalanjaona G: Endothelial cell seeding of a new PTFE vascular prosthesis. J Vasc Surg 2, 424, 1985.

8. Schmidt SP, Hunter TJ, Sharp WV, Malindzak GS and Evancho MM. Endothelial cell-seeded four-millimeter Dacron vascular grafts: effects of blood flow manipulation through the grafts. J Vasc Surg 1, 434, 1984.

9. Sharefkin J, Latker C, Smith M, Cruess D, Clagget P, Rich NM. Early normalization of platelet survival by endothelial seeding of Dacron arterial prostheses in dogs. Surgery 92, 385, 1982.

10. Whitehouse WM, Wakefield TW, Vinter DW, Ford JW, Swanson DP, Thrall JH, Froelich JW, Brown LE, Buirkel WE, Graham LM, Stanley JC. Indium-III-Oxine labelled platelet imaging of endothelial seeded Dacron thoracoabdominal vascular prostheses in a Canine model. Trans Am Soc Artif Intern Organs 29, 183, 1983.

11. Allen BT, Long JA, Clark RE, Sicard GA, Hopkins KT, Welch MJ. Influence of endothelial cell seeding on platelet deposition and patency in small-diameter Dacron arterial grafts. J Vasc Surg 1, 224, 1984.

12. Kempczinski RF, Ramalanjaona GR, Rosenman JE, Douville EC, Silberstein EB. Effect of Fibronectin-coating on endothelial cell kinetics in PTFE grafts. Abstract Society for Vascular Surgery 39th Annual Meeting June 1985. p 20.

13. Hunter GC, Carson SN. Arterial wall thromboxane: dominance after surgery predisposes to thrombosis. J Vasc Surg 1, 314, 1984.

14. Bourke BM, Roche WR, Appleberg M. Endothelial cell harvest for seeding vascular prostheses: the influence of technique on cell function, viability and number. J Vasc Surg 4, 257, 1986.

3. Endothelial Cell Lining

15. Bourke BM, Appleberg M, Reeve TS. Indium-III-Oxine platelet labelling for vascular graft assessment in the sheep model (In press).

16. Thakur ML, Walsh L, Malech HL and Gottschalk. Indium-III-Labelled Human Platelets: improved method, efficacy and evaluation. J Nucl Med 22, 381, 1981.

17. Hawker RJ, Hawker LM, Wilkinson AR. Indium (^{111}In)-labelled human platelets: optimal method. Clinical Science 58, 243, 1980.

18. Swinscow TDV. Statistics at Square One. British Medical Association. London. 1983.

19. Schmidt SP, Hunter TJ, Hirko M, Belden TA, Evancho M, Sharp WV, Donovan DL. Small-diameter vascular prostheses: two designs of PTFE and endothelial cell-seeded and non-seeded Dacron. J Vasc Surg 2, 292, 1985.

20. Sauvage LR, Berger KE, Wood SJ, Yates SG II, Smith JC, Mansfield PB. Interspecies healing of porous arterial prosthesis. Observations 1960-1974. Arch Surg 109, 698, 1974.

21. Plate G, Hollier LH, Fowl RJ, Sande Jr, Kaye MP. Endothelial seeding of venous prostheses. Surgery 96, 929, 1984.

22. Richardson JV, Wright CB, Hiratzka LF. The role of endothelium in the patency of small venous substitutes. J Surg Res 28, 556, 1980.

23. Herring MB, Dilley R, Peterson G, Wiggans J, Gardner A and Glover J. Graft material, length and diameter determine the patency of small arterial prostheses in dogs. J Surg Res 32, 138, 1982.

24. Herring M, Gardner A, Peigh P, Madison D, Baugham S, Brown J, Glover J. Patency in canine inferior vena cava grafting: Effects of graft material, size and endothelial seeding. J Vasc Surg 1, 877, 1984.

25. Schmidt SP, Hunter TJ, Sharp WV, Malindzak GS, Evancho MM. Endothelial cell-seeded four-millimeter Dacron vascular grafts: effects of blood flow manipulation through the grafts. J Vasc Surg 1, 434, 1984.

26. Weskler BB, Marcus AJ, Jaffe EA. Synthesis of Prostaglandin I_2 (Prostacyclin) by Cultured Human and Bovine Endothelial Cells. Proc Natl Acad Sci USA 74, 3922, 1977.

27. Gross JL, Moscatelli D, Jaffe EA, Rifkin DB. Plasminogen activator and collagenase production by cultured capillary endothelial cells. The Journal of Cell Biology 95, 974, 1982.

28. Thorgeirssen G, Robertson AL. The vascular endothelium - pathobiologic significance. A Review. Am J Pathol 93, 803, 1978.

29. Glimelius B, Busch C and Hook M. Binding of Heparin on the surface of cultured human endothelial cells. Thrombosis Research 12, 773, 1978.

30. Castellot JJ, Addonizio ML, Rosenberg R, Karnovsky MJ. Cultured endothelial cells produce a heparinlike inhibitor of smooth muscle cell growth. The Journal of cell Biology 90, 372, 1981.

3. Endothelial Cell Lining

3.4.3. Endothelial Cell Seeding with Microvessel Endothelial Cells - Animal and Human Studies

*SP Schmidt, WV Sharp, MM Evancho, TR Pippert,
SO Meerbaum, D Monajjem*

*Vascular Research Laboratory, Akron City Hospital,
Akron, Ohio, USA*

Abstract

The derivation of endothelial cells (EC) from fat microvessels circumvents familiar objects to the use of large vessel endothelium for prosthetic vascular graft seeding. These microvascular EC (MVEC) can be derived in abundant numbers by collagenase treatment of fat. In addition, it is likely that all patients would have available subcutaneous and/or omental fat for cell derivation. The ability of MVEC to surface on prosthetic grafts in vivo has not been extensively reported, however. This research summarizes our experience seeding MVEC onto 4 mm id Dacron and PTFE grafts which were evaluated in canine carotid arteries. In addition, our experience seeding human vascular grafts with MVEC in eight patients is also included.

Three experiments were performed using dogs to evaluate vascular graft performance. In Experiment I, 6 cm lengths of 4 mm id Microvel double-velour knitted Dacron grafts (Meadox Medicals, Inc) were implanted bilaterally in the paired carotid arteries of nine dogs. One of each pair of grafts was seeded with MVEC (mean number of seeded cells = 8.4×10^6 isolated by collagenase incubation of 2 grams of omental fat from which all grossly visible blood vessels had been dissected; the contralateral graft was non-seeded (NS). The protocol described in Experiment I was repeated in Experiment II with the exception that 4 mm id polytetrafluoroethylene (PTFE) grafts (Impra, Inc) were employed as the grafting material. Eleven dogs were utilized in Experiment II and the mean number of cells seeded per graft in this study was 6.41×10^6. The objective of Experiment III was to compare the performances of endothelial cell seeded (ECS) vascular grafts interposed bilaterally in the dog's carotid circulation when one graft was seeded with EC derived from the dog's external jugular vein (JVEC) and the contralateral graft was seeded with EC derived from omental fat microvessels. Ten dogs were evaluated in Experiment III. In five of these dogs, equal numbers of JVEC and MVEC were seeded onto 4 mm id Microvel Dacron grafts (1×10^6 cells/graft). In the remaining five dogs each graft was seeded with the maximal number of cells derived from each source (JVEC = 1.02×10^6 cells/graft; MVEC = 4.62×10^6 cells/graft). In all three animal experiments, the grafts were harvested at five weeks postoperatively, the patencies of the grafts determined, thrombus-free surface (TFS) areas calculated, and the grafts were processed for histologic and electron-microscopic evaluation.

At five weeks postoperatively, eight out of nine of both the ECS and NS Dacron grafts were patent in Experiment I. The mean TFS area for ECS grafts was 95% ± 11% which differed significantly from the mean TFS area of NS grafts in this experiment which was 54% ± 19%. Scanning electron microscopy of graft luminal surfaces revealed well-connected, flattened cells on the luminal surfaces of seeded grafts. Some midgraft regions of seeded grafts were completely covered with confluent, cobblestoned patterns of cells. Nonseeded midgraft regions were composed of a fibrin meshwork with embedded blood borne cells and platelets. Six of the ten ECS PTFE grafts were patent at five weeks postoperatively in Experiment II; seven of ten NS PTFE grafts were patent at this time. Once again, however, there were significant differences in TFS areas between the groups. ECS PTFE grafts averaged 55.1% ± 22.5% TFS areas which differed significantly from the TFS areas of NS controls (13.8% ± 11.6%). The lumina of the ECS PTFE grafts contained islands of EC, but the surface coverage was not extensive. All of the Dacron grafts evaluated in Experiment III were patent five weeks postoperatively, and the luminal surfaces of these seeded grafts occupied by endothelium. When equal numbers of cells were seeded, the mean TFS areas were approximately 80% in both groups. When the maximum numbers of derived cells were seeded, the grafts seeded with MVEC had mean TFS areas of 94% ± 8.2%; grafts seeded with the maximum number of JVEC had mean TFS areas of 78% ± 9.3%.

Between January and October 1987, nine ECS procedures were performed in eight patients requiring peripheral vascular surgery. These patients were grafted with PTFE grafts seeded with MVEC. Between 2-10 grams of fat were processed to derive the EC for graft seeding. The mean number of seeded cells was 4.01×10^6/graft. The grafts remain patent in six of the eight patients to date. The relative thrombogenicities of the grafts are being evaluated in the postoperative period by indium-111-oxine platelet scans.

Introduction

Researchers in the field of vascular graft development have long been intrigued with the notion that an interface of endothelial cells (EC) between an artificial graft material and the blood would improve the graft's performance. The intuitive logic underlying the development of an endothelialized vascular prosthesis is that, in vivo, under homeostatic conditions, the endothelium is the most nonthrombogenic biologic surface known. As perspectives on the biology of the EC have enlarged, it is now appreciated that the mechanisms of this nonthrombogenicity are active and that the endothelium is a much more complex biologic tissue than previously recognized.

Endothelialization of vascular grafts as a consequence of endothelial cell seeding (ECS) in experimental animal models has been extensively reported. Herring et al [1] pioneered research in ECS with an early description of techniques for seeding mechanically-derived venous endothelium into the interstices of Dacron grafts implanted in dogs. Additional reports by Graham et al [2] of successful seeding of polytetra-

3. Endothelial Cell Lining

fluoroethylene (PTFE) prostheses and Schmidt et al (3) evaluating low flow-induced thrombogenicity in EC seeded versus nonseeded (NS) Dacron grafts firmly established the technology of ECS. Subsequently, many authors have contributed to the literature of ECS (4,5). Preliminary results of ECS of vascular prostheses in patients are now being reported (6).

As the technology has evolved, several potential limitations of ECS in patient populations requiring vascular grafting procedures have been recognized. Of primary concern is an appropriate origin of the EC for graft seeding in patients. Animal research protocols have typically utilized jugular veins from healthy animals for derivation of EC for seeding. Patients presenting for vascular grafting procedures may not, however, have available healthy, non-essential vessels for derivation of EC for seeding. In our experience, venous EC have been very difficult to enzymatically harvest and maintain viable from patients requiring vascular surgery. Even if a suitable autologous vessel were available, it has been estimated that enough cells would need to be harvested to cover 45% of the surface area of the prosthesis being seeded to promote surface endothelialization. (7). It is unlikely that such a large number of cells could be derived to achieve successful endothelialization of femoropopliteal bypass grafts from available autologous large-vessels. Alternatively, a small aliquot of harvested human large-vessel EC could theoretically be cultured in vitro to derive a suitable number of cells for graft inoculation (8). However, tissue culture of harvested EC would require the patient to undergo two surgeries, one for derivation of cells for tissue culture and a secondary surgery at a later date for implantation of the seeded prosthesis. In addition, the artificial environment of tissue culture might induce chromosomal aberrations and/or phenotypic modulation of the endothelium which would predict graft failure. It is obvious that a suitable alternative to large-vessel endothelium must be defined if ECS of vascular prostheses in patients is to be of practical utility.

EC derived from fat microvessels may be the alternative to large-vessel endothelium for vascular graft seeding in humans. Extensive in vitro studies describing the suitability of MVEC for vascular graft endothelialization have recently been reported (9,10). Pearce et al (11) also recently reported their results seeding MVEC into the interstices of a porous PTFE graft. We, too, have accumulated extensive in vivo data using MVEC for vascular graft seeding. This report summarizes our animal studies in which MVEC was seeded onto 4 mm id Dacron and PTFE grafts. In addition, we present data comparing graft performances when grafts were seeded bilaterally with MVEC or vein-derived EC and evaluated in the same animal. We also report our preliminary experience seeding MVEC onto PTFE grafts implanted in patients undergoing peripheral vascular bypass grafting.

Materials and Methods

Animal Studies

The care of animals used in this research complied with the "Principles of Laboratory Animal Care" and the "Guide for the Care and Use of Laboratory Animals" (NIH Publication No 80-23, revised 1978). Three experiments were performed.

3. Endothelial Cell Lining

Experiment I -
Dacron graft seeding

Nine random-source adult mongrel dogs weighing 20-30 kg were conditioned and acclimatized in our laboratory. Six cm lengths of 4 mm id Microvel, double-velour knitted Dacron grafts (Meadox Medicals, Inc, Oakland, NJ) were microsurgically implanted into their paired carotid arteries utilizing the following procedures. Each dog was medicated with dipyridamole (50 mg b.i.d.) beginning four days preoperatively and aspirin (5 grains q.d.) beginning one day preoperatively. This protocol of antiplatelet therapy continued until graft harvest at five weeks postoperatively. Each dog was anesthetized initially with IV sodium pentothal (20-25 mg/kg), intubated and maintained during surgery with a mixture of oxygen and halothane. Both the neck and abdomen were sterilely prepped and draped.

Eight to ten grams of omental fat were removed from a 3 cm midline incision. The fat was placed in a sterile bag containing physiological saline and transported to the tissue culture laboratory. The sample was processed for endothelial cell derivation from the fat microvessels following procedures modified from Jarrell et al (12). The excised fat was trimmed to approximately 2 grams and washed vigorously with phosphate buffered saline (PBS). This 2 gram sample was as free from large, grossly visible vessel fragments as possible. Subsequently the sample was minced into pieces that could be aspirated into a 10 ml pipet and transferred to a 50 ml Erlenmyer flask containing 4 ml of collagenase (ICN Biochemicals, Cleveland, OH) at a concentration of 4 mg/ml. The collagenase/fat suspension was incubated in a 37°C water bath with continuous mixing for 20 minutes. Following incubation, the solution was transferred to a 15 ml centrifuge tube and PBS was added to a volume of 14 ml. The solution was spun at 100 x g for 6 minutes. The supernatant, which consisted primarily of adipose, was aspirated and the remaining cell pellet resuspended in 2.2 ml of PBS. From this solution 0.2 ml were diluted 1:10 in citric acid/crystal violet and the cells were counted on a hemocytometer. The mean number of cells derived per gram of omental fat using this technique was $3.0 \times 10^6 \pm 8 \times 10^5$; the mean number of cells seeded onto each graft was 8.4×10^6.

Both carotid arteries were isolated through a 6 cm midline incision over the trachea while the EC were being harvested from the excised fat. Following isolation the grafts were prepared for implantation using a preclotting procedure modified from Yates, et al (13). A 20 ml aliquot of blood was drawn from one carotid artery via a catheter. Clamping one end of the graft the remaining 15 ml aliquot of blood was injected into the lumen of the graft such that the blood was forced through the interstices of the Dacron. After five passes, one half of the prepared EC suspension was injected into the graft lumen followed by two more passes of whole blood. The graft was flipped, clamped at the opposite end, and the procedure repeated with the second half of the EC suspension. The preclotting procedure for the NS graft was identical except that the EC injections were omitted. The preclotted grafts were then placed in the beaker of heparinized blood and set aside during final preparation of the arteries for graft interpolation.

3. Endothelial Cell Lining

The carotid arteries were prepared by excision of a 3 cm segment bi-laterally. The exposed ends of the arteries were cleared of connective tissues with care to avoid damage to the intimal surfaces. Following a rinse in lidocaine, the grafts were anastomosed end-to-end to the host carotids using 7-0 Prolene suture with the aid of 2.5X magnifying loops. All bleeding was controlled prior to the return of the grafted vessels to their correct anatomical locations and muscle and skin closure.

At the fifth week postoperatively, each dog was sacrificed. The grafts were extirpated and processed using the following procedure. The grafts were isolated with minimal manipulation through a 20 cm midline incision over the trachea. All grafts were isolated and palpated for patency, and the dogs were systematically heparinized with 5000 units of heparin. The grafts and adjacent arteries were cleared of surrounding connective tissue and a clamp was placed proximal to each graft on the carotid artery allowing plenty of arterial tissue between the graft and the clamp. The arteries distal to the grafts were then clamped and the grafts resected and placed immediately into a physiological saline rinse. The extirpated grafts were subsequently cut longitudinally and photographed. The graft was then divided for histologic and electron microscopic processing.

Graft thrombus-free surface areas (TFSA) were calculated by projecting the photographic slides of the entire luminal surface onto tracing paper and outlining those areas where thrombus existed. Those portions were cut from the paper, weighed on an analytical balance, and compared to the total weight of the luminal outline.

An assessment of EC surfacing on each graft luminal surface was accomplished by scanning electron microscopy (SEM). Segments of each graft were fixed in 2% glutaraldehyde and 0.1 M cacodylate buffer for at least two hours. After fixation each sample was washed with buffer three times for 15 minutes per wash. Subsequently the tissues were placed in a solution of 2% osmium tetroxide and 0.1 M cacodylate buffer for one hour and washed with distilled water. The samples were then serially dehydrated in acetone and critical point dried in CO_2. In order to increase tissue conductivity each sample was sputter-coated with gold-palladium alloy. The tissues were scanned using a JOEL1-jsm-35C model electron microscope. Portions of intact carotid arteries served as positive controls for this procedure.

Experiment II

The protocol described in Experiment I was essentially repeated in Experiment II with the exception that 4 mm id PTFE grafts (Impra, Inc) were employed as the grafting material. Eleven conditioned adult mongrel dogs were utilized in this study. The ECS protocol for these PTFE grafts differed somewhat from that used in previous studies. A one-way valve was placed in one end of an 8 cm length of PTFE graft; the opposite end of the graft was clamped using a small hemostat. Three cc of autologous serum was used to precoat the graft for 30 minutes. The use of a serum precoat was based upon our previous experience in which serum worked as well as fibronectin in retaining cells seeded onto PTFE grafts (14). Serum was repeatedly added to the graft to replace serum loss through the graft internodal spaces. After 30 minutes, the serum was drained from the graft. Subsequently a 0.5 cc aliquot of harvested omental MVEC suspended in tissue culture media was injected through the valve into the graft. The mean total number of cells seeded per graft in this study was $6.41 \times 10^6 \pm 1.1 \times 10^6$. These cells had been derived from 2 grams of processed omental fat. Following inoculation of the cells, the graft was slowly and continuously rotated for 10 minutes. Subsequently the graft was rotated in quarters for 10 minutes/turn. The total cell inoculation time was, therefore, 50 minutes. Following inoculation, the clamp on the end of the graft opposite the valve was released and the graft was gently rinsed so that the effluent was collected and the number of cells flushed from the graft lumen counted. The mean number of cells retained on each graft was $3.61 \times 10^6 \pm 5.57\ 10^4$ which translated into 4.13×10^5 cells retained/cm^2 of graft material implanted in each dog.

All other procedures previously described in Experiment I were repeated in Experiment II including the medication protocol, length of postoperative graft implantation and methods of graft evaluation at necropsy.

Experiment III

The objective of Experiment III was to compare the performances of ECS vascular grafts interposed bilaterally in the dog's carotid circulation when one graft was seeded with EC derived from the dog's external jugular vein (JVEC) and the contralateral graft was seeded with EC derived from omental fat microvessels (MVEC). Ten dogs were evaluated in this experiment. In five dogs, equal numbers of JVEC and MVEC (1×10^6 cells/graft) were seeded onto 4 mm id Microvel Dacron grafts as previously described and the grafts were evaluated at 5 weeks postoperatively. In the remaining five dogs, each graft was seeded with the maximal number of cells derived from each source. The mean number of JVEC seeded onto these grafts was $1.02 \times 10^6 \pm 0.30 \times 10^6$, the mean number of MVEC seeded per graft was $4.62 \times 10^6 \pm 1.36 \times 10^6$. The graft seeding and evaluation process followed that described above in these dogs as well. All dogs in the experiment were maintained on antiplatelet therapy for the entire length of the experiment.

Human Studies

To date, nine peripheral revascularization procedures have been performed in eight patients using MVEC derived from omentum for graft seeding. None of these patients presented with a suitable autogenous vein for use in bypass grafting. All of the patients were bypassed using 6 mm id PTFE grafts. The nine surgical procedures that were performed include the following: Femoral-popliteal bypass grafting - above the knee (1); Fermoral-popliteal bypass grafting - below the knee (3); Femoral-anterior tibial bypass grafting (2); Femoral-posterior tibial bypass grafting (1); Iliac-anterior tibial bypass grafting (1); Iliac-profunda - profunda-peroneal bypass grafting (1). The MVEC seeded onto the grafts of these patients were derived from 10 grams of omental fat. Each fat sample was obtained as the first surgical event. The samples were dissected free of grossly visible blood vessels, finely minced and incubated in collagenase (1500 U/ml) for 20 minutes at 37°C in a shaking water bath. Between 40-90 minutes elapsed between the time the fat sample was received for processing and the time the EC were returned to

3. Endothelial Cell Lining

the surgical suite for seeding. The mean number of cells that were obtained from the fat processing in these nine procedures was 5.67×10^6; the mean number of cells seeded graft was 4.01×10^6. The cells were inoculated onto the PTFE grafts by mixing the aliquot of MVEC with 20-30 cc of autologous serum or plasma and forcing the mixture through the interstices of the grafts and coating the luminal surfaces with this mixture. The relative thrombogenicities of these grafts are being monitored in the postoperative periods by uptake studies of indium-111-oxine labelled platelets on the grafts.

Results

Animal Studies

The patencies and mean TFS areas of all grafts evaluated as animal implants are shown graphically in Figures 128 and 129. Figure 130 is a composite of gross appearances of representative grafts from each experiment.

Experiment I

At the time of graft harvest 88% (8/9) of the Dacron grafts seeded with MVEC were patent. In addition, 88% (8/9) of the NS grafts were also patent. Although these patency rates between the two groups revealed no difference, the gross appearances of the luminal surfaces of the grafts at the fifth week post-implantation differed markedly. Of the nine grafts seeded with MVEC, seven displayed no adherent thrombus along their entire lengths. NS grafts displayed red, non-elevated thrombus in midgraft segments with approximately 0.5 cm of pannus ingrowth of arterial endothelium from each anastomosis. One ECS graft

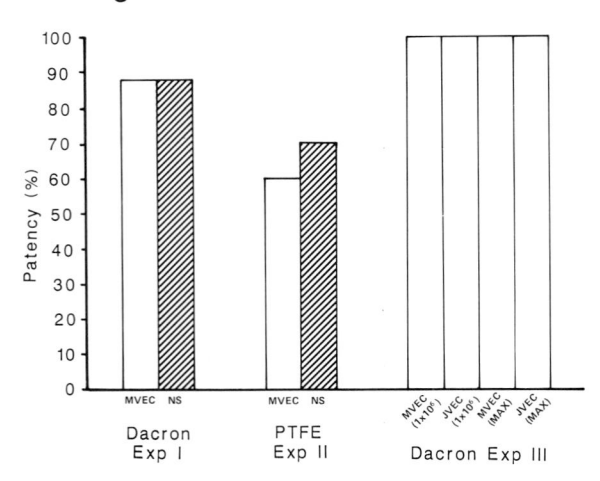

Fig. 128 Experiment I - Patencies of microvascular endothelial cell (MVEC) seeded 4 mm id Dacron grafts compared with nonseeded controls at 5 weeks postoperatively; Experiment II - Patencies of MVEC seeded 4 mm id PTFE grafts compared with nonseeded controls at 5 weeks postoperatively; Experiment III - comparative patencies of 4 mm id Dacron vascular grafts seeded with MVEC and jugular vein-derived endothelial cells (JVEC) at 5 weeks postoperatively.

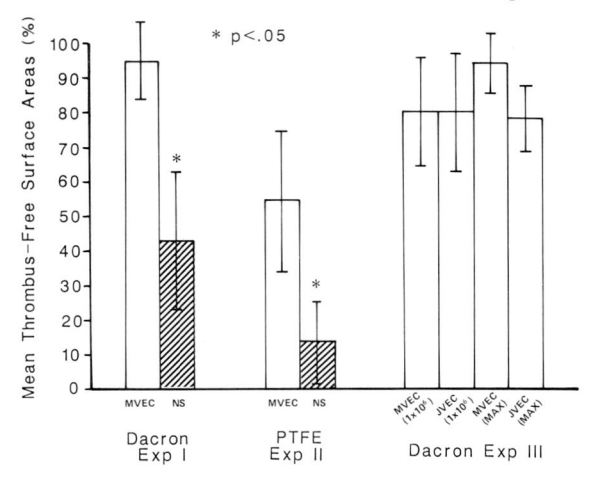

Fig. 129 Experiment I - Mean thrombus-free surface areas of MVEC seeded 4 mm id Dacron grafts compared with nonseeded controls at 5 weeks postoperatively; Experiment II - Mean thrombus-free surface areas of MVEC seeded 4 mm id PTFE grafts compared with nonseeded controls at 5 weeks postoperatively; Experiment III - comparative thrombus-free surface areas of 4 mm id Dacron vascular grafts seeded with MVEC and JVEC at 5 weeks postoperatively.

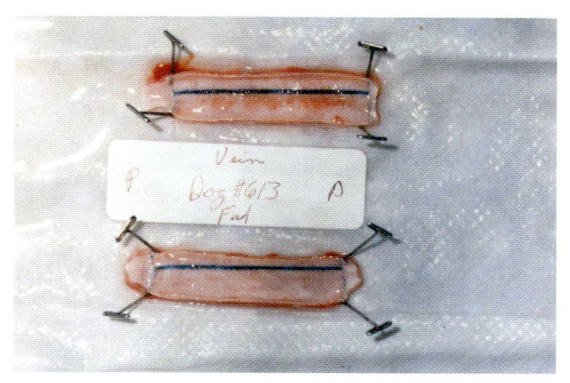

3. Endothelial Cell Lining

Fig. 130 a
Comparison of gross appearances of 6 cm lengths of 4 mm id Dacron vascular grafts seeded with jugular vein-derived endothelial cells (JVEC) [top] and microvascular-derived endothelial cells (MVEC) [bottom] at 5 weeks postoperatively. Each graft was seeded with the maximal number of endothelial cells derived from their respective origins.

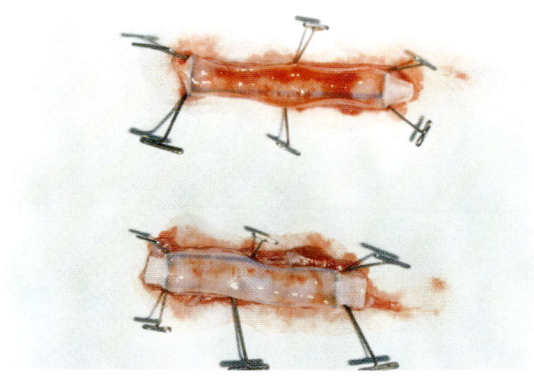

Fig. 130 b
Comparison of gross appearances of 6 cm lengths of 4 mm id PTFE vascular grafts seeded with MVEC (bottom) and nonseeded (top) at 5 weeks postoperatively.

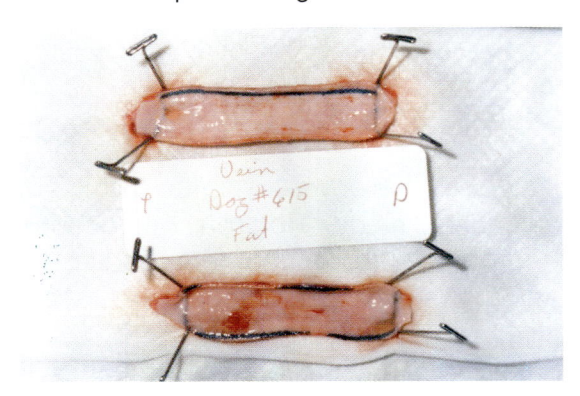

Fig. 130 c
Comparison of gross appearances of 6 cm lengths of 4 mm id Dacron vascular grafts seeded with JVEC (top) and MVEC (bottom) at 5 weeks postoperatively. Each graft was seeded with 1×10^6 endothelial cells derived from their respective origins.

showed red, non-elevated thrombus along its entire length with no pannus ingrowth; the contralateral control graft in this animal was quite similar. One pair of grafts was occluded bilaterally. The mean TFS area calculated for ECS grafts was 95.0% ± 11%. This value differed significantly from the mean thrombus-free surface area of non-seeded grafts in this study which was 43% ± 19% ($p<0.05$).

Figure 130 illustrates the gross comparison of seeded and nonseeded Dacron grafts from this experiment.

Haematoxylin and eosin stained histological sections of Dacron grafts seeded with MVEC are depicted in Figure 131. ECS grafts possessed smooth, cellular luminal surfaces adhered to the artificial graft material via connective tissue. NS graft sections revealed no evidence of cellular growth in the midgraft region. Clumps of thrombus overlayed an irregular layer of blood elements. Scanning electron microscopy of graft luminal surfaces revealed well-connected, flattened cells in the luminal surface of seeded grafts. Some midgraft regions of seeded grafts were completely covered with confluent, cobblestone patterns of cells reminiscent of EC in culture (Figure 132). NS midgraft regions were composed of a fibrin meshwork with embedded blood borne cells and platelets.

Experiment II

One of the dogs included in Experiment II experienced bilateral graft infections and was removed from the study. From the ten dogs remaining, six of the

3. Endothelial Cell Lining

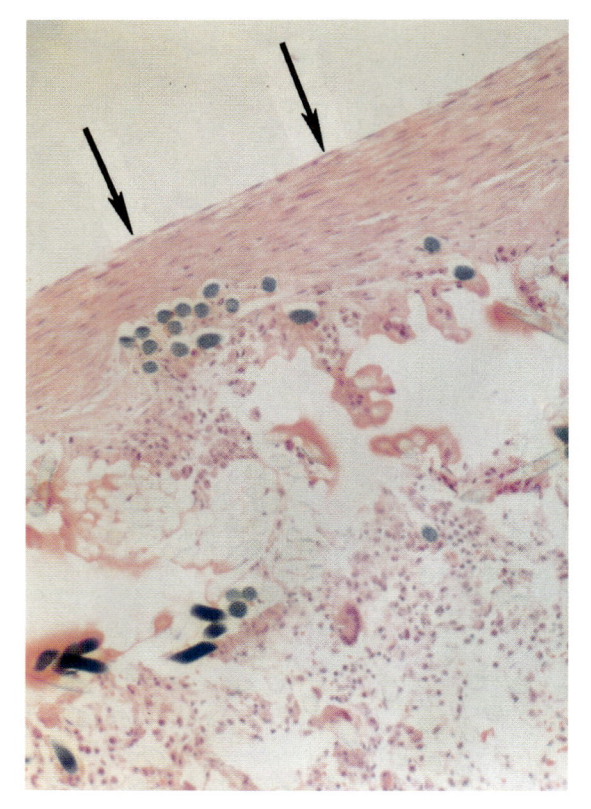

Fig. 131 Haematoxylin and eosin stained histologic section of a Dacron graft seeded with microvascular-derived endothelial cells. The arrows point to the nuclei of luminal endothelium (100 x).

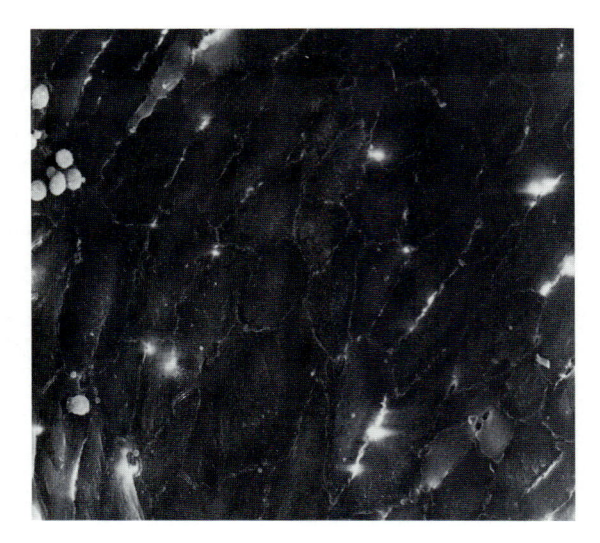

Fig. 132 Scanning electron micrograph of a midgraft region of a Dacron graft seeded with microvascular-derived endothelial cells at implantation and harvested 5 weeks postoperatively. The luminal endothelial cells are flattened with a cobblestone morphology (600 x).

MVEC-seeded grafts remained patent at 5 weeks postoperatively; seven of the NS grafts were patent at this time. The gross comparisons of seeded and NS PTFE grafts from this study are represented in Figure 130. In spite of the slightly higher patency rate in NS grafts from this study, MVEC-seeded PTFE grafts had significantly greater mean TFS areas. ECS PTFE grafts averaged 55.1% ± 22.5% TFS; NS PTFE graft mean TFS area averaged 13.8% ± 11.6%. A representative histologic section of a midgraft region of a PTFE graft seeded with MVEC is shown in Figure 133. In general, the coverage of the luminal surfaces by EC on these PTFE grafts was not as extensive as that seen on the Dacron grafts in Experiment I.

However, there were isolated clumps of cells visible by electron microscopy (Figure 134) in all patent seeded grafts and some midgraft regions were extensively covered by endothelium. It was presumed that the grafts that failed in this experiment were early failures in that the thrombus occupying the lumina of these grafts was very well organized.

Experiment III

All of the Dacron grafts evaluated in Experiment III were patent at 5 weeks postoperatively. The luminal surfaces of these grafts were extensively covered by endothelium, and there were no differences in mean TFSA between those grafts seeded with MVEC and grafts seeded with JVEC. All TFSA were greater than 80%. We were unable to distinguish any morphologic differences between the JVEC- and MVEC-seeded graft surfaces at 5 weeks postoperatively.

3. Endothelial Cell Lining

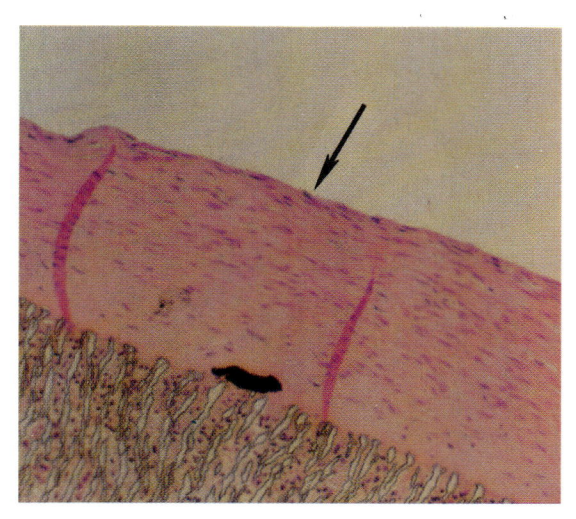

Fig. 133 Haematoxylin and eosin stained histologic section of a PTFE graft seeded with microvascular-derived endothelial cells. The arrow points to a nucleus from a luminal endothelial cell (100 x).

Human Studies

To date six of the nine grafts seeded with MVEC and implanted in patients remain patent. There have been no immediate postoperative complications in these grafts. One below-the-knee femoral-popliteal graft failed at 2 months postoperatively, and the leg was eventually amputated. The indium-111-oxine labelled platelet scan from this patient is shown in Figure 135 indicating the high thrombogenicity of this graft just prior to thrombosis. A second below-the-knee femoral-popliteal graft thrombosed at 5 months postoperatively, as did one femoral-tibial graft. We have not been able to retrieve samples of these failed grafts for histologic or SEM evaluations. The grafts in the remaining patients are functional with minimal platelet uptake visible in their grafts.

Discussion

The short-term performances of 4 mm id Dacron and PFTE grafts seeded with MVEC and evaluated in the canine carotid artery model have been excellent as inferred from the patency and TFS area data. All of the dogs included in our animal studies were medicated with antiplatelet agents throughout the entire postoperative period. Our continuing philosophy is that endothelial cell seeding combined with antiplatelet medication results in optimal long-term prosthetic graft function (15,16). However, because of the antiplatelet medications, inherent differences that may evolve in patencies between ECS and NS prosthetic grafts may be obscured.

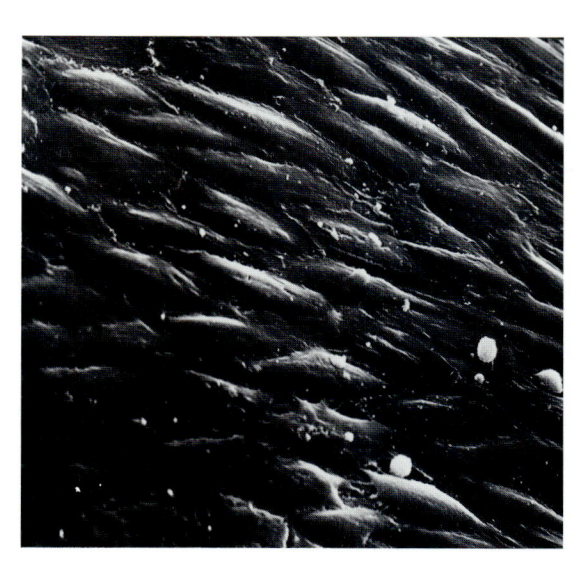

Fig. 134 Endothelial cells forming a clump on a midgraft section from a PTFE graft seeded with microvascular-derived endothelial cells at implantation and harvested 5 weeks postoperatively (600 x).

As expected, therefore, there were no significant differences in patencies of ECS and NS grafts evaluated in Experiments I and II. We prefer to carefully evaluate differences in TFS areas as indicators of the eventual graft fates. TFS areas were significantly greater in the ECS Dacron and PTFE grafts in Experiments I and II compared with respective

319

3. Endothelial Cell Lining

NS grafts. Only 13% of the surfaces remained thrombus-free in NS PTFE grafts at 5 weeks postoperatively, even in the presence of antiplatelet agents,

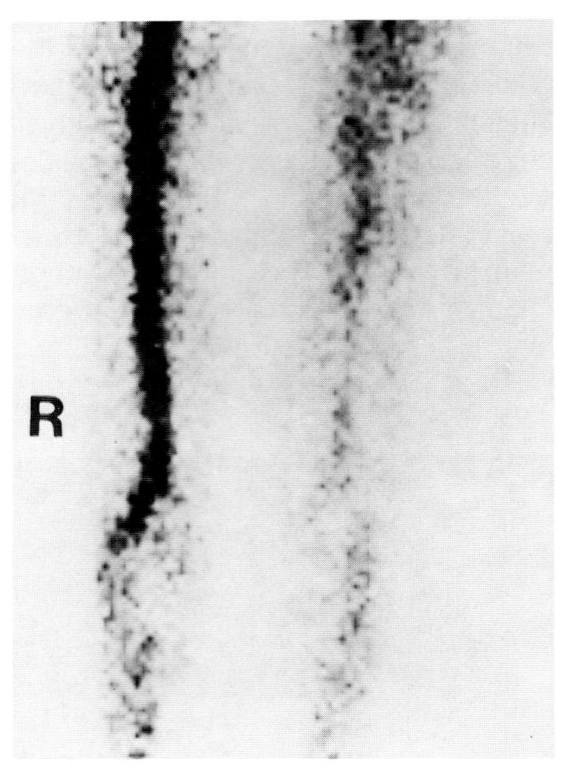

Fig. 135 Indium-111-oxine labelled platelet scan of a highly thrombogenic PTFE femoral-popliteal bypass graft (R) just prior to graft occlusion.

and it is postulated these grafts would soon occlude. In contrast, MVEC presumably remained functional when seeded onto the prosthetic grafts and the relatively high TFS area would suggest that active mechanisms of antithrombogenicity were operative.

There was virtually complete coverage of all Dacron grafts evaluated in the animal studies with surface EC. At 5 weeks postoperatively, the luminal surfaces of Dacron grafts seeded with MVEC were identical in appearance to those seeded with JVEC. There may conceivably be differences in the rates of establishment of the confluent neo-intima relative to the size of the inoculum of seeded MVEC. If these differences exist, however, they are complete before the fifth postoperative week. Grafts seeded with 1×10^6 MVEC appeared identical at this time to grafts seeded with the maximal number of derived MVEC. Surface coverage of PTFE grafts by MVEC at 5 weeks postoperatively was significantly less than that of Dacron. This probably reflects, at least in our opinion, the suboptimal methodologies available for seeding EC onto standard commercially-available, 30u PTFE graft material. Nevertheless, islands of EC were visible on all grafts and apparently conferred a distinct advantage to the graft in terms of retarding thrombus accumulation. The cells that were derived by collagenase incubation of omental fat were not pure collections of MVEC. We did not separate contaminating cells - including pericytes, mesothelial cells and fibroblasts - from the MVEC via passage through a Percol gradient. Our preliminary observations suggest that the inoculum of seeded cells may consist of 20-35% non-endothelial cell types. The theoretical debate regarding the optimal purity of the inoculum of cells for graft seeding remains unresolved. We chose to use the crude collection of cells rather than the purified MVEC from Percol separation because of our observations of the lethargic nature of percolled EC in culture. The in vitro viability and vitality of these cells, at least in our hands, is greatly reduced. In the final analysis, it doesn't appear to us, based upon our short-term animal implants, that inclusion of these contaminating cells was detrimental to graft performance.

Our initial experiences seeding MVEC onto human vascular grafts have also been very positive although we do not have any direct confirmation that the cells have indeed surfaced on these implanted prostheses. The patients have been very willing to donate omental fat, the length of time of derivation of the cells has been acceptable to the vascular surgeons, and the numbers of cells inoculated onto the grafts have been far greater than could be anticipated using immediate seeding of vein-derived EC. There have been no immediate postoperative complications following seeding of these MVEC. Postoperative evaluation by indium-111-oxine platelet labelling continues to offer information regarding the relative thrombogenicities of these grafts.

References

1. Herring MB, Gardner AL, Glover J. A single staged technique for seeding vascular grafts with autogenous endothelium. Surgery 84, 498, 1978.

2. Graham LM, Burkel WE, Ford JW, Vinter DW, Kahn RH, Stanley JC. Expanded polytetrafluoroethylene vascular prostheses seeded with enzymatically derived and cultured canine endothelial cells. Surgery 91, 550, 1982.

3. Schmidt SP, Hunter TJ, Sharp WV, Malindzak GS, Evancho MM. Endothelial cell seeded 4 mm Dacron grafts; effects of blood flow manipulation through the grafts. Journal of Vascular Surgery 1, 434, 1984.

4. Herring M, Glover J (eds). Endothelial seeding in vascular surgery. Grune & Stratton, Inc, Orlando, 1987.

5. Zilla PP, Fasol RD, Deutsch M (eds). Endothelialization of vascular grafts. Karger, Basel, 1987.

6. Herring MB, Gardner A, Glover J. Seeding human arterial prostheses with mechanically derived endothelium. The detrimental effect of smoking. Journal of Vascular Surgery 1, 279, 1984.

7. Herring M, Dilley R, Cullison T, Gardner A, Glover J. Seeding endothelium on canine arterial prostheses - the size of the inoculum. Journal of Surgical Research 28, 35, 1980.

8. Watkins MT, Sharefkin JB, Zajtchuk R, Maciag TM, D'Amore PA, Ryan US, Van Wart H,, Rich NM. Adult human saphenous vein endothelial cells. Assessment of their reproductive capacity for use in endothelial cell seeding. Journal of Surgical Research 36, 588, 1986.

9. Williams SK. Isolation and culture of microvessel and large-vessel endothelial cells: their use in transport and clinical studies. In McDonagh (ed), Microvascular perfusion and transport in health and disease. Karger, Basel, pp 204, 1987.

10. Radomski JS, Jarrell BE, Williams SK, Koolpe EA, Greener DA, Carabasi A. Initial adherence of human capillary endothelial cells to Dacron. Journal of Surgical Research 42, 133, 1987.

11. Pearce WH, Rutherford RB, Whitehill TA, Rosales C, Bell KP, Patt A, Ramalanjaona G. Successful endothelial seeding with omentally derived microvascular endothelial cells. Journal of Vascular Surgery 5, 203, 1987.

3. Endothelial Cell Lining

12. Jarrell BE, Williams SK, Stokes G, Hubbard FA, Carabasi RA, Koolpe E, Greener D, Pratt K, Moritz MJ, Radomski J, Speicher L. Use of freshly isolated capillary endothelial cells from the immediate establishment of a monolayer on a vascular graft at surgery. Surgery 100, 392, 1986.

13. Yates SG, Barros AAB, Berger KE, Fernandez LG, Wood SJ, Rittenhouse EA, Davis CC, Mansfield PB, Sauvage LR. The preclotting of porous arterial prostheses. Annals of Surgery 188, 611, 1978.

14. Schmidt SP, Boyd KL, Pippert TR, Hite SA, Evancho MM, Sharp WV. Endothelial cell seeding of ultralow temperature isotropic carbon-coated polytetrafluoroethylene grafts. Preliminary experiments and observations. In Zilla PP, Fasol RD, Deutsch M (eds). Endothelialization of vascular grafts. Karger, Basel, pp 145, 1987.

15. Schmidt SP, Hunter TJ, Falkow LJ, Evancho MM, Sharp WV. Effects of antiplatelet agents in combination with endothelial cell seeding on small-diameter Dacron vascular graft performance in the canine carotid artery model. Journal of Vascular Surgery 2, 898, 1985.

16. Hirko MK, Schmidt SP, Hunter TJ, Evancho MM, Sharp WV, Donovan DL. Endothelial cell seeding improves 4 mm PTFE vascular graft performance in antiplatelet medicated dogs. Artery 14, 137, 1987.

3.5. Improved Harvest Technique

3.5.1. Human Endothelial Cell Derivation Using the Neutral Protease Dispase

JC Stanley, BG Ruefer, WE Burkel, DW Haack,
LM Graham, JL Fisher, NJ Sharber

*Department of Surgery and Anatomy – Cell Biology,
University of Michigan Medical School, Ann Arbor, Michigan, and
Medical Products Division, WL Gore & Associates,
Flagstaff, Arizona, USA*

Dispase Derivation of HEC

Considerable research has been directed toward development of antithrombogenic linings in vascular prostheses by seeding synthetic grafts with autologous endothelial cells (1). Theoretic advantages of such hybrid conduits are well known, but the optimal method of deriving endothelial cells and the best means of their seeding remain to be defined.

Mechanical means of procuring endothelial cells have been abandoned because medial smooth muscle cells are often removed with the endothelium, and if seeded into a graft they may proliferate and contribute to unacceptable inner capsule thickening. Enzymatic derivation of cells has become the standard for seeding vascular grafts, since sequential incubation of donor vessels with collagenase and trypsin was first reported (2-5). Collagenase is the proteolytic enzyme used most often in studies related to endothelial cell seeding of vascular prostheses. Unfortunately, most investigators use crude preparations of bacterial collagenase that contain a number of nonspecific proteases whose biologic activity frequently varies from one batch to another. Problems regarding the impurity of collagenase are compounded by the fact that it is relatively toxic to cells (6), and in its more pure form is less active (7). Similar problems exist regarding the heterogeneic composition and cytotoxicity of trypsin (8).

Five particular characteristics of Dispase make it preferable to other proteolytic enzymes for laboratory and clinical use (9, 10). First, crystalline Dispase is a very pure and stable enzyme. Second, unlike other proteolytic enzymes, Dispase maintains a high degree of activity in the presence of serum. Approximately 5% of Dispase's activity is lost over 24 hours in the presence of bovine serum at 37°C, and less than 1% activity is lost over 24 hours at 4°C. Third, its activity persists in the presence of Ca^{++} or Mg^{++}. Fourth, at low levels Dispase does not appear to influence cell attachment to

3. Endothelial Cell Lining

substrate or subsequent cellular proliferation. Lastly, when conventionally used, Dispase exhibits no cytotoxicity. In this regard, cells have been observed to actually grow in solutions of this enzyme for considerable periods of time.

The paucity of specific information in the literature regarding the effectiveness of Dispase for derivation of macrovascular HEC provided the impetus for a series of studies by the authors (11), that are summarized in this present report.

Materials and Methods

Temperature Effects on Dispase Derivation of HEC

Enzymatic influences on chemical reactions usually proceed without temperature related deviations. However, in biologic systems the tissue's responsiveness to enzymes may be modified by temperature changes. This appears to be the case with Dispase derivation of HEC.

In the first portion of this study, HEC were grown in tissue culture to confluence on a gelatin substrate, providing a relatively constant number of cells. Exposure to Dispase at 20 units/ml activity for 20 minutes was then carried out at 25°C, 28°C, 31°C, 33°C and 36°C. The total cell yield as well as cell viability, determined by plating efficiency at 24 hours, was then determined. In general, increases occurred with higher temperatures, although the yield of viable HEC was not greater above 31°C (Table 39).

Thus, Dispase derivation of HEC seems best with temperatures in the 31°C to 36°C range. However, it is known that exceeding 37°C will be injurious to cells, and incubation tem-

Effect of Temperature on HEC Derivation from Cultured Endothelium Grown to Confluence[a]

	Mean Number of Cells (% of Total[b])	Plating Efficiency
Temperature[c]		
25°C	17,733 (3.1%)	83%
28°C	20,960 (3.6%)	62%
31°C	51,040 (8.9%)	72%
33°C	32,733 (5,7%)	67%
36°C	38,573 (6.7%)	63%

a - incubation with Dispase, 20 units/ml for 20 minutes
b - total number of cells averaged 577,000/chamber
c - observations n4 at 25°C, and n5 at 28-36°C

Table 39

peratures approaching 37°C do not appear to offer any advantage regarding numbers or viability of derived HEC.

In the second portion of this study, fresh human saphenous vein remnants were obtained following coronary artery bypass operations. Vein segments, 4 cm in length, were filled with Dispase having activity of 20 units/ml and incubated for 20 minutes. During the incubation, veins were immersed in a liquid-filled tray having temperatures of 25°C, 29°C, 33°C and 37°C. At the end of incubation, the enzyme solution was flushed from the vein and centrifuged to derive a pellet of endothelium. The cells were then rinsed, and a portion removed for counting, with the remainder being plated on a gelatin substrate. These latter cells were then incubated for 24 hours at 37°C. Total numbers of HEC harvested and their viability were established for the differing temperatures tested (Table 40). Although the greatest HEC yield occurred at 33°C, cell viability at this temperature was slightly lower than at 29°C or 37°C.

Effects of Enzyme Concentration on Dispase Derivation of HEC

An evaluation similar to that regarding temperature was performed in assessing the importance of enzyme concentration. In this portion of the study, known numbers of HEC were grown on gelatin coated plates and exposed to Dispase with activities of 5, 10, 15, 20, 25, 30, 40 and 50 units/ml for a period of 20 minutes at 32°C. Greater cell yields occurred with higher enzymatic concentrations (Table 41). In fact, nearly twice the number of HEC were obtained with Dispase activities of 50 units/ml compared to 40 units/ml.

Viability was also greater with higher enzyme concentrations. This is most likely a reflection of more efficient harvesting of healthy cells exposed to higher concentrations, and the possibility that lower concentrations were less efficient at detaching normal cells but more effective in deriving less viable HEC populations.

The second portion of enzyme concentration studies assessed HEC isolation from 4 cm segments of fresh human

Effect of Temperature on HEC Derivation from 4 Cm Saphenous Vein Segments[a]

Temperature	Mean Number of Cells	Plating Efficiency
25°C	18,933	54%
29°C	51,600	76%
33°C	95,200	66%
37°C	55,111	74%

a - incubation with Dispase, 20 units/ml for 20 minutes

Table 40

3. Endothelial Cell Lining

Effect of Dispase Concentration on HEC Derivation from Cultured Endothelium Grown to Confluence[a]

	Mean Number of Cells (% Total[b])		Plating Efficiency
Enzyme Concentration[c]			
5 units/ml	16,733	(2.9%)	57%
10 units/ml	17,813	(3.1%)	64%
15 units/ml	29,653	(5.1%)	66%
20 units/ml	18,613	(3.2%)	66%
25 units/ml	32,253	(5.6%)	70%
30 units/ml	57,866	(10.0%)	69%
40 units/ml	123,200	(21.4%)	80%
50 units/ml	234,773	(40.7%)	86%

a - incubation with Dispase at 32°C for 20 minutes
b - total number of cells averaged 577,000/chamber
c - observations n4 with 5 units/ml, and n5 with 10-50 units/ml

Table 41

saphenous veins using Dispase concentrations of 40, 50 and 60 units/ml. Not surprisingly, cell yields and viability paralleled those obtained in our experiments with cultivated cells (Table 42). In comparison to direct harvests from intact veins, the low percentage of cultured cells removed by proteolytic enzymes, as noted in our studies on both enzyme concentrations and temperature, is a

Effect of Dispase Concentration on HEC Derivation from 4 cm Saphenous Vein Segments[a]

	Mean Number of Cells	Plating Efficiency
Enzyme Concentration[b]		
40 units/ml	1,800,000	37%
50 units/ml	3,490,000	40%
60 units/ml	2,040,000	88%

a - incubation with Dispase at 32°C for 20 minutes
b - observations n7 with 40 and 50 units/ml, and n6 at 60 units/ml

Table 42

well recognized phenomenon. Indeed, such has been previously reported with the effects of Dispase in detaching human umbilical vein endothelium being much more efficient from whole vessels than from culture plates (12).

Identification of Dispase Derived Cells.

In an additional study enzymatically derived saphenous vein cells were grown to confluence on gelatin-treated cover slips. Peroxidase anti-peroxidase (PAP) immunocytochemical staining was then undertaken for factor VIII-related antigen. These studies demonstrated an almost universal presence of factor VIII-related antigen in the cytoplasm, confirming that the cells were endothelium. Similarly, scanning electron microscopy, with few exceptions, revealed the typical cobblestone appearance and characteristic microvilli of HEC.

Additional cell cultures underwent three passages, and were then subjected to studies defining the presence or absence of smooth muscle cells. Specific immunocytochemical assays included mouse-anti-human alpha-actin (HHF 35) to identify smooth muscle. Among all cultures studied, no smooth muscle cells were evident. Thus, Dispase appears to offer a high degree of selectivity in detaching and disassociating HEC from the internal elastic lamina of saphenous vein, without violating the media and contaminating harvests with other cells.

Discussion

Dispase appears to be a relatively unique proteolytic enzyme. It is a bacterial neutral protease obtained from culture filtrates of aerobically grown Bacillus polymyxa. The process of deriving Dispase was developed by Yoshio Irie in 1975 (9,10). Dispase is currently produced by the Godo-Shusei Company, Matsudo, Chiba, Japan.

Two forms of this neutral protease exist, a highly purified crystalline form, Dispase I, and a partially purified form referred to as Dispase II. Gel permeation chromatography of crystalline Dispase reveals two peaks (Figure 136). The first represents the active enzyme with a molecular weight of approximately 36 000, and the second represents the inactivated form of the enzyme with a molecular weight of approximately 10 000. Crystalline Dispase may be reconstituted for use with common solvents such as Hanks' balanced salt solution, as was the case in the studies described in this report, or with a number of other media, including Dulbecco's phosphate buffer solution and Eagle's minimal essential medium. Its persistent biologic activity in the presence of serum, as well as Mg^{++} and Ca^{++}, differentiate Dispase from many other enzymes used for cell disaggregation.

Although Dispase is not dramatically more effective in deriving cells compared to collagenase or trypsin (9,10, 14), exceptions do exist. In fact, Dispase has been found superior to trypsin in enzymatic derivation of rat epidermis, yielding nearly four times as many cells with a high degree of cell viability (13).

Dispase appears less injurious to cells at the time of harvest compared to other enzymes and chelating agents, and may allow for their greater growth potential following harvest (9,10,14). In this regard, Dispase dissociated human fibroblasts in culture exhibited growth within 48 hours, with greater substrate attachment and wheat germ agglutination than occurred following

3. Endothelial Cell Lining

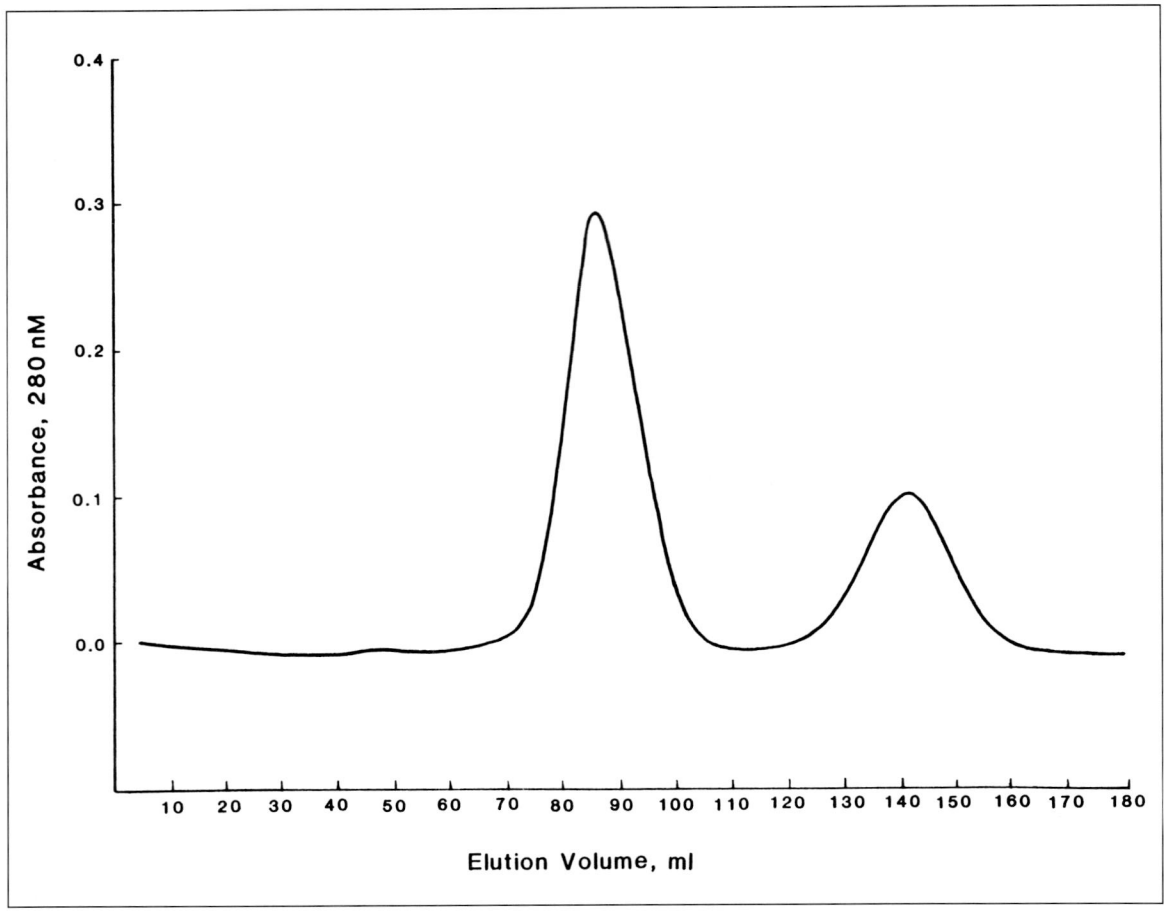

Fig. 136 Gel permeation chromatography of crystalline Dispase exhibiting high peak of active enzyme and low peak of inactive enzyme (Sephadex G-100, Hanks' BSS flow of 20 ml/hr at 4°C).

cellular dissociation with trypsin (16). Cell survival and function, when chronically exposed to dispersion with Dispase for 2 weeks, has also been noted in a number of sophisticated immunologic studies of pancreatic islet cells (15). Similarly, fibroblasts have maintained their viability when dispersed in a similar manner with constant exposure to Dispase for 4 months (9,10). Clearly, cytotoxicity is not a relevant issue with customary usage of Dispase.

In addition to the lack of injury to derived cells, Dispase is unlikely to produce adverse systemic effects in an intact animal or person. It is inhibited on nearly an equal molar basis by alpha-2 macroglobulin present in circulating blood (17). Although an exceedingly small amount of Dispase might remain associated with derived HEC following washing in Hanks' balanced salt solution or culture media, a few ml of blood would certainly neutralize any proteolytic activity accompanying such cells during their implantation as part of an endothelial cell seeded vascular prosthesis. This conclusion is consistent with experiences using Dispase to disperse cultured epithelial cells to cover extensive burn wounds, a situation in which no clinical evidence of systemic toxicity or untoward proteolytic activity has been reported (18). Mycoplasma and bacterial contamination of crystalline Dispase prepared by conventional means has not been observed. Similarly, pyrogenicity has not been ascribed to this particular neutral protease.

The role of temperature during proteolytic isolation of cells has received little attention in the literature, although in most laboratory settings harvesting has occurred with temperatures near 37°C. An exception has been the derivation of intact epidermal tissue in the form of sheets, including intact sweat glands, at temperatures of 4°C (14, 19). Dispase acts on cellular surface proteins or extracellular matrix, causing cell separation. It is speculated that cell-to-cell separations are more likely to occur at warmer incubation temperatures, whereas cell-to-basement membrane separations may be more likely to occur at colder incubation temperatures.

In regard to the site of cell separation, keratinocytes exposed to trypsin-EDTA exhibited a loss of cell-substratum as well as intercellular adhesion, whereas only the cell-substratum adhesion was disrupted following incubation with Dispase, suggesting that the surface glycoprotein responsible for intercellular adhesion was less likely to be affected by the proteolytic activity of Dispase (18). The action of Dispase on epithelial cells appears to be at the level of their hemidesmosome-basement membrane attachment. Sheets of corneal epithelium derived with Dispase exhibit intact basal cells and desmosomes, with their free basal cell surface exhibiting cytoplasmic blebs (21). Although Dispase affects surface membranes of cells, the functional sequelae may be less than noted with other enzymes such as trypsin (22). This would appear to be the case with better glucoreceptor preservation in pancreatic islet cells isolated with Dispase (23).

Perhaps the most important fact regarding the enzymatic derivation of endothelium for seeding of vascular prostheses is the realization that despite certain obligatory membrane effects caused by proteases, these effects are not exhibited by the progeny of the initially affected cells. In fact evidence suggests that the antithrombogenic character of endothelium derived by proteolytic enzymes is not impaired in subsequent generations of endothelial cells populating vascular graft surfaces (1).

If enzymatic derivation of HEC for use in seeding of vascular prostheses is to be of major importance as clinical trials evolve (24-26), then necessary attributes of any proteolytic substances used must include enzyme purity, stability, and biologic activity without cytotoxicity. In this regard, crystalline Dispase appears to be the most suitable of existing enzymes for the derivation of human endothelial cells.

3. Endothelial Cell Lining

References

1. Stanley JC, Burkel WE, Graham LM and Lindblad B. Endothelial cell seeding of synthetic vascular prostheses. Acta Chir Scand Suppl 529, 17, 1985.

2. Burkel WE, Vinter DW, Ford JW, Kahn RH, Graham LM, Stanley JC. Sequential studies of healing in endothelial seeded vascular prostheses. Histologic and ultrastructure characteristics of graft incorporation. J Surg Res 30, 305, 1981.

3. Graham LM, Burkel WE, Ford JW, Vinter DW, Kahn RH, Stanley JC. Expanded polytetrafluoroethylene vascular prostheses seeded with enzymatically derived and cultured canine endothelial cells. Surgery 91, 550, 1982.

4. Graham LM, Vinter DW, Ford JW, Kahn RH, Burkel WE, Stanley JC. Endothelial cell seeding of prosthetic vascular grafts. Early experimental studies with cultured autologous canine endothelium. Arch Surg 115, 929, 1980.

5. Stanley JC, Burkel WE, Vinter DW, Ford JW, Kahn RH, Whitehouse WM JR, Graham LM. Enhanced patency of small-diameter, externally supported Dacron iliofemoral grafts seeded with endothelial cells. Surgery 92, 994, 1982.

6. Hefley T, Cushing J, Brand JS. Enzymatic isolation of cells from bone: cytotoxic enzymes of bacterial collagenase. Am J Physiol 240, C234, 1981.

7. Striker GE, Harlan J, Schwartz SM. Human endothelial cells in vitro, methods in cell biology, vol 21A, Academic Press, New York, 1980, p. 146.

8. Weymouth C. To disaggregate or not to disaggregate. Injury and cell disaggregation, transient or permanent? In Vitro 10, 97, 1974.

9. Matsumura T, Yamanaka T, Hashizume S, Irie Y, Nitta K. Tissue dispersion, cell harvest and fluid suspension culture by the use of bacterial neutral protease. Japan J Exp Med 45, 377, 1975.

10. Matsumura T, Nitta K, Yoshikawa M, Takaoka T, Katsuta H. Action of bacterial neutral protease on the dispersion of mammalian cells in tissue culture. Japan J Exp Med 45, 383, 1975.

11. Ruefer BG, Stanley JC, Burkel WE, Haack DW, Fisher JL, Sharber NJ, Graham LM. Derivation of human endothelium using the neutral protease Dispase for seeding of ePTFE vascular prostheses (unpublished observations).

12. Thilo DGS, Muller-Kusel S, Heinrich S, Kaufer D, Weiss E. Isolation of human venous endothelial cells by different proteases. Artery 8, 259, 1980.

13. Takahashi H, Sano K, Yoshizato K, Shioya N, Sasaki K. Comparative studies on methods of isolating rat epidermal cells. Ann Plast Surg 14, 258, 1985.

14. Kitano Y, Okada N. Separation of the epidermal sheet by Dispase. Br J Dermatol 108, 555, 1983.

15. Wright JR Jr, Lacy PE, Unanue ER, Muszynski C, Hauptfeld V. Interferon-mediated induction of Ia antigen expression on isolated murine whole islets and dispersed islet cells. Diabetes 10, 1174, 1986.

16. Cassiman JJ, Brugmans M, van den Berghe H. Growth and surface properties of Dispase dissociated human fibroblasts. Cell Biol Int Rep 5, 125, 1981.

17. Starkey PM and Barrett AJ. α_2-Macroglobulin, a physiological regulator of Proteinase activity. In: Proteinases in Mammalian Cells and Tissues, Barrett AJ (ed), North-Holland, Amsterdam, p. 633 (1977).

18. Gallico GG III, O'Connor NE, Compton CC, Kehinde O, Green H. Permanent coverage of large burn wounds with autologous cultured human epithelium. N Engl J Med 311, 448, 1984.

19. Okada N, Kitano Y, Morimoto T. Isolation of a viable eccrine sweat gland by Dispase. Arch Dermatol Res 275, 130, 1983.

20. Roberts GP, Brunt J. Identification of an epidermal cell adhesion glycoprotein. Biochem J 232, 67, 1985.

21. Gipson IK, Grill SM. A technique for obtaining sheets of intact rabbit corneal epithelium. Invest Ophthalmol Vis Sci 23, 269, 1982.

22. Kohnert KD, Hehmke B. Preparation of suspensions of pancreatic islet cells: a comparison of methods. J Biochem Biophys Method 12, 81, 1986.

23. Ono J, Takaki R, Fukuma M. Preparation of single cells from pancreatic islets of adult rat by the use of Dispase. Endocrinol Japan 24, 265, 1977.

24. Herring MB, Compton RS, LeGrand DR, Gardner AL, Madison DL, Glover JL. Endothelial seeding of polytetrafluoroethylene popliteal bypasses. A preliminary report. J Vasc Surg 6, 114, 1987.

25. Ortenwall P, Wadenvik H, Kutti J, Risberg B. Reduction in deposition of Indium-III-labelled platelets after autologous endothelial cell seeding of Dacron aortic bifurcation grafts in humans: a preliminary report. J Vasc Surg 6, 17, 1987.

26. Zilla P, Fasol R, Fischlein T, Minar E, Hammerle A. Endothelial cell seeding of polytetrafluoro-ethylene vascuar grafts in humans: a preliminary report. J Vasc Surg 6, 535, 1987.

3. Endothelial Cell Lining

3.6. Modification of Graft Surfaces

3.6.1. Surface Modulation of Endothelial Cell Seeded PTFE Vascular Grafts

RB Patterson, RF Kempczinski

*Division of Vascular Surgery, University of Cincinnati
Cincinnati, Ohio, USA*

Background

Vascular prostheses implanted in humans do not form a biologically active flow surface, but are linked with an amorphous layer of compacted fibrin (1). This surface is highly thrombogenic in the presence of low blood flow. In experimental studies, endothelial cell (EC) seeding vascular prostheses prior to implantation improves both short and long term patency of small-diameter grafts, and reduces the risk of graft infection in the early post-implantation period (2-6). Seeding an uncoated PTFE prostheses is inefficient, with only 20% of harvested cells adherent immediately after seeding and only 17% of those cells remaining adherent 24 hours after implantation (7). If EC coverage is to become confluent, the retained cells must replicate and migrate until adjacent colonies merge.

Various cells grown in culture adhere poorly to plastic surfaces. They appear to require a biologic substrate and the addition of specific factors that are present in serum for optimal attachment and subsequent growth and migration (8). In vivo, ECs rest upon a basement membrane composed of collagenous and non-collagenous glycoproteins arranged in a randomly oriented granular matrix (9). The cells elaborate fibronectin (FN) which promotes cell adhesion and migration along the naturally occurring substrate. These observations of cell behaviour in culture suggest that application of similar substrates to vascular prostheses prior to EC seeding might improve both cell retention and cell migration with more rapid growth to confluence.

Previous Discoveries and Work in Progress

Fibronectin

Fibronectin is a ubiquitous glycoprotein, first characterized in 1948 by precipitation from its plasma component (10). Subsequently, it has been found to exist in a variety of related forms both as an intracellular and extracellular compound (11). FN is not found as a component of developmentally mature basement membranes (12,13), although its association with the basement membrane during proliferative activity suggests it may be incorporated early in angiogenesis, to be replaced at a later

3. Endothelial Cell Lining

stage with more stable collagen compounds (8). FN has been identified as the serum factor necessary for cell attachment and spreading in tissue culture. This activity is enhanced by coating the dish with collagen, for which FN has a specialized affinity. Cell-specific binding sites are present in the central portion of the FN molecule which appear to interact with the "adhesion patches" (14) present at the cell-substratum interface. Binding of FN to free cells does not occur prior to its complexing with the substratum, whether it is collagen or plastic. FN (both autogenous and exogenous) first complexes to the substratum and then forms a bridge to the specific binding sites on the cell surface.

Since successful seeding of vascular prostheses has similar requirements for cell attachment and spreading as in vitro culture, there has been extensive study of graft pretreatment with FN to improve initial EC adherence and subsequent coverage of the luminal surface. Using an in vivo seeding kinetics model developed in our laboratory (7), ePTFE viability grafts coated with FN were compared to similar but uncoated grafts (15). Initial EC retention was more than twice as great for FN coated grafts. Following restoration of blood flow through the grafts, EC loss occurred at three distinct rates: an initial rapid loss over 30 minutes, a gradual continuing loss over the first 24 hours and a plateau over the remaining time of implantation, with no significant loss of cells after 24 hours (Figure 137). Although the kinetics curves for both uncoated and FN coated

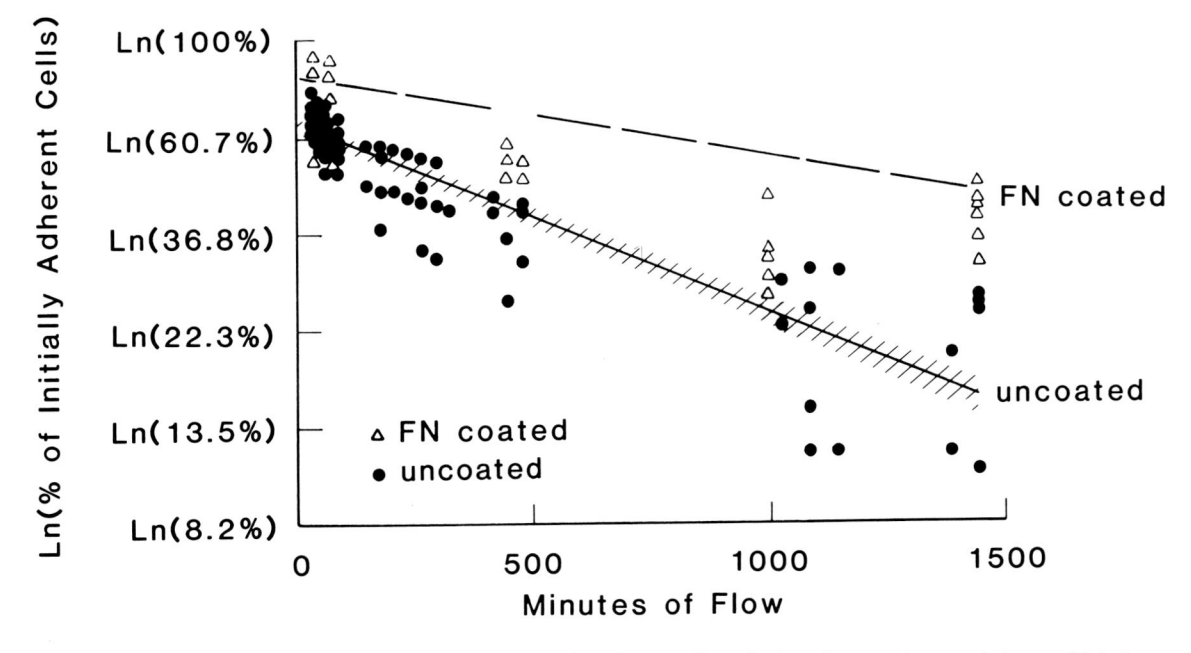

Fig. 137 Logarithmic percentage of endothelial cell retention during first 24 hours (phase 2) following restoration of flow for both uncoated and Fibronectin-coated polytetrafluoroethylene grafts. (Reprinted from Ramalanjaona G, Kempczinski RF, Rosenman JE, Douville EC, Silberstein EB: The effect of Fibronectin coating on endothelial cell kinetics in polytetrafluoroethylene grafts. J Vasc Surg 3: 264-272, 1986. With permission).

3. Endothelial Cell Lining

grafts were similar, the advantage of FN coating persisted at each interval, with a final retention of 21.3% vs. only 3.4% (P< 0.01) for untreated grafts.

Endothelial cells in culture, when grown to confluence, are capable of synthesizing their own FN and incorporating it into their extracellular matrix. The stability of seeded cells after 24 hours may be accounted for by the ongoing synthesis of endogenous FN of the attached and spreading cells. Thus the provision of exogenous FN on the graft surface may be necessary only for the critical period of initial cell attachment when the ECs are devoid of adhesive matrix.

Unfortunately, FN has an equal affinity for platelets and other formed blood elements (16). Seeger and Klingman (17) demonstrated improved seeding efficiency of grafts coated with FN. Although their data did not achieve statistical significance, they also found an increase in platelet deposition along the graft's entire luminal surface. They suggested that the benefits of improved seeding efficiency in low flow situations might be offset by this increased tendency to platelet adhesion.

An increase in platelet adherence to FN coating grafts was confirmed in a second series of experiments in our laboratory (18) in which FN coated increased platelet deposition by a factor of 3-5. This correlated with a statistically significant increase in graft thrombosis. Inhibition of platelet activity with ASA/dipyridamole (Figure 138) reduced total adherence of radiolabelled platelets to FN coated grafts three-fold during the first 24 hours, and was associated with a comparable increase in graft patency (80% vs. 27%). Although a dramatic reduction, this was still more than twice the number of platelets adherent to uncoated control grafts. The identification of a selective segment of FN responsible for cellular attachment (19) suggests that the desirable properties of FN may be available without increasing platelet adhesiveness.

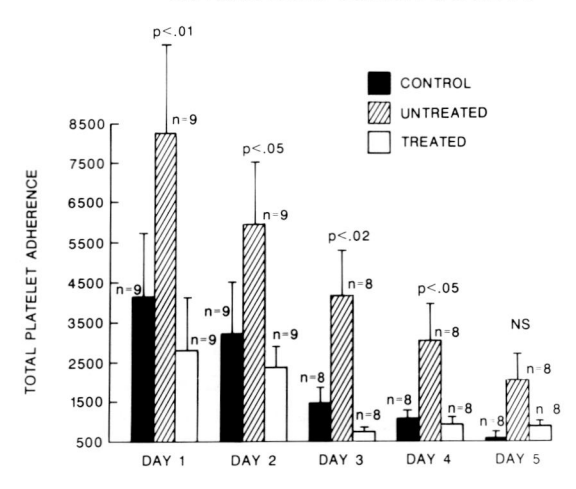

Fig. 138 A graph shows mean (SEM) total platelet adherence (counts/min) to FN grafts in both treated and untreated animals. Control animals had uncoated grafts and did not receive antiplatelet treatment. (Reprinted from Kempczinski RF, Ramalanjaona GR, Douville C, Silberstein EB: Thrombogenicity of a Fibronectin-coated, experimental polytetrafluoroethylene graft. Surgery 101, 439-444, 1987. With permission).

Matrix Compounds

The search for a more specific substrate to enhance seeding efficiency without the attendant drawbacks of FN has led to investigation of a wide variety of compounds found in native subendothelial layers. Certain matrix components are ubiquitous in basement membranes, although differing in relative amounts between various tissues and species (20). Collagen, types I, III and IV, gelatin, and laminin have been extensively studied in vitro, both as isolated substrates and as graft coating materials.

Macarak and Howard (8) isolated the cell - substrate interaction by studying EC adhesion, growth and "sprout cell" formation when cultured on various substrates in serum-free medium.

By eliminating serum from the culture medium, they avoided contamination with FN and other growth factors, thus helping to isolate the contribution of the target substrate. The most striking differences in cell behaviour was between cells plated directly onto plastic surfaces, and those plated on any of the substrates tested. Cells plated on treated surfaces rapidly flattened and spread radially, assuming a plate-like morphology. Cells seeded on untreated plastic in a serum-free medium spread slowly, and did not assume the confluent pattern of cells on a coated surface. Comparison of adhesion to collagen types I and III, basement membrane extract (collagen type IV), FN, and laminin favoured FN and type I collagen after 1 hour of incubation, but there was no significant difference at 8 hours between the various substrates. Differences in ability of cells to spread were not quantified, but qualitatively appeared similar for each substrate.

To study cellular migration as a property distinct from adherence, Hasson et al (21) developed a model for the investigation of the influence of isolated matrix components on the migration of cells in culture. They were able to demonstrate an increased rate of migration for cells plated on FN and gelatin coated dishes when compared to uncoated dishes. Laminin and a biologically synthesized extracellular matrix did not provide a statistically significant improvement over plain dishes. Since they included serum in their culture medium, FN was present in solution and may have contributed to some of the observed cellular activity.

Although these studies help to define the influence of matrix compounds on EC activity, arterial graft surfaces are distinctly different from tissue culture plates. Dacron surfaces are irregular, and provide difficult terrain for the adhesion and spread of ECs (22). PTFE, with its precise internodal distances, still presents an irregular framework for the attachment of EC. This results in a limited contact area for the ECs, even when grown to confluence, which is not present with the smooth surfaces of cell culture dishes. Recently, Zacharias (23) and Clowes (24) have suggested that the inability of Dacron grafts to form an endothelial surface, even after long-term implantation, may be related to an inherent inhibition of endothelial proliferation on the graft surface. PTFE did not exhibit this same resistance to endothelialization in their in vivo model. To be applicable to clinical EC seeding of vascular prostheses,therefore, studies of substrate compounds must be performed with graft material as their foundation.

In vitro culture of cells on graft material precoated with matrix compounds has produced results that are somewhat at variance with those observed in EC culture on plastic coated dishes. The unifying finding is the confirmation that coated grafts support cell attachment and growth better than uncoated grafts, regardless of their composition. The role of coating with isolated components (laminin, gelatin, collagen types I, III and IV, as well as FN) has failed to demonstrate consistent superiority of one compound over another (20-22, 27, 28). The collagen compounds, particularly in the

3. Endothelial Cell Lining

presence of bound FN, hold the most promise as coating materials.

A model of EC growth on graft surfaces in vitro has been developed by Williams et al (25). Using graft material immobilized in a plastic ring, they have been able to assess the effects of graft pre-treatment with various compounds (FN, collagen, and gelatin) on EC adhesion and growth. In a related series of experiments, pretreatment of Dacron grafts with either platelet rich plasma or a basement membrane-like compound derived from treated human amnion was studied (26). The control group of untreated Dacron exhibited gradual adherence in vitro, with 80% of ECs adherent in one hour. Despite satisfactory adherence (as measured by radioisotope labelling), cellular attachment, spreading, and growth to confluence was not observed. By contrast, adherence was much more rapid to the grafts pretreated with either platelet rich plasma or applied amnion. Morphologic differences in cell growth were striking between the plasma treated grafts and the amnion-derived collagen substrate. ECs on the plasma coated grafts assumed a stellate morphology, with poorly defined cell-cell junctions. When seeded on the Dacron surfaces with applied amnion, initial adherence was somewhat delayed, but the resultant monolayer achieved a typical cobblestone appearance with cell-cell attachments that resembled those of normal endothelium. These findings emphasize that reliance upon improved adhesion as the only endpoint in the evaluation of a graft surface modification may be overly simplistic. Rather, the growth characteristics and physiologic behaviour of ECs cultured on a substrate must also be assessed.

Foxall et al (27) compared the morphology of ECs grown in culture using Dacron and PTFE as a culture surface. They found that uncoated graft material was incapable of supporting cell attachment and growth, a finding at variance with others (2-4,29). Pretreating the graft material with collagen and FN resulted in cell attachment and growth, although only coated PTFE promoted growth to confluence with tight cell-cell junctions. When PTFE collagen/FN grafts were subsequently studied in a non-pulsatile perfusion system (28), EC loss over 60 minutes was minimal (7-11%). If these kinetics are confirmed in an in vivo model, this combination of coatings will prove significantly better than FN coating alone (15).

In an elegant series of in vitro experiments, Anderson et al (29) compared the growth in culture of ECs derived from umbilical vein in PTFE grafts of varying internodal distance and coated with a variety of matrix proteins, both alone and in combination. They found that collagen and a complex biologic matrix (Matrigel) coating resulted in statistically significant improvement in cell attachment. The authors concluded that the improvement seen with graft pre-treatment was due both to the mechanical properties of the compounds, preventing the seeded cells from penetrating the graft interstices, and to the biologic properties of the compounds themselves.

The behaviour of seeded cells on these individual substrates remains to be defined in grafts under in vivo physiologic conditions. Initial attachment and growth in culture media does not translate to the ability of cells to adhere under conditions of stress present in the circulation. Also, the complex interaction with circulating host factors cannot be adequately replicated in vitro.

3. Endothelial Cell Lining

Basement Membrane Gel

One obvious explanation for the lack of uniformity seen in previous experiments using individual basement membrane components is the complex nature of the membrane that is being mimicked. The interaction of the extracellular matrix proteins and the intracellular and serum proteins (i.e. FN) are not static and unidimensional. In response to injury, senescence, and stress, the agents responsible for vascular repair interact in an everchanging environment. Those components responsible for cellular attachment may be different from those responsible for cellular migration and cell-cell interaction. This is supported by the failure of cellular attachment to substrate when FN activity is blocked with antibodies (8). Although the coating of graft material with individual components improves the adherence and coverage of ECs when compared to untreated grafts, a proportionately balanced matrix may provide the proper biologic environment for the expression of physiologic cell functions.

Form et al (30) have demonstrated that the improvement in cell proliferation seen with laminin as a substrate is modulated by the binding of laminin with type IV collagen, and was further dependent upon the relative amounts of these two factors. As noted above, combinations of collagen and FN (either as a coating or free in serum-rich media) are superior to collagen alone.

In extensive work with the basement membrane matrix of mouse EHS tumor, Kleinman et al (31) have shown that the individual components (type IV collagen, laminin, heparin sulphate proteoglycan, nidogen and entactin) reconstitute in constant proportions to form a gel which is ultrastructurally similar to native basement membrane (Figure 3). They subsequently cultured melanoma cells (B16C3) with improved morphology, and have found prolonged survival of hepatocytes grown in culture. The reconstituted basement membrane gel supports cell adhesion, growth, and differentiation better than any of its individual components.

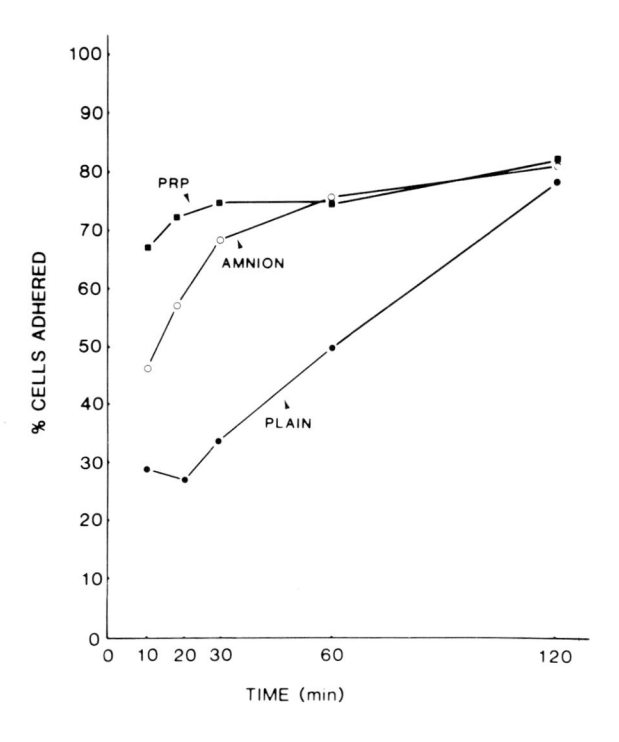

Fig. 139 Comparison of human adult endothelial cell adherence to untreated Dacron and Dacron treated with either platelet-rich plasma or human amnionic membrane. Establishment of a protein surface on Dacron accelerates the adherence of endothelial cells to the surface. PRP = surface resulting from clotting platelet rich plasma on Dacron. AMNION = surface resulting from the bonding of acellular amnionic membrane to the Dacron surface. The basement membrane surface of the amnion was oriented away from the Dacron surface. PLAIN = untreated Dacron weave. (Reprinted from Jarrell BE, Williams SK, Solomon L, et al: Use of an endothelial monolayer on a vascular graft prior to implantation. Ann Surg 203: 671-678, 1986. With permission).

3. Endothelial Cell Lining

Future Directions

Our current line of investigation is directed at the coating of a porous (45µ) PTFE prostheses with reconstructed basement membrane gel. We plan to compare its performance in vitro and in vivo to FN coating of this graft. Although the material evenly coats a plastic culture dish, the uniform coating of ePTFE grafts for in vivo applications is problematic (29). Incubation of the gel-filled graft holds the most promise for establishing a smooth luminal surface on ePTFE.

It remains to be seen if this surface will improve the adhesion and growth of cells in vitro, as well as improve the retention of seeded cells in vivo. Platelet adhesiveness, in the absence of von Willebrand factor and FN, may also be diminished (32).

3. Endothelial Cell Lining

References

1. Berger K, Sauvage LR, Rao AM, Wood SJ. Healing of arterial prostheses in man: its incompleteness. Ann Surg 175, 118, 1972.

2. Herring M, Gardner A, Glover J. A single-staged technique for seeding vascular grafts with autogenous endothelium. Surgery 84, 498, 1978.

3. Graham LM, Burkel WE, Ford JW, Vinter DW, Kahn RH, Stanley JC. Immediate seeding of enzymatically derived endothelium in Dacron vascular grafts. Early experimental studies with autologous canine cells. Arch Surg 115, 1289, 1980.

4. Kempczimski RF, Rosenman JE, Pearce WH, Roedersheimer LR, Berlatzky Y, Ramalanjaona G. Endothelial cell seeding of a new PTFE vascular prostheses. J Vasc Surg 2, 424, 1985.

5. Douville EC, Kempczinski RF, Birinyi LK, Ramalanjaona GG. Impact of endothelial cell seeding on long-term patency and subendothelial proliferation in a small-calibre highly porous polytetrafluoroethylene graft. J Vasc Surg 5, 544, 1987.

6. Birinyi LK, Douville EC, Lewis SA, Bjornson HS, Kempczinski RF. Increased resistance to bacteremic graft infection after endothelial seeding. J Vasc Surg 5, 193, 1987.

7. Rosenman JE, Kempczinski RF, Pearce WH, Silberstein EB. Kinetics of endothelial cell seeding. J Vasc Surg 2, 778, 1985.

8. Macarak EJ, Howard PS. Adhesion of endothelial cells to extracellular matrix proteins. J Cell Phys 116, 76, 1983.

9. Kefalides NA, Alper R, Clark CC. Biochemistry and metabolism of basement membranes. Int Rev Cyto 61, 167, 1979.

10. Morrison PR, Edsall JT, Miller SG. Preparation and properties of serum and plasma proteins. XVIII. The separation of purified fibrinogen from fraction I of human plasma. J Am Chem Soc 70, 3103, 1948.

11. Pearlstein E, Gold LI, Garcia-Pardo A. Fibronectin: a review of its structure and biological activity. Mol Cell Biochem 29, 103, 1980.

12. Boselli JM, Macarak EJ, Clark CC, Brownell AG, Martinez-Hernandez A. Fibronectin: its relationship to basement membranes. I. Light microscopic studies. Collagen and Related Research 5, 391, 1981.

13. Martinez-Hernandez A, Marsh C, Clark CC, Macarak EJ, Brownell AG: Fibronectin: its relationship to basement membranes. II. Ultrastructural studies in rat kidney. Collagen and Related Res 5, 405, 1981.

14. Shields R, Pollock K. The adhesion of BHK and PyBHK cells to the substratum. Cell 3, 31, 1974.

15. Ramalanjaona G, Kempczinski RF, Rosenman JE, Douville EC, Silberstein EB. The effect of fibronectin coating on endothelial cell kinetics in polytetrafluoroethylene grafts. J Vasc Surg 3, 264, 1986.

16. Plow EF, Ginsberg MH. Specific and saturable binding of plasma fibronectin to thrombo-stimulated human platelets. J Biol Chem 256, 9477, 1981.

17. Seeger JM, Klingman N. Improved endothelial cell seeding with cultured cells and fibronectin-coated grafts. Surg Res 38, 641, 1985.

3. Endothelial Cell Lining

18. Kempczinski RF, Ramalanjaona GR, Douville EC, Silberstein EB. Thrombogenicity of a fibronectin-coated, experimental polytetrafluoroethylene graft. Surgery 101, 439, 1987.

19. Pierschbacher MD, Ruoslahti E. Cell attachment activity of fibronectin can be duplicated by small synthetic fragments of the molecule. Nature 309, 30, 1984.

20. Hasson JE, Wiebe DH, Sharefkin JB, Abbott WM. Migration of adult human vascular endothelial cells: Effect of extracellular matrix proteins. Surgery 100, 384, 1986.

21. Hasson JE, Wiebe DH, Sharefkin JB, D'Amore PA, Abbott WM. Use of tritiated thymidine as a marker to compare the effects of matrix proteins on adult human vascular endothelial cell attachment: Implications for seeding of vascular prostheses. Surgery 100, 884, 1986.

22. Jarrell BE, Williams SK, Solomon L, Speicher L, Koolpe E, Radomski J, Carabasi RA, Greener D, Rosato FE. Use of an endothelial monolayer on a vascular graft prior to implantation. Temporal dynamics and compatibility with the operating room. Ann Surg 203, 671, 1986.

23. Zacharias RK, Kirkman TR, Clowes AW. Mechanism of healing in synthetic grafts. J Vasc Surg 6, 429, 1987.

24. Clowes AW, Zacharias RK, Kirkman TR. Early endothelial coverage of synthetic arterial grafts: porosity revisited. Am J Surg 153, 501, 1987.

25. Williams SK, Jarrell BE, Friend L, Radomski JS, Carabasi RA, Koolpe E, Mueller SN, Thornton SC, Marinucci T, Levine E. Adult human endothelial cell compatibility with prosthetic graft material. J Surg Res 38, 618, 1985.

26. Jarrell BE, Williams SK, Solomon L, Speicher L, Koolpe E, Radomski J, Carabasi RA, Greener D, Rosato FE. Use of an endothelial monolayer on a vascular graft prior to implantation. Temporal dynamics and compatibility with the operating room. Ann Surg 203, 671, 1986.

27. Foxall TL, Auger KR, Callow AD, Libby P. Adult human endothelial cell coverage of small-calibre Dacron and polytetrafluoroethylene vascular prostheses in vitro. J Surg Res 41, 158, 1986.

28. Sentissi JM, Ramberg K, O'Donnell Jr. TF, Connolly RJ, Callow AD. The effect of flow on vascular endothelial cells grown in tissue culture on polytetrafluoroethylene grafts. Surgery 99, 337, 1986.

29. Anderson JS, Price TM, Hanson SR, Harker LA. In vitro endothelialization of small-calibre vascular grafts. Surgery 101, 577, 1987.

30. Form DM, Pratt BM, Madri JA. Endothelial cell proliferation during angiogenesis. In Vitro modulation by basement membrane components. Lab Invest 55, 521, 1986.

31. Kleinman HK, McGarvey ML, Hassell JR, Star VL, Cannon FB, Laurie GW, Martin GR. Basement membrane complexes with biological activity. Biochemistry 25, 312, 1986.

32. Houdjik WPM, Groot PG de, Nievelstein PFEM, Sakariassen KS, Sixma JJ. Subendothelial proteins and platelet adhesion: von Willebrand cactor and Fibronectin, not thrombospondin are involved in platelet adhesion to extracellular matrix of human vascular endothelial cells. Arteriosclerosis 6, 24, 1986.

3.6.2. Surface Covering Precoating Procedures Enhance Adherence and Spreading of Seeded Endothelial Cells on PTFE Vascular Prostheses

*J Kähler [1], P Zilla [2], R Fasol [2], M Deutsch [3]

[1] Department of Surgery 2, Univ of Vienna, Austria
*(This is the MD thesis of Jan Kähler, University of Saarland, Homburg/Saar, Federal Republic of Germany)
[2] Department of Cardio-Thoracic Surgery, Groote Schuur Hospital, Medical School, University of Cape Town, South Africa
[3] Department of Cardiovascular Surgery, Provincial Hospital Wels, Austria.

In arterial vessels the high shear stress on endothelial cells is successfully resisted by a mechanical and a statical principle. The mechanical principle is the optimal relation between attachment and resistance area - which is in vivo ideally solved by the flattened, longitudinal alignment of spread endothelial cells (1). The statical principle is the well-differentiated intracellular cytoskeleton, which guarantees better surface attachment as well as anchorage within the monolayer formation. If new endothelium develops on a blood exposed surface, the two principles do not simultaneously apply. In contrast to cell spreading, the differentiation of the cytoskeleton only begins after confluent monolayer growth is achieved (2,3).

For this reason cell spreading remains a primary principle of cell attachment during the period of pre-confluence. However - prior to spreading - endothelial cells must find specific binding sites at the surface of the substrate which are a prerequisite for the primary adherence (4). Therefore, an ideal underlying substrate must facilitate both - primary adherence and cell spreading.

In spite of the importance of these two principles, they were only partially considered in endothelial cell seeding of vascular prostheses. Although the requirement for a protein precoating of the prosthetic surface was often demonstrated (5,6,7,8) only a small number of comparative studies is available (6,9,10,11). Therefore, after more than ten years of attempts to create an endothelial cell lining on synthetic vascular grafts there is still uncertainty concerning the ideal precoating substrate. In vivo, endothelial cells are known to rest on the complex connective tissue structure of the subendothelium. This basement membrane has been shown to be composed of several macromolecules such as collagens, glycosaminoglycans and the two glycoproteins fibronectin and laminin (12). For endothelial

3. Endothelial Cell Lining

cell seeding the ideal combination of these substrate should result in a high 'effective cell innoculum' as well as limited thrombogenicity. The 'effective innoculum' represents those endothelial cells which remain on the graft surface after the initial cell loss. This determinant is mainly dependent on the number of seeded cells, the primary adherence immediately after seeding and the shear stress resistance after reconstitution of blood flow. While the primary adherence seems to be a matter of adhesive glycoproteins (13,14), the shear stress resistance might also be influenced by the surface structure. A number of experiments indicate that a negligible cell loss occurs on smooth covered substrates (15,16,17), while a high detachment rate is found on uncovered glycoprotein coated prostheses (6,8,18). In the majority of experiments, smooth surfaces were achieved by whole blood preclotting (6,10) because surface-covering basement membrane compounds like different collagen types had for a long time the stigma of potential thrombogenicity. However, the increased number of comercially available collagen grafts might have encouraged some research groups to investigate the properties of collagen for seeding purposes (9,10, 16,17,19). Since one possible explanation for better cell attachment in smooth surfaces might be a larger initial attachment area, a comparative study should consider both, the attachment rate and the extent of endothelial cell spreading. For this reason we determined the primary adherence together with the average cell area on a variety of substrate combinations. To include fibrin without the negative effect of cellular blood compounds (20,21) in this study, we used a special dilution of a clinically approved fibrin glue (15,22). Standardized seeding conditions were provided by using a microprocessor controlled seeding device which guaranteed a constant rotation speed, a constant temperature of 37°C, and a 5% CO_2 atmosphere for the bicarbonate buffer (15,18,22).

Seeding Experiments on Various Precoating Substrates

A standard enzymatic harvest technique using 0.1% collagenase (CLS II; Cooper) was applied for the establishment of primary cultures from umbilical vein endothelial cells (23). Primary cultures were grown to confluence in 75 cm^2 tissue culture flasks and fed three times a week.

Six millimeter reinforced PTFE grafts (GORE Ges mbH, FRG) of 10 cm length were used for each experiment.

Precoating with fibronectin, laminin, collagen type I/III, and fibrin glue was performed by forcing these substrates through the interstices of the PTFE graft. A special design of a glass plug was inserted into the graft at one end and fixed from the outside by means of a Teflon ligament; the other end of the graft was clamped. A standard luer syringe which fitted exactly into the glass plug contained the various substrate solutions. For fibronectin precoating, 1 mg human fibronectin (HFN) was diluted in 25 ml calcium/magnesium free PBS to achieve a final concentration of 40 ug/ml. After the HFN solution was forced through the interstices of the PTFE material, the graft was incubated in this solution for another 60 minutes at room temperature (rt). The same precoating procedure as for HFN was applied for laminin, which was also diluted to a final concentration of 40 ug/ml. A smooth surface covering collagen matrix was achieved by forcing a commercially available mixture of type I (95%) and type III (5%) collagen through the graft interstices. After the procedure was repeated 3 times, excess collagen was removed from the graft lumen by using a size 3 fogarty catheter. Following a 60 minutes incubation at 37°C, the whole procedure was repeated twice. Subsequently the graft was airdried for 20 hours at rt. At the end of the air-drying procedure these grafts were either post-coated with HFN, laminin or type IV collagen. Type IV collagen surfaces were additionally post-treated with either HFN or laminin.

As an alternative approach to achieve a smooth surface, a special dilution of clinically approved fibrin glue was used as previously described (15, 22). After the fibrinogen compound was repeatedly forced through the inter-stices of the PTFE material, this low viscosity solution was allowed to run out and the whole graft was subsequently placed into the thrombin solution for 30 minutes at rt. Subsequently the graft was twice rinsed with calcium/magnesium free PBS (Flow) before the whole procedure was repeated.

Prior to cell seeding - during the centrifugation of the trypsin/serum suspension - an initial cell count was performed to allow the adjustment of the cell suspension to the seeding density of 3×10^4 EC/cm^2. To guarantee an even distribution of EC a rotation device (17) was used. After the cell suspension was filled into the graft, twelve 10 cm samples of each group were rotated for 60 minutes at 4 rph.

Immediately after rotation the graft was briefly rinsed in complete medium (37°C) and sliced into 4 equal pieces. One of them was incubated in 0.1 M citric acid/crystal violet solution (30 min) (24), and a second one was processed for scanning electron microscopy, using the method of Schroetter (25). The remaining two samples were incubated for another 3 hours in complete medium at 37°C. At the end of that period, one sample was treated with 0.1 M citric acid/crystal violet solution (30 min) and the other was processed for scanning electron microscopy (SEM). After incubation in the citric acid/crystal violet solution, 3 crystal violet portions of each sample were counted in the haemocytometer. The reliability of this procedure was previously assessed by SEM investigations of untreated and crystal violet treated grafts (15,26).

From each sample processed for SEM, scanning electron micrographs were taken from 8 random sites of the specimen at a magnification of 5×10^2. 13×18 cm prints of these micrographs were then used for the determination of the percentage of spreading cells and for the morphometric analysis of the spreading area of endothelial cells. Cells were considered as non spread when they were spheroid without a visible cell margin. The morphometric measurement of the cell area was done by means of a MOP-device (Kontron).

Surface Characteristics of Precoating Substrates

Since both glycoproteins - fibronectin and laminin - were molecularly bound to PTFE, the SEM appearance of the graft surface was unchanged after precoating with one of these substrates.

The two interstices filling matrices - the collagen type I/III mixture as well as the fibrin glue - produced similar surface

3. Endothelial Cell Lining

structures: both materials formed a densely woven mat that completely covered the underlying PTFE material. In a few areas the nodular structure of the PTFE graft could be recognized where the feltwork was thinner, but the majority of the graft area showed a grossly even distributed layer. In a blind study no clear distinction between the two substrates was possible. Both surfaces were characterized by alternating areas of an extremely fine meshwork of thin fibrils, a coarser meshwork filled with amorphous smooth structures or smooth amorphous sections where no fibrillar structures were present at all. Under low magnification the SEM appearance of the surfaces was generally smooth, only occasionally showing shallow folds parallel to the nodes of the graft material. When the type I/III collagen matrix was subsequently treated either with type IV collagen, HFN or laminin, the ultrastructural appearance was unaltered.

Primary Adherence of Seeded Endothelial Cells (Figure 140a)

After 60 minutes of microprocessor controlled seeding of 3×10^4 EC/cm^2 the significantly best cell adherence of $55.6 \pm 13.5\%$ was found on HFN coated type I/III collagen (p<0.5) (Figure 140a). In analogy the second best attachment rate of $50.2 \pm 16.1\%$ was found, when the same type I/III collagen matrix was coated with the other major glycoprotein laminin. Endothelial cell adherence on this substrate was significantly (p<0.05) better than on the remaining substrates with the exception of fibrin glue and purely fibronectin coated PTFE. On fibrin glue, an adherence rate of $43 \pm 14\%$ was still at least 10% higher than on 4 of the other substrates.

Quantification of Spreading Cells (Figure 140c,d)

After 60 minutes of graft rotation fibrin glue showed by far the highest percentage of spreading cells ($84 \pm 12\%$) which was significantly higher than on any other substrate (p<0.05) (Figure 140c). If either PTFE alone or the type I/III collagen matrix was coated with one of the two glycoproteins fibronectin or laminin, the mean percentage of spreading cells ranged between 72 and 54%. The significantly lowest percentage of spreading cells was found on substrates which contained type IV collagen. On these substrates more than 72% of adherent endothelial cells were not spreading at that point of time.

After a further incubation period of 3 hours fibrin glue still showed the highest percentage of spreading cells ($97 \pm 2\%$), but the difference from the other substrates was much less distinct than immediately after seeding. Even on surfaces containing type IV collagen more than 62% of adherent cells showed criteria of spreading (Figure 140d).

Morphometrical Analysis of the Spreading Area and Morphology of Seeded EC (Figure 140b)

Immediately after 60 minutes of rotation the average cell area ranged from 177 ± 121 um2 on type I/III collagen + laminin to 258 ± 127 um2 on fibrin glue (Figure 140b). No significant differences were found between the various substrates, with the exception of a far lower spreading area on substrates containing type IV collagen.

In contrast to the cell area the morphological appearance of spreading cells distinctly differed between smooth surfaces and uncovered glycoprotein

3. Endothelial Cell Lining

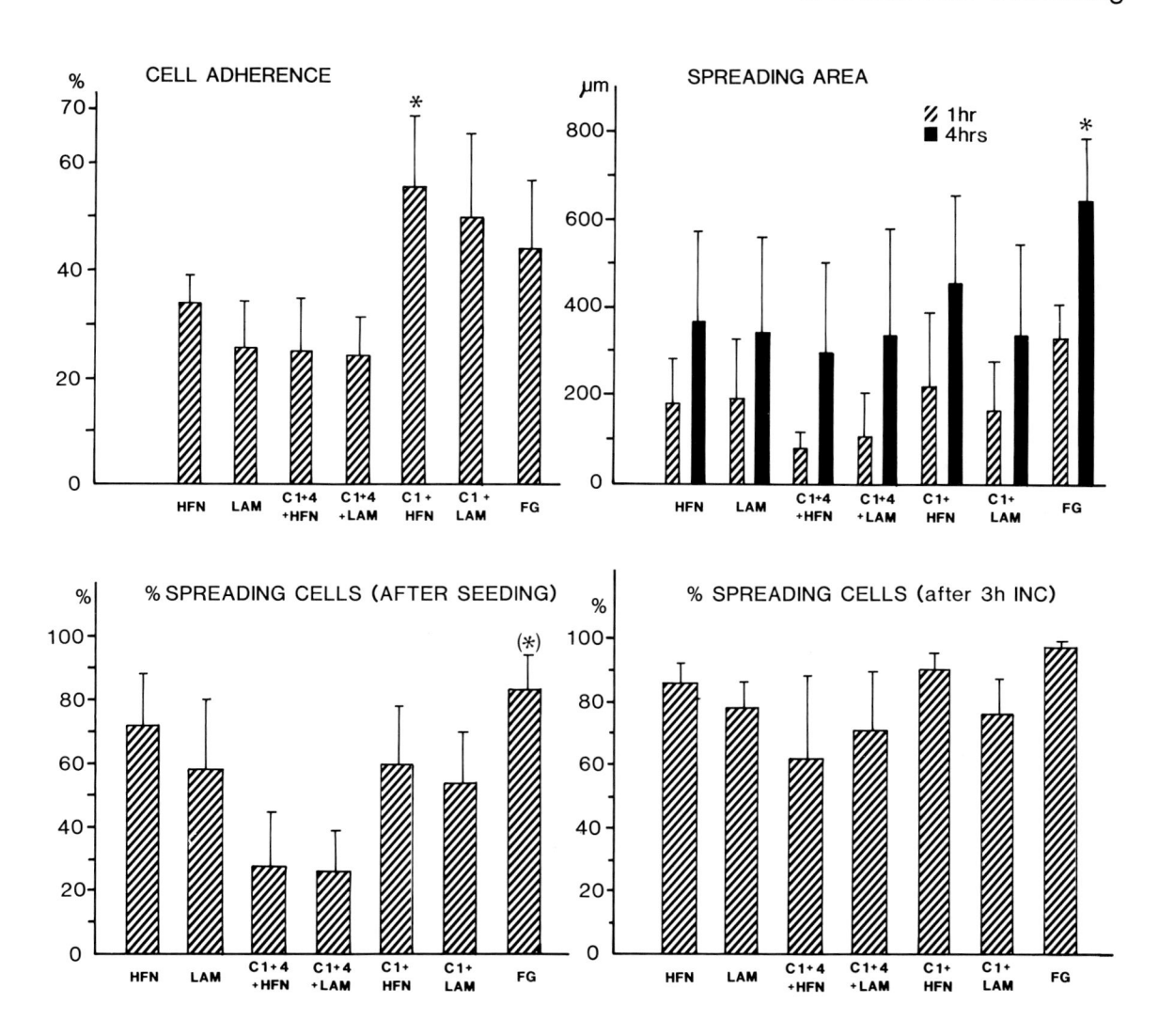

Fig. 140 Comparison of primary attachment and cell spreading of HUVEC after microprocessor controlled seeding onto PTFE grafts, precoated with 7 different substrates or substrate combinations.

a) (top left) Primary attachment after 60 minutes of seeding: the significantly highest percentage of seeded cells adhered to type I/III collagen, postcoated with human fibronectin (*) = $p<0.05$). Type I/III collagen postcoated with laminin was significantly better than all remaining substrates, with the exception of PTFE plus fibronectin (*) = $p<0.05$, HFN excluded). The far worst result were achieved on type IV collagen postcoated with the one of two glycoproteins fibronectin or laminin. **b) (top right)** Cell area after 60 minutes of seeding (1 hour) and after 3 hours of subsequent incubation (4 hours). After seeding (1 hour), the best cell spreading was found on fibrin glue, but none of the differences was statistical significant. After 3 hours of subsequent incubation (4 hours), the average cell area on all substrates was increased by 135%. With the exception of fibronectin coated type I/III collagen, the spreading area on fibrin glue was now significantly larger than on the other substrates ($p<0.05$).

c) (bottom left) left Quantification of spreading cells after the 60 minutes seeding procedure. At that time the highest percentage of spreading cells was by far found on fibrin glue ($p<0.05$). **d) (bottom right)** Quantification of spreading cells after an incubation period of 3 hours shows a much less distinct difference between the various substrates. None of the differences proved statistically significant.

coated PTFE surfaces: while endothelial cells were evenly distributed and ubidirectionally spreading on smooth surfaces, they were predominantly found to adhere to the nodes of the PTFE structure, along which they spread to an elongated shape.

After 3 hours of incubation the spreading area on fibrin glue was 623 ± 218 um2. With the exception of HFN coated type I/III collagen - where the average cell area was 467 ± 208 um2 - this value was significantly higher than on all other substrates.

Overall, the cell area of endothelial cells increased in average by 135 ±70% during the three hours of incubation.

In summary, the best primary adherence was found on fibronectin and laminin coated type I/III collagen, followed by fibrin glue. Considering fibronectin as the major principle of cell adhesion (27), the high primary adherence of endothelial cells on HFN coated type I/III collagen and on fibrin glue is understandable. In contrast to the non-specific, hydrophobic protein-substratum interaction between fibronectin and PTFE (21), fibrin and type I collagen form specific, covalent bonds with fibronectin (21,28).

The factor XIIIa mediated covalent binding of fibronectin to fibrin was previously achieved by whole-blood preclotting. The disadvantage of that form of fibrin application was the entrapment of cellular blood elements which were shown to reduce the prostacyclin production (20) and the attachment of endothelial cells (21). Therefore, we used clinically approved fibrin glue which was cell-free but contained sufficient amounts of factor XIII and fibronectin.

In collagen matrices, almost exclusively type I collagen binds fibronectin covalently, while type IV collagen binds the other glycoprotein laminin (29). The specificity of these reactions is high and the crossreactivity is therefore poor (30). In comparative studies between the two glycoproteins, the cell adherence on laminin was worse than on fibronectin (10,31). This confirms our results where the primary adherence was lowest on laminin coated type IV collagen. The underlying type I/III collagen had only surface smoothing purposes. The very low specificity of HFN to type IV collagen explains the low cell adherence on HFN coated type IV collagen and the equally low specificity of laminin to type I collagen could in turn explain the high adherence rate on laminin coated type I/III collagen: since the HFN binding sites of type I collagen were not occupied by laminin, they were free for that fibronectin, which was applied with the serum containing cell suspension. This would mean that the laminin coated type I/III collagen surfaces were effectively HFN coated type I/III collagen surfaces. This is in accordance with previous studies (9,31) which also achieved highest adherence rates on type I collagen. Since these studies used serum containing cell suspensions too, there was enough fibronectin available to produce fibronectin coated type I collagen as well.

Our quantitative determination of the percentage of spreading cells significantly favoured the fibrin glue matrix immediately after seeding. However, after 3 hours of incubation the differences between the various substrates were far less distinct and not significant, although, the highest percentage of spreading cells was also found on fibrin glue followed by HFN coated type I/III collagen.

The morphometric measurement of the attachment area of adherent cells again showed the best spreading on these two substrates, but only after 3 hours of further incubation was the superiority of fibrin glue statistically significant, followed by HFN coated type I/III collagen.

However, the fact that a 135% increase in the attachment area could be achieved by 3 hours of incubation should lead us to reconsider the single-staged procedure of seeding. The vein harvest might easily be performed a few hours prior to the operation under local anesthesia. A prolonged seeding procedure would then result in apparently better cell adherence.

When both types of surface structures were investigated under the scanning electron microscope (SEM), endothelial cells were evenly distributed on smooth surfaces while they were almost exclusively found on the nodal structure of uncovered PTFE. The fact that cell adherence rarely occurred in the internodal spaces could explain the relatively low initial cell adherence on uncovered PTFE. Moreover, cell spreading occurred ubidirectionally on smooth surfaces but also primarily along the nodes on uncovered PTFE. This resulted in elongated cells which were aligned at 90° to the theoretical blood stream. It seems likely that this cell orientation has a diminished shear stress resistance. However, a better shear stress resistance of endothelial cells on smooth surfaces was already indicated in earlier studies. In a comparative study, the cell loss from HFN coated PTFE was far higher than from a smooth polyester surface (6) or from a smooth whole blood clotted surface (18), and our own group found an almost complete cell loss after 16 hours of shear stress exposure of in vitro lined, only fibronectin-coated PTFE grafts (17). In contrast we found an intact monolayer even after 48 hours of pulsatile shear stress exposure, if the underlying substrate was smooth fibrin glue (15). Other groups found shear stress resistant monolayer after in vitro lining of smooth, HFN coated type I collagen matrices (16,17).

In summary, the results of our study indicate that on the one hand a smooth surface alone is not sufficient enough to provide a large spreading area, if the substrate type is not favouring cell adhesion. This was apparent on the smooth type IV collagen containing matrices. On the other hand, the cell spreading is much more advanced on smooth surfaces, if the substrate type enhances cell adhesion. This was the case with fibrin glue and HFN coated type I/III collagen.

Thus, endothelial cell seeding should preferably be performed on smooth surfaces which were shown to provide excellent adhesion and spreading properties. According to the present study the most suitable substrates seem to be fibrin glue and HFN coated, denatured type I/III collagen. The disadvantage of fibrin glue might be a fibrinolytical degradation. Although we could demonstrate that the inhibition of fibrinolysis by epsilon-amino-capronic-acid guarantees undegraded fibrin layers even 11 days after endothelial cell confluence is reached (15), the proof for longterm persistence is outstanding. The HFN coated type I/III collagen matrix might probably be therefore the better choice. Since the drying process denatures the collagen, its own thrombogenicity is expected to be reduced (32), while the thrombogenicity of the fibronectin post-treatment (33) was shown to be tolerable (5).

3. Endothelial Cell Lining

References

1. Langille BL, Adamson SL. Relationship between blood flow direction and endothelial cell orientation at arterial branch sites in rabbits and mice. Circ Res 48, 481, 1981.

2. Wong MKK, Gotlieb AI. Endothelial cell monolayer integrity: characterization of dense peripheral band of microfilaments. Arteriosclerosis 6, 212, 1986.

3. Schnittler HJ, Franke RP, Fuhrmann R, Petermeyer M, Jung F, Mittermayer C, Drenckhahn D. Influence of various substrates on the actin filament system of cultured human vascular endothelial cells exposed to fluid shear stress. In: Endothelialization of vascular grafts, Zilla P, Fasol R, Deutsch M (Eds), Karger, Basel, pp 183, 1987.

4. Shields R, Pollock K. The adhesion of BHK and PyBHK cells to the substratum. Cell 3, 31, 1974.

5. Seeger JM, Klingman N. Improved endothelial cell seeding with cultured cells and fibronectin coated grafts. J Surg Res 38, 641, 1985.

6. Kessler KA, Herring MB, Arnold MP, Glover JL, Park Hee-Myung, Helmus MN, Bendick PJ. Enhanced strength of endothelial attachment of polyester elastomer and polytetrafluoro-ethylene graft surfaces with fibronectin substrate. J Vasc Surg 3, 58, 1986.

7. Fasol R, Zilla P, Groscurth P, Wolner E, Moser R. Experimental in vitro cultivation of human endothelial cells on artificial surfaces. Trans Am Soc Artif Intern Organs 31, 276, 1985.

8. Ramalanjona G, Kempczinski R, Rosenman JE, Douville EC, Silberstein EB. The effect of fibronectin coating on endothelial cell kinetics in polytetrafluoroethylene grafts. J Vasc Surg 3, 264, 1986.

9. Williams SK, Jarrell BE, Friend L, Radomski JS, Carabasi A, Koolpe E, Mueller SN, Thornton SC, Marinucci T, Levine E. Adult human endothelial cell compatibility with prosthetic graft material. J Surg Res 38, 618, 1985.

10. Koeveker GB, Graham LM, Burkel WE, Sell R, Magill T, Stanley JC. PTFE grafts in an AV shunt model: influence of different precoating and blood preclotting procedures on endothelial cell attachment. In: Endothelialization of vascular grafts, Zilla P, Fasol R, Deutsch M (Eds), Karger, Basel, pp 177, 1987.

11. Radomski JS, Jarrell BE, Williams SK et al. Initial adherence of human capillary endothelial cells to Dacron. J Surg Res 42, 133, 1987.

12. Hay ED. Extracellular matrix. J Cell Biol 91, 205S, 1981.

13. Kleinman HK, Klebe RJ, Martin GR. Role of collagenous matrices in the adhesion and growth of cells. J Cell Biol 88, 473, 1981.

14. Yamada KM and Olden K. Fibronectins - adhesive glycoproteins of cell surface and blood. Nature 275, 179, 1978.

15. Zilla P, Fasol R, Preiss P, Kadletz M, Schima H, Tsangaris S, Groscurth P. Use of fibrin glue as a substrate for in vitro endothelialization of PTFE vascular grafts. Surgery (in press)

16. Foxall TL, Auger KR, Callow AD, Libby P. Adult human endothelial cell coverage of small-caliber Dacron and Polytetrafluoroethylene vascular prostheses in vitro. J Surg Res 41, 158, 1986.

17. Shindo S, Takagi A, Whittemore AD. Improved patency of collagen-impregnated grafts after in vitro autogenous endothelial cell seeding. J Vasc Surg 6, 325, 1987.

3. Endothelial Cell Lining

18. Kadletz M, Moser R, Preiss P, Zilla P, Fasol R. In vitro lining of fibronectin coated PTFE grafts with cryopreserved saphenous vein endothelial cells. Thorac Cardiovasc Surg 35, 143, 1987.

19. Hasson JE, Wiebe DH, Abbott WM. Adult human vascular endothelial cell attachment and migration on novel bioabsorbable polymers. Arch Surg 122, 428, 1987.

20. Hope W, Martin TJ, Chesterman CN, Morgan FJ. Nature 282, 210, 1979.

21. Klebe RJ, Bently KL, Schoen RP. Adhesive substrates for fibronectin. J Cell Physiol 109, 481, 1981.

22. Zilla P, Fasol R, Deutsch M, Fischlein T, Minar E, Hammerle A, Krupicka O, Kadletz M. Endothelial cell seeding of PTFE vascular grafts in humans: a preliminary report. J Vasc Surg 6, 535, 1987.

23. Jaffe EA, Nachman RL, Becker CG, Minick CR. Culture of human endothelial cells derived from umbilical veins. Identification of morphologic and immunologic criteria. J Clin Invest 52, 2745, 1973.

24. Watkins MB, Sharefkin JB, Zajtchuk R, Maciag TM, D'Amore P, Ryan UN, van Wart H, Rich N. Adult human saphenous vein endothelial cells: assessment of their reproductive capacity for use in endothelial seeding of vascular prostheses. J Surg Res 36, 588, 1984.

25. Schroetter D, Spiess E, Pawletz N. Benker R. A procedure for rupture free preparation of confluently grown monolayer cells for scanning electron microscopy. J Scan Electr Microscop Techn 1, 219, 1984.

26. Grimm M, Zilla P, Fasol R, Preiss P, Groscurth P, Krupicka O, Krausler S. Growth properties of cultured human endothelial cells on differently treated artificial heart materials. (manuscript submitted)

27. Pearlstein E, Gold LI, Garcia-Pardo A. Fibronectin: a review of its structure and biological activity. Mol Cell Biocrson JS, Price TM, Hanson SR, Harker LA. In vitro endothelialization of small-caliber vascular grafts. Surgery 101, 577, 1987.

28. Engvall E, Rouslathi E. Binding of soluble form of fibroblast surface protein, fibronectin to collagen. Int J Cancer 20, 1, 1977.

29. Murray JC, Liotta LA, Rennard SI, Martin GR. Collagen adhesion: characterization of murine metastatic and non-metastatic tumor cells in vitro. Canc Res 40, 347, 1980.

30. Aumailley M, Timpl R. Attachment of cells to basement membrane collagen type IV. J Cell Biol 103, 1569, 1986.

31. Anderson JS, Price TM, Hanson SR, Harker LA. In vitro endothelialization of small caliber vascular grafts. Surgery 101, 577, 1987.

32. Vlodavsky I, Eldor A, HyAm E, AQtzmon R, Fuks Z. Platelet interaction with the extracellular matrix produced by cultured endothelial cells: a model to study the thrombogenicity of isolated subendothelial basal lamina. Thromb Res 28, 179, 1982.

33. Kempczinski RF, Ramalanjona GR, Douville EC, Silberstein EB. Thrombogenicity of a fibronectin-coated, experimental polytetrafluoroethylene graft. Surgery 101, 439, 1987.

3.6.3. Cell Attachment Forces Regulating the Immediate Establishment of Endothelial Cell Monolayers

BE Jarrell, SK Williams, K Pratt, J Radomski, RA Carabasi

Department of Surgery, Jefferson Medical College, Philadelphia, Pennsylvania, USA

The establishment and maintenance of an endothelial cell monolayer upon a blood-contacting surface might prevent activation of the coagulation system and avoid long-term vascular implant dysfunction. Understanding the processes involved in establishing and maintaining such a monolayer requires separating the attachment process into individual steps and examining variables that might affect each of these steps. The initial steps that must be understood relate to basic physical and chemical mechanisms inherent in endothelial cell interactions with polymeric surfaces. Once these initial mechanisms are elucidated, factors that affect monolayer maintenance on the surface of a long-term implant can be examined. Because monolayer maintenance depends initially upon establishment of the monolayer, the steps leading to the formation of a monolayer will be examined in this chapter.

Establishment of a monolayer is primarily affected by the type of endothelial cell, the molecular composition of the surface, and environmental conditions that control interactions between the cell and the surface (1-4). All three factors can be manipulated to select for conditions felt to be optimal and examined using both in vitro and in vivo models. We have evaluated EC-polymer interaction using transmission electron microscopy, which has provided us with a morphological understanding of monolayer formation. For the purposes of understanding these events, we propose a general hypothesis to explain the events that take place in an in vitro model when human adult endothelial cells interact with a surface.

When endothelial cells with a specific gravity greater than the suspending medium are placed in a liquid medium overlying a surface, the force of gravity pulls the cells toward the surface. As the cells approach the surface, a variety of surface electrical and physico-chemical phenomena are present and regulate cell-surface interaction (5-7). These forces may reach equilibrium for a cell at a given distance from the surface and suspend the cell in a static position above the surface (Figure 141). To overcome this surface barrier, the human endothelial cell extends a foot process of small dimensions toward the surface (Figure 142). Once contact is made, a bond is generated between the cell and the surface (Figure 143). Cell-surface contact initiates a series of events that is associated with a message to the cell cytoskeletal structure to initiate further cell shape change. This occurs initially by a broadening to the point of attachment

3. Endothelial Cell Lining

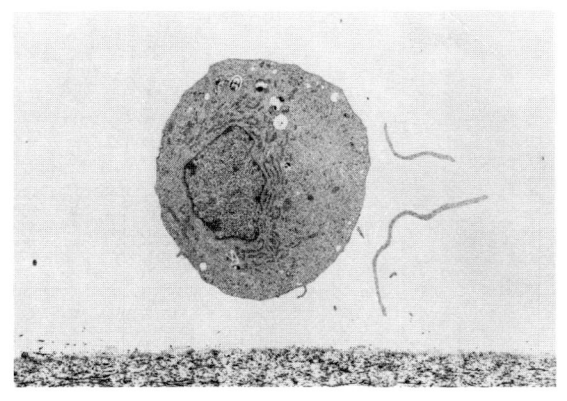

Fig. 141 Transmission electron microscopy illustrating a human endothelial cell associating with human amnion. This cell was incubated with the surface for five minutes, and resisted the shear force produced when the surface was washed with culture medium.

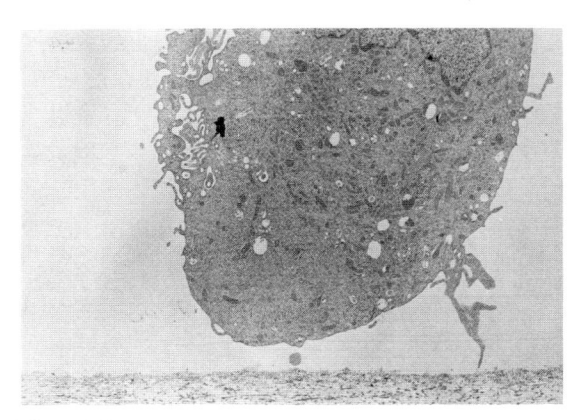

Fig. 142 The direct association of human endothelial cells with amnion is initiated by the formation of membrane pseudopodia as seen in this transmission electron micrograph.

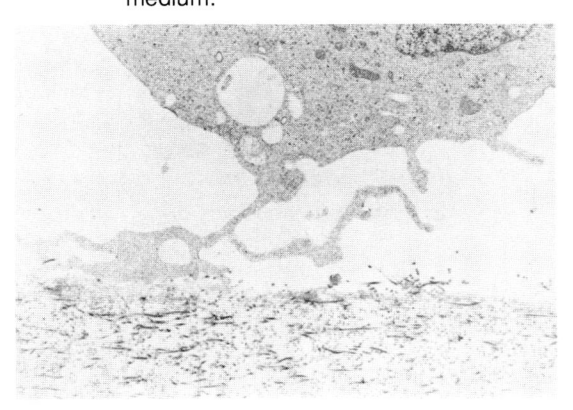

Fig. 143 Transmission electron micrograph of a human endothelial cell extending a foot process onto a human amnion surface. Direct interaction of the cell and amnion is now achieved.

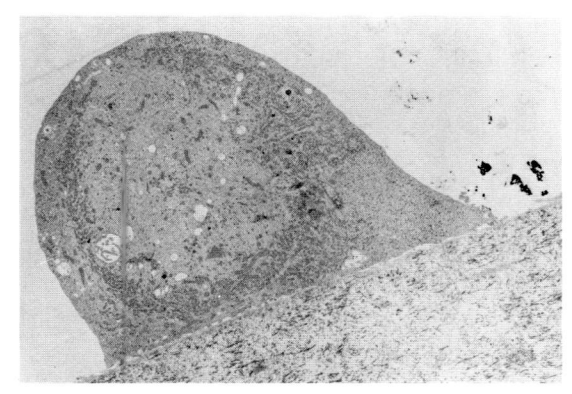

Fig. 144 Transmission electron micrograph of a human endothelial cell interacting with human amnion. This morphology is typical for cells in contact with amnion for approximately 20 minutes.

followed by a general cell shape change with spreading and flattening of the cell upon the surface (Figure 144). Cellular cytoskeletal machinery maintains cell spreading while further attachments to the surface occur. Once attached and spread, the endothelial cell extends pseudopodial processes laterally to initiate contact with neighboring cells, most likely using the same mechanisms involved in surface contact (Figure 145). Cell-cell contacts stimulate a specific junction to occur between the cells as well as inhibition of further spreading or growth.

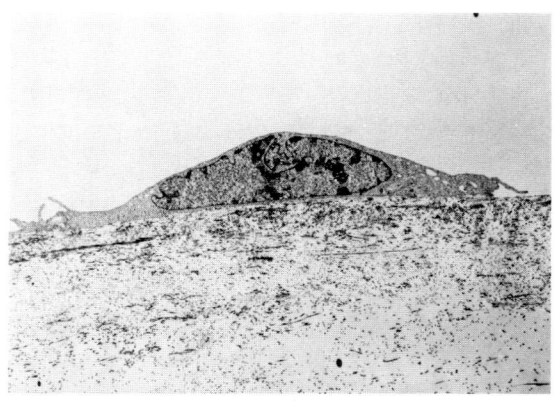

Fig. 145 Transmission electron micrograph of a human endothelial cell incubated with human amnion for 30 minutes. At this time, cells are highly shear resistant and exhibit a very close perinuclear association with the basement membrane. Cell to cell junctional associations are also visible.

3. Endothelial Cell Lining

The net result of these processes is to allow the cell to approach a surface, to attach and spread, ultimately producing complete coverage of the surface with a single layer of cells.

The morphological observations and the hypothesis suggest that there may be five different cell populations present during cell interaction with a surface (Figure 146). These populations might be identified by their relative degree of attachment to the surface at any specific point in time. The first population of cells is suspended within the liquid phase of the system. These cells are in the process of gravitating toward the surface. The time required for a cell to gravitate to a surface can be estimated using the Stoke's equation (8). In that equation the force of gravity opposes both buoyant forces and the viscous forces created during motion through the fluid. One calculation suggested that only brief times (< 5 minutes) were required for the cell to gravitate 3 mm through culture medium to a surface (9). Actual measurements have not been precisely performed, but another study suggested that up to 30 minutes may be required for this process to be complete (10).

A second population of cells is entrapped near the interface between the solid and liquid phases of the system. At this interface a force field exists for a short distance from the surface and is composed of both repulsive and attractive forces. When these forces are at equilibrium for a cell approaching the surface, the cell may stabilize in a static position close to the surface (5-7). This group of cells exists in a reversible position in that any shift of the force balance will result in movement relative to the surface. Thus changes in polymer surface, in proteins adsorbed upon the surface, in suspending fluid composition or in cell characteristics may greatly affect this equilibrium distance.

A third group of cells is composed of cells that are able to penetrate this force field by extending a foot process to the surface. These cells are presumably able to perform this task by generation of a microdomain of plasma membrane that is attractive with respect to the surface. In addition, this process may depend on cellular metabolism, requiring a chemical mediator or cytoskeletal message because of the directed nature of this foot process. The initial bond that forms between this cell and surface is undoubtedly tenuous but involves a stronger force of attachment than the

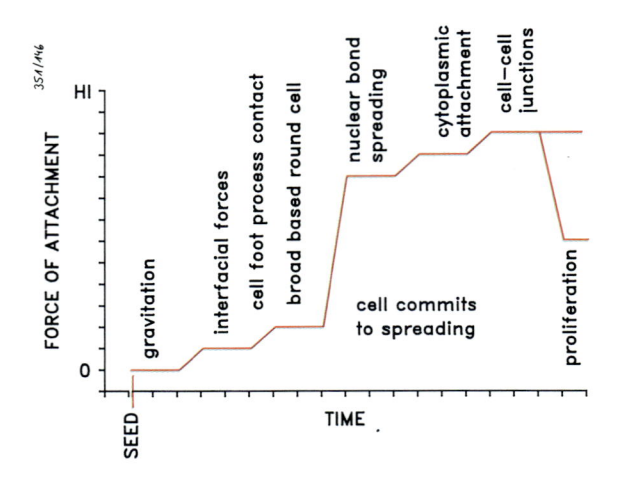

Fig. 146 A hypothetical sequence of human adult endothelial cell attachment to a surface based upon the sequence observed by electron microscopy and the force of attachment quantitated by the rotating disc assay. The principal mechanism in effect at each stage of attachment is stated above the curve. At the latest time point following cell-cell junctions, the cell can become quiescent or can undergo proliferation. If it remains quiescent, little change in attachment force will occur. If it fails to undergo contact inhibition or proliferates, a decrease in attachment force most likely occurs.

previous population. This step is also most likely reversible, although to a lesser degree than in the previous step. Directed messages from the cell surface to the cytoskeletal system are probably involved because the cell must either commit to further attachment to the surface, which involves major cytoskeletal and other changes, or detach after a finite contact time.

If the cell commits to spreading upon the surface, a fourth population of cells will be present. These cells will demonstrate a relatively strong force of attachment and will appear flattened and spread morphologically with major cytoskeletal rearrangement. Whether this process requires metabolic activity is not clear, but it undoubtedly allows the cell to greatly increase its surface area of contact with the surface. This may improve cellular ability to form specific attachment bonds as well as increase nonspecific attractive forces such as those involved with ionic bonds and interface forces.

Once spread, a fifth population of cells is composed of cells that have formed cell-to-cell junctions. During this stage, cell-surface adhesion would undergo a "maturing" process where specific cell-surface bonding occurs. In addition, adherent junctions between cells occur. These junctions serve as anchors and probably increase cellular ability to resist detachment.

In an attempt to identify these cell populations, we designed an experimental system that would allow quantitation of the force of attachment for large numbers of cells in a variety of experimental conditions and that allowed rigorous statistical evaluation of the results (9,11). The system employed a flat disc of a given surface material that allowed cell attachment to occur. Following a specified period of incubation, the disc was placed in culture medium and rotated under carefully controlled conditions. The rheology of the rotating disc has been described elsewhere by Levich (12). The shear stress at the surface of the disc is well-defined and is a linear function of the radial distance from the disc center. The center of the disc is exposed to stagnation flow that produces minimal shear stress. Thus under our current conditions, the shear stress varies from zero at the center to 90 dynes/cm^2 at a position 2 cm from the center. Edge effects are present in this model and turbulence or unspecified flow patterns can occur if certain conditions relative to the Reynold's number, boundary layer thickness, disc wobble or volume of suspending fluid are not controlled (13). In the data presented in this chapter, laminar conditions have been present. In addition, the control surface that has not been exposed to flow has yielded data essentially identical to data obtained from the center of the disc. Thus we have normalized shear stress data from radial positions on the disc to the no shear stress center of the disc.

The shear stress generated by the rotating disc is a drag force exerted upon the cells attached to the disc surface. This force is not normal to the surface and therefore does not quantitate the absolute value of the force required to detach the cell from the surface. Rather, it is a force exerted upon the elevated position of the cell that is perpendicular to the direction of flow. Shear flow over an object protruding from a surface has been evaluated (14). The drag on such a protrusion is proportional to the square of the protrusion radius when the protrusion has been idealized as a hemispherical object. In addition the object experiences

3. Endothelial Cell Lining

a torque in the direction of the flow. Thus, when cells are predominantly flattened and spread, the rotating disc system produces a relatively uniform drag tending to pull cells off the surface. Before a cell has fully flattened and is attached in a rounded condition, the drag is significantly increased compared to that seen with a fully flattened cell. In interpreting data, therefore, attachment forces can only be rigorously compared for cells with an equal degree of spreading.

Experiments were performed using the following sequence. A round piece of surface material was mounted upon a standardized disc apparatus. A tight-fitting collar was placed over the disc, creating an incubation well with the disc as its base. Any surface treatment, such as fibronectin coating, was performed and allowed to incubate for at least 12 hours to create a stable surface environment. Cultured endothelial cells were incubated with the surface of one disc for 5, 10, 15, 20 or 30 minutes within an incubator. Following incubation, the collars were removed and the discs rotated in culture medium for 30 minutes at 700 RPM. The surface was then stained with hematoxylin and the remaining cells counted using computer assisted techniques. Data for number of adherent cells was recorded as a function of incubation time as well as the radial position and hence, the corresponding shear stress conditions and detachment force on the disc.

We have used this system extensively using various types of endothelial cells, polymer surfaces and protein substrate coating. Conditions have been chosen to allow examination of the early events that occur following initiation of the incubation process. An incubation density of 2.5×10^4 cells/cm^2 was additionally chosen to minimize the formation of cell-cell junctions and thereby eliminate that population of adherent cells from the analysis. Thus the system as currently devised analyzes the force of attachment for the first four populations. Initial studies were directed at the relationship between the attachment force development as a function of time and number of cells attached. A typical example is shown in

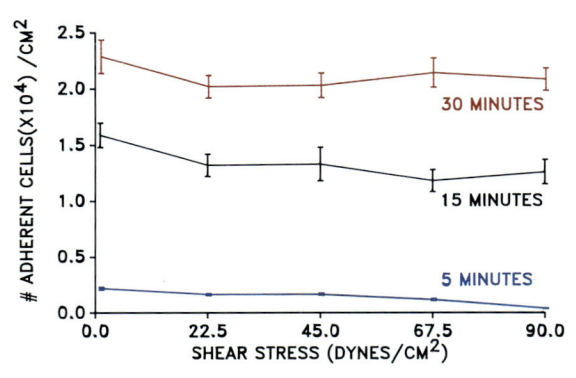

Fig. 147 Human adult endothelial cells were incubated upon fibronectin-precoated polystyrene for 5, 15 or 30 minutes followed by exposure to a shear stress ranging from 0 to 90 dynes/cm^2 for 30 minutes on the rotating disc apparatus. Cells remaining attached (mean ± standard error) to the surface were counted and recorded as a function of shear stress and incubation time.

Figure 147, where the relative attachment force is expressed as shear stress in dynes/cm^2. EC were incubated with fibronectin coated polystyrene for either 5, 15 or 30 minutes, and then exposed to the detachment force. Remaining attached cells were counted and photographed. A significant fall in adherent cell number is seen for short incubation times indicating that a population of cells exists that is weakly attached and becomes detached at high detachment forces. For cells incubated for 30 minutes, the slope of the line obtained by regression analysis does not differ significantly from zero, indicating that

3. Endothelial Cell Lining

the cells have attained a force of attachment that is uniformly expressed by all cells. Attachment rate dynamics are shown in Figure 148. A sigmoid-shaped curve is generated and is suggestive of an equilibrium process such as a Langmuir adsorptive process (15). Although time points earlier than five minutes were not obtained, it would appear that significant numbers of cells are transported to the polymer surface by five minutes. Furthermore, the curve becomes flat by 30 minutes at an equilibrium value of approximately 85% of the initial inoculation density.

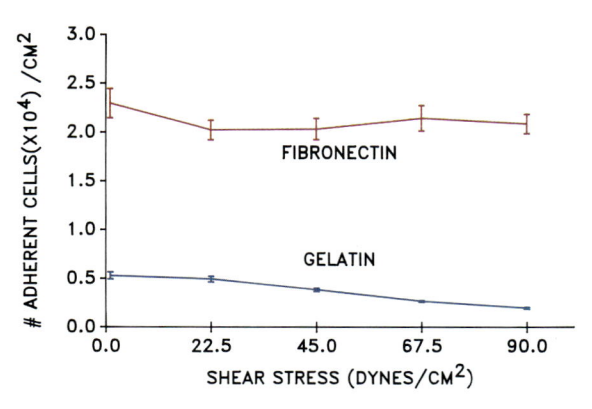

Fig. 149 Human adult endothelial cells were incubated upon fibronectin or gelatin precoated polystyrene for 30 minutes followed by exposure to shear stress ranging from 0 to 90 dynes/cm^2 for 30 minutes on the rotating disc apparatus. Cells remaining attached (mean ± standard error) to the surface were counted and recorded as a function of shear stress. Linear regression analysis and analysis of variance suggest that the slope of the curve of a fibronectin coated surface is not different from zero. For the gelatin coated surface, the slope is statistically less than zero, indicating significant cell detachment as shear stress increases.

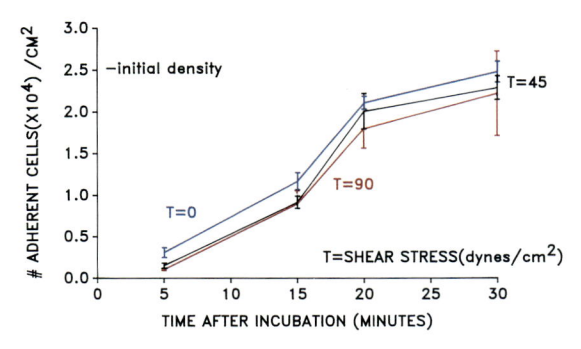

Fig. 148 Human adult endothelial cells were incubated upon fibronectin-precoated polystyrene for 5, 15, 20 or 30 minutes followed by exposure to a shear stress of 0, 45 or 90 dynes/cm^2 (T) for 30 minutes or the rotating disc apparatus. Cells remaining attached (mean ± standard error) to the surface were counted and recorded as a function of incubation time and shear stress. Rapid cell attachment occurs with a brief lag time. No difference in cell number was seen for the three shear stress regimes, suggesting a uniform force of attachment for cell populations at each time point.

The force of attachment that develops is very surface-dependent. In Figure 149, fibronectin-coated polystyrene allows firm cell attachment to occur. This firm attachment is typical of all cells attached to the surface. In contrast, gelatin-coated polystyrene allows fewer cells to attach over the same period of time. In addition, a continuum of attachment forces exists in contrast to that seen on fibronectin-coated polystyrene. Although approximately 40% of the cells are firmly attached, the remaining 60% of the cells demonstrate detachment over the range of shear stress examined, suggesting that they are in various stages of attachment. In Figure 150, the effect of underlying polymer surface was determined with respect to the number of adherent cells and their force of attachment. Although fewer cells attach to the polyethylene terephthalate (PET or Dacron) surface, the attached cells demonstrate firm attachment parameters over all shear stresses examined. This suggests that the early

3. Endothelial Cell Lining

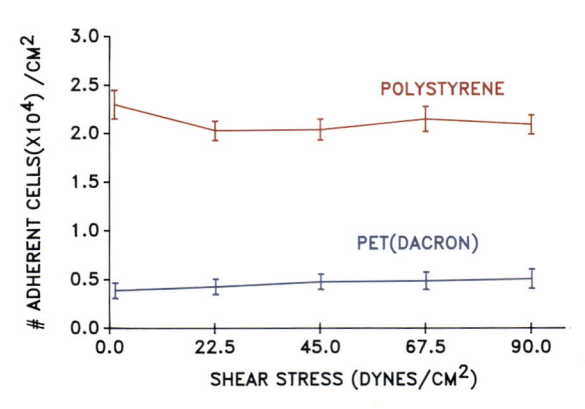

Fig. 150 Human adult endothelial cells were incubated on fibronectin coated polystyrene or polyethylene terephthalate (PET) for 30 minutes followed by exposure to shear stress ranging from 0 to 90 dynes/cm² for 30 minutes on the rotating disc apparatus. Cells remaining attached (mean ± standard error) were counted and recorded as a function of shear stress. In both cases, no significant fall in cell number was found as determined by linear regression analysis and analysis of variance.

stages of cell attachment, such as the approach to the surface and low surface area contact phases are impaired, but that once sustained contact occurs, attachment behavior is similar to that seen on fibronectin-coated polystyrene.

In order to gain insight into what these different stages of attachment might be for various cell-surface combinations, we examined cellular morphology of cells following exposure to the detachment force. Several observations are of interest in that they most likely demonstrate different aspects of cell attachment for different surfaces. For cells incubated with fibronectin-coated polystyrene, where there was no significant decrease in cell number with increasing detachment force, no reproducible change in cell shape was seen with increasing shear stress. Cell alignment in the direction of the net shear vector did not occur during the 30 minute exposure to shear stress (Figure 151). In Figure 152, cells incubated with Collagen IV/V-coated polystyrene demonstrate a significant number of rounded (e.g. not fully spread) cells in addition to spread cells. After exposure to shear stress, there was a small but statistically significant decrease in cell number. Of more interest is the observation that there are few rounded cells present at the highest shear stress position and, in fact, the cells are much more spread than at the lower shear stress position. This most likely indicates that focally adherent, rounded cells may undergo an increased rate of cell spreading if they are attached firmly enough to resist detachment. Thus a fully spread cell is not a prerequisite for the development of firm attachment forces. The opposite effect is also true in certain instances. For example, when cells are incubated on gelatin-coated polystyrene, they demonstrate a fully spread morphology. However, when they are exposed to shear stress, large numbers detach (as seen in Figure 149). Thus the presence of marked cell spreading does not guarantee firm cell adherence. Finally we have noted that although some cells demonstrate firm adherence as seen in Figure 153 at no shear stress, they display marked morphologic changes as shear stress increases. This change is marked by persistent peri-nuclear cell attachment but cytoplasm membrane streaming within the peripheral part of the cell. This suggests that there exists a differential force of attachment in different cellular regions during the process of attachment. This is not necessarily surprising in that it is well known that endothelial cells in vivo partially round up during mitosis but presumably

3. Endothelial Cell Lining

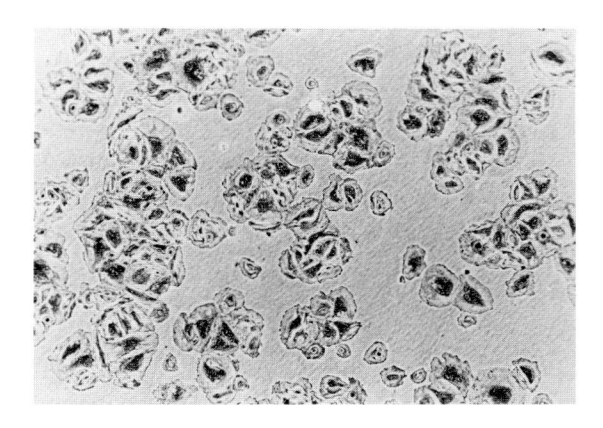

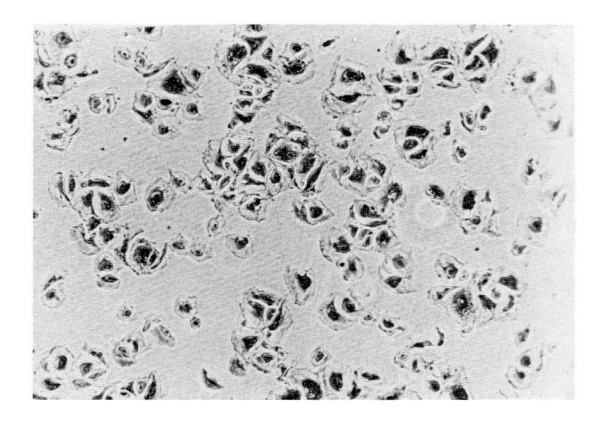

Fig.151 a **Fig.151 b**

Human adult endothelial cells were incubated on fibronectin coated polystyrene for 30 minutes followed by exposure to shear stress. In panel **a**, the cells were exposed to no shear stress and demonstrate a spread morphology. In panel **b**, the cells were exposed to a shear stress of 90 dynes/cm^2 for 30 minutes and demonstrate a morphology similar to panel **a**.

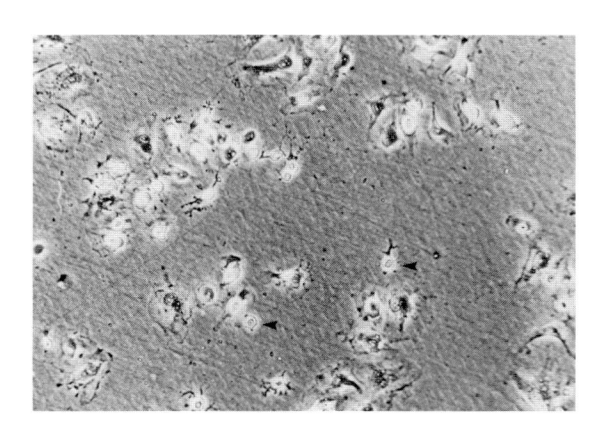

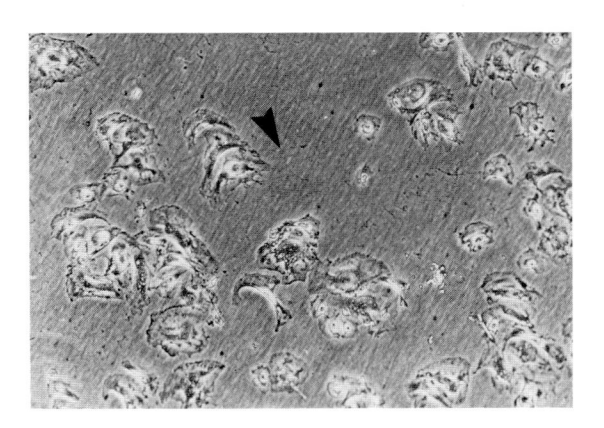

Fig.152 a **Fig.152 b**

Human adult endothelial cells were incubated on type IV/V collagen coated polystyrene for 30 minutes followed by exposure to shear stress. In panel **a**, the cells were exposed to no shear stress and demonstrate a large number of non-spread cells. The arrows depict several typical non-spread cells. In panel **b**, the cells were exposed to a shear stress of 90 dynes/cm^2 for 30 minutes. Although a small decrease in cell number was present, the morphology of those cells was quite different from the non-shear stress cells. Almost all cells were fully spread. The large arrow indicates the net shear vector.

remain attached at certain parts of the cell membrane to the vessel wall during this event. In addition, this cytoplasmic "loosening" probably occurs during the process of endothelial cell flow related reorientation. Thus the rotating disc device allows us to compare the relative difference of attachment force between the peri-nuclear and cytoplasmic part of the cell under certain conditions.

In summary, the rotating disc apparatus exerts a relative but quantifiable detachment force or drag upon cells attached to a surface. This force is less for fully spread cells but increases as the cell height protruding into the flow regime increases. Cells may be incubated for various periods of time and evaluated with respect to the force of attachment and cell morphology. Based upon these

3. Endothelial Cell Lining

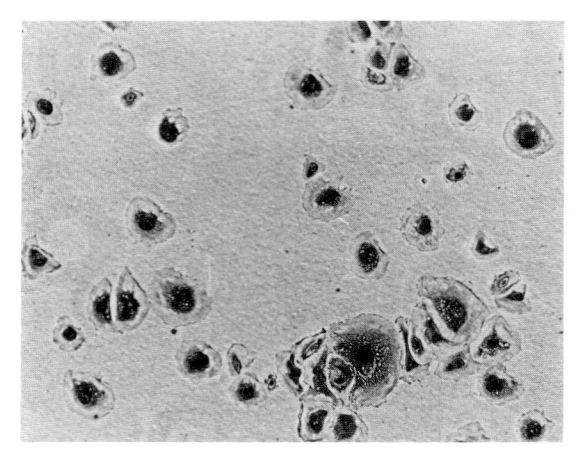

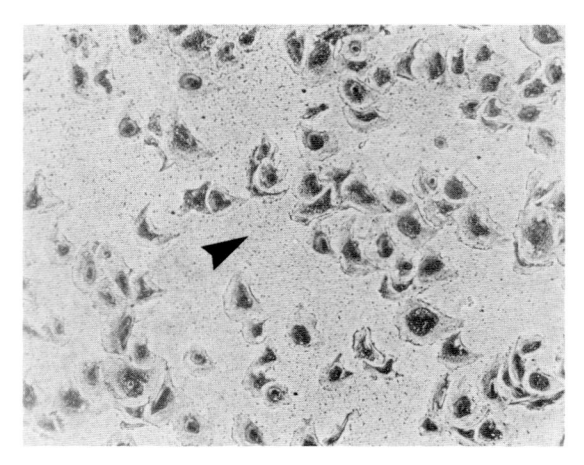

Fig. 153 a **Fig. 153 b**

Human adult endothelial cells were incubated with fibronectin-coated polystyrene for 30 minutes and exposed to shear stress for 30 minutes. In panel **a**, fully spread, symmetrical cells are present. In panel **b**, the cells demonstrate marked cytoplasmic "streaming" in the direction of the net shear stress vector, denoted as the large arrow.

evaluations, cell attachment appears to occur in discrete stages from the initial approach to the surface through cell spreading and monolayer formation. These stages can be separated based upon morphological appearances and measurements of the relative force of attachment. Different variables related both to cell differences and surface structure may affect the overall process of cell attachment by influencing certain stages of the attachment process. Understanding these variables may provide insight into the mechanism of attachment and the influence of surface protein conformation on this process.

Acknowledgements

We would like to thank M Litt and V Turitto for their advice and assistance and J Crouch for the preparation of this manuscript.

References

1. Jarrell BE, Shapiro S, Williams S et al. Human adult endothelial cell growth in culture. J Vasc Surg 1, 757, 1984.

2. Baker KS, Williams SK, Jarrell BE et al. Endothelialization of human collagen surfaces with human adult endothelial cells. Am J Surg 150, 197, 1985.

3. Jarrell BE, Williams SK, Carabasi RA et al. Use of an endothelial monolayer on a vascular graft prior to implantation. Temporal dynamics and compatibility with operating room. Ann Surg 203, 671, 1986.

4. Radomski JS, Jarrel BE, Williams SK et al. Initial adherence of human capillary endothelial cells to Dacron. J Surg Res 42, 133, 1987.

5. Prieve DC and Alexander BM. Hydrodynamic measurement of double-layer repulsion between colloidal particle and flat plate. Science, 231, 1269, 1986.

6. Bell GI. Models for the specific adhesion of cells to cells. Science 200, 618, 1978.

7. Hammer DA, Lauffenburger DA. A dynamical model for receptor-mediated cell adhesion to surfaces. J Biophys 52, 475, 1987.

8. Bird RB, Stewart WE, Lightfoot EN (eds): Transport Phenomena, John Wiley & Sons, Inc,, New York, NY, 1966.

9. Smith LM, Doctoral Thesis. Cell adhesion as influenced by substrate surface properties. Univ of Utah, 1979.

10. Weiss L, Harlos JP. Some speculations on the rate of adhesion of cells to coverslips. J Theor Biol 37, 169, 1972.

11. Pratt KJ, Jarrell BE, Williams SK et al. Kinetics of endothelial cell (EC) - surface attachment forces. J Vasc Surg, in press.

12. Levich VG. Physiochemical Hydrodynamics, Prentice-Hall, 2nd Edition, Chapter 2, p. 60, 1962.

13. Daily JW, Nece RE. Chamber dimension effects on induced flow and frictional resistance of enclosed rotating disks. Transactions of the ASME, 217, March 1960.

14. Hyman WA. Shear flow over protrusion from a plane wall, J Biochem 5, 45, 1972.

15. Vogler EA, Bussian RW. Short-term cell-attachment rates: a surface-sensitive test of cell-substrate compatibility. J Biomedical Materials Research 21, 1197, 1987.

3. Endothelial Cell Lining

3.7. In Vitro Lining

3.7.1. In Vitro Lining of PTFE Grafts with Homologous Endothelial Cells

*P Zilla, R Fasol, P Preiss, U Dudeck, J Odell, D Sanan,
H Reichenspurner, B Reichart*

*Department of Cardio-Thoracic Surgery,
Department of Medical Biochemistry,
University of Cape Town,
Cape Town, South Africa*

Following the disappointing discovery that vascular prostheses do not acquire an endothelial cell lining except for the small area of perianastomotic pannus ingrowth, autogenous endothelial seeding (AES) was attempted to solve this problem. In canine experiments, such seeded endothelial cells needed 4 to 6 weeks to grow into a confluent monolayer (1,2,3) and initial human trials suggested an even longer delay before formation of a completely surface-covering endothelium (4). Whether or not this delay can be tolerated and result in improved patency rates seems to depend on the graft diameter. If vascular prostheses have a diameter of 6 mm or more, their occlusion occurs progressively over the years and early thrombosis plays a minor role (5). Therefore, single-staged seeding seems to be a suitable method to improve the overall patency of these grafts.

However, the situation is markedly different in small diameter vascular prostheses of 4 mm or less. Canine experiments (6) as well as human trials (7) confirmed that the patency rate of these prostheses distinctly drops during the initial few weeks of implantation while it remains almost unchanged over the following months. This unsatisfactory high percentage of short term failure of small diameter vascular prostheses makes an instant surface coverage with haemocompatible endothelium much more desirable than in other grafts. For this reason, single stage endothelial seeding is not expected to distinctly improve graft performance.

One approach to achieve a confluent endothelium prior to implantation is the in vitro lining with cultured endothelial cells (8,9,10,11). In contrast to freshly seeded cells (12) the differentiated cytoskeleton of cultured cells enables them to withstand haemodynamic shear forces (9,11,13). Initial experiments with in vitro lining, however, required high seeding densities of up to 5×10^5 EC/cm^2 (8,9,14). In order to improve this unsatisfying seeding efficiency we used a pH and temperature controlled rotation dev-

3. Endothelial Cell Lining

ice (4,10,15,16). This technique made a low inoculum of 2×10^5 EC/cm^2 graft possible and produced an instant confluent monolayer (10,15). In a subsequent study we demonstrated that this method allowed an even further reduction of the EC inoculum to the physiological vascular density of 1.2×10^5 EC/cm^2 (11). Although only 43% of seeded cells became attached, all grafts showed confluent EC coverage right after seeding. This reduction of the required cell number results in a shorter cultivation-related delay.

Another problem for in vitro endothelialization is cell damage, primarily caused by exposure to proteases (17). Introducing an in situ harvest technique together with low density seeding of first passage cells, we were able to establish a culture technique that resulted in 1.4×10^7 first passage EC after 3 weeks (18). Moreover, other groups demonstrated that the application of microcarrier techniques (19), to mass cultures of adult endothelial cells (20) can completely avoid trypsinization.

Apart from improved culture conditions and better seeding techniques, a crucial point of in vitro lining remains the precoating substrate on the prosthetic surface. A comparative study of various substrates favored smoothly covering materials like collagen matrices or fibrin glue (16). Shear stress experiments with cultured saphenous vein endothelial cells on fibrin glue coated PTFE grafts confirmed that fibrin glue represents a highly suitable underlying substratum (15). Moreover, the inhibition of the fibrinolytic activity of endothelial cells by adding epsilon-amino-capronic-acid to the fibrin glue achieved a preservation of this underlying layer (11).

In Vitro Lining with Homologous Endothelial Cells

Even if various advances simplified the techniques of autologous in vitro endothelialization and shortened the time span between vein harvest and graft implantation, the method is still limited to non-acute cases and to big centres which can afford an expensive cell culture laboratory. Thus, an ideal solution would be the availability of homologous, cryopreserved in vitro-lined grafts. Such a concept is supported by seeding studies with allogenic endothelial cells from siblings (21). These experiments have shown that, in spite of the low antigenicity of sibling donor cells, the surface covering endothelium consisted of host cells 4 weeks later. However, although these seeded cells were not the cells that ultimately lined the grafts, they facilitated autologous endothelialization (21). Previous studies with cryopreserved cultured endothelial cells for in vitro lining (10), as well as two other successful seeding studies with homologous (22) and heterologous (23) endothelial cells further encouraged us to evaluate the possibility of homologous in vitro lining with cryopreserved endothelial cells.

Due to the well-known role of endothelial cells in the immuneresponse (24,25,26), rejection of homologous endothelium appears likely. Therefore, we established a multi-donor cell pool, aiming at a gradual rather than a complete acute rejection. Furthermore, to prevent a hyperacute rejection, all donors and recipients were blood-group identical. Since species differences might reduce the value of the results, our experiments were performed in primates.

361

3. Endothelial Cell Lining

In a first step, a multidonor endothelial cell pool was established. For that purpose, the right external jugular vein from 13 male chacma baboons - all blood group B - was taken, before the baboons were used for a different project. To guarantee smooth muscle cell free cultures, an 'in situ' harvest technique was applied (18) together with a microgrid follow up (18, 27) to determine the ideal point of time for splitting and seeding. In light microscopy, none of the 13 cultures showed any smooth muscle cell contamination. Immunohistochemical staining of AcLDL and F VIII rAg confirmed the purity of the cultures. First passage endothelial cells were then trypsinized at a cell density of 8×10^4 EC/cm^2 when the population doubling time was at the onset of exponential increase (18). Subsequently, 20 separate portions of 6×10^5 EC were cryopreserved from each culture (10). The duration of cryopreservation ranged between 5 and 58 days.

Ten days prior to implantation, one vial of each of the 13 donors was thawed and cells were mixed in a 150 cm^2 tissue culture flask. These pooled EC were trypsinized after two days for graft seeding.

For all experiments, 24 cm long completely reinforced 4 mm PTFE grafts were specially manufactured by W L Gore (Flagstaff, AZ). Following a preclotting procedure with a dilution of clinically approved fibrin glue (4,11,16) 1.2×10^5 EC/cm^2 were seeded (11) using a microprocessor controlled seeding device which guaranteed a constant rotation speed of 4 rph, a temperature of 37°C and a 5% CO_2 atmosphere for the bicarbonate buffer (10). The grafts were rotated for 3 hours prior to a 9 days cultivation period in a specially designed filterprotected culture glass (11). We decided on a 9-day period of graft cultivation, since it was previously shown that the formation of the dense peripheral band of microfilament bundles - which is thought to be the site of strong cell adhesion (29) - requires a cultivation period of 8 to 12 days after confluence is reached (13). After the 3 hours seeding procedure, all grafts showed a confluent endothelial cell monolayer in the scanning electron microscopy (SEM). Until cultivation day 9 an increase in cell density was obvious and the nuclear regions appeared less prominent than after seeding. In none of the samples areas of incomplete cell coverage were found. Subsequently, 18 male baboons, 29 ± 7 kg, all blood group B, received such in vitro endothelialized grafts as 12 cm long femoro-femoral interpositions. Fibrin glue precoated, non-endothelialized control grafts were regularly implanted contralaterally. None of the animals was a donor baboon. Beginning 2 days prior to the implantation and continuing for the duration of the experiment, all baboons received the same antiaggregatory treatment of 3.5 mg dipyridamole/kg/day and 20 mg acetyl salicyclic acid kg/day. Since single-stage seeding experiments in primates indicate that the endothelialization process is also not accomplished before the 4th week after implantation (29) we selected a 16 day period to assess the success of homologous in vitro lining for short-term performance. Therefore, the explantation of both grafts was performed on day 16.

Graft Performance and Loss of Homologous Endothelial Cells

Of the total number of 36 implanted grafts, 8 of the 18 endothelialized grafts

3. Endothelial Cell Lining

and 7 of the 18 control grafts were occluded as illustrated in Table 1. Thus, the patency rate for experimental grafts was 55.6% compared to 61.1% for control grafts, a difference which proved statistically not significant (P<0.1) (Table 43).

In scanning electron microscopy (SEM) the surfaces of the 8 occluded experimental grafts and of all control grafts were free of endothelial cells. They were either densely covered by platelets and some white cells, or by a loose meshwork of fibrin, entrapping platelets and single white cells. In a few areas the unchanged appearance of the fibrin glue layer was visible with a few adherent platelets.

The 10 in vitro endothelialized grafts which were patent showed a 34.4 ± 17.1% EC coverage (Table 44). It was highly significant that all patent experimental grafts showed endothelial cell islands, while not even one endothelial cell was found on the surfaces of the 8 occluded grafts of the same group. Since it was previously shown that EC coverage can still be found in grafts which are occluded (30) the occlusion per se cannot be the reason for de-endothelialization of these grafts.

Occasionally, remaining endothelial cells formed almost confluent areas with a diameter of up to 600μm. In some of these cell patches, only single cells were missing and their former attachment area was densely covered by spreading platelets. However, most of these EC formations were smaller, consisting either of single cells or groups of only a few cells, which were separated by platelet- and fibrin-covered interspaces (Figure 154). The majority of endothelial cells showed ad-

	Patency		
Graft	**Patent Grafts**	**Occluded Grafts**	**Patency Rate**
Control (n=18)	11	7	61.1%
Endothelialized (n=18)	10	8	55.6%

Table 43 Patency rates of endothelialized and non-endothelialized 4 mm x 12 cm fibrin glue coated PTFE grafts after 16 days of implantation.

	Percent Endothelial Cell Coverage	
Graft	**Patent Grafts**	**Occluded Grafts**
Control (n=18)	0%	0%
Endothelialized (n=18)	34.4 ± 17.1%	0%

Table 44 Percentage of endothelial cell surface coverage of endothelialized and non-endothelialized 4 mm x 12 cm fibrin glue coated PTFE grafts after 16 days of implantation.

3. Endothelial Cell Lining

herent white blood cells, most of which resembled granulocytes or monocytes in their surface morphology. They had mostly a sperical configuration with no signs of spreading. Only a few adherent white cells were either distinctly polarized or had the flattened appearance of spread cells.

It was characteristic that the endothelial cell islands showed no fibrin or platelet adherence. The fibrin meshwork or platelet appositions always sharply began at the margin of EC formations, independent of whether the cell groups were almost confluent or only consisted of a few single cells. Only two of the 10 patent experimental grafts had a preconfluent EC coverage. These endothelial cells formed large confluent areas with a cobble-stone relief and much lower white cell or platelet adherence. At the anastomotic site, only 11 of the experimental and 3 of control grafts showed anastomotic pannus ingrowth, which was in average 1.6 ± 0.7 mm and 1.3 ± 0.4 mm, respectively.

In summary, the attempt to use homologous, blood-group identical, pooled endothelial cells for the in vitro endothelialization of 4 mm PTFE grafts failed to achieve the goal of improving the short-term patency of small diameter vascular prostheses. However, it was interesting that all denuded grafts were occluded while all grafts with remaining EC were patent. On the one hand this difference indicates that a gradual rejection of endothelial cells would allow the remaining donor cells to maintain the early graft patency via their prostacyclin secretion. Unfortunately, such a gradual rejection could not be achieved uniformly, when only blood group antigens were considered for EC pooling. On the other hand, the distinctly high initial cell

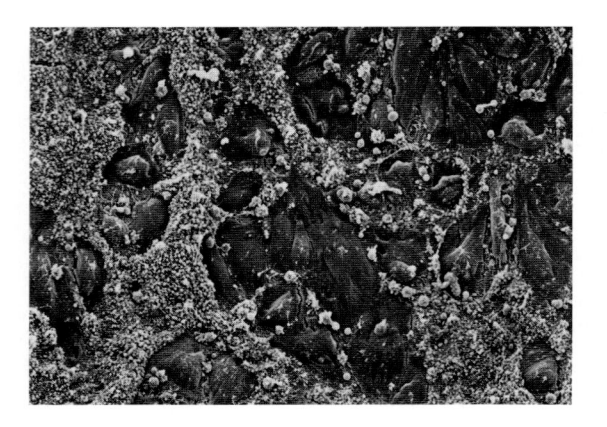

Fig. 154 Scanning electron micrograph of the mid-segment of an endothelialized PTFE graft 16 days after implantation. Residual cell islands, free of thrombotic depositions, are separated by endothelial cell free areas which are covered by a layer of fibrin and platelets.

loss underlines the key role endothelial cells play in the immune-response. Normally, an immune-answer to foreign antigen is initiated by antigen recognition by T helper cells. This process can only take place when the antigen is presented together with class II products of the major histocompatibility complex (MHC) (31). This dual recognition signal is provided by 'antigen presenting cells' (APC), which were, until recently, believed to belong exclusively to the monocyte/macrophage series. The discovery that endothelial cells are also APC (24,25,26) together with the fact that in allogenic transplantation MHC antigens are able by themselves to provide the dual recognition signal of MHC plus antigen, makes endothelial cells a highly probable target of immune-response (32).

The rejection speed, however, is dependent on where the genetic differences lie. A hyperacute rejection is entirely caused by cytotoxic antibodies, usually those to blood-group antigens. Since EC contained blood group antigens appropriate to the tissue donor's blood type (33), all homologous donor cells in our experiments were bloodgroup compatible. Therefore, it is very unlikely that endothelial cell rejection was caused by a hyperacute immuneresponse. In contrast, acute rejection is primarily mediated by T-cell immunity against MHC class II antigens like HLA-DR, HLA-DC and HLA-SB, but to a minor degree also by humoral antibodies. On the one hand an acute T-cell mediated rejection would be easily possible within our 16 days implantation period. The expression of HLA-DR antigen by EC begins to appear at 24 hours and reaches a maximal level after 4 to 5 days (34). On the other hand, a period of 16 days would theoretically also allow a specific humoral response like that one of cytotoxic anti-EM (endothelial-monocyte) antibodies (35), which are independent of HLA-DR antigens (36). Such a humoral component should be considered, since our ultrastructural investigations did not show the dense lymphocyte adherence which could be expected in acute T cell mediated graft rejection: at the time of explantation, endothelial cells were densely covered by white cells which in their majority showed the surface morphological features of granulocytes or monocytes. One interpretation for this phenomenon might be the expression of the intercellular adhesion molecule ICAM-1 (37,38) after induction by gamma interferon from immuno-stimulated T-cells. Another explanation for the massive leukocyte adherence might be interleukin-1 (IL-1) secretion by endothelial cells, which was previously found to increase granulocyte adherence in a time and dose dependent manner (39). The secretion of this cytokine could either be caused by a local inflammatory response to the prosthetic graft or by platelet derived thrombin (40) following the initial detachment of single EC. The previous finding that IL-1 stimulated granulocytes are metabolically non-activated and thus non-spreading (39) would correspond with our observation of primarily non-spread leukocytes. Since surface applied cytotoxicity is closely associated with the degree of granulocyte-spreading (39), participation of granulocytes in the destruction of the homologous endothelium is questionable. The possibility that leukocyte adherence is mediated by IL-1 is supported by the reports of other groups who found large numbers of adherent non-spread polymorphonuclear neutrophils in autologous seeded (31) and in vitro lined grafts (42). In these autologous experiments, thrombin- or inflammation-caused IL-1 secretion seems to be more reasonable than gamma interferon secretion as a consequence of an immune-response. However, if IL-1 secretion is the reason for granulocyte adherence, EC should also be expected to express procoagulant activities (40,43). When partially endothelialized grafts were investigated, no surface-morphological evidence for such an altered EC function was found, but a procoagulant activity of those grafts which were rapidly de-endothelialized and subsequently occluded, cannot be ruled out. Scanning electron microscopy showed that all remaining endothelial cell islands were not only free of adhering platelets but also free of fibrin. These fibrin formations - which covered a majority of the non-endothelialized surface - strictly ended at the margins of the endothelial cell islands. While the lack of platelet adherence could be explained by an immune-induced increase in the pros-

3. Endothelial Cell Lining

tacyclin production of endothelial cells (44) - IL-1 activated endothelial cells could still generate fibrin via the expression of a procoagulant molecule on the endothelial surface (40,43).

However, although the morphological appearance of the remaining cell islands indicates the persistence of their anti-aggregatory and anti-coagulant potential, the overall short term thrombogenicity of in vitro endothelialized PTFE grafts with non-MHC matched, homologous endothelial cells was not better than in the control group. It is likely that the majority of these EC were rejected by an acute immune-response with the concomitant expression of leukocyte-adhesive molecules on the endothelial cell surface. Moreover, it demonstrates that the previously described facilitation of autogenous endothelial cell coverage by pre-existing homologous EC (21) was rather a species specific event in pigs than a generally applicable phenomenon.

Therefore, if the concept of in vitro endothelialization of prosthetic grafts with cryopreserved allogenic cells shall be continued, further experiments must answer the question whether the EC loss was due to cytotoxic granulocytes or to an acute lymphocyte mediated rejection.

An approach to elucidate this key question would be a comparative study with both cell types - MHC matched allogenic EC sub-pools and autogenic EC.

3. Endothelial Cell Lining

References

1. Herring MB, Baughman S, Glover J, Kesler K, Jesseph J, Campbel J, Dilley R, Evan A, Gardner A. Endothelial seeding of Dacron and polytetrafluoroethylene grafts: the cellular events of healing. Surgery 96, 745, 1984.

2. Schmidt SP, Hunter TJ, Hirko M, Belden TA, Evancho M, Sharp W, Donovan DL. Small-diameter vascular prostheses: two designs of PTFE and endothelial cell-seeded and nonseeded Dacron. J Vasc Surg 2, 292, 1985.

3. Sharefkin J, Latker C, Smith M, Cruess D, Clagett GP, Rich N. Early normalization of platelet survival by endothelial seeding of Dacron arterial prostheses in dogs. Surgery 92, 385, 1982.

4. Zilla P, Fasol R, Deutsch M, Fischlein T, Minar E, Hammerle A, Krupicka O, Kadletz M. Endothelial cell seeding of PTFE vascular grafts in humans: a preliminary report. J Vasc Surg 6, 535, 1987.

5. Veith FJ, Gupta SK, Ascer E, White-Flores S, Samson RH, Scher LA, Towne JB, Bernhard VM, Bonier P, Flinn WR, Astelford P, Yao JST, Bergan JJ. Six-year prospective multicenter randomized comparison of autologous saphenous vein and expandet polytetrafluoroethylene grafts in infrainguinal arterial reconstructions. J Vasc Surg 3, 104, 1986.

6. Hancock JB, Forshaw PL, Kaye MP. Gore Tex (polytetrafluoroethylene) in canine coronary artery bypass. J Thorac Cardiovasc Surg 80, 94, 1980.

7. Sapsford RN, Oakley GD, Talbot S. Early and late patency of expandet polytetrafluoroethylene vascular grafts in aorto-coronary bypass. J Thorac Cardiovasc Surg 81, 860, 1981.

8. Foxall TL, Auger KR, Callow AD, Libby P. Adult human endothelial cell coverage of small-caliber Dacron and polytetrafluoroethylene vascular prostheses in vitro. J Vasc Surg 41, 158, 1986.

9. Sentissi JM, Ramberg K, O'Donnell TF, Connolly RJ, Callow AD. The effect of flow on vascular endothelial cells grown in tissue culture on polytetrafluoroethylene grafts. Surgery 99, 337, 1986.

10. Kadletz M, Moser R, Preiss P, Deutsch M, Zilla P, Fasol R. In vitro lining of fibronectin coated PTFE grafts with cryopreserved saphenous vein endothelial cells. J Thorac Cardiovasc Surg 35, 143, 1987.

11. Zilla P, Fasol R, Preiss P, Kadletz M, Schima H, Tsangaris S, Groscurth P. Use of fibrin glue as a substrate for in vitro endothelialization of PTFE vascular grafts. Surgery (in press).

12. Roseman JE, Kempczinski R, Pearce WH, Roedersheimer LR, Berlatzki Y, Ramalanjona G. Kinetics of endothelial cell seeding. J Vasc Surg 2, 778, 1985.

13. Schnittler HJ, Franke RP, Fuhrman R, Petermeyer M, Jung F, Mittermeyer Ch, Drenckhahn D. Influence of various substrates on the actin filament system of cultured human vascular endothelial cells exposed to fluid shear stress. In: Endothelialization of vascular grafts, Zilla P, Fasol R, Deutsch M (Eds), Karger, Basel, pp 183, 1987.

14. Anderson JS, Price TM, Hanson SR, Harker LA. In vitro endothelialization of small caliber vascular grafts. Surgery 101, 577, 1987.

3. Endothelial Cell Lining

15. Zilla P, Fasol R, Kadletz M, Preiss P, Groscurth P, Schima H, Tsangaris S, Moser R, Herold Ch, Griesmacher A, Mostbeck G, Deutsch M, Wolner E. In vitro lining of PTFE grafts with human saphenous vein endothelial cells: physiological shear stress exposure in: Endothelialization of vascular grafts. Zilla P, Fasol R, Deutsch M (Eds), Karger, Basel, pp 195, 1987.

16. Kaehler J, Zilla P, Fasol R, Deutsch M, Kadletz M. Precoating substrate and surface configuration determine adherence and spreading of seeded endothelial cells on PTFE grafts. J Vasc Surg 1989, (in press).

17. Watkins MB, Sharefkin JB, Zjatchuk R, Maciag T, D'Amore P, Ryan U, van Wart H, Rich NM. Adult human saphenous vein endothelial cells: assessment of their reproductive capacity for use in endothelial seeding of vascular grafts. J Surg Res 36, 588, 1984.

18. Zilla P, Fasol R, Hess D, Dudeck U, Siedler S, Preiss, Sanan D, Reichart B. In vitro endothelialization of ardiovascular prostheses. Part I: Rapid mass culture of autologuous endothelial cells. (manuscript in preparation).

19. Ryan U, Mortara M, Whitaker C. Methods of microcarrier culture of bovine pulmonary artery endothelial cells avoiding the use of enzymes. Tissue Cell 12, 619, 1980.

20. Vaccaro PS, Joseph LB, Titterington L, Stephens RE. Methods for the initiation and maintenance of human endothelial cell culture. J Vasc Surg 21, 391, 1987.

21. Hollier LH, Fowl RJ, Pennell RC, Heck CF, Winter KAH, Fass DN, Kaye MP. Are seeded endothelial cells the origin of neointima on prosthetic vascular grafts? J Vasc Surg 3, 65, 1986.

22. Zamora JL, Navarro LT, Ives CL, Weilbaecher DG, Gao ZR, Noon GP. Seeding of arteriovenous prostheses with homologous endothelium. J Vasc Surg 3, 860, 1986.

23. Pennell RC, Hollier LH, Solis E, Kaye MP. Xenograft seeding of Dacron grafts in dogs. J Surg Res 40, 332, 1986.

24. Burger DR, Vetto RM, Hamblin A, Dumonde DC. T-lymphocyte activation by antigen presented by HLA-DR compatible endothelial cells. In: Pathobiology of the endothelial cell, Nossel HL and Vogel HJ (Eds), Academic Press Inc, New York, p 387, 1982.

25. Hirschberg H, Braathen LR, Thorsby E. Antigen presentation by vascular endothelial cells and epidermal Langerhans cells: the role of HLA-DR. Immunol Rev 65, 57, 1982.

26. Pober JS, Collins MA, Gimbrone MA Jr, Libby P, Reiss CS. Inducible expression of class II major histocompatibility complex antigens and the immunogenicity of vascular endothelium. Transplantation 41, 141, 1986.

27. Herring MB, Evans D, Baughman S, Glover J. The quantitation of cultured cellular surface coverage: applications for transparent and opaque surfaces. J Biomed Mat Res 18, 567, 1984.

28. Gottlieb AI, Spector W, Wong MKK, Harker LA. In vitro reendothelialization: microfilament bundle reorganization in migrating porcine endothelial cells. Arteriosclerosis 4, 91, 1987.

29. Shepard AD, Raymond JC, Connolly J, Callow AD, Ramberg-Laskaris K, Foxall TL, Libby P, Keough EM, O'Donnell TF. Endothelial cell seeding of small-caliber synthetic vascular prostheses in the primate: sequential indium 111 platelet studies. CS Surg Forum 35, 432, 1984.

30. Shindo S, Takagi A, Whittemore AD. Improved patency of collagen-impregnated grafts after in vitro autogenous endothelial cell seeding. J Vasc Surg 6, 325, 1987.

31. Unanue ER, Allen PM. The basis for the immunoregulatory role of macrophages and other accessory cells. Science 236, 551.

32. Galumbeck M, Hagen PO, Saeber A, Urbaniak J. Inhibition of vascular allograft rejection by removal of the endothelium. Circulation 76, IV-55, 1987.

33. Sulzman AE. The histological distribution of the blood group substances in man as disclosed by immunofluorescence. J Exp Med 115, 977, 1962.

34. Collins TA, Korman A, Wake C, Boss J, Kappes D, Fiers W, Ault K, Gimbrone M, Strominger J, Pober J. Immune interferon activates class II major histyocompatibility complex genes and the associated invariant chain gene in human endothelial cells and dermal fibroblasts. Proc Natl Acad Sci USA 81, 4917, 1984.

35. Cerilli J, Brasile L. Endothelial cell alloantigenes. Transplantation Proc 12, 37, 1980.

36. Stastny P. Endothelial-monocyte antigenes. Transplantation Proc 12, 32, 1980.

37. Rothlein R, Dustin ML, Marlin SD, Springer TA. A human intercellular adhesion molecule (ICAM-1) distinct from LFA-1. J Immunol 137, 1270, 1986.

38. Dustin ML, Rothlein R, Bhan AK, Dinarello CA, Springer TA. Induction by IL-1 and interferon-gamma: tissue distribution, biochemistry and function of a natural adherence molecule (ICAM-1). J Immunol 137, 245, 1986.

39. Moser RS, Mansour K, Fehr J. Granulocyte-endothelium interaction on seeded grafts. In: Endothelialization of vascular grafts, Zilla P, Fasol R, Deutsch M (Eds), Karger, Basel, p. 42, 1987.

40. Stern DM, Bank I, Nawroth PP, Cassimeris J, Kisiel W, Fenton II KW, Dinarello C, Chess L, Jaffee EA. Self-regulation of procoagulant events on the endothelial cell surface. J Exp Med 162, 1223, 1985.

41. Callow AD. Perspectives on arterial graft function and failure. In: Endothelialization of vascular grafts, Zilla P, Fasol R, Deutsch M (Eds), Karger, Basel, p. 10, 1987.

42. Herring MB, Emerick S, Ashworth E. Perfusion-induced losses of cultured endothelium from vascular prostheses. In: Endothelialization of vascular grafts, Zilla P, Fasol R, Deutsch M (Eds), Karger, Basel, p. 38, 1987.

43. Bevilacqua MP, Pober JS, Majeau GR, Fiers W, Cotran RS, Gimbrone MA Jr. Recombinant tumor necrosis factor induces procoagulant activity in cultured human vascular endothelium. Characterization and comparison with the actions of interleukin-1. Proc Natl Acad Sci USA 83, 4533, 1986.

44. Goldsmith JC, McCormick JJ. Immunologic injury to vascular endothelial cells: effects on release of prostacyclin. Blood 63, 984, 1984.

45. Zilla P, Siedler S, Fasol R, Sharefkin J. Reduced reproductive capacity of freshly harvested endothelial cells in smokers - a possible shortcoming in the success if seeding? J Vasc Surg (in press).

3.7.2. Small Diameter Vascular Prosthesis with Highly Purified, Functional Autologous Venous Endothelial Cells

[1] W Müller-Glauser, [1] KH Lehmann, [1] P Bittmann, [1] U Bay, [2] P Dittes, [1] L von Segesser, [1] M Turina

[1] Clinic of Cardiovascular Surgery, University Hospital of Zürich, Gebrüder Sulzer AG, Winterthur, Switzerland; [2] IMS-BIOPUR, Freienbach, Switzerland

Introduction

Compliance, permeability, and antithrombogenicity are known to be typical properties of normal arteries. The compliance is due to a network of elastic and collagenous fibres as well as smooth muscle cells (1). These constituents of the vessel wall also allow an exchange of fluids and metabolites. Inner surfaces of walls are covered by a continuous barrier between blood and tissue.

The compliance determines the elastic properties of the arterial wall (2,3). The elasticity is necessary for non-turbulent blood flow (4) which is responsible for low thrombus deposition and minimal damage of the endothelium (5).

The antithrombogenicity is an active function of the endothelial cells (6), as demonstrated by their production of prostacyclin (7,8). The endothelial cells are also involved in the exchange of fluids and metabolites through the wall and are known to have specific cellular interactions with the smooth muscle cell of the media (6). These various exchange phenomena are supported by the extracellular matrix of the vessel wall.

Replacement of small arteries is still an unresolved problem in surgery. Efforts to develop an antithrombogenic material providing long-term patency of small diameter prostheses are still unsuccessful (9). Available small diameter non-biologic grafts are also lacking a compliance comparable to that of the native arteries (4). Flow conditions in these grafts are unfavourable and may cause thrombus deposition. Mismatch in compliance at the anastomoses results in a haemodynamic discontinuity which may contribute to excessive pannus formation (5). These effects are known to result in unsatisfactory long-term patency rates of small vascular grafts compared to autologous saphenous vein (10).

The present achievements suggest that neither the development of new materials nor the endothelial cell lining of available prostheses alone can substantially improve the long-term patency. It is therefore proposed that a more sophisticated graft concept, that takes into account both compliance and active thrombogenicity, is necessary (Table 45). Consequently, our aim was to develop a vascular prostheses with 4 mm id. consisting of a compliant syn-

3. Endothelial Cell Lining

New Concept of Small Diameter Vascular Prosthesis

Component	Property	Constituents
Artificial Vessel Wall	Compliance Permeability	Porous Polyurethane Polyester Network
Inner Surface	Long Term Antithrombogenicity	Intact Autologous Endothelial Cell Lining

Table 45

thetic material lined with autologous endothelial cells. *In vitro* and *in vivo* results show that small diameter vascular prostheses which are compliant, porous and nonthrombogenic are feasible.

We report here on the wall of the prostheses, the endothelial cell culture and the lining of experimental grafts. Short- and long-term implants are in progress to elucidate the behaviour of autologous-cell-lined grafts in contact with flowing blood.

Wall of the Prosthesis

A porous polyurethane matrix, reinforced by a polyester network, was chosen as the artificial vessel wall (Figure 155) and was demonstrated to meet the following structural and mechanical properties which appear to be necessary for a substantial improvement of the graft performance.

Structure

In analogy to the native vessel wall, the prosthesis was made of elastic and inelastic components. The elastic matrix is a polyurethane-siloxane-copolymer and conveys compliance. As protection against uncontrolled dilatation, a special polyester texture allowing only a defined radial expansion is combined with the polyurethane matrix. The structure of the wall is made highly porous to allow exchange of fluids and metabolites.

The porosity of the wall was demonstrated by a fluorescence test. The graft was filled with a fluorescein solution and placed in a water tank. After apply-

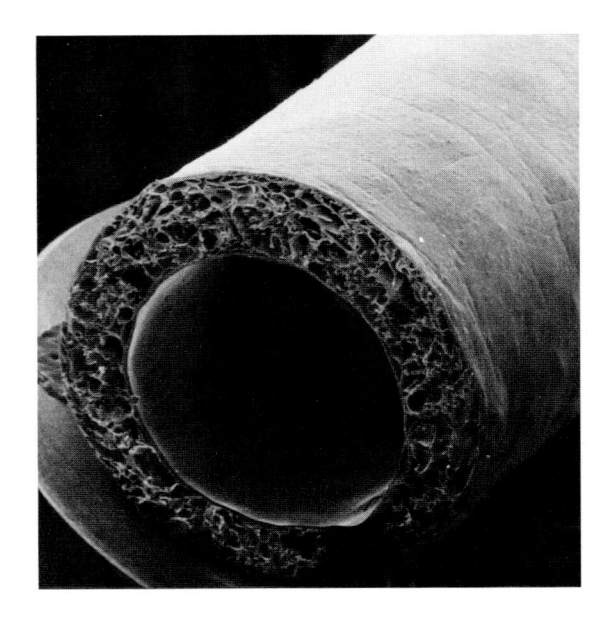

Fig. 155 New compliant vascular prosthesis with 4 mm id of porous polyurethane, reinforced by a special polyester texture. Scanning electron micrograph of a cross-section at low magnification. 1 white bar = 1 mm.

371

3. Endothelial Cell Lining

ing an internal pressure of 30 millibars, the dye was evenly distributed around the graft, demonstrating prosthesis porosity. A homogeneous dye distribution was also observed in tests of the inner parts of the graft wall without the textile reinforcement.

Mechanical Characteristics

Compliance was determined from readings of pressure, indicated by a pneumatic calibrator (Thommen, Switzerland) and optical measurements of the corresponding graft diameter using a laser micrometer (Zygo, USA). The mean compliance was 6.4×10^{-4} mmHg^{-1} (Table 46) which compares well with values for native dissected dog femoral arteries which are in the range of 10 to 20×10^{-4} mmHg^{-1} (3).

The relation between external diameter of the graft and arterial pressure is shown by graph 2 (Figure 156). Above a static pressure of 80 mmHg (about 110 mbars) an approximate similarity between the graph for native small arteries and our graft can be demonstrated. In contrast, ePTFE grafts are essentially non-elastic as demonstrated by graph 3.

Mechanical properties of our graft are summarized in Table 46. This new prosthesis is practically non-kinkable. The value for the minimal radius of curvature is about 5 mm. The minimal cut-out force was 7.4 N or slightly higher than with 4mm id. reinforced, thin-walled ePTFE grafts. Remaining deformation after exposure to 200 mbars for 60 minutes was less than 1%, i.e. well below the limit of 10% given in the report of Mortensen (11). Bursting pressure was above 5 bars, or much higher than 0.4 bar, the limit given in the report of Mortensen (11). Longitudinal resistance was demonstrated to be above 80 N. A corresponding limit of the tensile strength requirements has not been established in the UBTL study (11). Accelerated durability testing is in progress using an oscillating pressure pulse duplicator (Dynatek, USA).

Endothelial Cell Culture

It has been repeatedly proposed that an antithrombogenic inner surface of the prosthesis is best achieved by a complete monolayer of functional endothelial cells (12,13). This requires purified cell populations and an efficient lining technique.

Isolation of Highly Purified Venous Endothelial Cells

The isolation of human and canine venous endothelial cells was performed by means of a "vein holder" using 0.1% Clostridium collagenase (Serva, Heidelberg) (14). Cultures of the isolated cells (15) resulted in highly purified endothelial cell lines as demonstrated by immunochemistry of factor-

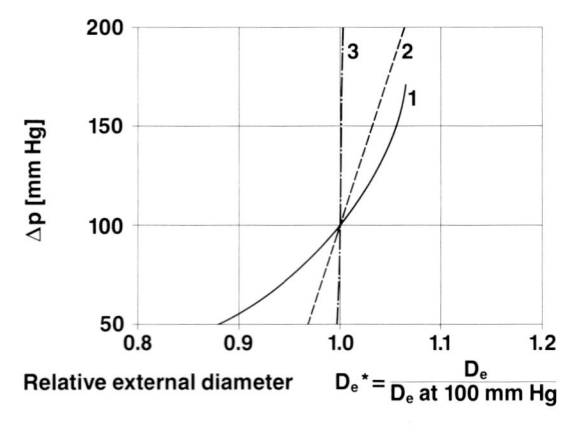

Fig. 156 Relative external diameter as a function of intraluminal pressure (Δp) for canine femoral arteries (graph 1) determined from Megerman et al (1986), the new compliant prosthesis (graph 2), and reinforced thin-walled ePTFE vascular graft (graph 3).

Mechanical Properties of Synthetic Prostheses with 4 mm Id

Parameter	PUR-Graft x̄ ± SD (N)	ePTFE a)	Dimensions
Compliance	6.4 ± 1.2 (7)	0.5	10^{-4} mmHg^{-1}
Kinking	5	5	mm
Cut-out Force	7.4 ± 3.0 (3)	5.0	N
Bursting Pressure	>5	[0.4] b)	bar
Remaining Deformation c)	<1	[< 10] b)	%
Longitudinal Resistance	>80	d)	N

a) reinforced thin-walled ePTFE vascular graft
b) from (11)
c) difference in diameter after 60 min exposure to 200 mbar
d) tensile strength requirements not established (11)

Table 46

VIII-related antigen (14) and uptake of acetylated low density lipoprotein labelled with a fluorescent probe (DiI-Ac-LDL) (16).

In an 18th passage of a human endothelial cell line, a high percentage of cells marked for the factor-VIII-related antigen, indicating the high purity of the endothelial cell population.

DiI-Ac-LDL uptake was tested in cultures of smooth muscle cells and fibroblasts. Fluorescence microscopy showed a very low uptake of lipoprotein by these cell types using phase-contrast and fluorescence microscopy of the same area of the cultures. By contrast, cultures of endothelial cell lines presented high percentages of marked cells.

Function of the Endothelial Cells

The functional integrity of the cultured endothelial cells is necessary for the success of the endothelial lining (17,18). Prostacyclin production was measured to demonstrate the antithrombogenic activity of the cells using a biochemical parameter (19). It was found to be about 0.3 ng/cm^2 for native dog veins, for confluent monolayers of cultured dog endothelial cells in the first passage, and for lined grafts. Comparable values were reported by other authors (20,21).

Extracellular matrix formation was demonstrated using fluorescence immunocytochemistry for fibronectin. Positive reaction was present in an extensive network of fibrous material formed by the endothelial cells *in vitro*.

3. Endothelial Cell Lining

Basal lamina equivalents and fibrillar constituents of the extracellular matrix were demonstrated by transmission electron microscopy of cultured human endothelial cells fixed in the presence of ruthenium (III) hexammine trichloride (22). This extracellular material may be important to adhesion of the endothelial cells on a prosthesis.

The shear stress resistance of the cultured endothelial cells was tested in a flow chamber *in vitro*. A confluent monolayer of human endothelial cells on a standard culture substrate (Biofolie, Haereus) was exposed to a flow of 75 pulses per minute. A peak velocity of 50 cm/sec corresponding to a shear force of 42 dynes/cm^2 was measured. These conditions are compatible with those found in human femoral arteries (23). The monolayer remained intact for 19 days under these flow conditions. The initial random orientation of the cells changed partially into an alignment with flow direction. Exfoliation of single cells, followed by closing of the defects and cell divisions were observed.

Endothelial Cell Lining

Our compliant graft was lined *in vitro* with cultured canine venous endothelial cells. The inner graft surface was coated using human fibronectin and filled with cell suspension. It was then rotated in horizontal position in an apparatus. Cultivation was performed for periods of 18 hours or 6 days. In 4 mm id. grafts, a coverage in excess of 95% has been repeatedly achieved. The coverage was checked by light microscopic examination after haemalaun staining of prostheses which were cut longitudinally for inspection of the internal surface. The light microscopic observations were confirmed by scanning electronmicroscopy (Figure 157).

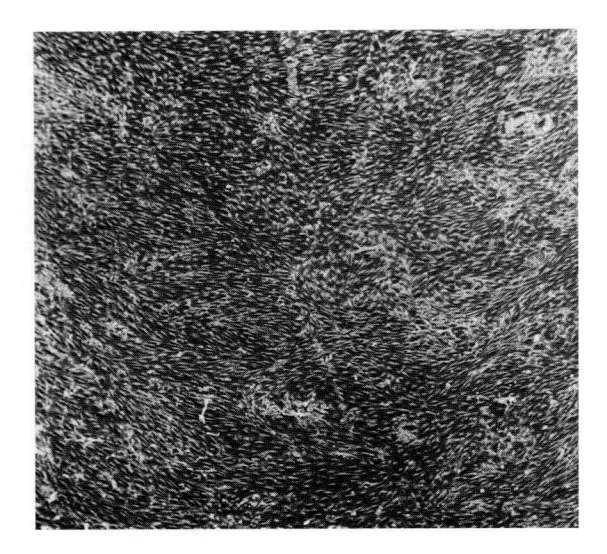

Fig. 157 Complete coverage of the inner surface of the new compliant prosthesis lined in vitro with autologous venous endothelial cells after 20 minutes in the flowing blood in a canine arteriovenous shunt. White bar = 1 mm.

Blood Contact

Ex vivo shunt studies and animal implants in short and long term experiments are in progress to elucidate the behaviour of autologous-cell-lined grafts in contact with flowing blood.

First results demonstrate lack of thrombus deposition on endothelial cells after exposure to flowing blood, indicating thromboresistance of the cultured cells (Figure 158). These observations are in agreement with findings of Mansfield et al (24).

Endothelial cell adhesion and intact monolayers were revealed by light microscopy after haemalaun staining in grafts exposed to the flowing blood for periods up to 24 hours. This was confirmed by scanning electronmicroscopy

3. Endothelial Cell Lining

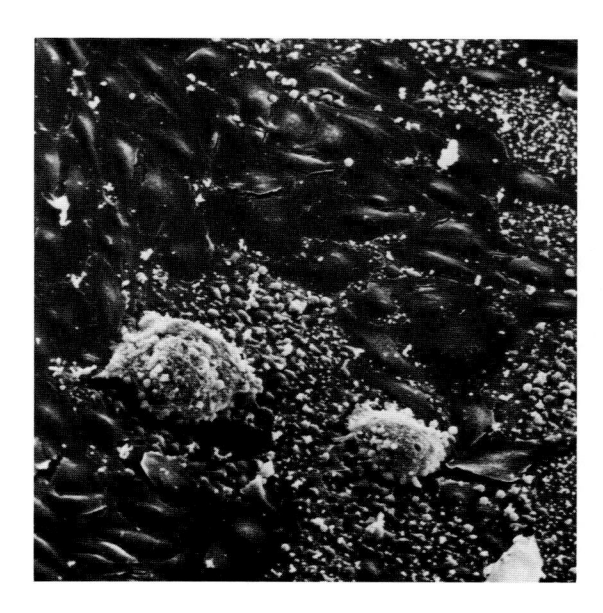

Fig. 158 Cultured canine autologous endothelial cells after 15 minutes of being exposed to flowing blood show thromboresistance in contrast to thrombogenic areas without endo-thelial cells. 1 white bar = 100 μm.

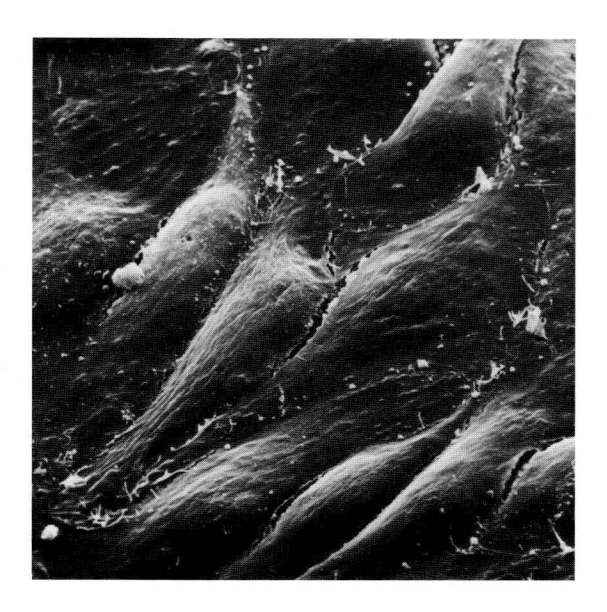

Fig. 159 Detail of complete monolayers from Figure 158 demonstrating marginal overlapping which is typical for endothelial cells. 1 white bar = 10 μm.

demonstrating the typical marginal overlapping of the cells (Figure 159).

Summary

1. A new compliant porous prosthesis, consisting of an elastic polyurethane matrix reinforced by a polyester network, was developed.
2. Highly purified and functional endothelial cells can be isolated from human and canine veins, multiplied in culture, and used for in vitro lining of the grafts. A coverage in excess of 95% was repeatedly achieved using canine endothelial cells.
3. *In vitro* and *in vivo* results from canine experiments show that small diameter vascular prostheses which are compliant, porous, and non-thrombogenic are feasible.

Acknowledgements

The authors thank Mrs MC Hensel for expert technical assistance with the cell culture; Mr A Huber for expert engineering assistance; Mrs D Meier for expert electronmicroscopic assistance.

Scanning electronmicroscopy was performed at the Institute of Anatomy, University of Zurich, Switzerland.

3. Endothelial Cell Lining

References

1. Bergel DH. The static elastic properties of the arterial wall. J Physiol 156, 445, 1961.

2. Megerman J, Abbott WM. Compliance in vascular grafts; in Wright, Vascular grafting: clinical applications and techniques. pp 344 (Wright-PSG, Boston, MA 1983).

3. Megerman J, Hasson JE, Warnock DF, L'Italien GJ, Abbott WM. Non-invasive measurements of non-linear arterial elasticity. Am J Physiol 250, H181, 1986.

4. Kidson IG, Abbott WM. Low compliance and arterial graft occlusion. Circulation 58 Suppl. 1, 1, 1978.

5. Nicolaides AN. Haemodynamic aspect of vascular grafting. In Skotnicki, Buskens, Reinaerts: Recent advances in vascular grafting. pp 43-57 (System 4 Associates, Buckinghamshire, England 1985).

6. Gimbrone MA Jr. Vascular endothelium: nature's blood container. In Gimbrone: Vascular endothelium in haemostasis and thrombosis. pp 1 (Churchill Livingstone, Edinburgh 1986).

7. Moncada S, Gryglewski R, Bunting S, Vane JR. An enzyme isolated from arteries transforms prostaglandin endoperoxides to an unstable substance that inhibits platelet aggregation. Nature (London) 263, 663, 1976.

8. Jaffe EA. Physiologic functions of normal endothelial cells. Ann NY Acad Sci 454, 279, 1985.

9. Callow AD. Presidential address: the microcosm of the arterial wall - a plea for research. J Vasc Surg 5, 1, 1987.

10. Veith FJ, Gupta SK, Ascer E, White-Flores S, Samson RH, Scher LA, Towne JB, Bernhard VM, Bonier P, Flinn WR, Astelford P, Yao JST, Bergan JJ. Six-year prospective multicenter randomized comparison of autologous saphenous vein and expanded polytetra fluoroethylene grafts in infra-inguinal arterial reconstructions. J Vasc Surg 3, 104, 1986.

11. Mortensen JD. Final report vascular replacements: a study of safety and performance. (UBTL Division of University of Utah Research Institute, Salt Lake city, UT 1981).

12. Herring M, Gardner A, Glover J. A single-staged technique for seeding vascular grafts with autogenous endothelium. Surgery 84, 498, 1978.

13. Graham LM, Burkel WE, Ford JW, Vinter DW, Kahn RH, Stanley JC. Immediate seeding of enzymatically derived endothelium in Dacron vascular grafts. Arch Surg 115, 1289, 1980.

14. Jaffe EA. Culture of human endothelial cells. Transplant. Proc 12 No. 3, Suppl 1, 49, 1980.

15. Thornton SC, Mueller SN, Levine EM. Human endothelial cells: use of heparin in cloning and long-term serial cultivation. Science 222, 623, 1983.

16. Voyta JC, Via DP, Butterfield CE, Zetter BR. Identification and isolation of endothelial cells based on their increased uptake of acetylated-low density lipoprotein. J Cell Biol 99, 2034, 1984.

17. Curwen KD, Gimbrone MA Jr, Handin RI. In vitro studies of thromboresistance: the role of prostacyclin (PGI_2) in platelet adhesion to cultured normal and virally transformed human vascular endothelial cells. Lab Invest 42, 366, 1980.

18. Libby P, Birinyi LK, Callow AD. Functions of endothelial cells related to seeding vascular prostheses: the unanswered questions; Herring, Glover, Endothelial seeding in vascular surgery, pp 17 (Grune and Stratton Inc, Orlando 1987).

3. Endothelial Cell Lining

19. De Groot PG, Brinkman HJM, Gonsalves MD, Van Mourik JA. The role of thrombin in the regulation of the endothelial prostaglandin production. Biochim Biophys Acta 846, 342, 1985.

20. Clagett GP, Burkel WE, Sharefkin JB, Ford JW, Hufnagel H, Vinter DW, Kahn RH, Graham LM, Stanley JC, Ramwell PW. Platelet reactivity in vivo in dogs with arterial prostheses seeded with endothelial cells. Circulation 69, 632, 1984.

21. Grabowski EF, Jaffe EA, Weksler BB. Prostacyclin production by cultured endothelial cell monolayers exposed to step increases in shear stress. J Lab Clin Med 105, 36, 1985.

22. Hunziker EB, Herrmann W, Schenk RK. Improved cartilage fixation by ruthenium hexammine trichloride (RHT): a prerequisite for morphometry in growth cartilage. J Ultrastruct Res 81, 1, 1982.

23. Mills CJ, Gabe IT, Gault JH, Mason DT, Ross J, Braunwall E, Shilling JP. Pressure-flow relationships and vascular impedance in man. Cardiovasc Res 4, 405, 1970.

24. Mansfield PB, Wechezak AR, Sauvage LR. Preventing thrombus on artificial vascular surfaces: true endothelial cell linings. Trans Am Soc Artif Int Organs 21, 264, 1975.

3.7.3. Cultivation of Human Endothelial Cells on Artificial Heart Materials

R Fasol, P Zilla, M Grimm, P Preiss, T Fischlein, O Krupicka

*Department of Surgery 2, University of Vienna,
Vienna, Austria*

Thromboembolism represents the major limiting factor for the clinical application of total artificial hearts (1).

One of the main reasons for this undesired complication is contact-induced platelet activation by the artificial surfaces of cardiac prostheses (2,3). This thrombocyte activation cannot be suppressed by anticoagulant therapy. Moreover, we recently demonstrated that anti-aggregatory drugs do not inhibit the entire cascade of platelet activation either. Despite therapeutic concentrations of anti-platelet substances, platelets are still able to undergo the so-called "shape change" (4), the initial morphological alteration during platelet activation (5). Therefore, attempts to find an ideal, non-thrombogenic material which prevents platelet, plasma protein, and red cell adhesion have proved disappointing. As a consequence, attention had turned to the formation of a so-called pseudo-neointima (PNI), a pannus-like cell formation, developing primarily on rough artificial surfaces (6, 7,8).

Even before it was clear that this PNI does not consist of genuine endothelial cells - at a time when most of the research groups were still involved in PNI studies - Adachi et al (10) reported, in 1971, the cultivation of bovine microvascular endothelial cells (EC) on silastic material, and Mansfield et al (11), in 1975, tried autologous lining of artificial surfaces with cultured endothelial cells in calves.

In artificial heart research, this idea was only taken up long after its initiation (12,13,14), but was successfully adapted to peripheral vascular surgery in 1978, when Herring introduced a single-stage technique, the so-called "endothelial cell seeding", for Dacron-velour vascular grafts (15). Many research groups have since performed seeding studies - including those with small diameter PTFE grafts. Various human trials have already been undertaken, but it is yet to be demonstrated that this technique will completely fulfil all expectations (16).

To offer endothelial cells a suitable substratum for adherence and spreading, the prosthetic surface of artificial implants must be either preclotted or precoated with protein substances. These preclotting procedures for porous vascular grafts differ markedly from the precoating procedures for the non-porous materials of artificial hearts.

However, a cell loss of up to 96% is found in the first 24 hours after implantation of "seeded" grafts (17), and the

3. Endothelial Cell Lining

creation of a confluent endothelium takes therefore several weeks. Thus, two-stage in vitro cultivation of endothelial cells on artificial surfaces - prior to implantation - seems to be a promising approach to provide a confluent and shear-stress-resistant endothelial lining for artificial hearts at the time of implantation. In order to evaluate the ideal material for this purpose, 11 different biomaterials were investigated concerning surface tension, influence of various precoating procedures and growth characteristics and durability of endothelium, cultivated on these surfaces.

Surface Tension of Artificial Heart Materials

For all experiments, glass cover slips (cs) (9 mm diameter) were coated with each material, except for Teflon, where we used thin discs in the size of the CS. In an initial step, the angle at the margin of a spreading droplet of distilled water was measured for each material to determine the surface tension, and thus the degree of hydrophobia (Table 47).

Influence of Precoating Procedures

In a subsequent study, the influence of precoating procedures on the proliferation rate and mitotic activity of endothelial cells was investigated. Following the initial seeding of 10 000 endothelial cells/cm^2 and a cultivation period of 7 days, fibronectin (HFN) - or glycosaminoglycane (GAG) - precoated surfaces were compared with uncoated control surfaces. The superiority of fibronectin coating turned out to be more significant after 7 days ($p<0.05$) of cultivation than after 2 or 3 days (13) (Figure 160).

H3-thymidine uptake was performed in order to compare the influence of different precoating procedures on the mitotic rate of endothelial cells. A 3 hour pulse of 1 µCi/20 000 cells yielded 10 216 ± 182 cpm 16 hours later, when endothelial cells were growing on fibronectin-coated surfaces. By contrast, only 8382 ± 182 cpm were counted after cultivation on GAG and 6862 ± 182 cpm in the control cultures ($p<0.05$) (Table 48).

Surface Tension of Artificial Heart Materials
(spreading angle)

Polyurethanes and PVC	1 Sec/30 Secs	Silicon-rubbers and Teflon	1 sec/30 secs
Biomer	88°/82°	Medical Adhesive	107°/104°
Cardiomat 610	70°/68°	3145 RTV	106°/103°
Lycra	87°/80°	Elasotosil E43	108°/106°
Mitrathane	72°/65°	Cardiothane 51	104°/10°
Pelethane	75°/72°	(PV + SR)	
PVC Tygon	88°/85°	Teflon PTFE	104°

Table 47

3. Endothelial Cell Lining

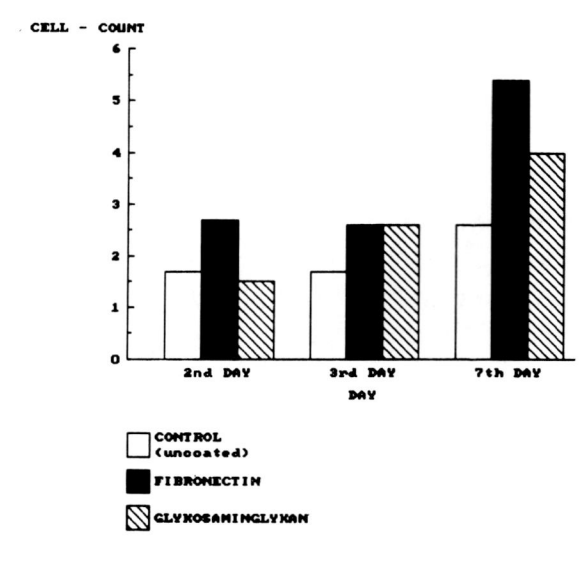

Fig. 160 Influence of different precoating procedures on the proliferation rate of human endothelial cells on polystyrene. The superiority of fibronectin precoating turned out to be significant in these short term experiments.

In Vitro Endothelialization of Artificial Heart Materials

Endothelial cells were obtained from human umbilical veins by the method of Jaffe (18). All biomaterials were then coated with fibronectin (3.3µg/cm^2) to improve adhesion and growth of endothelial cells (13). Following high density seeding (2 x 10^5/cm^2) three types of growth behaviour were found as a result of this preliminary study: endothelial cell monolayers, cell islands with sharply defined margins and single cells, which sometimes even displayed signs of cytotoxicity.

When we compared the different biomaterials 24 hours after seeding, we found an obvious dependence of cell adherence and initial morphology on hydrophobia: instant monolayer formation could be achieved more successfully on hydrophobic materials, while on hydrophilic surfaces, cell islands or unevenly distributed isolated cells were observed (13).

In a subsequent study, we cultivated adult human endothelial cells on the 2 most common polyurethanes and on 2 silicone rubber surfaces over the ensuing period of 11 days. Following high density seeding of 2 x 10^5 EC/cm, we investigated the durability of EC lining by means of light- and scanning electron microscopy as well as crystal-violet counting. On the silicone rubber surfaces, seeding of human endothelial cells produced an ideal cobble-stone monolayer (Figure 161-1) with a cell density of 62 ± 17 and 53 ± 18 x 10EC/cm^2 on day one. Although the day 1 cell count on polyurethane surfaces was even higher (98 ± 14 and 73 ± 11 x 10^3 EC/cm^2) the polyurethane surfaces displayed an uneven, patchy distribution of endothelial cells (Figure 161-4). After day 5, the cell count on the polyurethane surfaces had even increased (Figure 161-5), whereas the cell count on the silicone rubber surfaces decreased. Morphological investigations revealed that the ideally shaped cells initially found on

Influence of Precoating on H3-thymidine Uptake
(16 H after Seeding)

Fibronectin	Glycosaminoglycane	Uncoated Control
10216 ± 182 cpm	8382 ± 182 cpm	6862 ± 182 cpm

Table 48

3. Endothelial Cell Lining

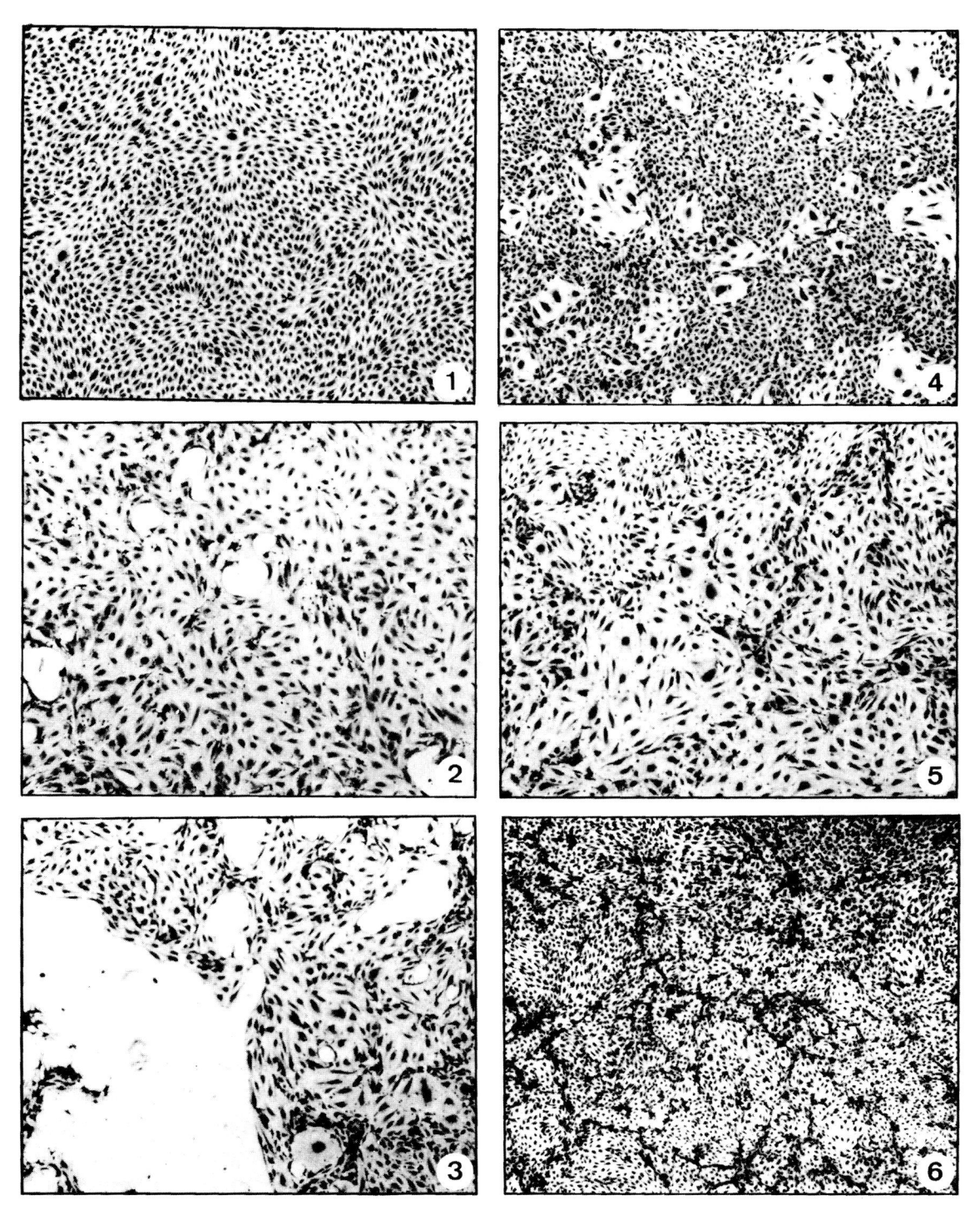

Fig. 161 Time course of the morphology of human saphenous vein endothelial cells on a silicone rubber ① - ③ (x 90). On day one after seeding, the silicone rubber surface showed an ideal cell morphology ①, whereas the polyurethane surface showed numerous giant cells unevenly distributed throughout the monolayer ④. On day five, the endothelial cells on both surfaces revealed overspreading ②, ⑤, and typical denuded areas on the silicone rubber were already visible ②. On day eleven, large areas of the silicone rubber appeared denuded; the remaining cells were overspread and sometimes displayed giant cells ③. The cell count on the Pellethane surface had increased markably, but the cell distribution was uneven and patchy ⑥. (Tex Heart Inst J 14: 119-126, 1987.)

3. Endothelial Cell Lining

the silicon rubbers had begun to detach, leaving small, denuded spheroid areas (Figure 161-2). By day 11, these cell free areas had increased to include a large percentage of the surface (Figure 161-3). In contrast, the cell counts on the polyurethane surfaces had further increased, but the cells frequently took the form of dense clusters (Figure 161-6). We then concluded that, despite the fact that materials with a high surface tension (such as silicone rubbers) seem to be ideal for the initial formation of an EC monolayer, the subsequent cultivation results in cell detachment. On materials with a lower surface tension (such as polyurethanes), the less differentiated monolayers do at least proliferate, although their morphology remains unsatisfactory.

In a further attempt to evaluate an "ideal" precoating procedure for the endothelialization of artificial heart materials, we investigated the proliferative capacity of EC and the influence of various precoating procedures on three different silicone rubbers (Medical Adhesive Silicone Type A Silastic; Elastosil E 43; 3145 RTV) and three different polyurethanes (Biomer; Enka; Pellethane) (14).

For these experiments, 9 mm glass coverslips were coated with the materials to be tested and all surfaces were individually precoated as follows:

Group 1: 3.3 µg/cm^2 human fibronectin (HFN) for 1 hour

Group 2: Fibroblast-derived extracellular matrix, by seeding murine fibroblasts (FB) L-929 onto the synthetics at a density of 1.5 x 10^4/cm^2, and lysing the FBs with hypo-osmolaric buffer after having achieved confluence

Group 3: 3.3 µg/cm^2 HFN (1 hour) prior to the seeding of 1.5 x 10^4/cm^2 L-929 FB onto the synthetic surfaces. On cultivation day 6, the fibroblast multilayer was briefly preserved by 2% glutaraldehyde, followed by a thorough rinsing procedure and an additional incubation with 3.3 µg/cm^2 HFN for 1 hour.

After seeding of 2.5 x 10^4 EC/cm^2 of second-passage human umbilical vein endothelial cells, the cell number was determined by using the crystal violet technique (19). Parallel series were performed on days 1, 5, 9 and 13. The results of these experiments are listed in Figure 162.

The morphological investigations of Group 1 specimens revealed that, up to day 5, endothelial cells reached confluence on both groups of materials if precoated with HFN. Between cultivation days 5 and 13, cell numbers on polyurethanes increased from 5 x 10^4 to 7 x 10^4/cm^2, but decreased on silicone rubbers from 5 x 10^4/cm^2 to 1 x 10^4/cm^2 due to the detachment of large spheroid areas (14).

In Group 2, the EC growth behaviour on fibroblast-derived extracellular matrix was similar to that in Group 1 as far as polyurethanes were concerned. However, neither an extracellular matrix nor any growth at all was found on silicone rubbers.

By contrast, prelining with glutaraldehyde-preserved fibroblasts (Group 3) resulted in the highest cell density (9-10 x 10^4 EC/cm^2) and the best differentiated cobble-stone morphology over the whole period of investigation. This was found almost equally on polyurethanes and silicone rubbers (14).

Summary of Results

Our initial experiments show that endothelial cells cultivated on fibronectin precoated artificial heart materials with a high surface tension detach after a

3. Endothelial Cell Lining

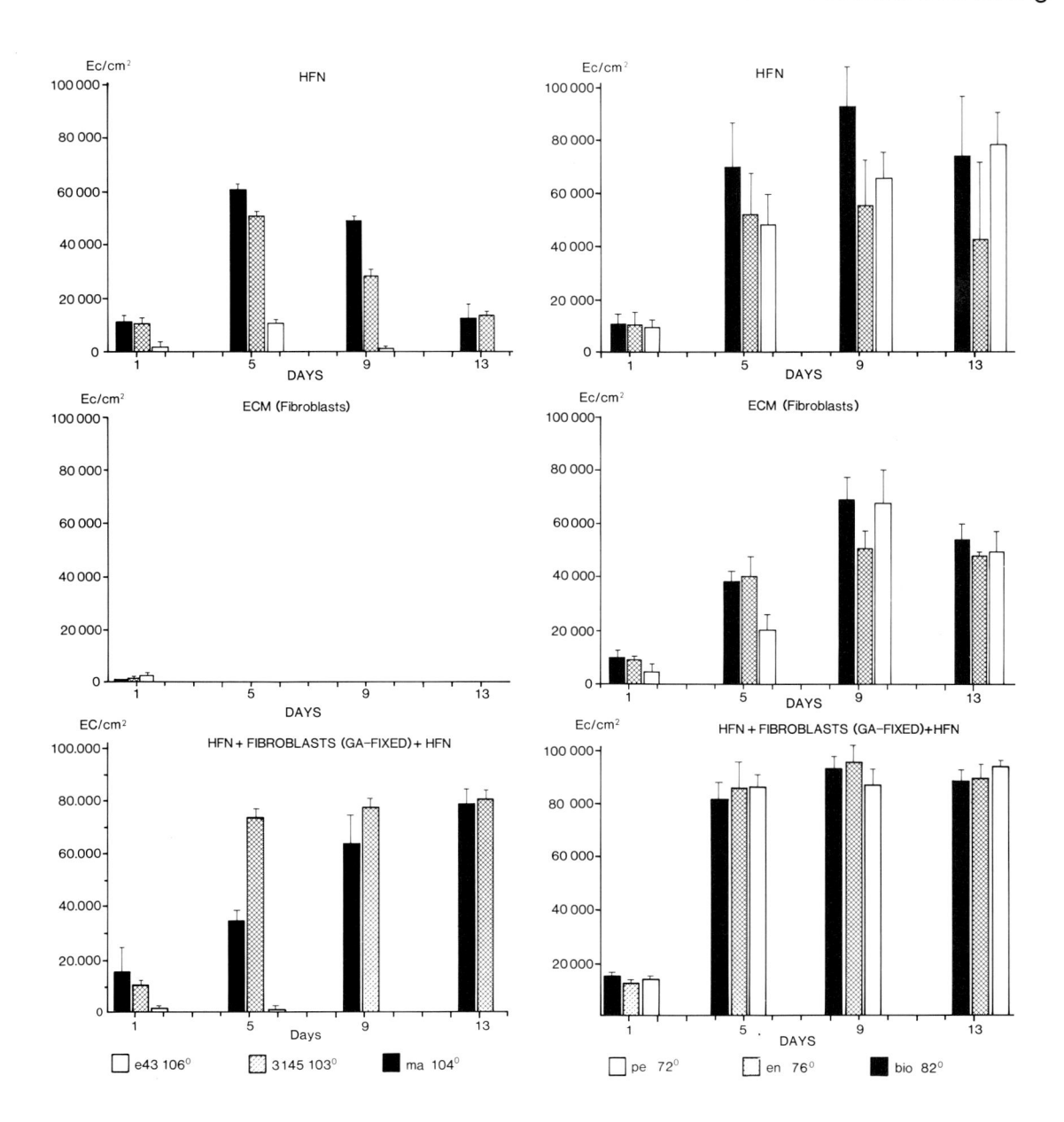

Fig. 162 Proliferative capacity of endothelial cells on the various precoating substrates: cell kinetic curves on hydrophobic silicone rubbers (Medical Adhesive Silicone Type A Silastic, 3145 RTV, Elastosil E43) and hydrophilic polyurethanes (Biomer, Enka, Pellethane). The materials were precoated with HFN, FB-derived ECM and with a glutaraldehyde-preserved cellular matrix + HFN.

On polyurethanes the growth behaviour was similar on fibroblast-derived extracellular matrix and on HFN coating. On silicone rubbers, no growth at all was found on FB-derived ECM.

Prelining with a glutaraldehyde-preserved cellular matrix and subsequent HFN postcoating resulted in the highest cell density and the best differentiated cobble-stone morphology over the whole period of investigation on both types of materials. No subsequent cell detachment was found on one of the three silicone rubbers (C).

383

few days, although the initial morphology and proliferation capacity seemed to be promising.

Our subsequent studies demonstrated that a glutaraldehyde-preserved and fibronectin postcoated cellular matrix enabled us to cultivate well-differentiated endothelial cell monolayers on both hydrophobic and hydrophilic synthetic materials.

Conclusion

Since endothelium has been shown to possess unrealized metabolic properties in the control of thromboembolism, we investigated the growth behaviour of endothelial cells on various artificial heart materials. In these experiments we were able to demonstrate that polyurethane materials - the standard biomaterial for artificial hearts - can be optimally lined with well-differentiated endothelial cell monolayers, provided that a glutaraldehyde-preserved cellular matrix is the underlying substratum. Thus, our experiments lead us to believe that long-term implantation of total cardiac prostheses could regain its attractiveness in modern cardiac surgery, if the cultured endothelium maintains its integrity and function in spite of the movement of the driving membrane and the turbulent flow conditions in artificial hearts.

References

1. Levinson MM, Smith RG, Cork RC, Emery RW, Icenogle TB, Ott RA, Burns GL, Copeland JG. Thromboembolic complications of the Jarvik-7 total heart: a case report. Art Organs 10, 236, 1986.

2. Mueller MM, Wohlfahrt A, Nowak H, Lee A, Trubel W, Buxbaum P, Zilla P, Fasol R. Observations of human thrombocytes during TAH replacement: effects of ASA on thromboembolism risk. Artif Organs, in print, 1988.

3. Fasol R, Zilla P, von Oppell U, Fischlein T, Deutsch M. Surface morphology of circulating platelets: a suggested parameter for the monitoring of endothelial cell-seeded grafts. J Cardiovasc Surg, in print, 1989.

4. Zilla P, Groscurth P, Varga G, Fischlein T, Fasol R. PGI 2 and PGE 1 induced morphological alterations in human platelets similar to those observed in the initial phase of activation. Exp Haematol 15, 741, 1987.

5. Zilla P, Groscurth P, Rhyner K, Felten A. Surface morphology of human platelets during in vitro aggregation. Scand J Haematol 33, 440, 1984.

6. Trono R, Hibbs CW, Fuqua JM, Edmonds CH, Holub DA, Brewer AM, Igo SR, Norman JC. Quantitative methods for testing pseudoneointima developing on textured blood-interfacing surfaces within left ventricular assist devices (LVADS). Trans Am Soc Artif Intern Organs 24, 352, 1987.

7. Trono R, Holub DA, McGee MG, Fuhrmann TM, Hibbs CW, Fuqua JM, Edmonds CH, Sturm JT, Bossart MI, Milan JD, Norman JC. Human pseudoneointimal (PNI) accretion kinetics during abdominal left ventricular assist device (ALVAD) utilization in man: a replication sequence. Trans Am Soc Artif Intern Organs 25, 311, 1979.

3. Endothelial Cell Lining

8. Harasaki H, Kambic H, Whalen R, Murray J, Snow J, Murabayashi S, Hillegass D, Ozawa K, Kiraly R, Nose Y. Comparative study of flocked versus biotized surfaces for long-term assist pumps. Trans Am Soc Artif Intern Organs 26, 470, 1980.

9. Mansfield PB, Wechezak AR. Tissue-cultured cells as an endothelial lining of prosthetic materials. Organ Perfusion and Preservation (Ed John C Norman), Appleton-Century-Crofts, New York, p 189 (1968).

10. Adachi M, Suzuki M, Kennedy JH. Neointimas cultured in vitro for circulatory assist devices: I - Comparison of cultured cells derived from autologous tissues of various organs. J Surg Res 11, 483, 1971.

11. Mansfield PB, Wechezak AR, Sauvage LR. Preventing thrombus on artificial vascular surfaces: true endothelial cell linings. Trans Am Soc Artif Intern Organs 21, 264, 1975.

12. Nichols WK, Gospodarowisz D, Kessler TR, Olsen DB. Increased adherence of vascular endothelial cells to Biomer precoated with extracellular matrix. Trans Am Soc Artif Intern Organs 27, 208, 1981.

13. Fasol R, Zilla P, Groscurth P, Wolner E, Moser R. Experimental in vitro cultivation of human endothelial cells on artificial surfaces. Trans Am Soc Artif Intern Organs 31, 276, 1985.

14. Grimm M, Zilla P, Fasol P, Preiss P, Groscurth P, Krupicka O, Krausler S. Growth properties of cultured human endothelial cells on differently coated artificial heart materials. (manuscript submitted)

15. Herring MB, Gardner AL, Glover J. A single staged technique for seeding vascular grafts with autologous endothelium. Surgery 84, 498, 1978.

16. Zilla P, Fasol R, Deutsch M, Fischlein T, Minar E, Hammerle A, Krupicka O, Kadletz M. Endothelial cell seeding of PTFE vascular grafts in humans: a preliminary report. J Vasc Surg 6: 535, 1987.

17. Rosenman Y, Ramalanjaona G. Kinetics of endothelial cell seeding. J Vasc Surg 2: 778, 1985.

18. Fehr J, Moser R, Leppert D, Groscurth P. Antiadhesive properties of biological surfaces are protective against stimulated granulocytes. J Clin Invest 76, 535, 1985.

19. Zilla P, Fasol R, Preiss P, Kadletz M, Schima H, Tsangaris S, Groscurth P. Use of fibrin glue as a substrate for in vitro endothelialization of PTFE vascular grafts. Surgery (in print).

4. Laser Treatment

4.1. Laser Treatment - Introduction

U von Oppell

*Department of Cardio Thoracic Surgery,
University of Cape Town, Medical School,
Cape Town, South Africa*

The laser (that is, light amplification by stimulated emission of radiation) was invented in 1958 and first used in medicine in 1962. Although extensively used since then in ophthalmology, it is only now making its appearance in the field of cardiac surgery. The paper by G Fasol introduces and explains the physics of lasers. The types of lasers from the more commonly used Nd:YAG laser to the Excimer laser, with their different delivery systems, advantages and disadvantages are mentioned.

Accepting the initial concept to use lasers to ablate biological tissue, research has been, and still has to be performed in a suitable experimental model. Dr H Breuer describes an effective method of producing atherosclerotic plaques in baboons by the use of electromagnetic stimulation and a cholesterol-rich diet.

The potential use of laser energy was recognized in the 1970s and thereafter suitable delivery and guiding systems have been produced. Most researchers accept the need of a fibreoptic system in the cardiovascular application of laser energy. However, whether lasers should be used in a contact - 'hot tip' probe - mode, utilizing transmitted thermal energy, or in a non contact mode, remains to be defined. The research performed by D Richens helps to define the difficulties with both these modalities. Further work on whether the laser should be used as a continuous or pulsed wave and the detection of free radicals is discussed by R Clarke.

The most troublesome complication in the vascular use of lasers is perforation of the vessel, and therefore some guiding system as described by D Richens is probably necessary. However, G Wollenek highlights the increased safety of the Excimer laser which will ablate tissue with predictable penetration and minimal neighbouring coagulative necrosis.

The attraction of using lasers to treat occlusive arterial disease stems from the belief that the removal of atheromatous material, as opposed to merely remodelling the vessel as performed by balloon angioplasty, will be more beneficial and long-lasting. B Höfling pursues this belief with an alternative to lasers, namely a mechanical percutaneous atherectomy catheter used in peripheral arterial vessels. Whether this can be adapted to the coronary arterial tree remains to be determined. Dr R Ginsburg, who performed the first percutaneous recanalization of a femoral artery, presents the Stanford experience. The formation of a centre for interventional vascular therapy in order to focus on treatment of the

4. Laser Treatment

artery, regardless of the end organ, will certainly help to accelerate and co-ordinate future research. Alternatives to lasers, in addition to the use of angioscopes, is described in his paper.

A significant amount of basic research in the intra-vascular use of lasers has been gained by their use in peripheral arteries. Finally, in 1983, Choy performed the first intra-operative laser angioplasty of the right coronary artery. F Hehrlein presents the first clinical results from the Justus Liebig University in Giessen, Germany, and furthermore discusses the reasons for their selection of the Argon laser.

I am in no doubt that future technology will produce the ultimate laser for intra-vascular use: a self-guiding, auto-analysing, percutaneous laser catheter that safely reopens occluded coronary vessels. The use of laser energy to 'weld' together tissue, as opposed to removing tissue, is also a distinct possibility in the future.

4.2. The Physics of Laser Light and its Interaction with Matter

G Fasol

Cavendish Laboratory, University of Cambridge, UK

Abstract

Lasers are used in rapidly increasing numbers for medical applications. The present article is an introduction to the principles of how lasers work, a simple discussion of how laser light differs from ordinary light, and an introduction to how laser light interacts with tissue.

Introduction

Lasers are used in such a large number of different medical applications today, that this article cannot even attempt to be comprehensive. The aim is rather, to give a simple introduction to how lasers work. The present article is biased towards applications in cardiovascular surgery to serve as a prologue to the later sections of this book.

The word "LASER" is an artificial word and stands for the first letters of "Light Amplification by Stimulated Emission of Radiation". These words describe the basic operating principle of every laser. Every laser works by using "stimulated emission" to produce a light beam, which is substantially different from the light of an ordinary lamp. The light of a laser can be made extremely parallel, of very high intensity, of precisely one colour, pulsed with a very short duration (the world record is down to a few femto seconds, 1 fs = 10^{-15} seconds) and it can be made to have a very precisely controlled cross profile.

Lasers are used for a large and increasing variety of applications - for processing of materials, for information handling (CD players, optical storage of information, etc) - and it is projected that the telecommunication system (including the telephone networks) will, in the near future, consist of lasers and optical fibres as the core components. It has been estimated (3) that 5 000 medical laser systems per year were installed in 1985 and that this number might increase to 15 000 per year by the year 1990.

For many surgical applications it is initially sufficient to consider a medical laser system as a "black box" producing a light beam at its output, which is characterized by the following properties:
- whether the laser light is continuous or pulsed
- in the case of a continuous laser beam:
  - the power (= light intensity)
- in the case of a pulsed laser beam:
  - repetition rate and pulse duration
  - the light energy delivered per pulse
- the divergence of the laser beam or the position and size of the focus
- the light wavelength (i.e. the colour)

4. Laser Treatment

- the cross section profile of the laser light beam

One aim of the present article is to explain what is inside the "black box" of a laser.

The traditional use of lasers in medicine is for cutting and removal of tissue, for application of heat, and for coagulation. The main fields where lasers are used today are ophthalmology and gynaecology - it is estimated (3) that more than 60% of medical laser systems are used in ophthalmology today. It is to be expected that in future lasers will be used for a great variety of new highly specific applications. One of them is laser angioplasty, with the possibility of using the laser system, not only for the removal of atherosclerotic plaque but also for spectroscopic control of the operation. Another application which is being studied currently is the use of lasers for suturing of arteries. Today's status of laser angioplasty research is covered by other articles in this volume. The present article focuses on the properties of laser light, the construction of laser systems, and the different interactions of laser light with tissue.

What is Light?

Light is electromagnetic radiation and is similar to radio waves, radar waves, infra-red radiation, X-rays, gamma rays, etc. A light wave fills the space in which it propagates with electric and magnetic fields which both oscillate with time and distance. If we could look in detail at a particular point in space through which a light wave passes, we would see an electric field and a magnetic field orientated perpendicular to each other, both oscillating in time with the frequency of the light wave (Figure 163).

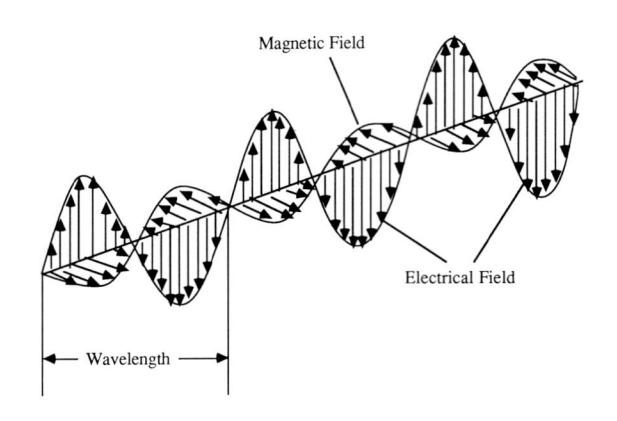

Fig. 163 Light is an electromagnetic wave. It consists of a periodic variation of electric fields and magnetic fields in space and time. Light waves propagate with the speed of light (300 000 km/sec in vacuum and somewhat slower in media).

The separation of the crests of the waves is the wavelength of the light wave. The light beams coming from a lamp or from a laser consist of a stream of different "wave packets". These are sections of continuous wave of a certain length. These wavepackets move with the velocity of light, which is 300 000 km per second in vacuum. In a medium, such as water, glass, or blood, the speed is typically a factor of 1.5 to 3 slower. This factor is the refractive index of the material.

Frequency and wavelength of a light wave are related by the following formula:

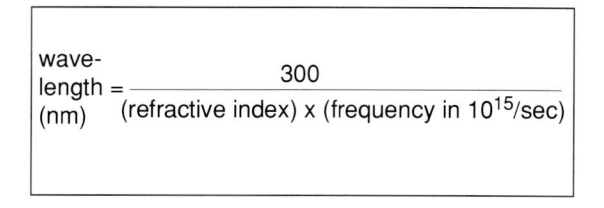

$$\text{wavelength (nm)} = \frac{300}{(\text{refractive index}) \times (\text{frequency in } 10^{15}/\text{sec})}$$

In a vacuum the refractive index is equal to 1.

For comparison: a sound wave (such as produced by the speaker of

4. Laser Treatment

stereo equipment) consists of a periodic variation of the pressure of the air. At every point which the sound wave reaches, the air pressure oscillates with time. Each of our ears monitors the variation of the air pressure as a function of time at the location of the ear. Since sound waves are pressure waves, they require a medium. Light waves, on the other hand, are able to propagate in a vacuum, since electric and magnetic fields do not need a medium to exist.

Light interacts with materials, because the oscillating electric field and the magnetic field of the light wave exert forces on the electrons, atoms, and molecules constituting the material.

Spectrum of Electromagnetic Waves

The difference between radio waves, radar, X-rays, light, and other electromagnetic waves, lies in the different wavelengths of the underlying electromagnetic radiation waves. Figure 164 shows the spectrum of electromagnetic radiation. When a light wave propagates from one medium to another (for example, from an optical fibre into blood), the velocity of the light wave and the wavelength change - but the frequency stays the same. Therefore, when the wavelength of a laser is given, it is its vacuum wavelength - the actual wavelength depends strongly on the medium in which the light travels.

Visible light has vacuum wavelengths ranging from around 400 nm (= 0.4 micrometer) for blue light, to around 700 nm (= 0.7 micrometer) for red light. The frequencies of visible light range from 0.75×10^{15} Hz for blue light to 0.4×10^{15} Hz for red light. This means that for blue light, both the electric and the magnetic field oscillate 0.4×10^{15} times per second. These frequencies are very

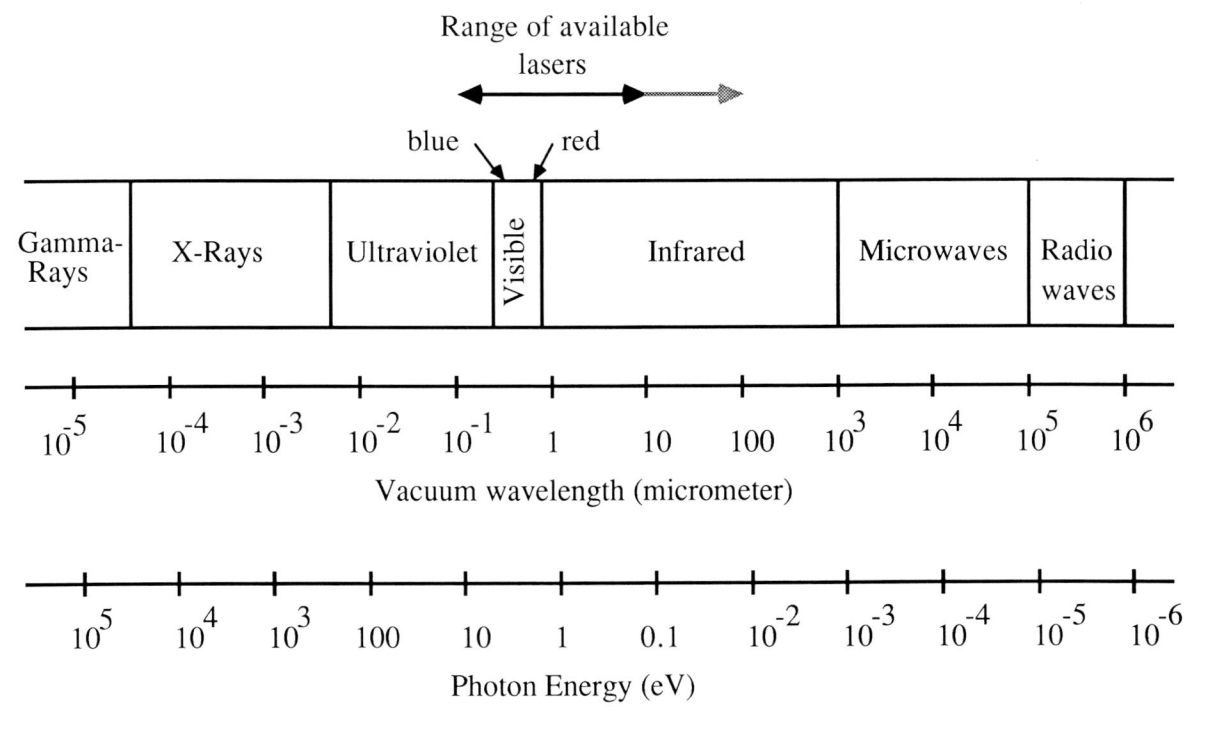

Fig. 164 The spectrum of electromagnetic radiation.

much higher than the frequencies of sound, which are of the order of 1 000 Hz. (1 Hz = 1 Hertz is the unit of frequency and is equal to 1 oscillation per second).

Laws of optics show that because of the diffraction of light the minimum spot size to which laser light can be focused is of the order of its wavelength. Therefore, ultraviolet light can be focused to considerably smaller spots than infrared light.

Light is a Stream of Light Particles, the Photons

When describing the interaction of laser light with tissue, and in particular when excitation of electrons or disruption of chemical bonds by laser light is described, it is not practical to consider laser light solely as a wave. In many situations it is necessary to take the quantum nature of light into account. I will not give explanations of the quantum character of light - I will just list the most important facts, and I hope that this will help to bridge a language gap between surgeons and "light engineers".

Light is "quantized": this means that light from a lamp or a laser consists of a stream of particles. These particles are called photons. Their existence was found by Max Planck and Albert Einstein early this century. Each such photon particle has an energy, which is uniquely related to the frequency of the light beam. The energy E of each photon in a light wave with frequency f is:

$$E(photon) = h.f$$

where h is a fundamental constant of nature, named "Planck's constant".

The value of h is:

$$h = 1 \text{ eV} / 2.418 \times 10^{14} \text{ Hz},$$

where $1 \text{ Hz} = 1 \text{ sec}^{-1}$ is the unit of frequency. This equation allows one to calculate the energy of its constituting photons from the frequency of a light wave. Physicists in fact commonly use the energy of the photons, when stating the frequency of a light wave. The energy of the photons of visible light ranges from 3.1 electron Volts per blue photon to 1.7 electron Volts per red photon. One "Electron Volt" (abbreviated 1 eV) is the energy required to accelerate one electron across a potential difference of 1 Volt - it's an energy unit used by physicists and chemists and is abbreviated "eV". It is a very useful measurement unit for energy, because the energies of the photons of visible light and of chemical bonds are in the range of a few eV's. Figure 2 shows the corresponding vacuum wavelength and photon energy.

In many processes (for example, when light interacts with chemical bonds) single light particles (= photons) interact on a one-to-one basis with the chemical bonds. Thus one single light particle (= one single photon from the light beam) breaks one single chemical bond in the molecule in a one-step process. Most interaction processes of light with electrons are such one-photon - one-bond or one-photon - one-electron processes. Sometimes, so-called non-linear or higher order processes are possible, where two light particles interact at the same time with one single electron or one single chemical bond. Such processes become par-

4. Laser Treatment

ticularly important at high light intensities.

It is very important to make a clear difference between the energy of each of the photons constituting the light beam (ie. its colour) and the intensity (ie. the number of photons per unit area per second) of the light beam. For most processes, it is the light power per unit area, together with the energy of the photons (and not the total power of the laser beam) which determines the details of the interaction of laser light with tissue. Thus, the same laser beam with the same total power might lead to evaporation of tissue when sharply focused, but only to mild heating when defocused.

Polarization of Light

The previous sections discussed some of the properties of light, which are at present important in medical applications. Physicists and engineers are interested in a range of further properties, such as the polarization state of the light. It was explained above, that a light wave consists of an electric field and a magnetic field, varying periodically in space. The magnetic field and the electric field are always perpendicular to each other. The direction of the electric field of a light wave may have a fixed orientation with respect to the propagation direction of the light wave. In this case the light is "linearly polarized". The polarization direction is defined as the direction of the orientation of the electric field. Another possibility is that both the electric and the magnetic fields rotate in a plane perpendicular to the direction of propagation. If the intensity of the electric field remains constant as it rotates, the light is termed "circularly polarized". If it varies in intensity during rotation, the light is termed "elliptically polarized". The polarization state of light is often important for the microscopic interaction of the laser light with a medium: e.g. when light is polarized in the same direction as the orientation of a chemical bond, the interaction will, in general, be stronger than if both are oriented perpendicularly to each other.

Comment

There are many other types of waves in the world besides electromagnetic radiation (light, X-rays, gamma rays, radio waves, radar): i.e. sound waves (wavelike oscillation of the pressure in the medium), neutron beams, alpha radiation (consisting of Helium nuclei), beta radiation (consisting of a beam of electrons), etc . . .

For a much more detailed introduction to the properties of light I would recommend an introductory book by one of the pioneers of this field (4).

How does a Laser work?

The basic operating components of every laser are

- a light amplifier and
- an optical resonance cavity, which consists basically of two extremely accurately aligned mirrors at opposing ends.

Light Amplification

A light amplifier is an active optical instrument, which has the following property: when a light wave enters on one side, a light wave of the same frequency (= colour) and the same phase (time relationship of the electric and magnetic field oscillations) as the incident light

4. Laser Treatment

Light Amplifier

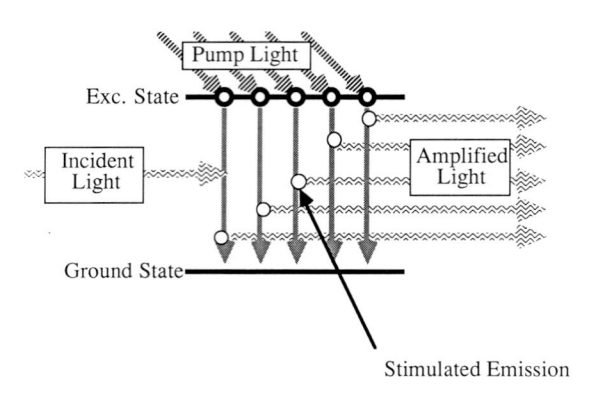

Fig. 165 a) An optical amplifier augments the intensity of an incident light beam by stimulated emission of light particles (photons) in phase and with the same wavelength as the stimulating light wave.

wave emerges on the other side. In addition to the input opening for the incoming light wave and the output opening for the amplified light wave, a light amplifier has a third input, the pump input, which provides the energy necessary to amplify the intensity (= the number of photons) of the light wave. The third input can be an electric current, laser light from a "pump laser" or an array of pump lasers or light from a pump lamp (Figure 165a).

Stimulated Emission of Light

A light amplifier increases the intensity of the incident light wave by "stimulated emission" of additional light quanta, which have the same wave-length and the same phase as the incident light wave. These additional light quanta augment the intensity of the incident light. A light amplifier contains an active medium in which stimulated emission may take place, provided that the active medium is brought to the correct conditions. Active media used for optical amplifiers are, for example, a gas column, filled with a Helium and Neon gas mixture, an Argon gas column, Carbon Dioxide gas column, a YAG crystal doped with Niodymium ions, a semiconductor diode prepared to certain specifications, a jet of a dye solution, etc.

Electrons in atoms, molecules, crystals or in glasses can occupy only certain allowed energy states. Electron states in atoms and in molecules, and some electron states in crystals, are called orbitals. In a particular system in equilibrium a range of allowed electron states will be filled with electrons, and another range of allowed states at higher electron energies will be empty. In a molecule, most bonding states will be filled with electrons, and most anti-bonding states will be empty. When electrons are excited from lower-lying, initially filled states, to previously empty, higher-energy states, these electrons will stay for a short time in the higher energy state. This time is usually in the range of 1 ns to 10 ns (1 ns = 10^9 seconds). Subsequently, the electrons will drop down again to the lower energy state, emitting exactly one light quantum (= one photon) per electron. The energy of the emitted photon (and therefore the wavelength of the emitted light) is determined by the separation of the initial and the final energy state of the laser medium. To achieve population inversion and laser action, a certain combination of electronic transition probabilities, energy pumping, and temperature must be fulfilled.

Optical Resonance Cavity

The second essential component of every laser system is an optical cavity, as shown schematically in Figure 165b.

4. Laser Treatment

It consists essentially of two mirrors. One of the two mirrors (the one on the left hand side in the schematic view of Figure 165b), is the so-called "high reflector". It is a mirror with a reflectivity very close to 100% for the wavelength of the laser. The other mirror is the "output coupler" - it is only partially reflective and transmits a small part of the light from within the cavity. Both the high reflector and the output coupler mirror of a laser cavity are sophisticated instruments. They consist of a high quality glass coated by evaporation in vacuum with a number of dielectric layers to achieve the required reflecting and transmitting properties. They usually only work for a narrow wavelength range, and they have to be changed if laser operation in a different wavelength range is required.

The optical resonance cavity has similar properties with respect to light waves as the string of a violin with respect to elastic vibrational waves, or as the acoustic resonance cavity of an organ pipe with respect to the sound waves in the gas column of the organ pipe. Light waves in the optical resonance cavity can have certain standing waves with very well-defined frequencies and spatial distributions. This is sketched in Figure 165b.

Laser = Optical Resonance Cavity + Optical Amplifier

The basic construction of every laser is the combination of an optical resonance cavity with an optical amplifier inserted as shown schematically in Figure 165c. The construction of many laser systems actually closely resembles the schematic view of Figure 165c. Most laser systems contain additional optical components. Sometimes the optical cavity is folded by additional mirrors -

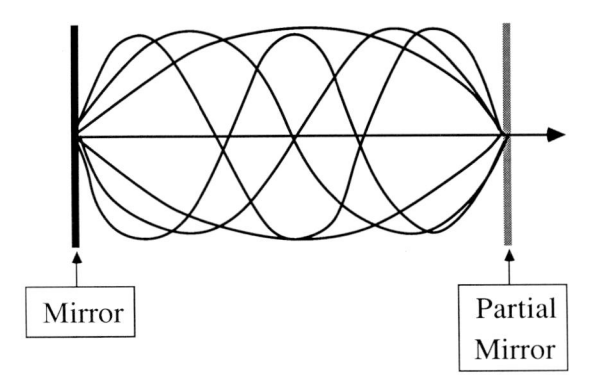

Fig. 165 b) Schematic view of an optical resonance cavity.

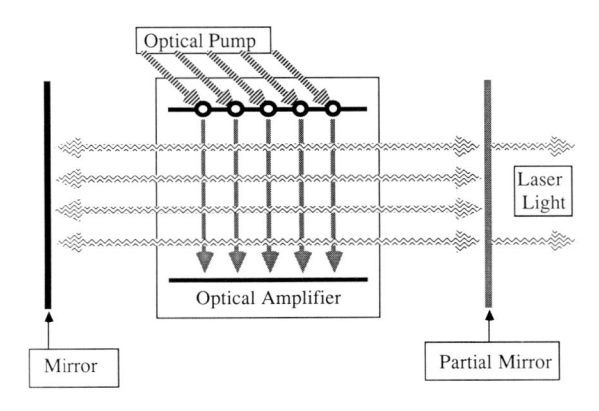

Fig. 165 c) The basic components of every laser are optical amplifier and optical resonance cavity.

but the basic operational principle is always as shown in Figure 165a,b and c. When a laser is constructed according to Figure 165c and the optical pumping is switched on, laser action will not be guaranteed. The main condition for laser action is the following:

- The optical amplifier must amplify the light wave during one round trip in the optical cavity by a factor greater than the losses due to absorption, scattering, due to losses at the mirrors and due to the light leaving the cavity at the output coupler.

397

4. Laser Treatment

Transverse and Longitudinal Light Modes of a Laser

A laser cavity has resonance modes for light waves in a similar way as a flute or an organ pipe has resonance for sound waves. In an organ pipe the vibrating lip excites sound waves in the gas column of the acoustic resonance cavity. The length of the acoustic cavity of a flute or an organ pipe defines certain wavelengths and certain distributions of the soundwave with which resonance can occur. The specific resonance frequencies are called the "eigenfrequencies" of the cavity. They are a specific property of the geometry of the organ or the flute, and will, in addition, depend on the properties of the air inside, the temperature, humidity etc. In an exactly analogous way, every laser cavity has certain resonance modes for the light. Each such resonance mode has a specific wavelength of light, and a specific light intensity distribution parallel and perpendicular to the axis of the laser. Each laser is, in principle, able to operate in several combinations of longitudinal and transverse resonance modes. The actual light modes which the laser emits, and the wavelength and the intensity parallel and perpendicular to the axis of the laser, depend on the construction and adjustment of both the optical cavity and the light amplifier. For most applications, operation in the TEM_{00} mode is necessary.

A few Limitations of the Previous Discussion

In the preceding section it was explained, that a laser relies on a standing light wave inside an optical resonance cavity excited by an optical amplifier. There are flaws in this argument:
- It was explained above that an optical amplifier can amplify an incident light wave that is already present in the cavity. However, when we switch on the optical amplifier of the simple theoretical laser described above, there is no initial light in the cavity. How does the laser get started?
- When the laser operates, the amplification must exceed the losses in the cavity. The light wave will be amplified on every return trip inside the cavity. Following the discussion the light intensity inside the cavity should increase without limit. Where is the limit?

In both cases the answers lie in the non-ideal behaviour of the laser. The optical amplifier always has a background emission of light due to spontaneous emission - this background emission starts the laser off. Secondly, the optical amplifier will only amplify up to a certain maximum light intensity; for higher intensities the energy provided by the pump will not be sufficient anymore. The actual intensity of the laser output will be a balance of the non ideal properties of the amplifier with the losses from the cavity.

Pulsed Lasers

There are many different ways of producing laser pulses:
- simply switching the laser on and off by a shutter outside the laser
- pumping by a flash lamp, or pumping by a pulsed laser (e.g. some pulsed Nd:YAG lasers, pulsed dye lasers)
- pumping by a pulsed gas discharge (e.g. excimer laser)
- Q-switching

For the discussion above we have assumed that the laser operates continuously. Many lasers operate in a pulsed mode - indeed pulsed lasers are

4. Laser Treatment

particularly important for angioplasty and many other medical applications. Pulsed laser light may have totally different interactions with tissue than corresponding continuous (CW) laser light of the same wavelength and the same average power.

The power of continuous lasers and the time averaged power of pulsed lasers as used in medicine lies in the range from a few Milliwatts up to around 50 Watts. The pulse length of many medical lasers is of the order of 1 to 1 000 ns (1 ns = 1 nanosecond = 0.000 000 001 second).

If we take a typical excimer laser with a pulse length of 10 ns, a repetition rate of 100 Hz, and a pulse energy of 10 mJ per pulse, the average power is 1 Watt. The peak power, i.e. the laser power during the short laser pulses, on the other hand is 10^6 Watt. Such high powers cannot be achieved with continuous lasers. The peak power is related to the strength of the electric field of the laser light. A pulsed laser with high peak power and high peak fields may interact entirely differently with tissue than a CW laser with the same average power output would.

During the time of a 1 nanosecond laser pulse, light propagates 30 cm, during the time of a 100 femtosecond pulse it propagates only 0.03 mm, which is much shorter than the length of typical lasers. Short light pulses therefore may not even be able to make a full round trip inside the laser cavity during this time. To understand the operation of lasers with very short pulse lengths, a more detailed analysis is necessary, which is beyond the scope of the present article.

Properties of Laser Light - What makes Laser Light Different from Ordinary Light?

Laser light has the following main properties:

- Laser light is collimated: i.e. Laser light can be produced as a highly parallel beam with very small angular spread. Laser light will remain almost parallel over very large distances. Fundamental laws of optics show that the amount of angular spread determines the minimum spot size to which laser light may be focused. Thus, as a consequence of the small angular spread, laser light may be focused to extremely small spot sizes. Thus, laser light energy can be delivered in extremely high intensity into a very small and well defined volume. Ultimately, the minimum angular spread and the minimum spot size of the focus is limited by diffraction.
- Laser light can be made to have an extremely high light intensity. It is important that high light intensity may be achieved with a laser in combination with a very small beam diameter, small angular spread, small wavelength range, etc.
- Laser light can be produced which is highly monochromatic, i.e. the beam will contain only wavelengths from a very narrow wavelength range. Indeed, sophisticated laser systems exist for special applications, where the wavelength spread is astronomically small.
- Laser light can be very highly coherent. This means that the oscillations in the light wave keep their regular behaviour over a very long distance and for a very long time, i.e. the wave

4. Laser Treatment

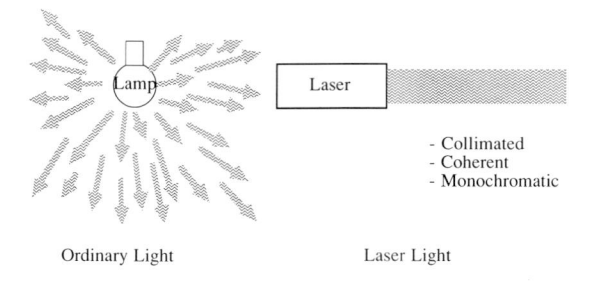

Fig. 166 Laser light versus ordinary light. Laser light is collimated, coherent and may be highly monochromatic.

packets are very long compared with those found in ordinary light.
- Lasers exist which make very short pulses of very high intensity with most of the properties above.

It is an essential property of lasers that many or most of the above properties, ie. collimation, coherence, beam diameter, monochromaticity, high intensity, etc. may be achieved concurrently.

Ordinary light as produced by the sun, light bulbs or fluorescent tubes, consists of a stream of very short light wavepackets with a broad frequency spectrum - it contains light with many different wavelengths. These wavepackets go in many different directions. Such ordinary light may be made to be collimated or monochromatic, but the intensity will be dramatically lower (i.e. many million times) than achievable with a laser.

Figure 166 schematically shows these essential differences between ordinary light and laser light.

Some Types of Lasers

The present section gives an overview of several laser systems which are at present relevant to the medical field. A large number of totally different types of lasers are available today. Table 49 lists some criteria which may assist the choice of a laser system for a particular application.

Different types of lasers together cover a broad wavelength range, intensity range, and pulse length range. Figure 167 gives a schematic view of the wavelengths of some common types of laser. The wavelengths of gas lasers (KrF, XeCl, Ar, Kr, CO_2, etc) and of lasers relying on atomic impurities in crystals (Nd:YAG, Er^{3+}, etc) are determined by atomic transitions. Such lasers therefore have one or more fixed laser lines, which have an extremely narrow wavelength distribution. The wavelengths will be exactly the same from one laser to another. Other lasers, such as semiconductor lasers, dye lasers, or the free electron laser, have laser emissions with a much broader wavelength range. The wavelength at which these lasers operate may be varied by changing the construction or the operating conditions of the laser. In the following section, a short introduction to some types of lasers will be given. Since a large number of different lasers exists, and since the development of lasers advances very rapidly today, this list is just an introduction, without aiming for completeness. Table 50 summarizes prop-

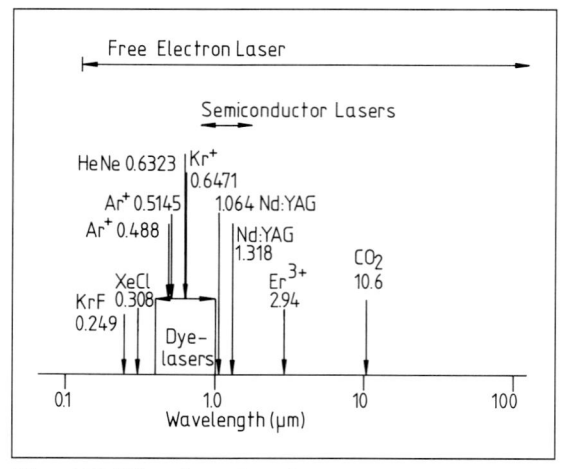

Fig. 167 Wavelengths of some common lasers.

4. Laser Treatment

Checklist for the Choice of a Laser System:

Wavelength	Tunable
	Fixed wavelength (= colour)
	- Single Wavelength
	- Multiple Wavelength
Time Domain	Continuous (CW)
	Pulsed →Pulselength
Light Intensity	
Interaction with the Tissue under Question	
Legal Requirements, Safety	e.g. FDA Approval
Delivery System	Fibre-optic System
	- Non-contact Delivery
	- Contact delivery e.g. Sapphire
	- Heat Conversion Probe
	Mirror System
Services required	- Cooling Water
	- Current Supply
	- Space (Separate Power Supply, etc)
Price	- System Cost
	- Cost of Replacement Components
	- Cost of Service Contract/Warranty
Reliability, Service	

Table 49

erties of some laser systems which are used in medical applications today.

Carbon Dioxide Laser

The carbon dioxide (CO_2) laser emits laser light at 10 600 nm in the far infrared. CO_2 laser light is very strongly absorbed in most materials, so that it is used for cutting and welding both organic and inorganic materials, including metals, in industry and medicine. CO_2 laser light is absorbed within a surface layer of 0.03 mm (= 30 micrometer) or less in tissue, almost independently of tissue type (5). The light is converted to heat within this thin layer and evaporates the tissue. Water within the cells is evaporated, leading to explosive evaporation of the cells.

Conventional CO_2 lasers emit continuous light. They produce cuts with extensive thermal damage in a layer beyond the cut (6). The TEA (transversely excited atmospheric pressure) CO_2 laser generates pulses of a duration between 50 and 1 000 ns with ener-

401

4. Laser Treatment

Properties of some Laser Systems, used in Medical Applications

Laser	Wavelength	Spectrum	Penetration in tissue	Mode
CO2	10 600 nm	Far Infra-red	appr. 30 um	CW, pulsed
Nd:YAG	(1319 nm) 1064 nm 532 nm) (355 nm)	infra-red Infra-red visible ultraviolet	up to 1mm up to 1mm	CW, pulsed
Argon	514.5 nm (488.4 nm) (+ other weaker lines)	green blue	deep, 1mm and more deep	CW
Krypton	647.1 nm (676.4 nm) (+ other weaker lines)	red red	deep, 1mm and more deep, 1mm and more	CW CW
Dye	tunable	infra-red visible ultraviolet		CW, pulsed down to a few fs
Excimer	193 - 351 nm	ultraviolet ultraviolet	a few micrometer a few micrometer	pulsed only 1 - 800 ns

Table 50

gies up to around 200 mJ per pulse, and a repetition rate of up to 500 Hz. The TEACO$_2$ laser can be used to ablate tissue without any observable thermal tissue damage. These results are similar to excimer laser ablation (7), which will be discussed below.

CO$_2$ laser light is strongly absorbed in water or blood. Therefore we may expect difficulties when applying CO$_2$ laser light in medical situations, where the light has to penetrate a layer of blood before reaching the tissue. This problem has been recently solved. It was found that focused CO$_2$ laser light pulses can propagate in blood through a channel in the liquid, which previous laser light pulses have created by evaporation (8,9).

Many medical applications require a fibre optic delivery system. Ordinary fused silica fibres are not suitable for CO$_2$ laser light. Today's delivery system for CO$_2$ lasers consist of articulate arms, constructed of metal tubes, where the laser light is guided by mirrors around the bends in the tube. Recently silverhalide (AgCl$_x$Br$_{1-x}$) fibres were found to be suitable for the transmission of CO$_2$ laser light (10). This development, together with the TEA. CO$_2$ laser, may make the CO$_2$ laser suitable for laser angioplasty.

Nd:YAG Laser

The optical amplifier of a Nd:YAG laser consists of an Yttrium Aluminium Garnet (YAG) crystal doped with Niodymium impurities. Pumping is by an arc lamp or a flash lamp. Future Nd:YAG lasers may be pumped by semiconductor laser arrays. The main Nd:YAG laser line is at 1.064 micrometer, in the near infra-red. In addition, frequency doubling and tripling achieves laser emission at 532 nm and at 355 nm, respectively. The intensity of these harmonics is lower than that of the principle line. An additional emission line, which is less frequently used, lies at 1.319 micrometer. Pulsed and continuous versions are available. Nd:YAG lasers have a large number of applications in medicine.

At the same intensity, Nd:YAG laser light has a deeper penetration depth in tissue than CO_2 laser light. The penetration depth is of the order of 1 mm, but depends strongly on the intensity of the light and the type of tissue. Because of deeper penetration, Nd:YAG laser light scatters markedly within the tissue.

The recent development of optical fibre delivery systems in combination with a variety of different contact laser probes, has opened a variety of surgical applications. Contact laser probes are made from ceramic sapphire, which is a very hard material with good heat conductivity, and which is transparent to Nd:YAG laser light. The direct contact of the probe with the tissue reduces scatter and reflection. Different probe profiles allow a variety of applications for precise cutting, tumor therapy, controlled heating, etc. (11). Typical power levels for these contact applications are pulses of 20 Watt with a 2 second duration.

The 1.319 micrometer Nd:YAG laser line, which shows deeper penetration depth, has been applied to tissue fusion and wound sealing (12).

Argon and Krypton Lasers

The main element of these lasers is typically a 1 meter long glass or ceramic tube containing Argon or Krypton gas through which a very high current (around 50 amps) is passed. Therefore, a high current power supply and a high throughput cooling water supply are required, which usually have to be specially installed for the laser. Argon gas is a more efficient laser medium than Krypton gas. As a consequence, an Argon laser needs a lower electrical current, less maintenance, and is less costly than a Krypton laser with the same light output power.

Both the Argon and the Krypton laser can lase at different wavelengths, ranging from the ultraviolet to the near infrared. The output power is highest at 514.5 nm (green) for the Argon laser at 647.1 nm (red) for the Krypton laser. Typical power levels for continuous Argon and Krypton lasers are 1 to 10 Watt. Both Argon and Krypton lasers can be operated in single line or multi-line mode by changing the mirrors of the laser cavity.

The penetration depth of low intensity continuous Argon and Krypton laser light in tissue is deep - of the order of millimeters. At high intensities, tissue ablation can be achieved. Because the main Argon and Krypton laser lines are transmitted into the eye, they are used extensively in ophthalmology. Argon and Krypton lasers are also used to pump dye lasers. These can produce pulsed and continuous light with wavelengths anywhere from the near infrared to the near ultraviolet.

A future application of the Argon laser is to replace suturing of anastomoses of blood vessels. The precise mechanism of tissue welding is an active area of research today (13,14,15,16).

Excimer Lasers

An excimer laser consists of a cavity filled with a mixture of a rare gas (such as Argon, Krypton or Xenon) and a halogen gas (Fluorine, Chlorine or

4. Laser Treatment

Bromine), with another rare gas as a background. During operation, excited states of rare gas - halogen molecules (the so-called excimer molecules) are formed and yield the laser light emission.

The excimer laser is operated by an electrical discharge between two electrodes inside the laser cavity and produces pulses of very high peak light intensity. The pulse length of conventional excimer lasers is of the order of a few nanoseconds (1 nanosecond = 0.000 000 001 second). Recently, however, excimer lasers have been developed with pulse lengths up to the 300 ns range and longer (17). Excimer lasers with such "stretched" pulse lengths have the advantage that transmission through optical fibres is easier, because of the reduced peak power.

Using different gas fillings, various emission lines in the ultraviolet can be achieved. As shown in Table 51, a large energy range can be covered.

Excimer laser light pulses are absorbed in a very thin surface layer (of the order of a few micrometers) in biological materials and in polymers. Thus, the excimer laser pulses deposit their energy in a small volume, during a time which is much smaller than the thermal relaxation time of the material. Secondly, the excimer laser pulses produce an extremely high electric field intensity during the pulse duration. The thin irradiated layer of the material is therefore subjected to very extreme conditions during the excimer laser pulse.

Provided that a certain threshold intensity is exceeded (which depends on pulse length and the type of tissue), polymers and biological tissues are "ablated". Tissue is removed with extreme precision. Consecutive pulses remove material, molecular layer by molecular layer - with complete absence of any detectable adjacent thermal damage. Ablation allows spectacular micromachining, such as holes drilled into human hair. The technique of ablation was pioneered by Srinivasan and collaborators from IBM research laboratories in Yorktown Heights (18). Srinivasan et al (19) also investigated excimer laser ablation of atherosclerotic plaque, which has become an active area of research today (20,21,22,23). For a review, see (24).

Fused silica optical fibres have been used for the longer wavelength excimer laser lines - for the XeCl (308

Emission Lines of Excimer Lasers

Excimer	Laser Emission Wavelength	Energy of Emitted Photons
ArF	193 nm	6.42 eV
KrCl	222 nm	5.58 eV
KrF	249 nm	4.98 eV
XeBr	282 nm	4.40 eV
XeCl	308 nm	4.03 eV

Table 51

nm) and the XeF (351 nm) excimer lasers (24,25,26). A difficulty is the tendency of excimer laser light to damage the optical fibre material, in particular at the point where the excimer laser light is focused into the optical fibre, or where it is coupled into a laser probe (26). The problems associated with fibre damage are easier to solve for the new excimer lasers with extended pulse length.

Dye Lasers

The active medium of a dye laser is a solution of dye molecules (such as Rhodamine, Coumarine or Oxazin) in a solvent. The dye solution is usually pumped through a carefully machined nozzle, such that a well-defined dye stream is formed. The pump laser is focused to a spot on the dye jet.

Although flashlamp pumped dye lasers exist, most dye lasers are pumped by a laser. For a particular laser dye, the wavelengths of the pump laser must lie within the absorption spectrum of the laser dye. The dyes used for laser operation have broad absorption and emission spectra. Laser action can only occur in wavelength ranges of sufficiently low self absorption of the dye solution. By adjusting optical components of the laser cavity, the emission wavelength of a dye laser can be tuned continuously over a range of wavelengths. This wavelength range depends on the dye being used. By changing the laser dye, a different tuning range is achieved. Thus, by changing the laser dye solution and by changing, if required, the pump laser or its wavelength, dye lasers covering the whole light wavelength range from the near infra-red to the near ultraviolet are available. Common pump lasers are the Argon and Krypton gas lasers, or harmonics of Nd:YAG lasers. Commercial medical dye lasers are available which are automated and require only periodic maintenance. Dye lasers exist for continuous and for pulsed operation. Pulse lengths can be made as short as a few femtoseconds (1 femtosecond = 10^{-15} seconds). The interaction of femtosecond dye laser pulses with the retina has recently been investigated (27).

Dye lasers offer the opportunity of tuning the wavelength of the laser accurately to the absorption properties of the tissue. Indeed, commercial medical dye lasers are used in ophthalmology. In this application, dye laser light can be made to affect particular cells in the retina, by tuning the wavelength of the dye laser light to the response of the particular cells targeted by the surgeon.

Laser Light Delivery Systems

One possible delivery system for laser light consists of an arrangement of mirrors reflecting the light to the point of application inside articulated tubes. This mode of application is found in commercial CO_2 lasers, or in a recent medical excimer laser system (29). At the end of the tube inside which the laser light is guided by a sequence of mirrors, there is a lens which focuses the laser light to a spot, to achieve the light intensity necessary for the removal of tissue.

In eye surgery, the laser light is usually delivered by a microscope system, so that precise focusing to a particular spot inside the eye is possible. Thus, very high precision, both parallel to the propagation direction of the light and laterally, can be achieved. The laser light in some applications is very sharply focused, so that the light intensity immediately before and after the point of

4. Laser Treatment

focus is not sufficient to cause any damage, therefore the intended damage is restricted to a very small area around the point of focus. Thus, in the minute region of the focus, a very high light density is achieved, leading to highly non-linear interaction with the material, including dielectric breakdown.

In contrast, for most internal applications, such as laser angioplasty, optical fibre delivery systems are necessary.

Most delivery systems include a Helium - Neon gas laser. The Helium - Neon laser sends a very weak but visible red light beam through the system in the same way as the main laser. Using this weak red light, the delivery system is aimed at and focused on the intended location.

Optical Fibre Delivery Systems

The nature of angioplasty and of many other medical applications requires optical fibre systems. An optical fibre laser light delivery system consists of:
- the input coupling component, where the laser light is coupled from the laser into the optical fibre
- the optical fibre conducting the laser light
- the output coupling component, where the laser light is coupled from the fibre into the output probe
- the probe
- additional components for guidance, control of temperature, or observation of the ablation and calibration components for measuring the light intensity.

Optical Fibres

Optical fibres are a result of research in the field of telecommunications over the last decade. Optical fibres are today capable of conducting laser light over many kilometers without any appreciable loss of intensity. Optical fibres for telecommunication systems operate in the infra-red. Optical fibre systems for medical applications need special construction for the wavelength required and for the usually high pulsed light intensities. Recently, optical fibre delivery systems have been developed even for CO_2 lasers (10) and excimer lasers (24, 25, 26).

An optical fibre consists of two concentric parts: the core and the cladding. Both usually consist of silica glass. The core of the fibre consists of optical material with higher refractive index than the cladding. Light which is incident from within the core of the fibre onto the interface between core and cladding with an angle smaller than the angle of total reflection is reflected back into the core of the fibre.

"Total reflection" is a physical phenomenon which will be well familiar to scubadivers. When the surface of water is viewed from below the water at a shallow angle, the surface looks totally silvery, exactly like a mirror. This effect is not seen when one looks perpendicularly onto the same water/air surface; nor is it observed when one looks onto the air/water surface from above the water. In the latter case there always is some transmission of light into the water. In the case of total reflection, there is no light propagation at all across the interface.

Since total reflection only occurs with sufficiently shallow angles, there is a certain acceptance angle of the optical fibre both on entrance and exit from the optical fibre. Because of the high collimation (parallelism) of the laser light, this requirement does not cause particular difficulties, but it does require special optics and care. Another consequence of the existence of a limiting angle for total reflection is that optical fibres have a minimum radius of curvature for bends. If an optical fibre is bent more strongly, light will be lost from the core of the fibre.

Laser light may damage the entrance or exit surface of the optical fibres if the laser is focused to spots with too high an intensity. Dielectric breakdown on either side of the fibre ending, due to the high peak pulse intensity, may also cause damage. Damage of the optical fibre poses a particular problem for excimer laser light. In order to solve this problem it has been proposed to use excimer lasers with extended pulse length and to use tapered fibre systems (24).

Light may, of course, be passed in both directions through optical fibre systems, so that the same fibre may be used both for application of the laser light and for spectroscopic observation of the tissue at which the probe is pointed. Laser angioplasty guided by observation of luminescence was pioneered by Ginsburg and collaborators (30) and is discussed in later articles in this book.

Probes

Several types of probes are in use today. In initial research, optical fibres have been introduced directly into the body or into arteries. This mode of operation has major problems. The optical surface of fibres is easily damaged, fibres may break, and broken parts of the fibre may remain in the body. The fibres themselves may cause unintended damage to the tissue.

Contact probes have been developed for medical application of the Nd:YAG laser for example, where the laser light is coupled from the end of the optical fibre into a ceramic sapphire probe, which is both hard and resistant to thermal damage. Such an optical probe may be constructed in different shapes, to obtain specific spatial distributions of the emerging light (11).

Solid metal probes have been used, where no optical path between the optical fibre and the surrounding tissue exists. The laser light is used solely as a means to transport energy to the metal "hot tip", which is heated by the laser light. The interaction of the probe with the tissue is both mechanical and through the high temperature of the metal tip (31). Constructions have been reported, where a combination of both heat and an additional optical emission is used.

One major problem in laser angioplasty is the danger of mechanically perforating the blood vessel, by pushing the probe through the wall, or by "optical" perforation occurring if the laser burns through the blood vessel. This problem could be solved by controlling both the mechanical movement of the probe and the operation of the laser light emission, by monitoring the tissue targeted by the probe.

Probes have been constructed which transport the laser light to the point of application and, in addition, contain control elements such as a thermocouple (to measure the temperature at this point). Thus, using a feed-back system, heating of the surrounding tissue to an accurately controlled temperature is possible.

Interaction of Laser Light with Tissue

For many applications it is sufficient to know that laser light deposits a certain amount of heat per pulse or per second in a certain volume. The amount of heat and the location and size of the volume are, in principle, ac-

4. Laser Treatment

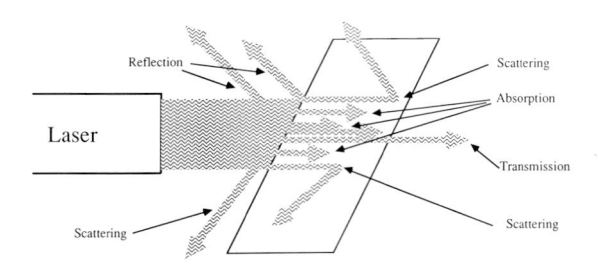

Fig. 168 Laser light may be transmitted, scattered or absorbed by materials.

curately controllable. In the following section, the interaction of laser light with tissue will be analysed in greater detail. Figure 168 shows the main interaction channels of laser light with tissue.

Reflection

When light falls onto a surface, part of the light energy is reflected back. This reflected part does not enter the tissue and is therefore lost for the application of cutting, etc. This is not harmful, unless the reflected laser light causes heating in uncontrolled areas. Reflection is a function of the mismatch of the indices of refraction, and is of the order of 5 to 10% between typical optical media. The amount of scattering can be reduced by using intermediate optical media to reduce the mismatch of the refractive index at the interface.

Scattering

Scattering is a result of fluctuations of optical properties of the tissue. Thus, the more inhomogeneities in the tissue, or the higher the roughness of an interface, the higher the scattering. When laser light is strongly absorbed, e.g. CO_2 laser light or excimer laser light, most photons will be absorbed by the tissue, before they get the chance to be scattered. Less strongly absorbed laser light (e.g. CW visible light, as from an Argon laser), on the other hand, is scattered substantially in biological tissue.

Scattering may actually become the dominant process determining the propagation of light in tissue.

The absorption depth is affected strongly by the scattering, as is the lateral size of the volume affected by laser light. A laser beam propagating in tissue, which is not strongly absorbing, will broaden substantially due to scattering. The broadening of a laser beam in the visible range due to multiple scattering, has been studied theoretically and experimentally (32,33,34).

Transmission

If a section of tissue is of a thickness comparable to, or thinner than the absorption length, some part of the laser light will be transmitted and emerge on the other side.

Absorption

The absorption of light in tissue leads to an exponential decrease of the light intensity in the tissue with increasing depth (though scattering will influence the precise depth profile of the laser light intensity). Thus there is a layer at the surface of the tissue with which the laser light interacts directly. This layer may be as thin as a few micrometers, as for CO_2 laser or excimer laser light. There may be an additional layer which is affected by heat conducted from the directly irradiated layer into the surrounding material. Thus, for continuous (CW) laser irradiation, a layer with varying degrees of thermal injury is usually found.

The detailed interaction of light with biological liquids (such as blood) and with tissue, depends on the light intensity. Thus, in general, the penetration of laser light in biological tissue cannot be determined from low intensity transmission measurements (8,9). Light can be

4. Laser Treatment

absorbed by tissue through the following mechanisms:

- absorption of laser light by excitation of thermal vibrations, leading to direct heating of the tissue
- absorption by excitation of electrons, leading either:
  - to bond breaking (only invoked to explain tissue ablation by high intensity laser pulses)
  - to subsequent heating by energy transfer from the excited electrons to thermal vibrations
- multi-photon absorption (only laser pulses of high peak intensity) leading to direct bond breaking and heating.

The interpretations of experiments by different researchers concerning direct bond breaking differ at present, so that it is not clear whether this complicated process has to be invoked. All other processes lead to heating of the material. At low laser intensities the heating of the tissue will be reversible. For example, if the tissue is heated to 40° C, the tissue may not show any damage after cooling down. When the laser-tissue interaction is investigated as a function of the laser intensity, there will be a threshold for the laser intensity, above which irreversible thermal damage occurs.

The microscopic character of irreversible damage is found to depend strongly on the type of tissue and on the type of illumination (i.e. wavelength and whether the light is pulsed or continuous). Examples of different types of laser damage found experimentally are:

- Irreversible damage of biological materials occurs when heating is above approximately 41° C. Parts of the cells are destroyed. These are the conditions used for vascular welding or suturing (15,16). Kopchok et al (16) determined a temperature of 44.2 ± 1.6° C for laser welding for anastomoses. Other experimental applications of controlled heating are in cancer therapy. Tumor cells have a lower temperature threshold for irreversible thermal damage than healthy cells, and this therefore can be exploited for the preferential distruction of tumour cells.
- When the cells are heated to 100° C, the water in the cells evaporates. Due to the drastically increased volume of the vapour, the cells explode. This is the effect used by CW lasers to achieve cutting and tissue removal. Charring and thermal damage usually also occur when a CW laser is used in this way.
- Ablation. Laser pulses of sufficiently high peak intensity and sufficiently short duration remove molecularly thin layers with each pulse, without any observable thermal damage (e.g. ablation using pulsed Nd:YAG, pulsed CO_2, or excimer laser).

There are two limiting cases (Figure 169):

- continuous irradiation
- pulsed irradiation

In the case of continuous irradiation, the illuminated volume is in thermal contact with the surrounding tissue. Thus, heat from the irradiated layer is conducted to the surrounding tissue. Thermal damage may be caused in surrounding tissue, even though it is not directly illuminated by the laser light - this is schematically shown in Figure 169a.

In the case of pulsed irradiation, however, the time of the laser pulse may be

4. Laser Treatment

Fig. 169 a) For continuous illumination, the irradiated volume of tissue is thermally coupled to its surroundings.

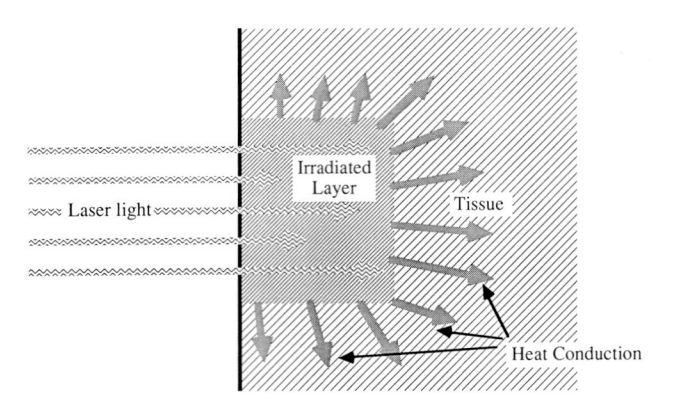

(a) Continuous Irradiation

Fig. 169 b) When the pulse length is shorter than the thermal relaxation time of the tissue, the relevant quantity is the capacity of the illuminated volume to absorb the light of the laser pulse.

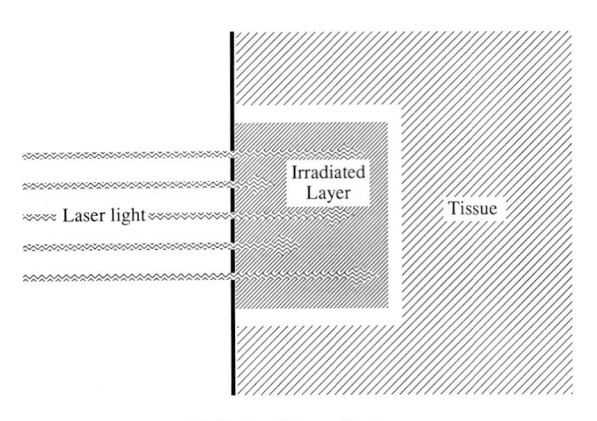

(b) Pulsed Irradiation

faster than the thermal relaxation time of the tissue. In this case the heat cannot be conducted away during the length of the laser pulse. Thus, the relevant quantity is the capacity of the irradiated volume to absorb the energy of the laser pulse in question, as shown schematically in Figure 169b.

It appears that cutting and tissue removal by lasers has similar limiting factors: cutting with continuous (CW) lasers involves thermal damage, as does ablation using pulsed lasers. The thermal damage caused by CW irradiation for cutting and tissue removal consists of a superficial zone of coagulation necrosis, and a deeper zone underneath of polymorphous lucunae, as described, for example, in (35).

Ablation

It is found experimentally that once the laser intensity per pulse exceeds a certain threshold, removal of tissue may be achieved without observable thermal damage. Microscopic studies show that, for subsequent laser pulses, each pulse removes subsequent molecularly thin layers of tissue. This removal of material, which is possible with very precise spatial control, has been discovered using ultraviolet pulsed excimer laser light by Srinivasan at IBM Research Laboratories in Yorktown Heights, and is called ablation (18,19, 20).

Recent studies (35), show that ablation can also be achieved by lasers with various other wavelengths: e.g. by visible lasers (36) (482 nm, 1 microsecond pulse duration, 40 - 80 mJ/pulse), pulsed TEA CO_2 lasers, pulsed Nd: YAG laser. The essential criterion to achieve ablation without thermal injuries, seems to be that the laser light has to be pulsed, and the energy per pulse has to exceed a certain threshold.

Detailed studies have been devoted to determine the microscopic mechanisms of ablation. Thus, the molecular units emerging from the point of ablation have been analysed. The competing explanations for the microscopic process are:

- nonthermal model: direct breaking of specific bonds by the laser light. (37, 38)

410

- thermal model: evaporation of tissue, with the possibility that a plasma is formed (35).

The precise microscopic process of ablation is still under investigation. It is interesting to note that the difficulties in understanding the microscopic processes underlying the ablationf tissue are somewhat similar to difficulties encountered in understanding "laser annealing". When impurities are implanted in single crystal silicon wafers for computer chip production, the zone of implantation is extensively damaged due to the implantation of the impurities. When the surface of the silicon crystal is irradiated by nanosecond excimer laser pulses, the silicon recrystallizes and the single crystal quality is restored without diffusion of the implanted impurities. It is extremely difficult to determine whether melting of the crystal takes place or whether an intermediate plasma state is produced. The main difficulty is to measure meaningful physical properties on the short time scale involved.

Details of the ablation process, as used for laser angioplasty, are discussed in several articles in this book.

Diagnostics and Imaging

In addition to the removal of tissue and to tissue ablation, laser light may also be used for characterization of tissue. Some possibilities are absorption spectroscopy, luminescence, and Raman spectroscopy. Work on spectroscopy to guide the laser beam for angioplasty is reported in other articles of the present volume - it was pioneered by Ginsburg et al (30).

In consequence of the demands of astronomy and of military applications, optical multichannel spectrometers have been developed recently, which allow one to measure extremely weak light with a spatial less than a micrometer. These developments enable optical spectroscopic techniques to provide new tools for medicine.

Both luminescence and Raman spectroscopy require essentially the same measuring configuration: a volume of tissue is illuminated by the laser. Both scattered, but otherwise unchanged laser light, luminescence and Raman light emerge from the illuminated tissue. All these types of scattered light are collected by an optical fibre or a collecting lens and analysed by a monochromator. A monochromator is an optical instrument, which, at its exit, separates the different wavelength components of the incident light. Thus the monochromator spreads the scattered light from the tissue into its different wavelength components. At the exit of the monochromator the spectrum of the light emerging from the illuminated tissue may be measured with an optical multichannel analyser instrument (OMA). An OMA usually has around 1 000 wavelength channels, so that the whole spectrum can be recorded in one step.

Luminescence Spectroscopy

Laser light lifts electrons to excited electronic levels in the tissue, e.g. into antibonding states of molecular bonds. These electrons subsequently fall back into lower electronic states - the light emitted during this relaxation process is luminescence. Most materials show luminiscence light emission under laser illumination. The spectrum of luminescence light emitted by a particular material is due to the characteristics of its electronic structure and therefore is characteristic of the material. In principle, the luminescence light emitted

4. Laser Treatment

may be used to characterize the tissue like a "finger print". However, there are difficulties to do so. One of the difficulties is that it is usually quite difficult to relate the luminescence spectrum to specific properties of the tissue. In addition, luminescence is usually very strongly dependent on impurities in materials, i.e. luminescence from possibly irrelevant impurities might dominate the luminescence spectrum. Still, despite these difficulties, luminescence may be a useful way of characterizing tissue in many circumstances. For angioplasty, the luminescence spectra of arteriosclerotic plaque and of arterial vessels have been investigated: (39) shows a clear difference of the luminescence spectra of normal as opposed to calcified human arteries, and uses these different luminescence properties for mapping the properties of a piece of artery.

Raman Spectroscopy

Raman Spectroscopy is named after the Indian physicist C V Raman, who discovered this effect. When laser light with photon energy E_L falls onto a tissue, the scattered light may contain components with photon energies different from that of the incident laser light. There may be light components with energies

$$E_L + E_{vib} \text{ and } E_L - E_{vib}$$

where E_L is the energy of the laser photons and E_{vib} is the energy of particular bond vibrations. The chemical bonds in a particular molecule have very sharp characteristic vibrational frequencies. The vibrational frequencies are characteristic of a particular bond. Molecular units and subunits, and crystals also have characteristic vibrational frequencies. The frequency shifts of the Raman scattered light have a spectrum, which directly correspond to vibrational frequencies of the tissue. It is often fairly straightforward to identify molecules and crystals from their vibrational spectra, as measured by Raman scattering.

It is possible that Raman spectra will find applications in medicine for the characterization of tissues - especially as optical multichannel instruments make measuring the usually very weak Raman spectra much easier than was previously possible.

Laser Safety

Lasers are usually reliable and safe to operate, as long as the safety regulations are observed. These safety regulations are stated by the manufacturers. There are also relevant safety laws and regulations which must be observed.

The main types of damage lasers can produce, if not handled carefully, are:

- damage to the eye, if laser light hits the eye or enters the eye
- high intensity laser light will damage exposed skin or clothing
- laser instruments usually contain high voltage power sources, which are dangerous when exposed
- some lasers use large amounts of cooling water. If leakage occurs in any part of the cooling water circuit, damage to the laser itself and its surroundings may occur as a consequence of flooding. Adequate protection against defects in the cooling water circuit is necessary
- the gases used in excimer lasers and the dye solutions in the dye lasers may be harmful. Thus the systems

4. Laser Treatment

must incorporate adequate protection against leakage.

Usually it is recommended to use appropriate safety spectacles which attenuate the laser light intensity to reduce the risk of accidental eye damage. Specific safety precautions are required for invisible (infra-red and ultraviolet) laser light.

Summary

The article gives an introduction to the nature of light and the differences between laser light and ordinary light. The physics of laser operation is introduced, and the interaction of laser light with tissue is discussed.

4. Laser Treatment

References

Two recent volumes (References 1 and 2) collect articles describing recent advances in laser applications in medicine:

1. "Lasers in Medicine", edited by SN Joffe, JA Parrish and RS Scott, Proceedings SPIE, 712, 1987.

2. "Special Issue on Lasers in Biology and Medicine", IEEE Journal of Quantum Electronics, Guest Editors: TF Deutsch and CA Puliafito, Volume QE-23, 1701, 1987.

3. Arons IJ. The outlook for lasers in medicine: markets and opportunities, in reference 1: 224, 1987.

4. Feynman RP. QED - the strange theory of light and matter. Princeton University Press, Princeton, 1985.

5. Wolbarsht ML. Laser surgery: CO_2 or HF, IEEE J Quantum Electron. QE-20: 1427, 1984.

6. Abela GS, Normann S, Cohen D, Feldman RL, Geiser EA, Conti CR. Effects of CO_2, Nd:YAG and Argon laser radiation on coronary atheromatous plaques. Amer J Cardiol 50: 1199, 1984.

7. Deckelbaum LI, Isner JM, Donaldson RF, Sylvie BS, Laliberete M, Clarke RH, Salem DN. Use of pulsed laser energy delivery to minimize tissue injury resulting from carbon dioxide laser irradiation of cardiovascular tissues. J Amer College Cardiol 7: 898, 1986.

8. Saar A, Gal D, Wallach R, Akselrod S, Katzir A. Transmission of pulsed laser beam through opaque liquids by a cavitation effect. Appl Phys Lett, to be published 1987.

9. Isner JM, Clarke RH, Katzir A, Gal D, DeJesus ST, Halaburka K. Transmission characteristics of individual wavelengths in blood do not predict ability to accomplish laser ablation in a blood field: inferential evidence for the "Moses Effect". Circulation 74: II 361, 1986.

10. Gal D, Katzir A. Silver halide optical fibres for medical applications. IEEE J Quantum Electron QE-23: 1827, 1987

11. For a review of several different applications of the Nd:YAG laser, see: J Aoki, S Suzuki, Y Shiina, T Miwa, N Daikuzono and SN Joffe. Experimental study and clinical application of new ceramic endoprobe with Nd-YAG laser; endoscopic hemostasis, pyroplasty and cutting biopsy, Ref 1: 2 (1987) and the following papers of Ref 1: papers 712-01, 712-02, 712-03, 712-04, 712-05, 712-07, 712-08, 712-09, 712-51, 712-52.

12. Dew DK. Review and status report on laser tissue fusion, Ref 1: 255.

13. Dew DK, Serbent R, Hart WS, Boynton C, Byrne JD, Evans, JG. Laser assisted microsurgical vessel anastomosis techniques: the use of argon and CO_2 lasers. Lasers Surg Med 3: 135, 1983.

14. Higginson LAJ, Farrell EM, Keaney MA, Walley VM, Singleton DS, Taylor RS, Nip WS, Keon WJ. Arterial response to laser irradiation. Ref 1: 250, 1987.

15. White RA, Donayre C, Kopchok G, White G, Abergel RP, Lyons R, Klein S, Dwyer R, Uitto J. Vascular welding using the argon laser. Ref 1: 252, 1987.

16. Kopchok G, Grundfest WS, White RA, Donayre C, Fujitani R, Litvack F, White GH, Klein SR, Morgenstern L. Argon laser vascular welding: the thermal component. Ref 1: 260, 1987.

4. Laser Treatment

17. Taylor RS and Leopold KE. Microsecond duration optical pulses from a UV-preionized XeCl laser. Appl Phys Lett 47: 81, 1985.

18. Srinivasan R. Ablation of polymers and biological tissue by ultraviolet lasers. Science 234: 559, 1986.

19. Linsker R, Srinivasan R, Wynne JJ, Alonso DR. Far-ultraviolet laser ablation of atherosclerotic lesions. Lasers Surg Med 4: 201, 1984.

20. Grundfest WS, Litvack F, Forrester JS, Goldenberg T, Swan HJC, Morgenstern L, Fischbein M, McDermid IS, Rider DM, Pacala TJ, Laudenslager JB. Laser ablation of human atherosclerotic plaque without adjacent tissue injury. J Amer Coll Cardiol 5: 929, 1985.

21. Isner JM, Donaldson RF, Deckelbaum LI, Clarke RH, Laliberte SM, Ucci AA, Salem DN, Konstam MA. The excimer laser: gross, light microscopic and ultrastructural analysis of potential advantages for use in laser therapy of cardiovascular disease. J Amer Coll Cardiol 6: 1102, 1985.

22. Farrell EM, Higginson LAJ, Nip WS, Walley VM, Keon WJ. Pulsed excimer laser angioplasty of human cadaveric arteries. J Vasc Surg 3: 284, 1986.

23. Bowker TJ, Cross FW, Rumsby PT, Gower MC, Rickards AF, Brown SG. Excimer laser angioplasty: quantitative comparison in vitro of three ultraviolet wavelengths on tissue ablation and haemolysis. Laser Med Sci 1: 91, 1986.

24. Singleton D, Paraskevopoulos G, Taylor RS, Higginson LAJ. Excimer laser angioplasty: tissue ablation, arterial response, and fiber optic delivery. IEEE J Quantum Electrom. QE-23: 1772, 1987.

25. Nevis EA. Alteration of the transmission characteristics of fused silica optical fibres by pulsed ultraviolet radiation. Proc SPIE 540: 421, 1985.

26. Taylor RS, Leopold KE, Michailov S, Brimacombe RK. Damage and transmission measurements of fused silica fibres using long optical pulse XeCl lasers. Opt Commun 63: 26, 1987.

27. Birngruber R, Puliafito CA, Gawande A, Lin Wei-Zhu, Schoenlein RW. Femto-second laser-tissue interactions: retinal injury studies. IEEE J Quantum Electron QE-23: 1836, 1987.

28. Danly BG, Temkin RJ, Bekefi G. Free-electron lasers and their application to biomedicine. IEEE J Quantum Electron, QE-23: 1739, 1987.

29. Caro RG, Muller DF. A medical excimer laser system for corneal surgery and laser angioplasty. In Ref 1: 95, 1987.

30. Ginsburg R, Kim DS, Guthaner D, Toth J, Mitchell RS. Salvage of an ischemic limb by laser angioplasty: description of a new technique. Clin Cardiol 7: 54, 1984.

31. Cumberland DC, Tayler DI, Welsch CL, Guben JK, Sanborn TA, Moore DJ, Greenfield AJ, Ryan JJ. Percutaneous laser thermal angioplasty: initial clinical results with a laser probe in total peripheral artery occlusions. Lancet 1: 1457, 1986.

32. Sinofsky E, Dumont M. Measurement of laser beam spreading in biological tissue scattering. In Ref 1: 58, 1987.

4. Laser Treatment

33. Yoon G, Welch AJ, Motamedi M, Van Gemert MCJ. Development and application of three-dimensional light distribution model for laser irradiated tissue. IEEE J Quantum Electron, QE-23: 1721, 1987.

34. Bolin F, Preuss LE, Taylor RC, Sandu TS. A study of the three-dimensional distribution of light (632.8 nm) in tissue. IEEE J Quantum Electron QE-23: 1734, 1987.

35. Isner JM, Steg PG, Clarke RH. Current status of cardiovascular laser therapy, 1987. IEEE J Quantum Electron QE-23: 1756,1987.

36. Prince MR, LaMuraglia GM, Teng P, Deutsch TF, Anderson R. Preferential ablation of calcified arterial plaque with laser-induced plasmas, IEEE J Quantum Electron, QE-23: 1783, 1987

37. Srinivasan R and Mayne-Banton V. Self-developing photoetching of poly(ethylene terephtalate) by laser radiation. Appl Phys Lett, 41: 576, 1982.

38. Srinivasan R and Braren B. Ablative photodecomposition of polymer films by pulsed far-ultraviolet (193 nm) laser radiation: dependence of etch depth on experimental conditions. J Polym Sci Polym Chem Ed 22: 2601, 1984.

39. Sartory M, Sauerbrey R, Kubodera S, Tittel FK, Roberts R, Henry PD. Autofluorescence maps of atherosclerotic human arteries - a new technique in medical imaging. IEEE J Quantum Electron, QE-23: 1794, 1987.

4.3. Coronary Artery Plaque Rapidly Induced by Local Electro-Magnetic Stimulation and Western Diet

H Breuer [1], J Fincham [2], P Hinrichsen [3], CJ Uys [4],
H Weich [5], B Reichart [1]

[1] Department of Cardiothoracic Surgery,
[2] Research Institute for Nutritional Diseases,
[3] Department of Medical Physics,
[4] Department of Pathology, University of Cape Town,
South African Medical Research Council, Tygerberg,
[5] Cardiology Unit, University of Stellenbosch,
South Africa

Abstract

A reliable method has been developed to produce atherosclerotic-like plaque in the right coronary arteries (RCA) of baboons. The stenoses develop as a consequence of electro-stimulation at the chosen position and feeding of a Western diet. Histologically the structure of the constrictions is similar to atherosclerotic lesions. The stenoses occupy, on average, 55% of the available lumen; total occlusion was also observed. The pulsed stimulus lasted for 30 min per day for an average of 16 days. This method can be utilized to create models of arterial disease relevant to man in order to develop and refine methods of recanalization.

Introduction

Recently, laser radiation has been guided via optical fibres along the interior of the blood vessels toward stenoses in these vessels. Absorbing the power of the laser radiation, the tissue making up the constriction evaporates or ablates, resulting in an unrestricted channel for the blood flow. This method is still in its experimental stage, however, Cumberland et al (1,2) and others (3) have already achieved remarkable results.

However, further progress is hampered by lack of a suitable animal model. A method is required which can produce an atherosclerotic plaque within the CA at a predetermined position relatively quickly in order to perfect safe surgical clearance of the arteries. This artificially produced stenosis should meet the following criteria:

- Resemble micro- and macroscopically as close as possible a naturally formed plaque from a human CA.
- Grow within a suitable time span, eg weeks or months.
- Be produced in a CA with a size resembling that of man's.

Feeding primates atherogenic diets containing high proportions of saturated fats and cholesterol does produce

4. Laser Treatment

suitable stenoses, but this method is slow and expensive (4). In addition, severity and position of the constrictions cannot be predicted.

Betz et al (5) fed rabbits a high cholesterol diet and, in addition, electrically stimulated a small section of the aortic wall. As a result, atherosclerotic plaques developed at the point of stimulation. The walls of the aorta and CA are morphologically different. In addition, rabbits are difficult to anaesthetize and the CA are very small.

We have modified and developed the method of Betz et al (5) and applied it to the CA of the baboon (Papio ursinus). As a result, we have succeeded in inducing the formation of atherosclerotic plaque within weeks at predetermined positions. Our method thus satisfies all three of the above criteria.

Methodology

Primates

Baboons (18-30 kg, male) served as experimental animals. The described procedure was approved by the Ethics Committee of the University of Cape Town. The primates were kept in individual cages. They were fed an atherogenic diet (AD) which has been described in detail by Fincham et al (6). This diet promotes progression of atherosclerosis to advanced disease in large and medium arteries of susceptible individual male and female Vervet monkeys (Cercopothecus aethiops) within 2-4 years.

The AD was provided as baked patties each weighing approximately 65 g. The baboons were fed twice per day, each receiving 4 patties daily. The diet was supplemented daily with baboon cubes, bread and fruit. The primates appeared to be strong and healthy. One week before entering the trial, each animal was weighed and checked for haemoglobin, HCT, MCH, MCV, RBC, WBC, salmonella, shigella; a differential blood count was included. Throughout the trial, the baboons were under veterinary supervision.

Electrodes (see Figure 170)

Material: (37% Au, 63% Ag). Two bent strips (each 9 mm long, 1.5 mm wide, 0.05 mm thick) formed two parallel brackets, tightly clamped around a 5 mm wide and 0.5 mm thick strip of GORE-TEX (Gore Inc, Flagstaff, USA). Both electrodes were separated by 2-3 mm on the GORE-TEX. To each electrode, a 35 cm long wire (Cu, 5 strands, 0.4 mm total diameter, PVC-insulated) was silver-soldered. All metal surfaces, except those adjacent to the vessel, were sprayed with a silicon-based inert

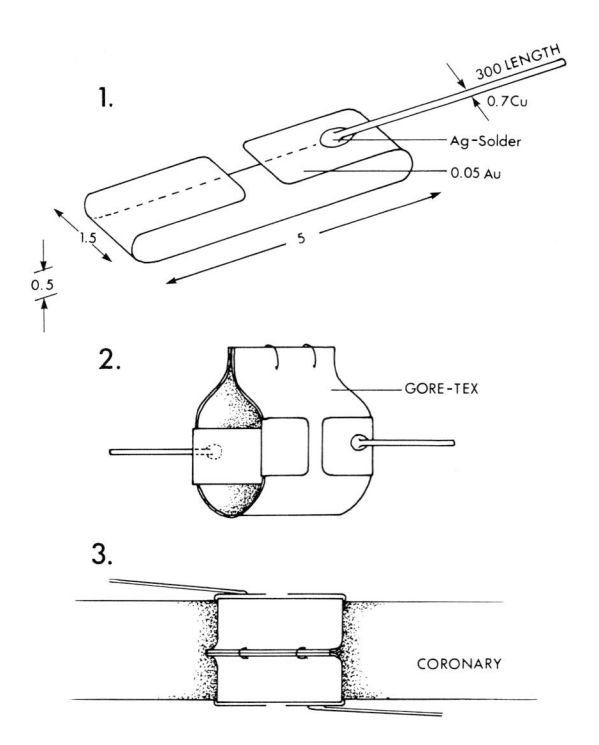

Fig.170 Electrodes for electrostimulation. All measurements in mm.

flexible coating. The electrodes and wires were sterilized by gas.

Implanting the Electrodes

The baboon was first immobilized with Ketamine-hydrochloride (5 mg/kg), then with Morphin, Pancuronium bro-mide (2 mg) and Atropine (0,25 mg) and ventilated (10-20 breaths/min) using a mixture of 40% oxygen and 60% nitrous oxide. ECG and blood pressure in the femoral artery were monitored. Subsequently, a median sternotomy was performed and the pericardium opened longitudinally.

The electrodes were wrapped around the dissected RCA approximately 3 cm from its origin. The arrangement formed a cuff, loose enough to avoid any pressure, but tight enough to prevent sliding.

Both wires were led away parallel to the vessel, but in opposing directions. Approximately 3 cm distal from its electrode, each wire was fixed to the myocardium by one suture. From this point, the wires were led through the thoracic wall and skin in the anterior axillary line through the third intercostal space. Before exiting through the skin, the wires were fixed with a suture to a suitable structure, and 2 cm protruded through the skin.

Stimulation Mode

During electromagnetic stimulation, the protruding wires were connected directly to a constant voltage square wave pulse generator. Pulse height: 9 V, pulse width: 10 ms, pulse separation: 100 ms.

Stimulation Procedure

Stimulation of the electrodes began 5 to 8 days after implantation. Approx. 5 min before stimulation each animal was immobilized and anaesthetized. Thereafter, the animal was moved onto the operating table and ventilated via an endotracheal tube. The protruding wires were connected to the electrical pulse generator. Each baboon was stimulated 5 x per week, at the same time of day, for a duration of 30 min. The ECG was initially monitored, but, as it was soon established that the electrical stimulation had no effect on it, this was abandoned. No side effects or complications were noticed during or as a consequence of stimulation.

Histology

After the end of the trial for each baboon, a section of the RCA centered around the implanted electrode was removed and fixed in neutral buffered 10% formalin (pH 7.2), at a fixative to tissue volume ratio of about 20:1. Subsequently the electrodes were removed, the artery processed, embedded in wax, and sectioned at 5 micron intervals for examination by light microscopy. Haematoxylin and eosin were used for staining. In some cases Verhoeffs/Giesen's stains were used to display connective tissues and alcian blue/periodic acid Schiff stains for acid mucopolysaccharides and proteoglycans.

Angiography and Catheterization

The RCA of each baboon was visualized by angiography once or twice during the experiment. The selected baboon was immobilized and transported to the Central Research Laboratory of the University of Stellenbosch, Tygerberg. There it was kept overnight and prepared the next morning for angiography. After angiography, the baboon was immobilized again and transported back to its cage at the Medical School. For this day, the animal's electrodes were not stimulated. If angiography indicated the

4. Laser Treatment

existence of stenoses, the animal was sacrificed within one to four days.

The baboons were catheterized using the Seldinger technique through the right femoral artery. A 7 French 8,5 cm soft tip Judkins right coronary catheter could be engaged in the ostium of the CA. Bolus injections of Conray 420 contrast medium (3-5 ml) were given into the artery under direct fluoroscopic vision.

In one baboon a 3F Gruntzig coronary infusion catheter was passed through the Judkins catheter which acted as a guiding catheter. A pressure gradient was measured over the electrode area, and the existence of a significant constriction (more than 30% of the vessel cross section) was demonstrated.

The baboon heart is electrically very unstable, and if ventricular fibrillation occurs, very difficult to defibrillate. The procedure could thus not be used routinely to determine the degree of stenosis. In addition, transstenotic pressure gradient measurement seems to be of limited value in cases of severe stenosis (7).

Results

Behaviour

All animals displayed normal behaviour throughout the trial. No side-effects due to the atherogenic diet, the implanted electrodes, the stimulation procedure, or from repeated anaesthesia was observed. Electrocardiograms, recorded before and during angiography and catheterization, remained normal.

External to Coronary Arteries; at Site of Electrodes

The diameter of the CA was approximately 2 mm. Most retained a circular shape. Some were compressed into an elliptical shape, most likely due to asymmetrical stress where one of the connecting wires broke. At the site of the implanted electrodes there was acute and chronic periarteritis of moderate severity. Morphologically the cellular reaction to the foreign material was restricted to a few extravascular erythrocytes, neutrophils, plasma cells, many lymphocytes and fibroblasts. Moderately dense connective tissue had formed around the electrodes. These reactions were observed, whether or not the electrodes were electrically stimulated during the experiment.

Inside the Coronary Arteries; at Site of Electrodes

a. Controls

Controls received electrodes without attached wires. They were kept about 6 weeks after implantation. All controls displayed normal CA, i.e. under the position of the electrodes. (There are indications that stenoses may also be produced by mechanical stimulation, e.g. repeated flexing at a position of the CA, caused by relatively stiff wires connected to the electrodes. This effect is currently under investigation.)

b. Electromagnetically Stimulated coronary Arteries

Proliferative intimal plaque, varying in extent, formed in the CA under the electrodes. It extended the full length of the implanted electrodes. Outside the electrode, the CA appeared to be normal (see Figures 171a and b). Typically the arteries showed a notable degree of intimal myofibroblast proliferation. In general, this presented as a cellular eccentric intimal plaque, resulting in a reduction of lumen size.

Histology of a typical artificial plaque: Medial smooth muscle cells are evenly separated by small to moderate

4. Laser Treatment

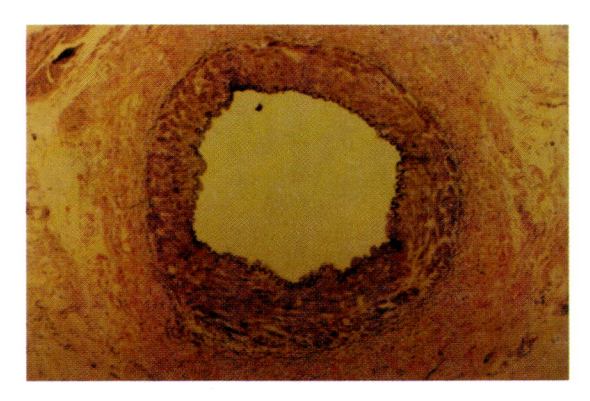

Fig. 171 a) Transverse section of CA from baboon (Ref: 011) selected at a site away from the electrode placement. The vessel appears normal and shows no intimal proliferation. Haematoxylin and eosin, x 70.

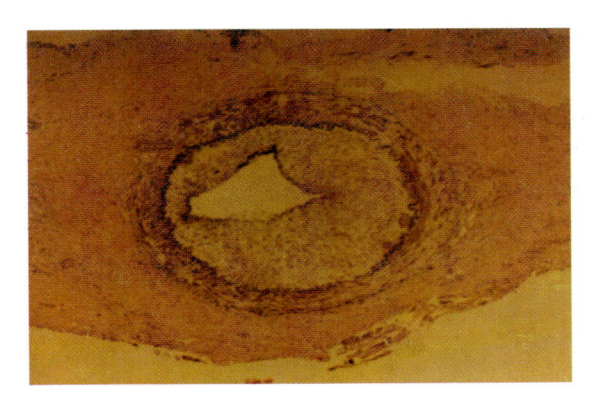

Fig. 171 b) CA section from same baboon (Ref: 011) selected at the site of electrode placement. Adventitial fibrosis is present and there is a notable degree of eccentric intimal thickening resulting in significant narrowing of the lumen. The plaque consists of myofibroblasts proliferating in a myxoid background. The media and internal elastic lamina are intact. Haematoxylin and eosin, x 70.

amounts of extracellular substance, a mixture of collagens and glycosaminoglycans. The intima is variably thickened by proliferation of myofibroblasts, separated by small to copious volumes of extracellular substance. Intimal thickening by plaque is circumferentially eccentric. The endothelium is usually intact and there is no thrombosis. No subendothelial foam cells, inflammatory cells, or plaque mineralisation is present. Disruption of the internal elastic membrane and disorientated secretion of elastin by smooth muscle cells is a marked feature. No cholesterol crystals are observed within the plaque.

Numerical Results

Thirteen baboons participated in the experiment, 2 served as controls, i.e. non-stimulated electrodes were implanted. Seven of the 8 stimulated baboons developed, after an average of 16 stimulations, intracoronary plaques. The produced stenoses occupied, on average, 55% of the available lumen. One baboon did not develop a plaque, probably because the connecting wire broke early after implantation. Three baboons died during the experiment (one acute heart failure, two infections).

From this trial it is not possible to correlate the size of the occluded cross-sections of stimulated RCA with the number of stimulating electrical pulses (i.e. the total electrical energy applied). The reason for this is the uncertainty of the time when a connecting wire to the electrodes may have broken. However, we can safely state that stimulation of approximately 30 minutes x 18 times leads to a sizeable plaque (ie. in excess of 50% of the cross section of the RCA is blocked).

Conclusion

The method described produces stenoses of CA lumens by intimal plaque formation within a few weeks. The results are significant and provide cardiovascular surgeons with a suitable and realistic model on which to practise laser surgery or other related techniques.

4. Laser Treatment

Acknowledgements

The support F Barends, Dr E Cornish, P Human, and F Snyders, is greatly appreciated. We thank Colin Woodroof (RIND) for preparing the sections for histology. The experiments were financially supported by a grant from the South African Research Council (MRC).

References

1. Cumberland DC, Taylor DI, Welsh CL, Guben JK, Danborn TA, Moore DJ, Greenfield AJ, Ryan TJ. Percutaneous laser thermal angioplasty: initial clinical results with a laser probe in total peripheral artery occlusions. The Lancet I, 1457, 1986.

2. Cumberland DC, Starkey IR, Oakley GDG, Fleming JS, Smith GH, Giotti JJ, Taylor DI, Davis J. Percutaneous laser-assisted coronary angioplasty. The Lancet 2, 214, 1986.

3. Crea F, Davies G, McKenna W, Pashazade M, Taylor K, Maseri A. Percutaneous laser recanalization of coronary arteries. The Lancet 2, 214, 1986.

4. Fincham JE, Woodroof CW, Van Wyk MJ, Capatos D, Weight MJ, Kritchevsky D, Rossouw JE. Promotion and regression of atherosclerosis in Vervet monkeys by diets realistic for westernized people. Atherosclerosis 66, 205, 1987.

5. Betz E, Schlote W. Responses of vessel walls to chronically applied electrical stimuli. Basic Res Cardiol 74, 10, 1979.

6. Fincham JE, Faber M, Weight MJ, Labadarios D, Taljaard JJF, Steytler JG, Jacobs P, Kritchevsky D. Diets realistic for westernized people significantly effect lipoproteins, zinc, vitamins C, E, B6 and haemotology in Vervet monkeys. Atherosclerosis 66, 191, 1986.

7. Ganz P, Abben R, Friedman PL, Garnic JD, Barry WH, Levin DC. Usefulness of transstenotic coronary pressure gradient measurements during diagnostic catheterization. Am J Cardiol 55, 910, 1985.

4.4. Excimer Laser - Tissue Interactions

*G Wollenek, G Laufer, W Klepetko,
F Grabenwöger, E Wolner*

2nd Surgical Department, University of Vienna,
Austria

The potential use of laser radiation in cardiac and vascular surgery has been recognized since the late 1970s. Recent studies have demonstrated the ability of laser radiation to recanalize severely stenotic or totally occluded arteries. Therefore the effect of argon, carbon dioxide and Nd:YAG laser energy on healthy and pathological vascular tissue underwent intensive in vitro (1,2,3,4) and even in vivo (5,6,7) examination.

A considerable amount of experimental work, as well as first clinical steps, have been carried out in the field of peripheral and coronary arteries, but the clinical role of lasers still remains to be evaluated.

The prerequisites for successful laser angioplasty are:
- Tissue ablation in the centre of the irradiated area corresponding to the diameter of the laser beam with no or minimal neighbouring coagulative necrosis.
- Prediction of the penetration depth with respect to the ablation rate (knowledge of the laser's ablative quality at different biological structures).
- Tissue ablation without significant differences in quality and quantity between normal tissue and their pathological alterations.
- Sufficient technical requirements, especially concerning the transmission system and its functional end, e.g. the shape of the fibre tip.
- Low risk of perforation: role of the sharp edges of the bare fibre, mechanical components, problem in maintaining an axial position of the fibre within the vessel, scattering.
- Low incidence of thrombosis and the role of drug therapy.
- Safety of the system for the patient as well as for medical staff.

During the last years, continuous wave lasers have mostly been used. These lasers are thought to ablate biological tissue by a thermal process with consecutive vaporization, causing substantial thermal injury, and they are not able to destroy heavily calcified plaques. Another problem of importance is the high rate of re-occlusion reaching up to 100%. In addition, questions concerning the high rate of perforation have not yet been answered.

The risk that the technology of laser angioplasty would fail due to these systemic limitations became apparent. More control, greater precision, and less thermic alteration of neighbouring tissues were principal demands in order to avoid perforation, wall destruction

4. Laser Treatment

with swelling and necrosis, and aneurysm formation (8). So the initial enthusiasm for curative applications has given way to a more realistic estimation of the clinical valence concerning the treatment of atherosclerotic disease.

Interrupted or pulsed mode laser energy minimizes this pattern of damage, as the surrounding tissue is not subjected to damaging heat. With further technical developments of conventional systems, an improvement in the utility may be expected. Steg et al (9) were able to demonstrate recanalization of human atheromatous coronary arteries in vitro with minimal thermal damage, using a nanosecond pulsed Nd:YAG laser. This pulsed Nd:YAG laser light resulted in precisely cut lesions with central tissue vaporization but minimal evidence of thermal injury, whereas pulsed Nd:YAG lasers with frequency-doubled and tripled wavelengths caused defects comparable to those of very mitigated continuous wave lasers. Most recent studies have suggested that Excimer laser radiation will be able to minimize these risks.

Excimer Laser

Compared with conventional lasers, the Excimer laser provides a very different type of material ablation. Excimer lasers are pulsed gas lasers that use a mixture of a rare gas and halogen as the active medium to generate pulses of short wavelength, high energy, ultraviolet irradiation. Depending on the gas mixture (argon-fluorine, krypton-fluorine, xenon-chloride) employed, the precise wavelength is 193, 248, or 308 nm. Basic mechanisms of Excimer laser action were investigated by Srinivasan et al (10). In his explanation, very high energy levels in the ultraviolet range cause a disruption of molecular bonds, suggesting a photochemical mechanism for tissue ablation. However, Murphy-Chutorian et al (11) published another interpretation, believing that the ablative effect of Excimer laser energy (at least in the case of 351 nm) on vascular tissue is predominantly a thermal process and is similar to that of other wavelengths: it is the manner in which laser energy is delivered and not the laser wavelength which allows precise ablation. This view correlates with our experience: in 1986 we performed temperature measurements of the substance in the vicinity of the lasered punched out defect (12). The incident energy density was measured using a powermeter, and the Siemens TMO thermoprobes were situated at distances of 50, 250, 500, and 1 000 micrometers from the defect to be created. These distances were later controlled by measuring the distance by light microscopic resolution. The irradiations were performed at different frequencies (5, 10, 15 pulses per second), at an energy fluence between 3 and 30 mJ/mm^2, and at different wavelengths (193, 248 nm). Figure 172 shows the results of the temperature measurements during radiation at 193 nm: the diagram demonstrates the interrelation between measured distance, duration of exposure, and local temperature. The problem with this investigation was the technical inability to register the ultrashort temperature peaks in the range of a few nanoseconds. The noticed longer-lasting mean temperature elevations though were produced in a series of tests, and appear to allow some comparison of the "effective thermic influence". At both investigated wavelengths, our study confirmed a significant dependence of the rise in

4. Laser Treatment

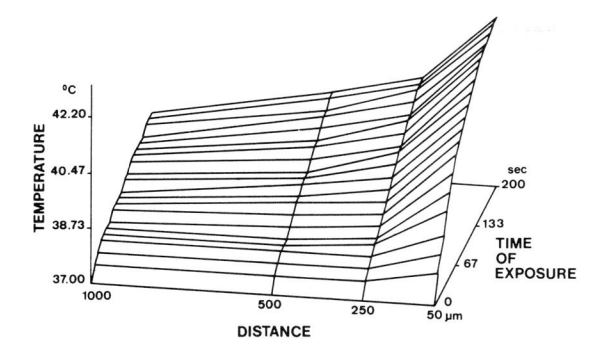

Fig. 172 Temperature measurements during radiation at 193 nm: diagram showing the interrelation between measured distance, duration of exposure and local temperature (10 Hz, 2.7 mJ/mm^2/ pulse).

temperature with the frequency. The increases with 248 nm radiation were similar to that of 193 nm, although the increase was greater. In general, a gaussian distribution was displayed in the target surroundings.

Only a small part of the original energy of the beam is transformed into thermal energy. The peak of the pulse energy achieved is ultra-short and most energy disappears at the moment of contact with the biological material, whereas the small amount of thermal energy absorbed is dissipated by the normal mechanism of heat conductivity. This is a relatively slow process with undoubtable tissue consequences. As this heat dissipation requires a certain "thermal relaxation time" between two pulses, local accumulation of heat will occur if the interval is too short. Murphy-Chutorian et al (13) calculated the "thermal tissue relaxation time" to be in the range of 50 to 100 milliseconds. This period is necessary to allow sufficient time for the tissue surrounding the area of incident laser radiation to dissipate its heat and return to its normal temperature. If the normal value is reached before the next pulse, no cumulative increase in temperature or subsequent thermal laseralization will occur. The same working group suggested that the radiation-free interval at 10 Hz should be 100 milliseconds, and did not observe any vacuolization of the border on histology. Though the influence of different power densities has to be taken into consideration, our studies showed a thin zone with lacunae and coagulation necrosis, even at 10 Hz in transmission electron microscopy. Consequently, there is thermal energy formation, and it seems impossible to avoid this heat generation. However, its accumulation can be controlled.

Nevertheless, the final explanation for the ablative effects of Excimer laser radiation in far ultraviolet has not yet been found. And, as there is a reaction at the surface of the irradiated tissue within a few nanoseconds, the question arises whether there are different mechanisms resulting in one similar end effect under these conditions.

This mechanism, although of some disclarity, leads to extremely precise ablation. The penetration depths by UV are extremely small, namely fractions of a micrometer, a few micrometres at most. This is due to the very strong absorption by most organic molecules when exposed to the ultraviolet range. Proteins, which constitute about 15-20% of all cells, also absorb in this spectral region, usually with a peak around 280 nm.

In Vitro Studies

The tests were carried out using an Excimer laser Lambda Physik EM 102 at 193 and 248 nm, and a Technolas Excimer laser MAX 10 at 308 nm. The power densities were varied between 3 mJ/mm^2/pulse (193 nm without a transmitting device) and 30 mJ/mm^2/pulse

4. Laser Treatment

(248 nm using a movable device constructed by Zeiss Germany, and 308 nm with flexible bare fibres with a diameter of 1 mm), the exposure time between 5 and 20 pulses per second was up to 200 seconds. Following the concept that lengthening the laser pulse would allow the same pulse energy to be delivered at a reduced peak power, we used a pulse length of 70 nanoseconds in the case of 308 nm in order to gain easier transmission through the fibres. At 193 and 248 nm radiation, the pulses had a duration of 14-16 nanoseconds.

Using Excimer laser radiation in the far (B with respect to C) ultraviolet region, the piercing action of the beam results in circumscribed, sharply defined borders with very smooth intimal topography. Even in light microscopic resolution, no thermal lesions were visible in the vicinity of the application site, and the architecture of the surrounding area was well preserved (Figure 173) using healthy or arteriosclerotic human vessel segments. Even in fibrous, cholesterol and of importance, severely calcified plaques, good results were obtained. With the exception of severe calcification, the ablation rate was similar, constant, pulse synchron and therefore, in reality, predictable. Under the conditions described, the 193 nm radiation caused an ablative progression of about 0.5 micrometres, in the case of 248 and 308 nm respectively, the observed ablation rate was about 20-30 micrometres.

Scanning electron microscopy showed no damage to the intima endothelial cells at the border of the vaporized area. The newly formed crater wall had a comparatively smooth surface without any residues of carbonization.

Transmission electron microscopy revealed a very thin zone, of about 4 micrometres, with signs of destruction or damage. Within this zone typical signs of thermal influences on biologic tissue could be observed: as a consequence of phase transitions, rare lacunae were embedded in coagulated substance. There was no evidence however of carbonization, therefore these findings indicate the presence of a low-degree of heating adjacent to the lost substance. Beyond this zone, no ultrastructural alteration of myocytes or fibres was found; even the cell organelles, which are very sensitive to thermal influences, were without visible changes with respect to their integrity and structure. Only in some specimens was the structural integrity of the border noticed to be torn up, which is likely to be an acoustic effect from plasma formation and plasma-related pressure waves (Figure 174).

In Vivo Studies

In 193 nm and even in 248 nm, transmission of far ultraviolet laser power remains the major problem when performing animal studies and clinical tri-

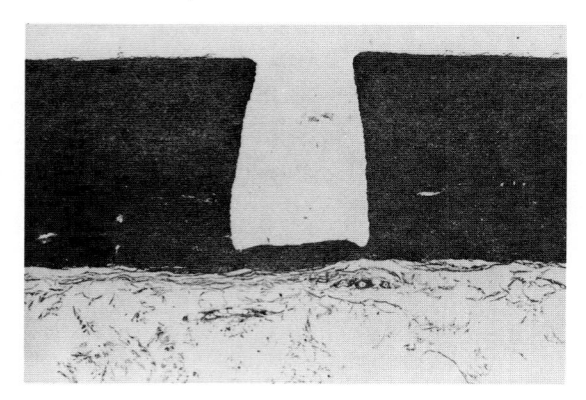

Fig. 173 Section of cadaveric aorta after argon fluoride irradiation in air. The margin of the laser-induced crater defect shows no evidence of carbonization or other thermal damage (193 nm, 10 Hz, 2.7 mJ/mm^2/pulse).

4. Laser Treatment

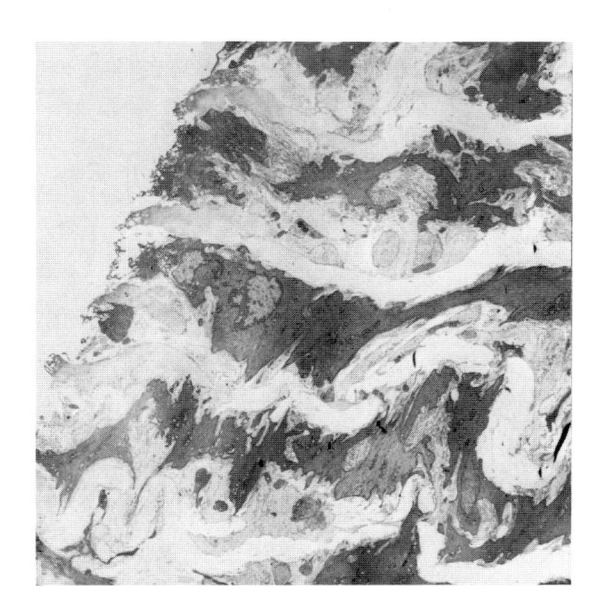

Fig. 174 Specimen of cadaveric aortic wall after 193 nm laser irradiation in air. There is a thin layer of protein coagulation with multiple lacunae due to phase transition phenomena (about 1 μm) and underlying zone of coagulation (about 3 μm) passing then into tissue without visible damage of its ultrastructural integrity (TEM, 194 nm, 10 Hz, 2.7 mJ/mm^2/pulse).

als. In the case of 193 nm, no flexible or rigid fibre with sufficient efficiency exists. For 248 nm, an energy transmitting device was designed in collaboration with ZEISS optical manufacturers and combined with the Excimer laser. This new transmission system allows movement in all directions and rotation in the long axis, thus permitting easy handling and guiding in the operative field. It consists of a rigid articulated arm, and the beam is directed by several mirrors. In the very distal part, rotation is possible, and the laser beam is focused by means of lenses. The most reliable of the Excimer lasers is the XeCl, which is well suited to medical applications since its 308 nm wavelength is readily absorbed by tissue.

In February 1987, Prevosti et al (14) reported in vivo experiences of healing in canine femoral arteries using a 308 nm Excimer laser. They found early platelet adhesion with rapid re-endothelialization without surface thrombus formation, late fibro-intimal ingrowth without surface damage or aneurysm formation.

Using the articulated arm with 248 nm radiation, we performed in vivo experiments on young rabbits. Following a laparotomy, the abdominal aorta having a diameter of about 2 mm, was opened longitudinally for 1 cm. The exposed intimal surface was then irradiated and the vessel thereafter closed with sutures. In ten animals there was good runoff, but 50% of them showed vascular spasm soon after completion of the suturing, and in these animals a consecutive thrombosis with plegia was observed. The reason for this observation is, as yet, unclear. Possibly some surgical shortcomings played a part. On the other hand, this local vascular spasm corresponds with Ginsburg's observations in seven patients, who experienced significant discomfort and intense vascular spasm during the delivery of laser energy (15).

In order to evaluate the feasibility of percutaneous Excimer laser angioplasty we attempted it on one patient. This was a 64 year old male with inoperable bronchial carcinoma and rest pain from a total occlusion of the superficial femoral artery. Using a Seldinger technique, the 7 cm long occlusion was recanalized. Only a thin channel corresponding to the diameter of the fibre used (1 mm), was created. The procedure therefore had to be completed with balloon dilatation. Three months later, the patient is without pain, showing satisfactory arterial perfusion.

According to the headline of the newspaper USA TODAY, December 16,

4. Laser Treatment

1987, Keon and his team from the Ottawa Civic Hospital heart institute are the first to have used an Excimer laser to successfully recanalize a coronary artery stenosis.

Discussion and Conclusion

To date, there are three main means for the treatment of occlusive disease: conservative, semiconservative (PTA-PTCA, streptolysis, eventually laser angioplasty and rotational thrombectomy devices) and surgical (bypass grafting and eventually laser angioplasty). These techniques may be used as a single method or by supplementing each other. In our opinion, use of the very expensive laser radiation should be limited to small vessels such as coronary arteries or crural vessels; where no other techniques are able to give similar or potentially better therapeutic results. Minor indications would be the crossing of total occlusions prior to balloon dilatation and, occasionally, sealing vessel wall defects by thermal fusion of intimal flaps following dilatation of stenosis.

Ultraviolet laser radiation especially, with an optimal combination of the parameters, frequency and energy fluency, promises radiation with improved preservation of tissue integrity and better healing conditions. Until now, the exact role for ultraviolet radiation and the part played by UV related interactive processes, such as mutagenesis, is unclear and poorly understood (16). There are indications that the pyrimidine dimers contribute strongly to the mutagenic effect. So far, no conclusive investigations with reproducible results are available to answer the questions concerning the laser related interaction with DNA in neighbouring biological structures. Nevertheless, greater risks are to be expected in biological areas with high reproductivity rates. In contrast to these regions, atheromatous plaques have fatty, hyaline, fibrous, and calcific components with low reproductivity.

In order to avoid tissue perforation, many questions have to be answered concerning the optical geometry of fibres and lenses, modifications of the delivery system, and the development of guiding or controlling systems. Perforation, the most troublesome complication of this method, is due to mechanical reasons, or arises as laser light is unable to differentiate between normal or pathological layers.

Using the technique of Excimer laser induced, simultaneous ablation and fluorescence spectral analysis, we have tried to evaluate the feasibility of real time tissue differentiation as a prerequisite to computer-guided laser angioplasty. We used the Technolas Excimer laser MAX 10 at 248 nm and a pulse length of 16 nanoseconds. The power was reduced so that an energy fluence of 50 mJ/mm^2/pulse was measured at the incident spot. As a repetition rate we choose 5 Hz. The fibre was coupled to a multichannel analyzer system OSMA (Spectroscopy Instruments), the fluorescence was analyzed by a 30 cm spectrograph with a 1 nanometer resolution range. Finally, the spectral pattern was processed by a computer system. One laser pulse produced one spectrum. Different samples of healthy and pathological material were irradiated. In human arteries, there were significant differences in the relative intensity of the peaks at 380 and 460 nanometres. However, in healthy examples, both peaks showed similar maximum intensities, whereas,

4. Laser Treatment

in atheroma, the peak at 460 nanometres was significantly smaller. These first results indicate that the pattern of specific peak intensity may be suitable to help to avoid perforation of vessel walls (17).

Excimer lasers offer pulsed ultraviolet sources with higher overall efficiency in combination with intense local absorption, good ablative qualities, and minimal thermal damage. The in vivo and in vitro experiences have documented the interesting potential of laser angioplasty. In general, Excimer lasers seem to be advantageous in some respects, but much basic research still has to be done prior to routine clinical Excimer laser angioplasty in patients.

4. Laser Treatment

References

1. Abela GS, Normann S, Choen D, Feldmann RL, Geiser EA, Conti CR. Effects of carbon dioxide, NdYAG, and Argon laser radiation on coronary atheromatous plaques. Am J Cardiol 50, 1199, 1982.

2. Choy DSJ, Stertzer SH, Rotterdam HZ, Bruno MS. Laser coronary angioplasty: experience in 9 cadaver hearts. Am J Cardiol 50, 1209, 1982.

3. Lee G, Ikeda RM, Kozina J, Mason DT. Laser dissolution of coronary atherosclerotic obstruction. Am Heart J 102, 1074, 1981.

4. Wollenek G, Laufer G, Wolner E. Qualitative und quantitative Auswirkungen der Neodym-YAG-Laserstrahlung auf Schweineaorten unter dem Gesichtspunkt der Angioplastik. Langenbecks Arch Chir 367, 3, 1958.

5. Ginsburg R, Wexler L, Mitchell RS, Profitt D. Percutaneous transluminal laser angioplasty for treatment of peripheral vascular disease. Radiology 156, 619, 1985.

6. Cumberland DC, Sanborn TA, Taylor DI, Moore DJ, Welsh CL, Greenfield AJ, Guben JK, Ryan TJ. Percutaneous thermal angioplasty: initial results with a laser probe in total peripheral artery occlusion. Lancet 1457, 1986.

7. Crea F, Davies G, McKenna W, Pashazade M, Taylor K, Maseri A. Percutaneous laser recanalization of coronary arteries. Lancet 214, 1986.

8. Lee G, Ikeda RM, Theis JH, Chan MC, Stobbe D, Ogata C, Kumagai A, Mason DT. Acute and chronic complications of laser angioplasty: vascular wall damage and formation of aneurysms in the atherosclerotic rabbit. Am J Cardiol 53: 290, 1984.

9. Steg PG, Astier R, Meyer G, Englender J, Lavergne A, Menasche PH, LeCarpentier Y. In vitro pulsed laser angioplasty of human atheromatous coronary arteries. Laser 2: 156, 1986.

10. Srinivasan R, Wynne JJ, Blum SE. Action of far ultraviolet light on organic polymer films: applications to semiconductor technology. J Radiat Curing 10, 12, 1983.

11. Murphy-Chutorian D, Selzer P, Wexler L, Kosek J, Quay ST, Huestis W, Shaw J, Ginsburg R. Cardiovascular laser research at Stanford University. Seminars Interven Radiol 3, 61, 1985.

12. Wollenek G, Laufer G. Thermal effects of far ultraviolet Excimer laser radiation in biologic tissue. Vol XXXII Trans Am Soc Artif Intern Organs 327, 1986.

13. Murphy-Chutorian D, Selzer PM, Kosek J, Quay SC, Profitt D, Ginsburg R. The interaction between Excimer laser energy and vascular tissue. Am Heart J 112, 739, 1986.

14. Prevosti LG, Leon MB, Dodd JT, Smith PD, Bonner RF, Rabinowitz M, Virmani R. Early and late healing responses of canine arterial wall to Excimer laser irradiation (Abstract). JACC 9/2, 85A.

15. Ginsburg R, Wexler L, Mitchell RS, Profitt D. Percutaneous transluminal laser angioplasty for treatment of peripheral vascular disease: clinical experience with sixteen patients. Radiology 156, 619, 1985.

16. Peak MJ, Peak JG, Moehring MP, Webb RB. Ultraviolet action spectra for DNA dimer induction, lethality, and mutagenesis in Escherichia coli with emphasis on the UVB region. Photochemistry and Photobiology 40, 613, 1984.

17. Laufer G, Wollenek G, Hohla K, Horvath R, Wuzl G, Wolner E. Excimer laser induced simultaneous spectral identification and ablation of human arterial tissue layers. Submitted to Circulation.

4.5. Peripheral Laser and Mechanical Angioplasty - The Stanford Experience

R Ginsburg

*Center for Interventional Vascular Therapies,
Stanford University Medical Center,
Stanford, California, USA*

Introduction

In January 1987 we established a new unit called the Center for Interventional Vascular Therapies (CIVT) at Stanford University Hospital. The impetus for its creation was the rapidly expanding number of devices being developed for the treatment of occlusive vascular disease. We believe that, in order to provide objective and scientific perspectives to this ever-growing and frenzied area of medicine, a new approach is needed.

The goal of the CIVT is to focus on the artery as an organ, regardless of the end-organ it ultimately supplies, and this approach is different from traditional medical teachings. The CIVT is composed of cardiologists, interventional radiologists, vascular surgeons, as well as cardiac surgeons engaged in a coordinated effort to care for patients. Moreover, this unit strives to offer the patient "one-stop shopping" for their vascular problems, and encourages second opinions and "failure analysis" of previous vascular interventions. Additionally, a full complement of diagnostic and therapeutic modalities is offered to the patient, including risk-factor modification, drug therapy, angioplasty, and surgery.

As part of our angioplasty program, we are presently evaluating the following devices: 1 mm angioscope (Machida), Laserprobe (Trimedyne), Rotablator (Biophysics International) and the Kensey catheter (Cordis). It is in the context of this brief overview of our program that our experience with these new devices is presented.

Angioscope

The device we are presently evaluating is a 1 mm flexible angioscope (Machida, Orangeburg, New York). The scope is ETO sterilized and reusable. It requires a xeon light source and a video camera, monitor, and tape recorder.

The scope is issued for viewing both peripheral as well as coronary arteries. A guiding catheter (5-8 FR) is first inserted to the most distal site of the area to be examined, using standard guidewires. Once in place, the scope is inserted through the guiding catheter to its most distal end. The guiding catheter is then flushed with saline. The flow rate is not fixed, and depends on the volume and the rate of flow of blood in the vessel being examined. Usually 100-200 cc's are infused during an examination. As with other non-vascular scoping procedures, a much better view is obtained when the catheter and angioscope together are withdrawn (retrograde) through the vessel. If the scope is advanced alone, there is a risk of perforation or dissection, but more importantly, the scope has the tendency not to remain coaxial, and only the wall is visualized.

As technology advances with the angioscope, so does our enthusiasm for this device. We believe its indications will be primarily for diagnosis and in therapeutic decision-making. As we are all acutely aware, an angiogram shows only shadows and can suggest, but not prove, underlying pathophysiology. On the other hand, the scope can rapidly and precisely determine what is occluding the lumen of the vessel. It is this new, readily attained information that has altered our approach to treating patients. We can now carefully choose the appropriate device or agent, depending on the visually observed disease state.

The limitations of the scope are their expense, especially the "start-up" costs needed for the video equipment and camera. The scopes are fragile and need care during use and sterilization. Most importantly, steering or guiding systems still need to be designed to permit their use to full potential.

Rotating-tip (Kensey Catheter)

We are presently participating in clinical trials using the Kensey catheter for the treatment of total occlusions of both the peripheral as well as coronary arteries. This device is described in detail in another chapter, but in brief, the catheter has a small rotating "cam"-like tip that spins at 45-90 K RPM and is perfused with saline or dilute contrast at 20-30 cc's/minute. This device is designed primarily for totally occluded vessels. It does not have a guidewire system and must be advanced carefully under fluoroscopic guidance. Because the tip is a fixed size, for most vessels balloon angioplasty is needed to further improve the luminal diameter.

The catheter is most effective on vessels occluded with thrombus or a semisolid "gruel"-like material. The device does not work well in areas of fibrous capped lesions where there is the tendency to seek the path of least resistance (most commonly, the subintimal plane).

A unique feature of the device is that contrast is ejected from the distal tip at high velocity. The contrast penetrates the wall of the vessel and can even extravasate. Not infrequently, during a procedure it appears that the device has perforated the vessel when, in reality, the contrast has extravasated along the subintimal plane within the boundaries of the vessel, giving the inexperienced operator a degree of anxiety.

Overall, this device is "user friendly", and the equipment needed to operate it is not complex and is physically small. The device requires patience and, unlike the Laserprobe, it is advanced very slowly and in most cases advances forward on its own power. The risk of perforation is small, unless it is manually pushed out of the vessel. Although excellent for total occlusions, it probably will not be useful to enlarge mildly stenotic vessels.

Simpson Atherectomy Catheter

The goal of lasers and other new angioplasty devices has been to actually remove, rather than merely remold, the lumen of the severely diseased arterial vessel. The only percutaneous device on the market today that removes atheromatous material is the Simpson Atherocath. This device is, in the truest sense, an atherectomy catheter, since it removes from the body the atheromatous material obstructing the vessel lumen.

The Simpson catheter is composed of a metallic capsule at the end of a catheter. The capsule is slit longitudinally, and in it is a rotating blade which spins at two thousand revolutions per minute. A low pressure balloon is attached longitudinally, and, when inflated, pushes the open slit of the capsule against the atheroma so it can be engaged by the rotating cutter. Through multiple passes of the cutting blade the atheroma is literally "shaved" off the opposing wall. The goal of this device is to provide a smooth luminal surface to decrease the potential of restenosis, as well as to remove material from the body.

The device is presently available in 7, 9, and 11 French sizes. Although experimental coronary studies are in progress, the device is presently only available for peripheral use. The catheter has a fixed guidewire at its terminal end, and does not allow the "over-the-wire" technique. Also, because the capsule is relatively long and inflexible, it is easier to use retrograde rather than antegrade. The catheter can accommodate four or five passes at an atheroma before the depository at the end of the capsule must be emptied.

The advantages of this device over standard balloons are that it removes material and permits the histologic study of the lesion. The disadvantages are that multiple passes must be performed, requiring a long procedure time and potential injury to the vessel wall, as well as inability to tract over a guidewire, expense, and lack of data to demonstrate less restenosis than balloons.

Laser Assisted Angioplasty

Percutaneous laser angioplasty for the treatment of occlusive vascular disease has been the goal for many investigative groups during the past decade. The immediate appeal to physicians for this new technology was that it removed rather than mechanically reshaped the lumen of a vessel. Moreover, unlike balloon angioplasty, it was potentially useful for the treatment of long total occlusions and diffuse diseases. The issue of restenosis, although now a major limiting factor of balloon angioplasty, was not appreciated ten years ago and was not a primary goal of lasers.

The basic question many ask is: Why use lasers in the first place? I think it is relatively safe to say that, for the majority of physicians, their first experience with lasers was not dissimilar to that of the lay public. In the late seventies, lasers became larger-than-life on the cinema screen, and these backlot fantasies were soon extrapolated into clinical medicine, particularly into cardiovascular medicine. However, anyone who was tempted to work in this area soon realized the many difficult technological hurdles which had to be overcome.

Laser energy, as described in other chapters in this book, can be delivered through fiberoptic transmission cables. The flexibility and size of these glass fibers permits their use through guiding catheters and therefore access to arterial vessels of almost any size and location. One of the major problems still

4. Laser Treatment

facing us today is, however, the delivery of this energy from a small diameter fiber to a large target site. Many ingenious and creative engineering designs and models have been developed over the years and implemented clinically, but, as yet, none solves all the problems we constantly face in the treatment of vascular disease. Some of the limiting factors include the size of the device which can be safely inserted into an artery (usually no greater than 9 FR or 0.118 inch), flexibility of the fiber, thermal injury to non-target tissue, and perforation through the wall of the vessel.

A critical problem in the design and testing of laser devices has been the lack of a suitable model of human atherosclerosis. Most animals do not spontaneously develop atherosclerosis. One of the most available animal models for vascular disease is the high cholesterol fed rabbit in whom the vessels are first mechanically debrided of their endothelial cells with a balloon. These vessels can appear angiographically to be similar to man, but histologically the vessels are not comparable since they are primarily comprised of foam cells and very soft non-calcified material. Moreover, other animals such as the pig or monkey can similarly develop disease, but these animals are not easy nor inexpensive to use for scientific study. Because of these less than ideal animal models, many of these new devices had to be tested directly in man to determine their efficacy. It became generally accepted to use the peripheral leg arteries for testing, because the arteries were in a less hazardous position than the carotid or coronary arteries. The peripheral arteries have now become a standard site for the development of new therapies.

More than a Test Bed?

In the United States, the treatment of peripheral vascular disease has primarily been under the purview of the vascular surgeon. Specialists in internal medicine generally had less of an interest in this clinical problem, possibly because there was little to offer therapeutically other than surgery, and therefore, most were of the persuasion that this was almost solely a surgical problem. More recently, with better understanding of the pathophysiology of vascular disease and the advent of balloon angioplasty, as well as the well-known limited long-term viability of bypass grafts, there has been renewed interest in alternative methods in the treatment of peripheral vascular disease.

At Stanford, our initial clinical studies with percutaneous laser angioplasty was done in the peripheral (leg) vessels of patients with severe end-stage vascular disease. We chose this route because the peripheral vessels offered us relatively straight arteries, variable complexity of lesions, accessibility to external compression in cases of perforation, relatively safe environment in case of distal emboli, and, most importantly, they were amenable and accessible to surgical bailout should it be required. This was our original rationale in using this cohort of patients.

In September 1985 we reported our initial experience with percutaneous transluminal laser angioplasty (Radiology 156:619, 1985). We made the following observation: First, laser energy could be successfully passed through silica fiber bundles and delivered into an arterial vessel. Second, the glass fiber could be passed in many (but not all) cases through atherosclerotic lesions in similar fashion to a guidewire.

4. Laser Treatment

Third, the procedure was painful if there was insufficient cooling by blood saline or contrast around the fiber tip to protect normal vessel wall. Fourth, if the vessel was severely diseased, the fiber could go subintimal and perforate, in similar fashion to, but more easily than, a guidewire.

Although we had demonstrated and contributed several important steps in the early development of laser angioplasty, we believed that there were many unresolved hurdles yet to be overcome. Most important was that our goal and the goal of others was to use the laser to debulk significant amounts of atheromatous material from the lumen of the vessel to improve hemodynamic flow. Also, it was desired that this procedure would replace and not be an adjunct to balloon angioplasty. Also, it became obvious to us that peripheral vascular disease was complex and unpredictable. Our goal was to use the peripheral vessels as a testing ground without the expectation that the then state-of-the-art was realistically sufficient to be a definitive treatment solution for this disease.

Do Lasers have a Role in the Treatment of Peripheral Vascular Disease?

The answer to this question, based upon the technology available to us in 1987, is a qualified maybe. We are witnessing two disciplines - angioplasty and peripheral vascular disease treatment undergoing rapid maturation and change. As previously pointed out, the disease process in the leg arteries is complex. How to determine the pathophysiology of the artery from a shadow seen angiographically is as yet undefined. Moreover, the approach in the health care system towards diagnosing and treating peripheral vascular disease is changing from a purely surgical disease to more of a medical problem. Many physicians are just becoming aware of the options available to them to treat their patients.

Patients with claudication need to be carefully evaluated to determine if this is due to ischemia and whether this is a result of inflow or distal disease. Patients with iliac, common femoral, or profunda disease need to be aggressively treated, since limb loss can occur. However, the most commonly diseased vessel in the leg, the superficial femoral artery, rarely needs to be re-opened if the other major vessels are open. A SFA occlusion can usually be best treated by an exercise program, medication, and having the patient stop smoking. The SFA usually first occludes Hunter's canal and then occludes retrograde. Even if it is re-opened, long term patency is not spectacular. This vessel is, however, long and straight and is ideal for devices such as the hot tip probe.

Overall, lasers in their present configuration can help, but are of limited usefulness in the overall therapy of peripheral vascular disease. The Laserprobe is a device manufactured and marketed in the United States by Trimedyne Inc, Santa Ana, California. At the time this paper was written (late 1987) this was the only laser-driven cardiovascular device clinically approved for general use by the FDA. The approval indications were the use of this device in otherwise impossible cases for the treatment of peripheral vascular disease. It was believed that the device would be useful in cases where standard "Dotter" or balloon procedures were determined to be unsatisfactory. Se-

4. Laser Treatment

veral other laser angioplasty devices are in early clinical trials.

In practice, the hot tip probe is primarily an assist device to be used in conjunction with balloon angioplasty. The above-knee peripheral vessels are quite large in diameter, ranging from 5 to 8 mm in diameter. This discrepancy in size almost mandates for most cases that balloon angioplasty be used along with the device. However, the peripheral vessels below the knee become quite small (down to 1.0 mm in size), and in these vessels the mismatch in size is less apparent, and, at least theoretically, the hot tip probe alone could be the primary angioplasty device.

The specific clinical situations where the hot tip probe is believed to be most useful is in totally occluded vessels. In the peripheral vessel, total occlusions are most common in the superficial femoral, popliteal, and tibio-peroneal trunk respectively. Atherosclerotic lesions develop in the adductor canal where the vessel crosses through interosseous membranes. The plaque becomes hemodynamically critical, totally occludes, and the thrombus begins to propagate in retrograde fashion. The overall composition of the totally obstructed vessel depends, in part, on the duration of the obstruction and the extent of involution that occurs along with calcium and fibrous tissue deposition.

Once heated, the hot tip probe travels along the path of least resistance. In vessels with a relatively soft thrombus core, the probe works well and has little opportunity to perforate or cause thermal injury to normal vessel wall. However, in the rock-hard, old solid atherosclerotic lesions, there is much greater chance for the probe as well as guidewires to enter into and traverse the endarterectomy or subintimal plane. If the probe can find its way back into the true lumen more distally, then this is not a major concern, but in most cases, it remains subintimal. The subintimal path is hazardous, and the risk of perforation or severe thermal injury is high. Therefore, the limitations of the probe are not necessarily the technology itself but the variable, complex nature of the vascular disease itself.

The Laserprobe has several configurations. One useful one is the "monorail" probe which has a small hole on the side of the head to permit use over a 0.018" or smaller guidewire system. Although the wire system doesn't help in total occlusion, sometimes there are tandem lesions with a tight proximal lesion and a total distal lesion. The ability to use the probe with a steerable guidewire is a great help to deliver the probe past tortuous, non-occluded lesions to the target site. However, the "monorail" system is presently only available on the 2.0 mm tip, limiting the guiding catheters that can accommodate it.

Technically there is a significant learning curve in the use of the probe, not dissimilar to balloon angioplasty. The fiberoptic cable itself is relatively flimsy and not easy to steer or direct. In peripheral vessels, we have developed a preference for the 1.5 mm probe. Using the Seldinger technique, we usually insert a 8 French Hemaquet sheath with check valve into the artery. Although one could insert the probe directly into the sheath, there is usually a tremendous amount of leakage around the small fiber cable at the check valve. Therefore, we prefer to insert through the sheath a multipurpose coronary guiding catheter and at its proximal end connect "Y" connector with adjustable "O" ring valve. This prevents back-leakage, but permits control and manipulation of the fiber cable. In practice, the guiding catheter is advanced to the target site. A saline or dilute contrast solution is infused through one arm of the "Y" connector and is then advanced through the distal end of the guiding catheter. The laser is activated and the hot tip advanced. The direction of the probe can be controlled in part by torquing the guiding catheter. The smaller 1.5 mm probe heats up quite rapidly and does not need a long warm-up time (usually a few seconds). We have found that intermittently pulsing the probe gives better thermal control of the tip as it is an "unforgiving" instrument. Once a tract is made, the probe commits itself to continuing to follow the path it creates. Not infrequently, this is an undesirable subintimal path. If the probe is successfully advanced through the lesion, the operator may not want to lose the lumen, which could occur if the probe is withdrawn. Therefore, the proximal end of the fiber can be cut and the fiber cable used as a guidewire, being careful to realize that the distal tip cannot be pulled back through the balloon catheter because of its size. Balloon angioplasty can now be performed, and when completed, the combined systems can be removed.

Potential Problems with the Probe

Clinical experience with the probe is not extensive, although it is now available for general clinical use in the therapy of peripheral disease. Therefore, questions such as long-term patency and untoward effects of thermal injury are unknown. However, preliminary experience suggests that this is not of much concern.

The primary difficulty in using the probe (or any other device) in totally occluded vessels, is in guiding tight instruments down the true lumen of the vessel. In patients with extensive and old disease, there is a high likelihood of the instrument entering the subintimal or endarterectomy plane. When this occurs, satisfactory long-term results can rarely be obtained. One disadvantage with the probe is that if it tracts subintimally, there is a greater risk of thermal injury to surrounding normal wall as well as perforation.

Another potential problem is in smaller distal vessels of the periphery. When the vessel diameter approaches the diameter of the probe itself, there is a greater risk of thermal injury. This occurs because there is less blood flow cooling the surrounding tissue. Also, more of the probe is in contact with the total surface of the vessel and, therefore, there is greater dissipation of the thermal energy to potentially normal vessel wall. Whether or not this will become a significant clinical problem is unknown.

What's Hot; What's Not

Due to unexplained electronic problems with our laser, it was not always operational when we were about to advance the Laserprobe. Therefore, we discovered by chance during one of these power failures that the probe works well even when cold. The "football" shape of the laserprobe evidently permits the probe to "snowplow" through the soft core of an obstructed vessel, and in many instances this is the true lumen.

Because of this early observation, we have randomized our patients to use of the hot or cold probe. To date we have found that the probes work well un-

4. Laser Treatment

heated, but there are specific situations when thermal energy is needed.

Other Devices: 1987

In 1987 there has been an "explosion" in new devices and technology. Which of these devices will survive or ultimately prove most effective is at present unknown. A list and a brief highlight of these devices is given below:

Laser Angioplasty

This year there are several delivery systems which employ free beam laser energy to remove atheromatous material. Some of these devices use Excimer laser energy, which can be carried through fiberoptic bundles over the wire catheters, with up to seven fibers extruded in their wall. Such devices are now being tested. Another system uses multiple fibers which are extruded in and over the wire catheter with a small sapphire protector at the end. This system is coupled to an argon laser source. A third device uses a sophisticated system to fire the laser energy only when a computer recognizes the target as plaque rather than as normal vessel wall.

Hot Tip Angioplasty

Lasers are not the only means to heat metal tips. Radio-frequency (microwave) energy can also be used to generate heat in a metal tip. The advantage of a RF generator is the low cost, maintenance, and ease of operation compared with a laser unit. However, the disadvantage is that the delivery system does not have the flexibility or the small diameter of small fiberoptic cables. If hot tip angioplasty has a future, then we suspect that lasers will be replaced by these more compact and convenient units.

Laser Balloon Angioplasty

One problem with balloon angioplasty is the formation of intimal flaps. These flaps can cause both acute closure, as well as be partly responsible for the initiation of chronic restenosis. Developed by Spears, LABA is a process whereby the flaps of the vessel are welded to the media during balloon angioplasty. This welding is accomplished by emitting laser energy (Nd:Yag) through a diffuser lens located in the angioplasty balloon. The welding is believed by Spears and co-workers to prevent restenosis, and intensive investigation is underway to document this hypothesis.

Rotablator

This is another mechanical angioplasty device just beginning clinical testing in the United States. This device is unique in that it operates co-axially over a guidewire. A small, football-shaped tip spins at 145,000 rpm and slides back and forth over this guidewire. The driver for this device is an air-turbine similar to a dental unit. The indications for the use of this device are diffuse disease and tight stenoses not approachable by balloons. The disadvantage of the device is that it is not suitable for total occlusions. Moreover, there is always the concern for emboli generation, although this does not appear to be a clinical problem.

Ultrasonic Catheters

Lithotripsy or shock-wave dissolution of stones is used more and more frequently for the treatment of gallstones and kidney-stones. This same concept is being explored for use in the lumen of atherosclerotic vessels. Prototype devices have been tested in which ul-

4. Laser Treatment

	Center for Interventional Vascular Therapies February - August 1987			
	Laserprobe Hot/Cold	Balloon	Kensey	Total
Iliac	5/1	5	4	15
SFA/TRI	8/5	16	17	46
Total	13/6	21	21	61
Success	16%/26%	95%	19%	52%

Table 52

trasonic energy is passed down fine cables and the delivered energy is able to shatter calcified material in the atherosclerotic plaque. The advantage of the device is its ability to remove calcium, but the disadvantage is the potential for large debris formation.

Summary

The results of our comparative trial of the Laserprobe, Kensey, and balloon for peripheral angioplasty are shown in Table 52.

From February to August 1987, 61 patients were entered into the study. All lesions were first approached with standard guidewires and catheters. If a wire could be passed, then primary balloon angioplasty was performed. If this was not successful, then either the Laserprobe or the Kensey catheter was used.

The data to date suggest that a successful procedure is directly related to the extent of the disease present. In the "impossible" lesions, the new devices are successful about 20% of the time.

Conclusion

Many new technologies are being developed for the treatment of occlusive vascular disease. At present, no one device is ideal for all clinical situations. The process of atherosclerotic vascular disease is complex and much still needs to be understood. These new devices are all complementary to one another and are needed for the high-volume complex angioplasty laboratory. However, because they are useful in only limited cases, we would not recommend them for general use until more studies have been completed.

4. Laser Treatment

4.6. Percutaneous Atherectomy: A New Method for Non-Operative Vessel Reconstruction

B Höfling [1], A von Pölnitz [1], D Backa [1], G Bauriedel [1],
L Lauterjung [2], KW Jauch [2], K Remberger [3]

[1]Department of Medicine,
[2]Department of Surgery,
[3]Department of Pathology, Klinikum Grosshadern,
Ludwig-Maximilians-Universität, Munich,
Federal Republic of Germany

Abstract

The use of percutaneous transluminal angioplasty has met with encouraging initial success rates, but the limiting factor is the high restenosis rate. Therefore alternatives (percutaneous laser or atherectomy) are under development; the peripheral Simpson Atherectomy catheter (p-SAC) was designed to allow the removal of plaque material from peripheral vessels and may result in a lower restenosis rate.

We used the p-SAC in 21 patients with symptomatic peripheral vascular disease. A total of 41 lesions were successfully reduced from 82.7 ± 14% to 21 ± 16%. Four lesions were totally occluded and 16 (39%) were calcified. Clinically, standardized walking distance increased from 79.9 ± 71.1 meters to 152.6 ± 89.7 meters (p<0.0001) and Doppler index improved from 0.58 ± 0.17 to 0.81 ± 0.16 (p<0.0001). Follow-up is now available up to 6 months, with no significant change in non-invasive parameters; at angiography (2-6 months; n=14 lesions) residual stenosis of 20.7 ± 13.7% was documented. There has been one restenosis and this patient has had repeat successful atherectomy.

In conclusion, percutaneous atherectomy appears to be a safe and effective technique for the treatment of patients with peripheral vascular disease. The immediate success rate, particularly in the superficial femoral and popliteal arteries, is high; long-term results to date are encouraging. The ability to remove obstructive material percutaneously may lead to improved long-term results as compared to balloon angioplasty or surgery, and provides access to plaque material for histologic evaluation. The atherectomy technique could be adapted to approach coronary artery disease.

Introduction

As the life expectancy of the population increases, diffuse vascular disease and its treatment will become even more important. Atherosclerotic plaque development is a continuous and recurring process, and therefore reliable alternatives to surgical intervention are desirable; of course the preventive approach with risk factor reduction and

4. Laser Treatment

medical therapy remains a major goal. In recent years, many new attractive percutaneous techniques have been developed. Balloon angioplasty is currently a commonly used procedure, although the long-term restenosis rate of 25 to 45% (1,2,3) is high. The more sophisticated various Laser techniques under development are still problematic because of energy control, vessel perforation, and acute reocclusion (4,5). Therefore, mechanical and better controllable devices are attractive. Several rotating systems are becoming available, but the risk of embolization and vessel wall damage are not yet sufficiently investigated. The atherectomy technique has the advantages of good catheter control with the "cutter" incorporated into a housing at the catheter tip, thus preventing vessel perforation. A further advantage with diagnostic implications is the ability to remove plaque material, and thereby lower the risk for distal embolization. The peripheral Simpson-atherectomy catheter (pSAC) (6) has undergone the largest number of clinical trials to date (7,8,9), although several other atherectomy catheters are now in development. We would like to report on the first 21 patients with symptomatic peripheral vascular disease treated with the p-SAC catheter at our institution.

Method

The atherectomy procedure is performed in the catheterization laboratory under heparinization. After baseline angiography and angioscopy (10) the p-SAC is advanced to the stenosis under flouroscopic control. The essential feature of the catheter is a cylindrical housing with an opening encompassing one-third its circumference at its tip. The

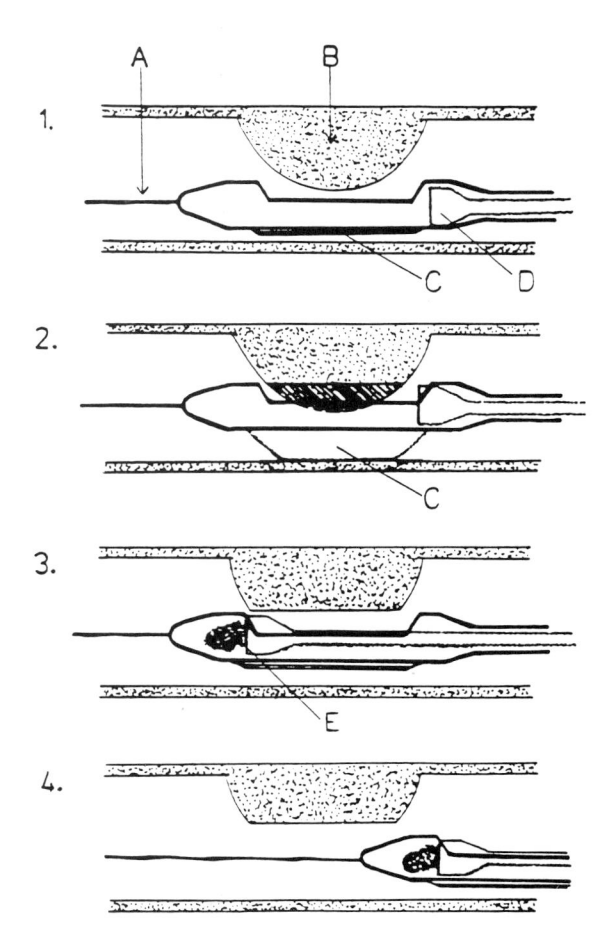

Fig. 175 Working principles of the p-SAC; housing is first positioned with the aid of an attached guiding wire (A) so that obstructing plaque (B) protrudes into the opening. A low pressure balloon (C) is then inflated, to secure the position. The integrated cutter (D) is then advanced, slicing off layers of plaque (E), which are trapped in the distal housing cup.

housing contains an integrated, externally controllable rotating cutter (2 000 reotations/min) which is used to excise slices of plaque. The working principle of the catheter is further explained in Figure 175. The p-SAC is first positioned so that the stenotic plaque protrudes into the window of the housing, and a low-pressure balloon (10-40 p.s.i.) is then inflated, maintaining the housing securely in place within the vessel. The motor-driven cutter is then advanced, excising

4. Laser Treatment

Patient Characteristics (n=21)

male/female	20 (95%) /1 (5%)
age (yrs)	64.9 ± 8.9
smoking	18 (86%)
hypertension	17 (81%)
hypercholesterolemia (>250mg/dl)	11 (52%)
diabetes	4 (19%)
coronary artery disease	15 (71%)
cerebral vascular disease	8 (38%)
previous peripheral surgery/PTA	33 (14%)

Table 53

up to 15 mm long and 1 mm thick slices of plaque, which are trapped within the distal housing cup. Captured material can then be submitted for histologic and biochemical evaluation.

Angioscopic evaluation was performed before, during, and after the intervention, using a flexible fiberoptic endoscope (d=1.5 mm, Miniflex Angioscope, American Edwards Lab). The angioscope is co-axially guided by a cut X-ray dense Cournand catheter inserted into the vessel through a 9F sheath. Constant saline irrigation delivered by a pressured bag inflated to 300 mm Hg prevents opacification of the field of view. A 250 Watt cold light source (American Edwards Lab) provides intravascular illumination. The endoscope is coupled to a miniature video camera (Endovision 553, Storz Inst, FRG) and images obtained are thereby relayed to a high resolution color video monitor. Permanent recordings are made, using a video cassette recorder (U-matic VO-5800 PS, Sony).

Histological evaluation was performed after initial fixation of excised specimens in 6% Formaldehyde, followed by embedment of alcohol-dried specimens in paraffin. Four to seven micron slices are then prepared with Hemotoxylin-eosin, as well as with Van Gienson stains.

Patients could be discharged 24 hours post-atherectomy. All were encouraged to modify their risk factors and maintain long-term therapy with aspirin. All results are reported as mean ± sd. The paired student-t-test was used to calculate significance of differences pre- and post-atherectomy; all p values are two-tailed.

Patients

Twenty-one patients with moderate to severe claudication underwent atherectomy, 7 had rest pain, and 2 had gangrene. Patient characteristics and risk factors are summarized in Table 53. More than 85% were smokers and over 80% had a history of hypertension; 2 patients had previous unsuccessful balloon angioplasty; and 1 had undergone a femoral-popliteal bypass, with a new stenosis just proximal to the bypass. All patients underwent baseline arteriographic study and were accepted for atherectomy if an 80% stenosis of the symptomatic side was found; co-existing stenoses greater than 60% were treated along with the target lesion. All patients also had baseline Doppler ultrasound evaluation and standardized walking distance measurement (3 km/hr with a 12.5% grade) which were repeated post-atherectomy and at 1 month, 3 months and 6 months. Control angiography was performed at 6 months.

Results
Angiographic Examples

In the following figures, we show some examples of lesions which can be handled by atherectomy. Figure 176 is of concentric superficial femoral stenosis pre- and post-atherectomy, which can be effectively treated by changing the rotational position of the catheter although an eccentric stenosis is probably better suited for atherectomy, since the plaque more easily protrudes into the opening of the catheter housing. In Figure 177 we show an example of bilateral atherectomy, performed during a single catheterization session; there are very irregular Type II eccentric stenoses of both superficial femoral arteries (Figure 177a) which were successfully atherectomized in 2 hours. In Figure 177b, the angiographic findings, pre- and post-atherectomy of the right artery are shown.

Angioscopic Examples

Angioscopy can be useful in optimizing the procedure. In Figure 178 we show an angioscopic image of a stenotic plaque pre- and post-atherec-tomy in which the vessel wall was relatively smooth post-procedure. How- ever, in another case as seen in Figure 179, the angioscopic picture revealed a large residual flap which we could then selectively remove with additional pas-ses of the catheter. The angioscope was also useful in exploring total occlusions.

Angiographic Results

Twenty-one patients with 41 stenoses (iliac n=5, SFA n=35, and popliteal n=1) underwent atherectomy. The mean baseline stenosis of 82.7 ± 14% was reduced to 21.0 ± 16.0%. Results according to vessel distribution are presented in Table 54. The effects of lesion morphology and the presence of calcification are presented in Table 55. There was immediate technical success (defined as residual stenosis less than 50%) in 93% of lesions; 2 failures were of iliac lesions and the third in an SFA lesion in an area of aneurysmal dilatation. Eight patients with a total of 14 treated stenoses were reangiogrammed 4.8 months (range 2-6 months) post-atherectomy. The mean residual stenosis was 20.7 ± 13.7% (not significantly changed from immediately post-atherectomy). In one patient, restenosis of an SFA lesion developed at 2 months and he underwent successful repeat atherectomy.

No major complications were seen. In particular, there were no instances of embolization or vessel rupture.

Clinical Results

Rest pain resolved in 7/7 cases and gangrene healed in 2/2 cases. Figure 180a is of a gangrenous extremity due to a 100% occlusion of the popliteal

4. Laser Treatment

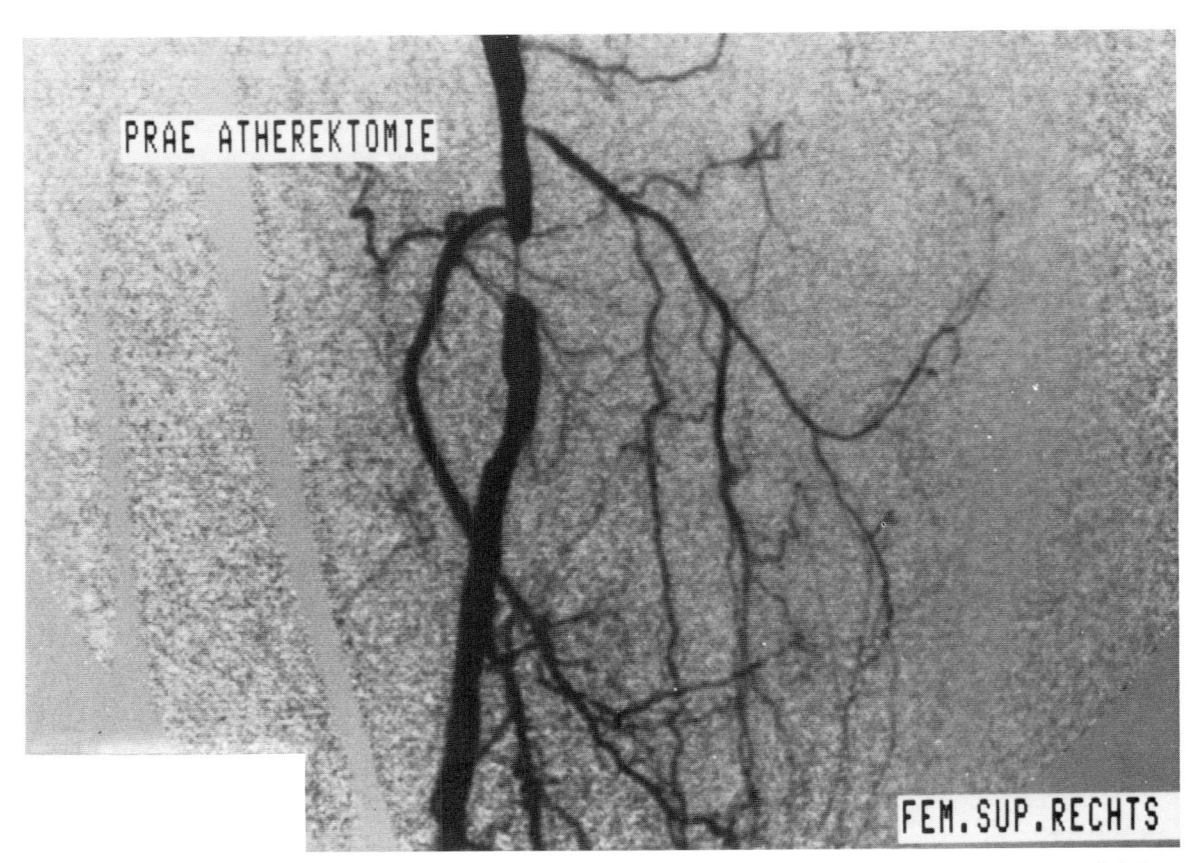

Fig. 176 a,b) Digital subtraction angiographic image of a concentric lesion of the superficial femoral artery pre-atherectomy (a, above) and after 5 passes of the cutter (b, below).

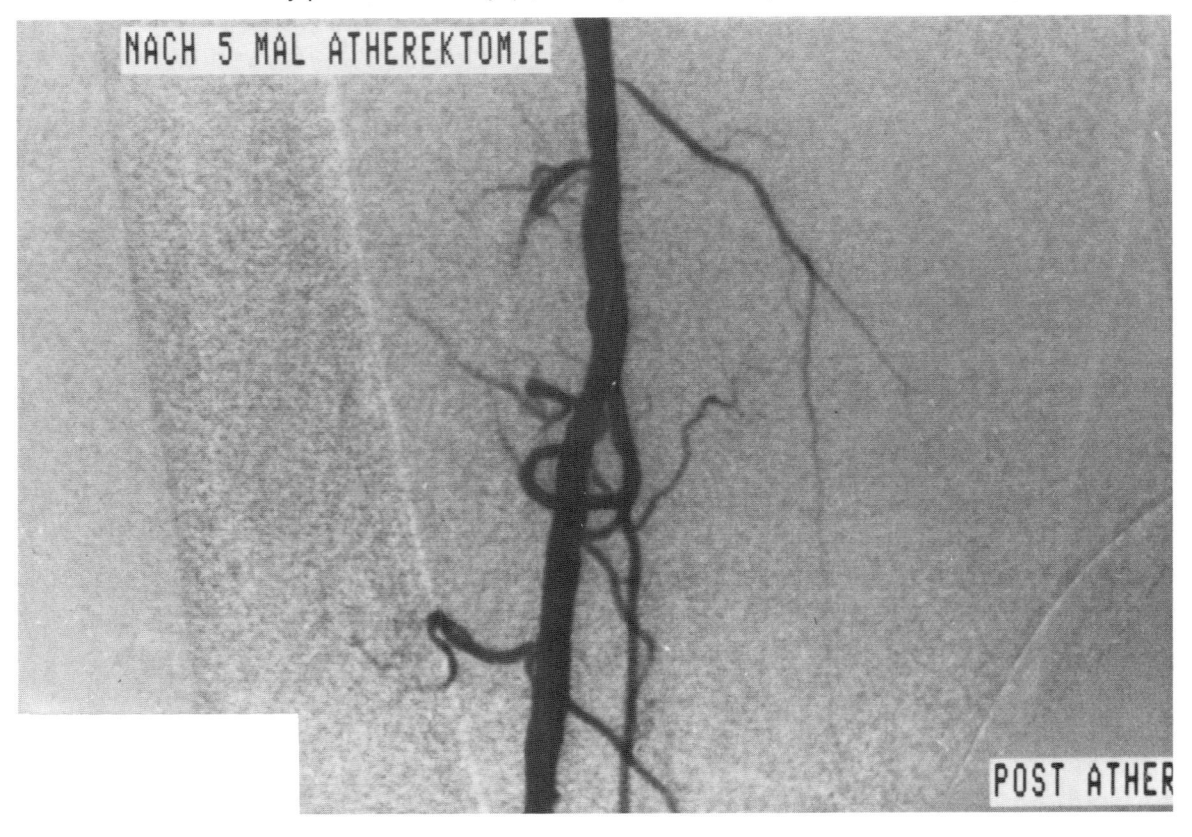

4. Laser Treatment

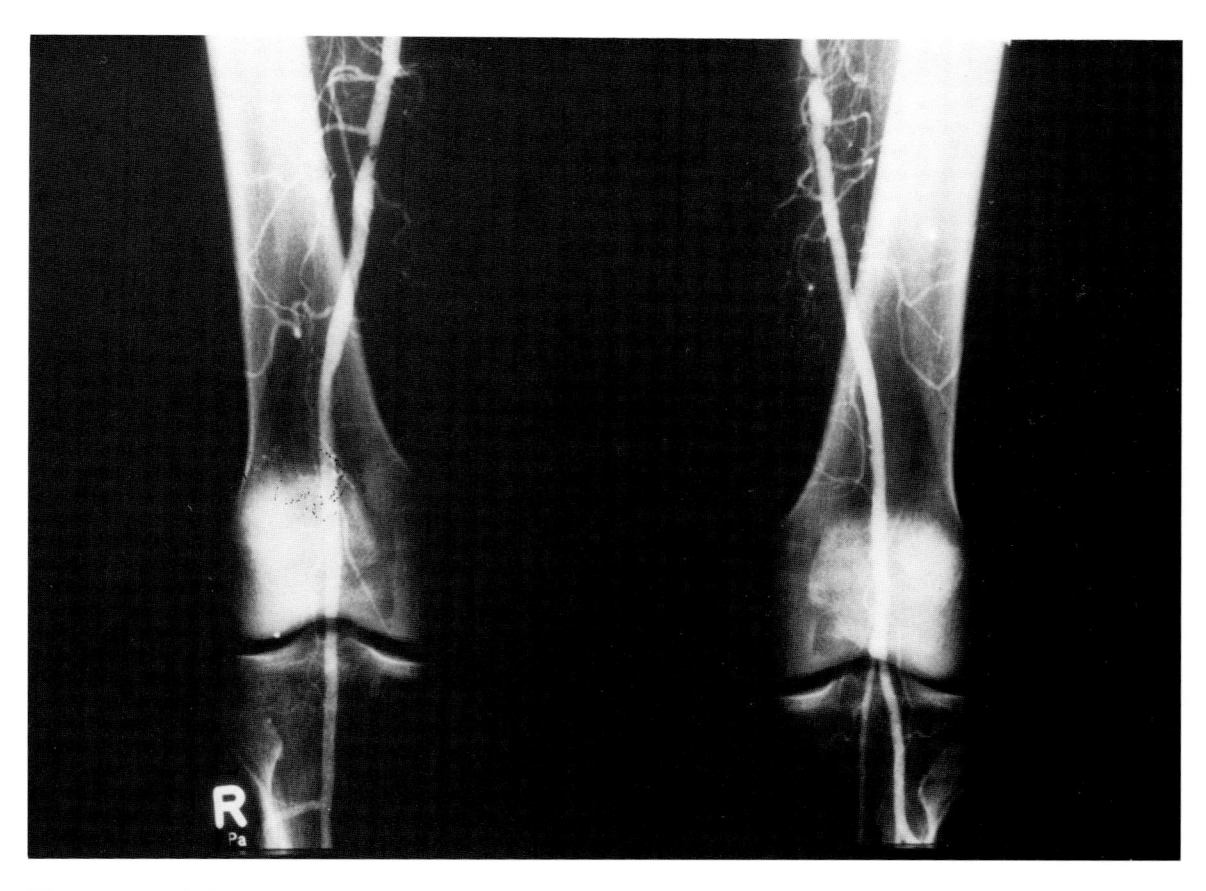

Fig. 177 a, b) Patient who in one session underwent bilateral atherectomy of eccentric lesions of the superficial femoral arteries (a, above); Right SFA pre- and post-atherectomy (b, below).

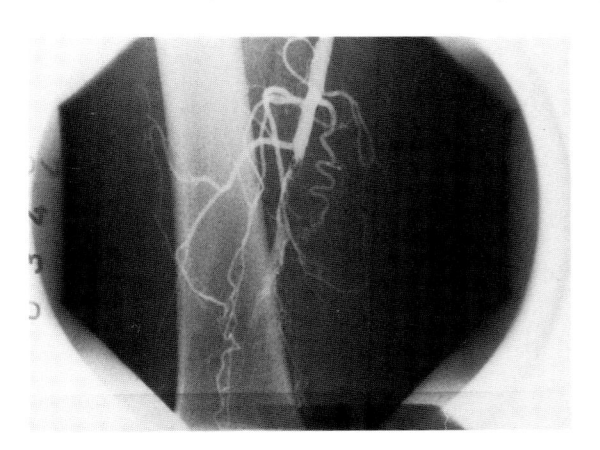

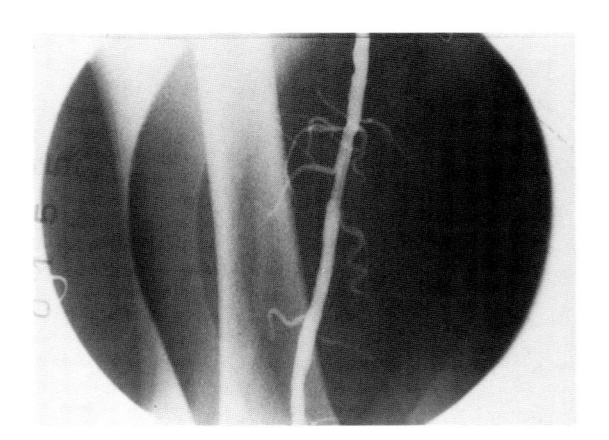

445

4. Laser Treatment

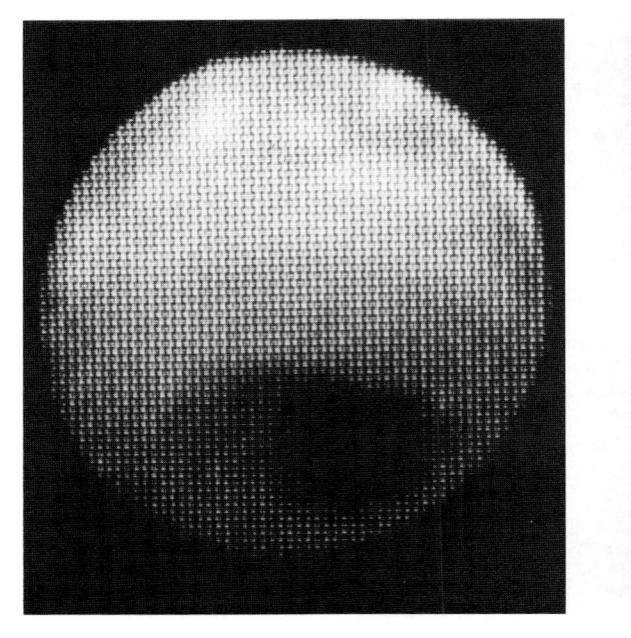

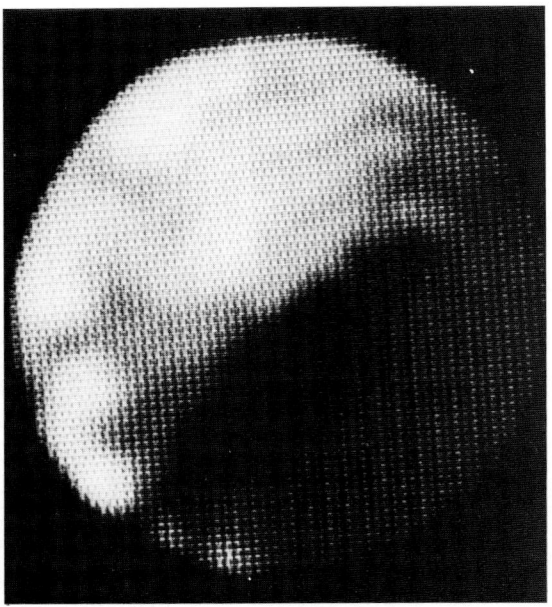

Fig. 178 a, b) Angioscopic picture of an eccentric stenosis pre-atherectomy (a, left) and post-atherectomy (b, right). On the post-image, one can appreciate a smooth residual surface.

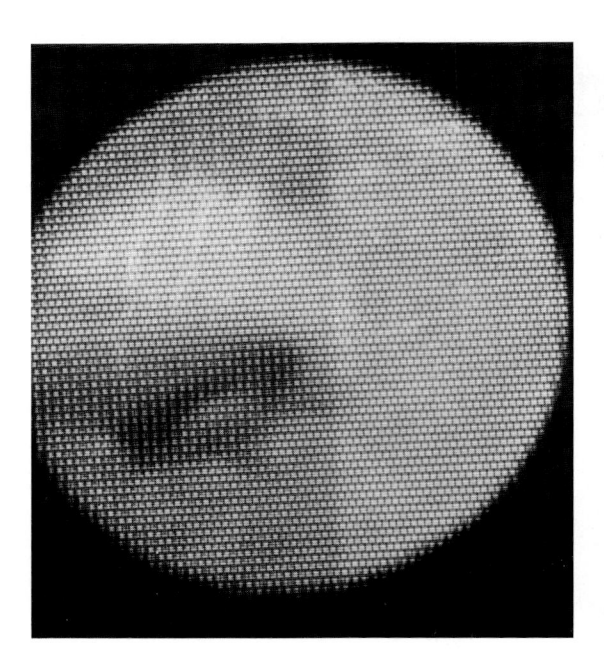

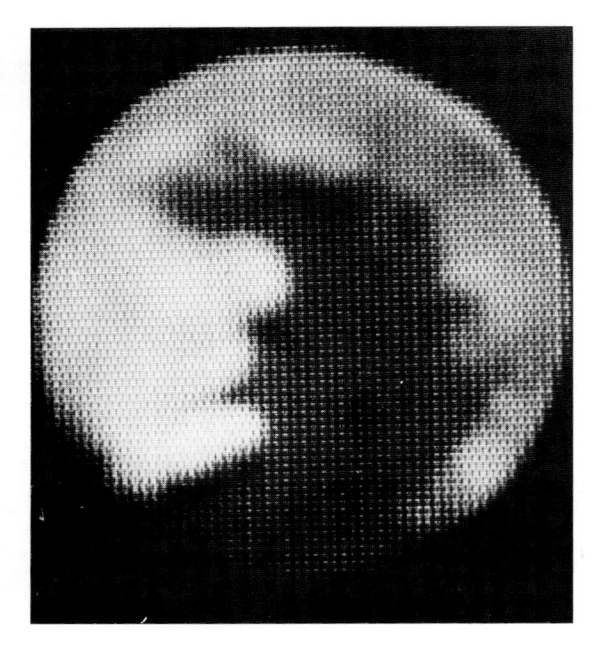

Fig. 179 a, b) Angioscopic picture of lesion pre-atherectomy (a, left). An irregular, obstructing flap was seen angioscopically post-atherectomy which was then selectively removed by further atherectomy (b, right).

artery, which was successfully atherectomized; at 3 months follow-up (Figure 180b) the gangrene has healed, and the patient's walking distance was up to 200 meters (m).

For the entire group, baseline walking distance (WD) increased from 79.9 ± 71.9m to 152.6 ± 89.7m (p<0.0001; n=20). The initial improvement has been maintained at follow-up, with a 6m

% Stenosis (mean ± s.d.) of all Lesions, with Vessel Distribution and Total Occlusions, Pre- and Post-Atherectomy and at 6 Months Follow-up

	pre	post	6mo
all	82.7 ± 14.0 n=41	21.0 ± 16.0* n=41	20.7 ± 13.7* n=41
iliac	81.7 ± 13.3 n=5	38.3 ± 22.3** n=5	25.0 ± 7.1 n=2
femoral	82.9 ± 14.3 n=35	18.0 ± 12.8* n=35	19.1 ± 14.9* n=11
popliteal	100.0 n=1	20.0 n=1	30.0 n=1
100% occluded	100.0 n=5	12.5 ± 9.6* n=5	30.0 n=1

* $p<0.0001$ vs. pre
** $p<0.02$ vs. pre

Table 54

% Stenosis (mean ± s.d.) According to Calcification and Morphology, Pre- and Post-Atherectomy and at 6 Months Follow-up

	pre	post	6mo
calcified	83.4 ± 14.8 n=16	25.0 ± 20.0* n=16	28.3 ± 7.5** n=6
non-calcified	82.3 ± 13.8 n=25	18.4 ± 12.6* n=25	15.0 ± 14.9* n=8
concentric	86.3 ± 12.9 n=12	16.9 ± 10.3* n=12	26.7 ± 11.6 n=3
eccentric	78.8 ± 13.6 n=25	24.4 ± 18.1* n=25	18.0 ± 14.6* n=10

* $p<0.0001$ vs. pre
** $p<0.001$ vs. pre

Table 55

4. Laser Treatment

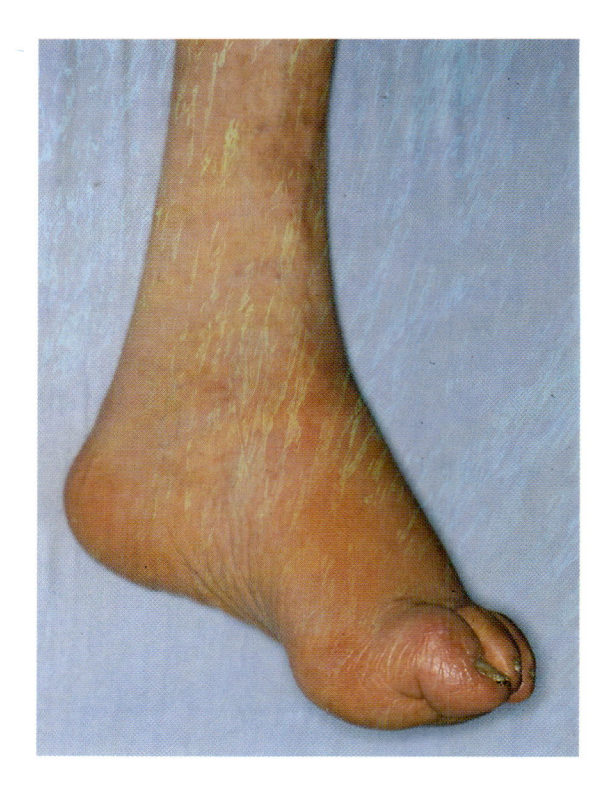

Fig. 180 a, b) Photograph of a patient with pregangrene of the lower extremity due to a 100% stenosis of the popliteal artery (a, above). Same extremity as in Fig a, 3 months post-atherectomy (b, below.)

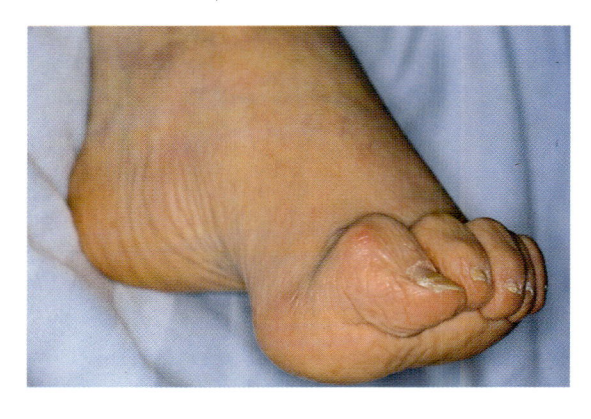

WD of 202.3 ± 70.4m measured (n=8). Baseline ankle/brachial index of the treated leg for the entire group was 0.58 ± 0.17 and rose significantly to 0.81 ± 0.16 (p<0.0001) post-atherectomy. This improvement has been maintained over 6m with an index of 0.86 ± 0.23 (n=8).

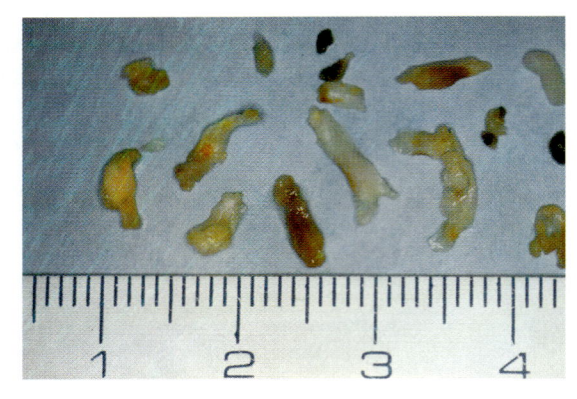

Fig. 181 Tissue specimens directly after removal via p-SAC; numeric scale in centimeters, divisions in millimeters.

Histologic Results

A total of 167 specimens taken from 41 stenoses (2-27 specimens per stenosis) 1-12 mm long and 0.2-2.0 mm thick were examined. Macroscopically (Figure 181) specimens consisted of either soft, white, shiny tissue, or brown-yellow thickened tissue; from formerly obliterated vessels, extremely calcified material was removed. Histologically, as seen in Table 56, intima was found in every stenosis, while media segments and thrombi were found in over 50%. Calcification was seen in 20% of stenoses, while neither external elastic lamina nor adventitia were recovered in any case.

Importantly, pathologic abnormalities, such as fibrous thickening of the intima, were found in 100% of stenoses, although more typical hallmarks of atherosclerosis, such as foam cells, organized thrombus, or atheroma with acicular cholesterol crystals and clefts within the intima, were less often found. Evaluation of a restenosis revealed non-specific fibroblasts infiltrating the intima without media or thrombus formation, which remained unchanged from the original histology.

4. Laser Treatment

Histological Findings in n=41 Stenoses (100%); all Specimens Removed via the p-SAC (Peripheral Simpson Atherectomy Catheter)

Intima
present	100%
fibrous thickening	100%
edema	97%
int elastic lamina	53%
pseudoelastic lamina	50%
capillarization	33%
inflammatory infiltrate	30%
calcification	20%
foam cells	20%
atheromatous plaque	3%

Media
present	50%
calcification	10%

Thrombus
present	53%
fibrin	53%
old/organized	30%
fresh	27%
inflammatory infiltrate	13%

Not Present
external elastic lamina
adventitia

Table 56

Conclusion

Atherectomy has been shown to be a safe and, in the relative short term follow-up to date, effective technique for the treatment of peripheral vascular disease, although the equipment currently available is best suited for the femoral or popliteal arteries. The presence of calcification does not preclude good results; although both concentric as well as eccentric lesions can be treated, the atherectomy catheter (at the present time) is better suited for eccentric lesions. Total occlusions can also be treated, usually after an initial Dotter technique to establish vessel patency.

The ability of the catheter to remove plaque material is valuable in several regards; firstly, by actually removing plaque material, the restenosis rate may be lower than that post-balloon angioplasty; secondly, the risk of distal embolization is largely eliminated; and thirdly, the removed specimens may be substituted for histologic and biochemical evaluation, useful both in studying the atherosclerotic process as well as for diagnostic purposes. In cases of restenosis, the histologic picture found may be useful in providing a theoretical basis for medical therapy (anti-platelet agents, cytotoxics or anti-thrombotics) of the chronic atherosclerotic process. Interestingly, however, the angiographic appearance after atherectomy is usually of a widely patent vessel, although often only fibrotic intima has been removed, theoretically suggesting that the bulk of plaque has been left behind.

Further study is needed, both to develop better catheter systems which are more ideally suited for a particular lesion and which safely remove more plaque material, and for application of these systems to the coronary circulation.

4. Laser Treatment

References

1. *Dotter CT, Grüntzig AR, Shoop W, et al (eds). Percutaneous Transluminal Angioplasy, New York, Springer Verlag, 1983.*

2. *Schneider E, Grüntzig A, Bollinger A. Langzeitergebnisse nach perkutaner transluminaler Angioplastie (PTA) bei 882 konsekutiven Patienten mit iliacalen und femoro-poplitealen Obstruktionen. VASA 11, 322, 1982.*

3. *Levine S, Ewels CJ, Rosing DR, Kent KM. Coronary angioplasty: clinical and angiographic follow-up. Am J Cardiology 55, 673, 1985.*

4. *Ginsburg R, Wexler L, Mitchell RS, Proffit D. Percutaneous transluminal laser angioplasty for treatment of peripheral vascular disease: clinical experience with 16 patients. Radiology 156, 619, 1985.*

5. *Fourrier J, Marache P, Brunetaud, Mordon S, Lablanche JM, Bertrand ME. Human percutaneous laser angioplasty with sapphire tips: results and follow-up. Circulation 76, IV-231, 1987 (abst).*

6. *Simpson JB, Johnson DE, Thapliyal HV et al. Transluminal atherectomy: a new approach to the treatment of atherosclerotic vascular disease. Circulation 72, III-146, 1985 (abst).*

7. *Höfling B, Simpson JB, Remberger K, Lauterjung L, Backa D. Percutaneous atherectomy in iliac, femoral and popliteal arteries. Klin Wschr 65, 528, 1987.*

8. *Simpson JB, Zimmermann JJ, Selmon MR et al. Transluminal atherectomy: Initial clinical results in 27 patients. Circulation 74, II-203, 1986.*

9. *Höfling B, Simpson JB, Backa B et al. Perkutane Transluminale Excision von okkludierendem Plaquematerial (Atherektomie) mit einem neuen Katheter. Z Herz-, Thorax-, Gefässchir 1, 124, 1987.*

10. *Höfling B, Backa D, Bauriedel G et al. Angioscopic controlled percutaneous atherectomy. Circulation 76, IV-232, 1987 (abst).*

4.7. Contact Laser Surgery - A Study of Five Different Laser Probes

D Richens, MR Rees, DA Watson

Cardiac Research Laboratories, Killingbeck Hospital, Leeds, England

Abstract

The ability to precisely control laser energy and to pass it down flexible glass fibres makes it an attractive means of performing angioplasty. Complications of its use may arise when the tip of the optical fibre is in contact with the wall of a coronary artery. Modified fibre tips have been developed to minimize these complications. We have tested five different laser probes when used in the contact mode. We compared three sapphire tip probes and one cooled glass fibre with a standard bare optical fibre. None of the five means of transferring laser energy appeared to be suitable for use in the coronary tree.

Introduction

Lasers are machines that can produce beams of high energy light. These light beams can be controlled very precisely and can be passed down flexible glass optical fibres (1). The first laser was developed in 1960 by The Howard Hughes Corporation in the United States, and lasers began to be used by the medical profession shortly afterwards (2,3). It was not until the 1980s, however, that people tried to use laser energy within the coronary tree to treat ischaemic heart disease (4,5). Early attempts at laser coronary angioplasty involved firing naked laser light from bare optical fibres, and these resulted in a high incidence of perforation of the vessel wall (6,7).

Many of the complications that occur from the use of lasers within closed blood vessels are due to contact between the tip of the fibre and the wall of the artery. When the laser is fired in the contact mode, light is reflected off the surface of the target tissue back down the fibre causing melting and burn back of the fibre tip (8). The tip of the fibre then produces a thermal effect on the tissue in its own right, independent of the laser beam, and this causes coagulation and adhesion of the surrounding tissue to the fibre.

A bare optical fibre has a sharp tip (Figure 182). This is capable of perforating the wall of the vessel or causing intimal damage due to mechanical trauma. These complications of perforation, tissue adhesion, and fibre burn back led to the development of a number of modified laser probes. Hot metal caps were devised where laser energy is discharged from the fibre into a metal tip at the end of the probe. This absorbs all the laser energy and creates a thermal effect on the surrounding tissue (9,10).

4. Laser Treatment

Other means of modifying the bare optical fibre included cooling of the fibre by infusion of saline and also attaching optically modified tips to the end (11, 12).

Sapphire-tipped probes are examples of optically modified tips. We compared the use of three different sapphire-tipped probes and a cooled bare optical fibre with a standard fibre 600 microns in diameter. All the probes were tested in the contact mode.

Methods

Laser

The laser used was a Pilkington Mark 2 Fiberlase. This emits continuous wave Nd:YAG laser energy with a wavelength of 1064 nm. Light of this wavelength is in the near infra-red part of the electromagnetic spectrum and, as such, is invisible to the naked eye. In order to aim the laser beam it is therefore necessary to use a second beam of light which is visible, and the machine emits a constant beam of red light from a low power laser (Helium-Neon). This aiming beam emerges from the tip of the fibre, allowing the operator to see where the Nd:YAG laser will pass.

Laser Catheters

Five types of laser catheters were used:

1. A bare 600 micron glass fibre. The fibre has an outer cladding of silicon and a further outer coating of clear PTFE producing an outer diameter of 1060 microns (Figure 182). The bare 600 micron optical fibre was the standard fibre used within all laser catheters tested.
2. Bare cooled fibre (Figure 183). The 600 micron optical fibre is surrounded by an outer PTFE jacket.

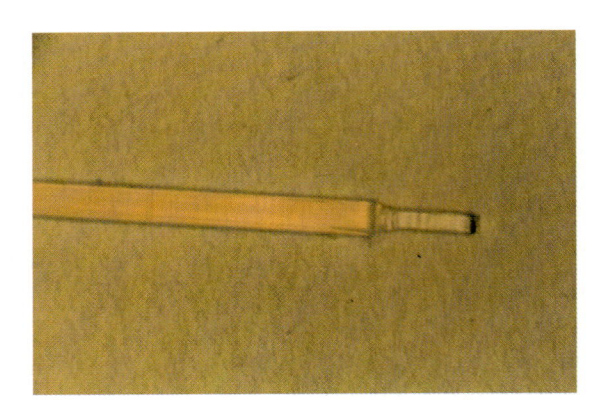

Fig. 182 Bare 600 micron optical fibre.

This has an outer diameter of 2.1 mm. In order to protect the target tissue from the sharp end of the optical fibre, and in order to maintain the optical fibre in the co-axial position within the outer cooling jacket, a distal ring of stainless steel is inserted into the outer plastic. Saline is infused down the fibre within the outer jacket around the optical catheter at a rate of 10 mls per minute, and this fluid emerges from the hole at the end of the probe.

3. Conical sapphire tipped probe. The sapphire is a physiologically neutral, synthetic sapphire, with a melting point of greater than 2000°C, and a high mechanical strength. It is held in a gold-plated, stainless steel holder which is screwed into a circular stainless steel adaptor, inserted at the distal end of a bare cooled fibre. Saline is infused within the outer 2.1 mm jacket and emerges from the side port of the metal holder (Figure 184).
4. Hemispherical sapphire-tipped catheter.
5. Blunt ended sapphire-tipped catheter.

In all cases the laser catheters were inserted at their proximal end into the continuous Nd:YAG laser. All fibres, apart from the bare 600 micron fibre,

4. Laser Treatment

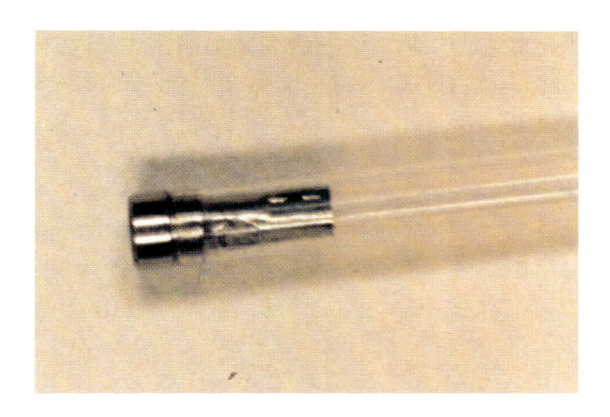

Fig. 183 Cooled 600 micron optical fibre. The stainless steel ring at the distal end maintains the central optical fibre in a co-axial position.

were cooled with saline pumped down the inside of the outer jacket at a rate of 10 mls per minute.

Beam Profiles

The beam profile of each probe was determined by still 35 mm photographs of the helium-neon aiming beam emerging from the catheter tip when in contact with a block of gelatin. Gelatin is animal protein which dissolves on heating in water and, on cooling, sets to form a jelly. This can be cut into 1 cm cubes and forms a useful standard medium of animal protein with which to assess laser tissue interactions. 25% gelatin was used throughout.

Microscopic Examination of Laser Craters

Each laser catheter was held by two flexible clamps at 90° to a piece of fresh porcine cadaveric aorta. These pieces were placed in a tissue bath of normal saline at room temperature, and the catheter was in all cases just touching the surface of the intima. A laser beam of 30 Watt power was fired for 5 seconds at each piece of aorta, producing an energy of 150 joules. The pieces of aorta were then transported in normal saline and examined grossly. Each experiment was repeated five times.

Histological Examination

Following gross examination, the tissue was placed in 10% neutral buffered formalin. Representative tissue blocks were obtained and embedded in paraffin. Sections were cut and stained with haematoxylin and eosin, and Van Gieson and elastin stains.

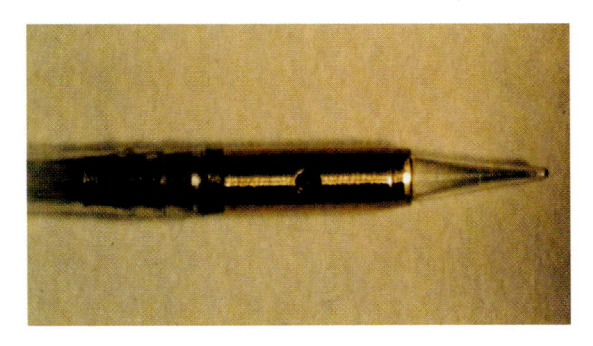

Fig. 184 Conical sapphire tip mounted on sapphire tip adaptor and attached to cooled optical fibre.

Use within Intact Vessel

Each catheter was inserted via the coronary ostia of a post-mortem intact human heart into coronary vessels. The catheter was introduced until the probe was in contact with an obstruction, and the laser was then fired at a power of 30 Watts for 5 seconds.

Results

Beam Profiles

The shape of the helium-neon aiming laser beam as it passes through the gelatin blocks is illustrated in Figure 185.

The light emerging from the bare fibre tip diverges with a half angle of 13°. The

4. Laser Treatment

light from the conically tipped sapphire probe is focused at the point of the probe and diverges with a half angle of 50°. The hemispherical sapphire tip acts as a lens with a focal length of 2 mm, the half angle of divergence from the focal point is 40°. The blunt-ended flat-tipped sapphire probe projects the light as a wide beam with a half angle of divergence of 20°.

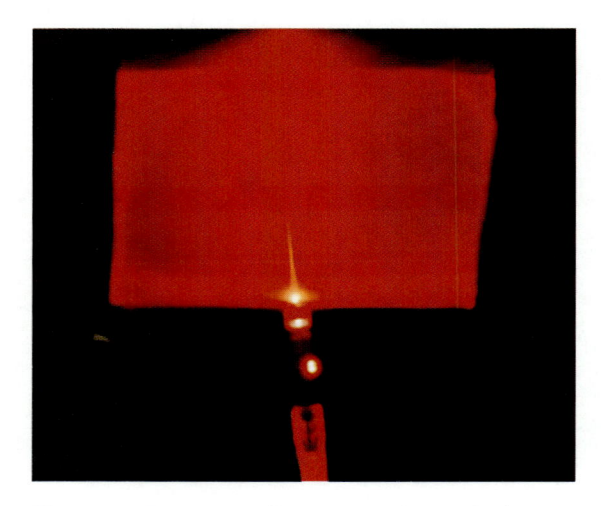

Fig. 185 Beam profile of hemispherical sapphire tip.

Microscopic Examination of Laser Craters

All the probes caused carbonization at the edge of the laser craters. In every case there was adhesion of the target tissue to the tip of the probe during application of the laser energy. Tissue adhesion could be prevented by removal of the probe whilst the laser was still being fired.

The bare and the bare cooled fibre created cylindrical laser craters penetrating into the wall of the aorta. Tissue adhesion to the bare cooled fibre was greater than that of the simple optical fibre.

Craters caused by passage of 150 joules down probes ending with sapphire tips were impressions within the wall of the vessel. There was some carbonization and alteration of the advential side of the aortic wall in all cases using the sapphire-tipped probes.

Histological Examination

Passage of laser beam from the bare and bare cooled fibre resulted in well-demarcated cylindrical craters in the aortic wall. These craters penetrated into the aortic media, tissue adhesion to the probes resulted in the avulsion of the intima of the aortic wall when the fibre was removed (Figure 186). The laser crater caused by vaporization of tissue was surrounded by a narrow adjacent rim of coagulation necrosis with vacuole formation. Coagulation necrosis was maximal around the deeper aspect of the laser crater. The controlled effect index of craters caused by the bare optical fibre (the ratio of the radius of the hole created and the extent of coagulation necrosis) was 3.0 (12).

None of the sapphire-tipped probes created laser craters by vaporization of tissue when 150 joules of energy was put into the proximal end of the fibres.

The conical laser probe caused an impression in the wall of the aorta; this was due to contraction of the vessel wall at this point. There was some separation of layers of media in adjacent tissue. There was coagulation necrosis at the advential surface of the aortic wall.

The hemispherical sapphire-tipped probe resulted in an impression in the wall of aorta. This was not due to vaporization of tissue, but due to contraction of the vessel wall at the point of contact. There was separation of the layers of the media in adjacent areas. There was marked coagulation necrosis with vacuole formation in the advential aspect of the aortic wall.

4. Laser Treatment

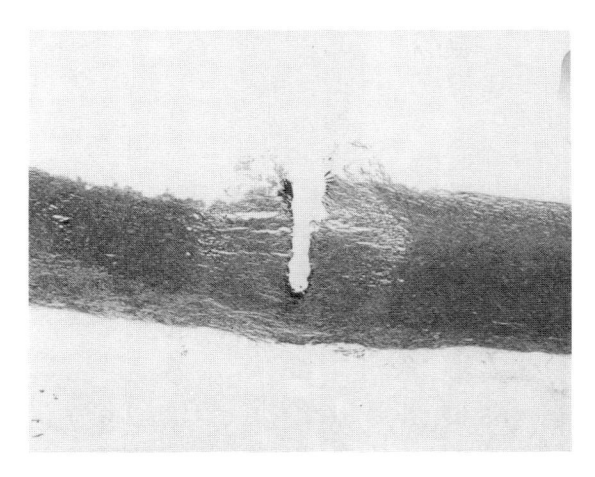

Fig. 186 A section of porcine aorta following exposure to 150 joules of energy from bare optical fibre in the contact mode. Magnification times 20, stained with haematoxylin and eosin.

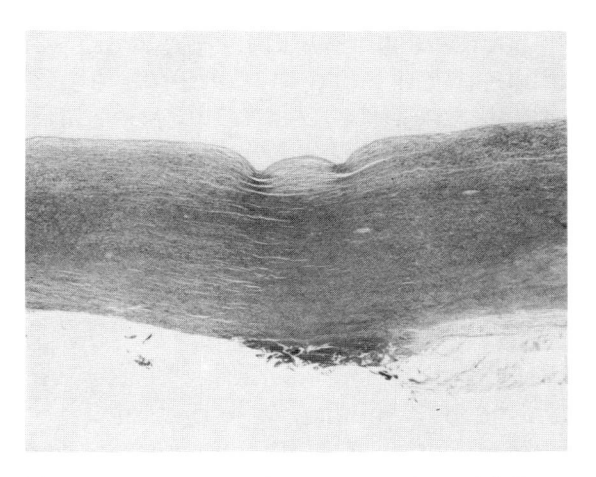

Fig. 187 A section of porcine aortic wall following exposure to 150 joules of laser energy from the blunt-ended sapphire tip in the contact mode. Magnification times 20, stained with haematoxylin and eosin.

The blunt-ended sapphire-tipped probe caused a doughnut-shaped impression in the aortic intima. In cross section this appeared as two craters (Figure 187). Each impression was due to contraction of the vessel wall with separation of medial layers in adjacent and intervening areas. There was coagulation necrosis of the advential surface of the wall.

Use within Closed Vessels:

Tissue adhesion occurred in each instance. After use, the bare optical fibre had undergone some changes due to heating. The outer PTFE cladding had melted and there was a rim of carbonization around the distal tip with distortion at its end. The sharp end of the bare fibre caused some damage to the artery during passage of the probe.

The bare cooled fibre exhibited marked tissue adhesion. After use, examination of the probe revealed oxidation of the stainless steel locating ring at the distal end with melting of the plastic PTFE sheath. This could cause embolization of the ring within the coronary tree. The stainless steel was distorted and the glass fibre extended from the end of the probe.

The combined length (8.8 mm) of the sapphire tip, sapphire tip holder, and sapphire tip adaptor on the end of the bare cooled fibres leads to an inflexible distal tip (Figure 184). Mechanical trauma occurs when these probes are passed through tortuous diseased coronary arteries. This is least with the hemispherical probe and most with the conical probe. The blunt-ended sapphire tip and the hemispherical sapphire tip showed marked oxidation of the metal adaptor following use within closed coronaries at energy levels of 150 joules. In all cases, a cuff of thermal damage to the intima in the coronary artery surrounding the metal adaptor, but proximal to the tip of the probe, occurred during firing of the laser.

Discussion

Tissue adhesion and carbonization of laser craters occurred regardless of the catheter used.

4. Laser Treatment

The bare fibre and the conical sapphire tip fibre led to intimal damage secondary to mechanical trauma when the probes were passed down intact coronary arteries.

Laser energy (150 joules) fired into the proximal end of a bare 600 micron optical fibre is sufficient to cause vaporization of tissue in the wall of fresh cadaveric porcine aorta. However, when an identical amount of laser energy is inserted into the proximal end of a fibre with a sapphire-tipped probe at its distal end, there is no vaporization of tissue. Instead we see an impression within the aortic wall created by contraction of the vessel wall at this point of contact.

Contraction as described above is due to thermal effects at temperatures lower than that necessary to cause vaporization (13). It is obvious that energy is lost at the interface between the laser fibre and the sapphire tip. This can be clearly seen as back reflection of light and emission of light from the side of the sapphire-tipped adaptor in Figure 4.

The shape of the sapphire tip determines the profile of the laser beam as it emits from the end of the probe. The conical sapphire tip focuses the majority of the light at its tip, creating high energy densities at the tip of the probe, but low energy densities a short distance away from the tip owing to the wide angle of divergence of the beam.

The hemispherical sapphire tip acts as a lens focusing the light approximately 2 mm from its tip (Figure 185).

The blunt-ended sapphire tip emits the beam as a wide column of light. It does not appear to focus the light.

The conical sapphire tip, by virtue of its ability to focus the light at the surface of the tissue, could be used for cutting, and the hemispherical tip could be used for cutting and vaporization of the tissue owing to its ability to focus the laser energy.

Because light is lost at the fibre optic sapphire tip interface, it is necessary to introduce higher powers than 30 Watts at the proximal end of the laser fibre if vaporization is to occur in the target tissue at the sapphire tip.

We measured the power of laser beams emitted from the end of the sapphire tip probes, using a power meter (OPHIR). We discovered that 20% of power is lost at this interface. When 50 Watts of laser power is fired, using a sapphire tip probe, for 5 seconds, it is possible to create holes in porcine aortic wall as shown in Figure 188.

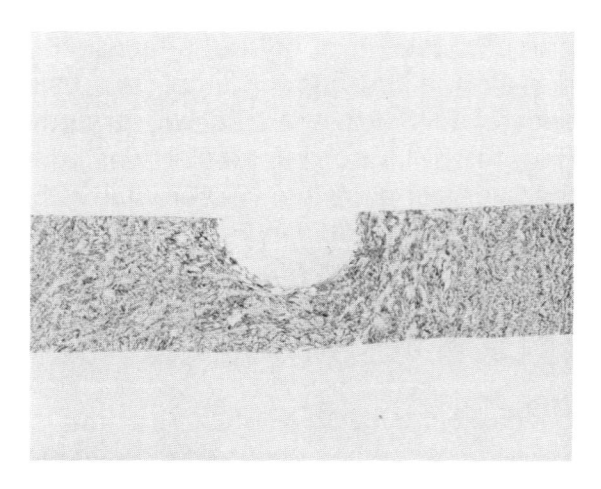

Fig. 188 A section of porcine aortic wall following exposure to 250 joules of laser energy from the hemispherical sapphire tipped probe. Magnification times 20, stained with van Giesen and elastin.

These higher powered laser craters have different shapes from that of the bare optical fibre. The different shape of the craters is due to the alteration of the beam profile by the sapphire tip. The hemispherical sapphire tip probe creates a smooth hemispherical crater with a controlled effect index of 7.0.

The conical sapphire-tipped probe creates a laser crater the shape of a truncated cone. The controlled effect index is 6.0.

We were unable to vaporize any tissue with a blunt-ended sapphire tip probe.

Scattered light lost at the fibre and optic sapphire interface causes heating of the metal sapphire tip adaptors. When the sapphire-tipped probes are used within the closed coronary arteries the heating effect of these metal adaptors causes burning of a cuff of intima adjacent to the adaptor but proximal to the tip of the sapphire probe. Metal components at the end of these laser probes heat up sufficiently to cause damage to the coronary artery before sufficient power is emitted from the tip of the probe to cause vaporization of the target.

Tissue adhesion, inflexibility of distal tips, and the heating effect of metal components are all complications of the probes that we have tested. We do not feel that any of the five probes is suitable for use within closed coronary arteries for contact laser coronary angioplasty.

Acknowledgements

The authors would like to thank Mrs Julie Brookes for preparation of the manuscript, Mrs Helena Wright for histological preparation and, Miss Anne Schofield for production of the illustrations.

4. Laser Treatment

References

1. Doiran DR, Profio AE. Laser instrumentation and safety. Clinics in Chest Medicine 6, 209, 1985.

2. Maiman TH. Stimulated optical radiation in ruby. Nature 187, 439, 1960.

3. Fox JL. The use of laser radiation as a surgical "light knife". Surg Res 9, 199, 1969.

4. Macruz R, Martins JRM, Tupinamba A, Lopes EA, Vargas H, Pennaaf DE, Carvalaho VB, Armelin E, De Court LV. Therapeutic possibilities of laser beams in atheromas. Arq Bras Cardiol 34, 9, 1980.

5. Choy DSJ, Stertzer S, Rotterdam HZ, Sharrock N, Kaminow IP. Transluminal catheter angioplasty. Am J Cardiol 50, 1206, 1982.

6. Choy DSJ, Stertzer SH, Myler RK, Marco J, Fournial G. Human coronary laser recanalization. Clin Cardiol 7, 377, 1984.

7. Choy DSJ, Stertzer SH, Rotterdam HZ, Bruno MS. Laser coronary angioplasty: experience with cadaveric harts. Am J Cardiol 50, 1209, 1982.

8. Ben-Schachar G, Spector ML, Morse DE, Adams ME, Sivakoff MC, Riemenschneider TA. Hazardous by-products of laser irradiation - a qualitative and quantitative study. Jacc 17, 46A, 1986.

9. Lee G, Chan MC, Rink DL, Beerline D, Lee MH, Reis RC, Mason DT. Coronary revascularization by a new coaxially-guided laser heated metal cap system. Am Heart J 113, 1507, 1987.

10. Abela GS, French A, Crea F, Conti CR. "Hot tip": Another method of laser vascular recanalization. Lasers in Surgery and Medicine 5, 327, 1985.

11. Geschwind HJ, Blair JD, Mongkolsmai D. Development and experimental application of contact probe catheter for laser angioplasty. J Am Coll Cardiol 9, 107, 1987.

12. Geschwind HJ, Morton JK, Vandormael MG. Efficiency and safety of optically modified fibre tips for laser angioplasty. J Am Coll Cardiol 10, 655, 1987.

13. Sliney DH. Laser-Tissue interactions. Clinics in Chest Medicine 16, 203, 1985.

4.8. Cardiovascular Applications of Laser Technology

RH Clarke, JM Isner

*Department of Chemistry, Boston University,
Boston, Massachusetts, USA
Department of Medicine, Tufts-New England Medical Center,
Boston, Massachusetts, USA*

That the laser is a unique tool for the treatment of cardiovascular disease seems to be an accelerating idea, one that requires careful development for safe application in the clinical arena, but with enormous potential for applicability as a percutaneous alternative to by-pass surgery. The attention focused on this field by the 1985 NHLB-sponsored workshop, "Laser and Fiberoptic Applications in Cardiovascular Research" supports this point, particularly in highlighting the need for co-operative effort to "bridge the gap" between the basic scientific aspects of the problem and the clinical development(1).

The mechanism by which laser light energy impacts and ablates cardiovascular tissue has been the subject of considerable speculation (2-6). The delivery of continuous wave (cw) or pulsed energy has quite different consequences in its effect on the tissue target site. In cases of excimer laser ablation, for example, several groups have reported ablation of the tissue site with no evidence of lateral thermal damage (2,3,7). In contrast, light delivered in a cw mode, or light delivered from a non-focused pulsed laser source produces extensive thermal damage to the surrounding tissue (7).

Our research group at Boston University and at the New England Medical Center has been actively involved in the problem of understanding laser light interactions with cardiovascular tissue for the past several years. Our initial efforts were in the treatment of hypertrophic cardiomyopathy with cw argon-ion lasers, ultimately successfully applied to three patients (5,6). We had continued studies of cw laser on cardiovascular tissue, noting, along with several other research groups, the tendency of cw lasers to produce extensive thermal damage in the surrounding tissue. Pathologic examination of cardiovascular tissue sites irradiated with cw lasers has consistently disclosed gross charring at the perimeter of the laser crater, and distinctive light microscopic findings: a superficial linear zone of coagulation necrosis, and a subjacent zone of polymorphous lacunae (5, 6). These findings have been interpreted as the result of thermal injury, an interpretation that has been supported by analyses from our laboratory of the photoproducts collected during cw argon laser irradiation of human atherosclerotic plaque (7).

Subsequent to these cw laser findings our group began an extensive investigation of the effects of pulsed laser sources on cardiovascular tissue (5,7). There are several reasons why pulsed lasers might be expected to eliminate

4. Laser Treatment

the thermal injury observed with cw lasers. First, the considerably greater peak powers at high photon energies, such as might be achieved with excimer nanosecond pulsed lasers, may be expected to initiate photoablation of tissue sites by direct electronic excitation and (nonthermal) bond-breaking photochemical reactions. Further, experiments by Anderson and Parrish (9), as well as work by Wolbarsht (10) and Welch (11), suggest that thermal injury of adjacent, non-target tissue sites may be avoided if exposure time utilized for each pulse is shorter than the thermal relaxation time away from the irradiated site. Consequently, if the peak power generated by the laser is great enough to accomplish a given volume of tissue ablation at suitably brief pulse durations and suitably brief cumulative exposures, such as is obtained with the nanosecond pulses of the excimer laser, then the energy impacting the tissue site is all taken up in ablation and kinetic energy of product release, avoiding energy release in the form of thermal damage to the surrounding tissue.

Srinivasan was the first to demonstrate that pulsed delivery of excimer laser energy could, in fact, ablate portions of organic polymer materials without causing thermal damage to surrounding areas (12); he subsequently extended these observations to tissue target sites. Excimer lasers use a mixture of rare and halogen gases as the active medium to generate pulses of short wavelength, high energy, ultraviolet light. Experiments in our laboratory (2,5) and in the group of Forrester et al (13) have demonstrated that a variety of excimer wavelengths can vaporize atherosclerotic plaque without apparent thermal injury. Elimination of thermal injury in residual laser-irradiated tissues could be potentially advantageous for several reasons. First, if tissue vaporization could be accomplished without heating non-target healthy tissue (e.g. arterial walls), then perforation of the underlying wall might be more readily avoided. Secondly, elimination of pathologic injury to the residual lumen surface might diminish the likelihood of thrombotic re-occlusion or atherosclerotic restenosis.

Why is the understanding of the details of the photoablation process important? For laser angioplasty to be successful, the process of photoremoval of the diseased site must be effected with minimal damage to the surrounding tissue; basically, it is an issue of controlled photoablation. And to control the process requires a full understanding of the photophysical process involved, specifically under conditions of energy dissipation and loss in the presence of a fluid field.

Our recent interest in this problem has led to the application of several experimental chemical and spectroscopic techniques aimed at elucidating the mechanism responsible for the tissue ablation process. We have examined the photoproducts released in cw vs. pulsed laser light energy delivery and have found that the same equilibrium products dominate the gas phase material released (7, 14). We have also investigated the emission properties, both fluorescence and plasma photoemission from the surface of tissue undergoing photoablation by both cw and pulsed laser sources (15,16). We have recently used laser Raman light scattering to probe the make-up of the atherosclerotic lesions as they are targeted for laser ablation (17). And in our most recent work we have found the first evidence for the presence of organic free

4. Laser Treatment

radicals by electron paramagnetic resonance (EPR) when both Cw and pulsed lasers impact on cardiovascular tissue. The results of our initial EPR studies are presented in the section below. It is the overall goal of this work to build up a full description of the mechanism of the laser ablation process. Such information is expected to be of importance in establishing the conditions required for the optimization and control of laser light energy in a percutaneous laser angioplasty procedure.

In an attempt to find direct evidence for the form of products released in the actual dominant photomechanism of photoablation, we have begun a series of investigations aimed at detecting and identifying the possibility of free radical formation as a consequence of photoablation of cardiovascular tissue by both cw and pulsed laser energy. The appearance of free radicals accompanying laser ablation is of importance in that the creation of such species implies specific bond breakage and subsequent release of distinct molecular fragments whose origin may lead to understanding the pathway of photoablation.

Since paramagnetic free radicals are extremely reactive, typically undergoing reaction to a stable, diamagnetic (all spins paired) form in times on the order of several hundred nanoseconds (18), we have utilized the method of spin trapping to intercept and detect any free radical formation accompanying laser photoreaction at a tissue site (19). In this method an organic intermediate is added to the reaction solution that will react with the free radicals present as they are formed; upon reaction with the unstable free radical, the intermediate is converted to nitroxide, a well-known stable paramagnetic species (19,20), which is detected in a conventional EPR spectrometer.

Detection of Free Radicals by Spin Trapping

In our initial experiments we used the method of spin trapping (19) to detect free radical formation upon laser interaction with tissue samples of myocardium, calcified aortic valves, and segments of coronary arteries, both disease-free and those containing extensive atherosclerotic lesions. Both argon-ion laser energy in the visible 514 nm and in the UV, 351-363 nm, and pulsed excimer laser energy at 351 nm and 308 nm, have been investigated.

Port-mortem tissue samples were rinsed with distilled water and mounted in the bottom of a quartz EPR tube. The size of tissue sample was approximately the diameter of the EPR tube (5 mm). The tissue sample was in contact with fused silica optical fiber connected to the laser, as indicated in Figure 189.

The spin trap used was a commercially available spin trap reagent: N-tert-butyl-∂-phenylnitrone (PBN) was purchased from Aldrich Chemical Co. PBN was chosen because of its stability and insensitivity to light. PBN was dissolved in cyclohexane to a concentration of 50mM and about 20 drops of this solution were added freshly in each experiment to cover the tissue sample mounted in the EPR cavity. All solutions were purged with a flow of nitrogen gas bubbled through the solution, and sample tubes were subsequently kept under nitrogen atmosphere.

The tissue sample was irradiated through the optical fiber by the output of a focused laser beam (Figure 189). A Coherent Innova 20 argon-ion and Questek series 2240 excimer laser

4. Laser Treatment

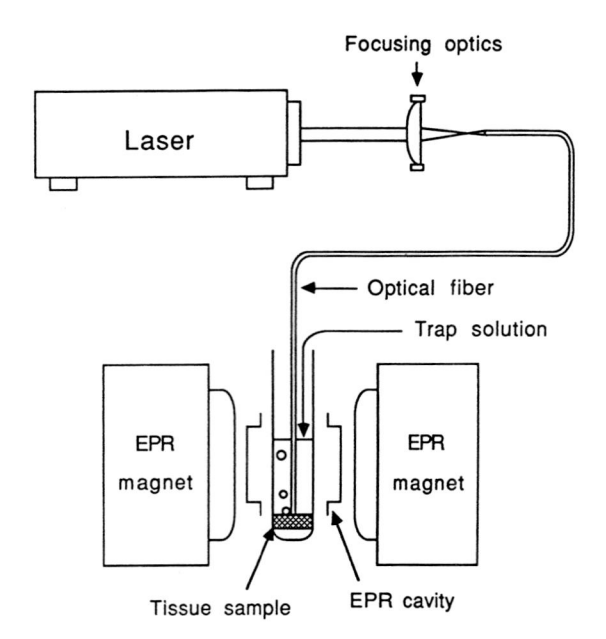

Fig. 189 Schematic description of experimental set-up for EPR of laser-generated radicals

were used to generate short-lived radicals. The laser output power was ~0.3 watts for 514 nm and 0.1~0.3 watts for the pulsed UV photoablation.

When myocardium samples mounted in cyclohexane solution at the bottom of an EPR tube are irradiated with the visible output of an argon-ion laser coupled to an optical fiber, short-lived radicals are trapped by the PBN in solution, and an EPR spectrum of the trapped complex is observed as shown in Figure 190. As the laser energy continues to irradiate the sample, a buildup of trapped radical concentration is observed with the signal intensity increasing with cumulative time of sample exposure to the laser light. When the tissue sample is absent and only the PBN solution is irradiated, no EPR signal is observed.

If this experiment is repeated with a sample of coronary artery segment exhibiting gross atherosclerotic disease and the laser energy is directed at the diseased site, an identical result is obtained, but with a lower EPR signal intensity. The lower intensity might be due to the lower efficiency of absorbance compared to myocardium of the argon visible wavelengths by the plaque material (4), although other explanations, such as lower rates of radical formation, may also be involved. An identical result is obtained when a piece of calcified aortic valve is placed in the EPR cavity and illuminated by the laser light.

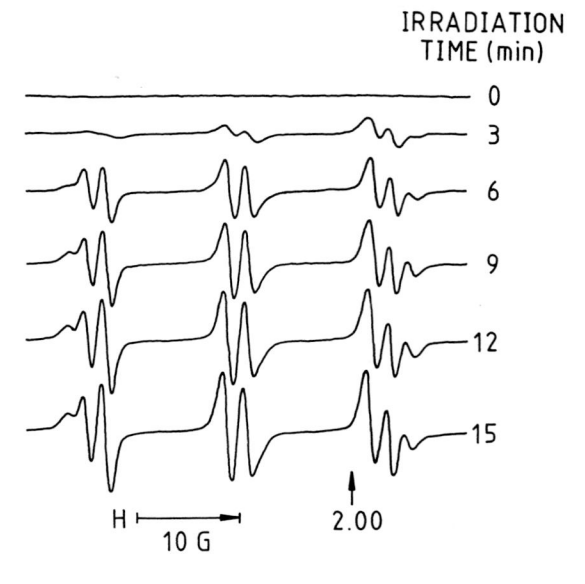

Fig. 190 EPR spectra observed for 514 nm argon

Free Radicals Produced with a Pulsed Laser Source

To compare effects produced when ablating tissue with a pulsed laser, a laser which has been reported by several groups to produce injury-free tissue removal, as compared with the typical thermal injury on cw laser ablation (4,7,21), we have examined the effects of excimer laser irradiation on the same sample series. The results observed are different in two respects from the cw experiments. First, a quali-

4. Laser Treatment

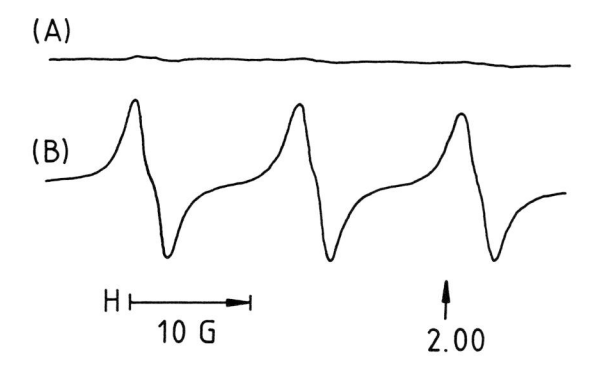

Fig. 191 EPR spectra observed for 308 nm excimer irradiation without myocardium (A) and with myocardium (B) in presence of PBN.

tatively different hyperfine pattern is observed on excimer ablation of myocardium; the pattern is shown in Figure 191. The doubling of the nitrogen triplet is clearly absent in the results with excimer laser ablation; the same result is observed with both 351 nm and 308 nm excimer laser wavelengths. A second difference on photoablation with the pulse excimer compared with cw argon-ion laser irradiation is in the intensity of the observed EPR signal. When equal amounts of total energy from the excimer laser at 308 nm (40 Hz, 7.5 millijoules/pulse, 20 second exposure; total energy delivered = 6 joules) was delivered to a myocardium sample through a 1000 μ optical fiber and compared with the same energy at 514 nm (0.3 watts for 20 seconds; total energy delivered = 6 joules) delivered cw through the same fiber to a second myocardium sample, the excimer EPR signal intensity was ~200 times that of the cw laser experiment. Since the EPR signal is directly proportional to the number of spins present in the EPR cavity, the result indicates a concentration of radicals produced by the excimer laser ~200 times that produced by the cw laser per unit energy delivered.

We have attempted a computer simulation of both the excimer and argon-ion laser results to determine the appropriate hyperfine constants as an indication of the nature of the radicals being trapped. Using a standard simulation program, the two sets of EPR spectra were matched to calculated spectra as the hyperfine parameters were adjusted. The most immediate difference in the excimer and argon simulations is the fact that it takes two distinct paramagnetic species to properly represent the EPR spectrum observed with the argon laser, as opposed to only a single species in the excimer simulation.

Although the results are presented for myocardium samples, there is no observable difference in the spin trapping ERP results of ablation of diseased coronary arteries. The spin trapping simulations are expected to be indicative of, and applicable to, all the cardiovascular tissue samples examined in these experiments.

The results presented here provide clear and direct evidence of free radical formation accompanying laser ablation for *both* cw and pulsed lasers. Whatever the significant differences are in the mechanism of laser action in the case of the excimer laser, postulated by some researchers to act via an excited state photochemical bond-breaking reaction (21), as compared with the expected thermal laser processes with the argon-ion laser (4), both lasers are operating by mechanisms which involve the production of significant radical fragments accompanying laser interaction with the tissue sample. Further, the results appear independent of laser wavelength and tissue composition within the limits of the present experiments.

4. Laser Treatment

Although both the pulsed laser and the cw laser produce free radicals, they are not the same radical in the two cases. That they are *not* the same radical is evident qualitatively in the difference in hyperfine structure in the two EPR spectra; this difference is confirmed quantitatively in the computer simulations in which the hyperfine splitting parameters are not only distinct in the two cases, but, further, the presence of more than one radical species is required to explain the hyperfine patterns observed with visible and UV argon laser ablation of tissue targets.

There appear to be no reproducible differences among tissue types in our experiments when a specific laser wavelength and type is selected to produce the free radical EPR spectra. Rather, the main difference is in pulsed laser action vs. cw. This is strikingly demonstrated when the 351 nm excimer-generated EPR spectrum is compared with the 353 nm argon-generated spin trap signal; here the laser wavelength is virtually identical in the two experiments, yet the hyperfine patterns are distinctive. However, it should be pointed out that the computer simulations indicate that the observed spin trap EPR spectra are dominated by hyperfine constants from the nitroxide unit itself; therefore, differences in radicals produced by different tissue targets might not be seen and might remain obscured by the nitroxide-dominated lineshapes.

What do the present results imply about the mechanism of laser action in the pulsed vs. cw configuration, a subject of much speculation in the literature (21-23)? The finding that radicals are produced in both cases makes the differentiation of mechanism of laser action in the two cases less clear; but it does seem to require significant direct bond breakage in both cases. That the excimer laser produces free radicals more efficiently may indicate the greater efficiency of this laser in direct bond cleavage, although several mechanistic steps may be involved in both cases, rendering discussion of relative efficiency somewhat inconclusive.

Comparison of Free Radicals by Laser and Ultrasound

In the above experiments we demonstrated that laser ablation of cardiovascular tissue is accompanied by the formation of short-lived organic free radicals. The nature of the radicals generated was dependent on whether the laser light energy was applied as a continuous wave (cw) or as a pulsed source.

We have also investigated the results of spin trapping experiments on cardiovascular tissue, using quite different energy sources for the tissue removal process. We have compared the EPR spectra of radicals obtained when an ultrasonic source is used to degrade segments of myocardium with the results of using an argon-ion and excimer laser to effect damage of the same tissue target.

Ultrasonic experiments on tissue were performed with a Heat System-Ultrasonics, Inc model W-225R operating at room temperature with a microtip probe which is ~3 mm diameter at the tip end. The ultrasonic frequency was 20 KHz which is determined by the size of the lead zirconate titanate crystal. The output power from the microtip probe in contact with the tissue sample was ~32 watts. The high ultrasound power was chosen to provide damage to tissue samples which are expected to be difficult to disrupt with ultrasound.

4. Laser Treatment

At the start of sonication of the tissue sample, the tissue solution turned milky and the solution exhibited foaming.

Ultrasonic-generated short-lived free radicals were trapped in a flow system depicted in Figure 192. The flow rates were adjusted by the drain size of the tissue container and the two valves which allowed mixing of the spin trap solution and the sample solution in any required proportion. The flow rate was normally no faster than 1.1 ml per minute. The solution temperature of the tissue container rose as high as 43°C towards end of the sonication. This flow system provided both the advantage of avoiding the sonic disruption of PBN and reduction of excessive temperature build-up at the tissue sample.

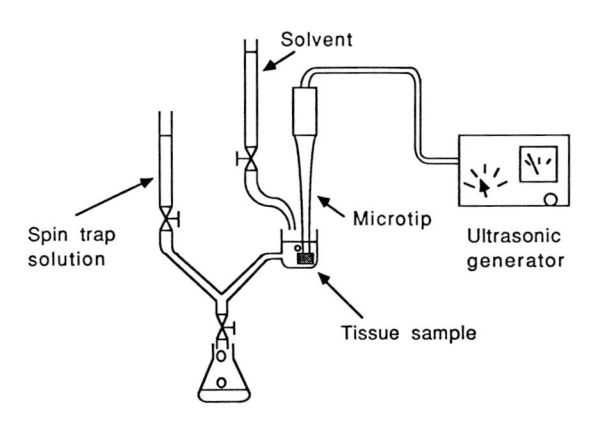

Fig. 192 Schematic representation of the experimental arrangement for ultrasonically producing and spin trapping of free radicals from myocardium with a flow system.

The trapped short-lived free radicals were measured on a Varian E104 X-band spectrometer operating in the TE_{102} mode. EPR spectra were recorded at room temperature. In the ultrasound flow experiments, EPR spectra were averaged - 5 hours with a Tracor Northern digital signal averager NS-570 connected directly to the EPR spectrometer. Typical EPR recording conditions were the following: microwave frequency 9.5 GHz; modulation frequency 100 Hz; time constant 0.5 second. The resonance field was measured relative to the standard free radical 2,2-diphenyl-1-picrylhydrazyl (DPPH). The EPR result of ultrasonication of myocardium is shown in Figure 193.

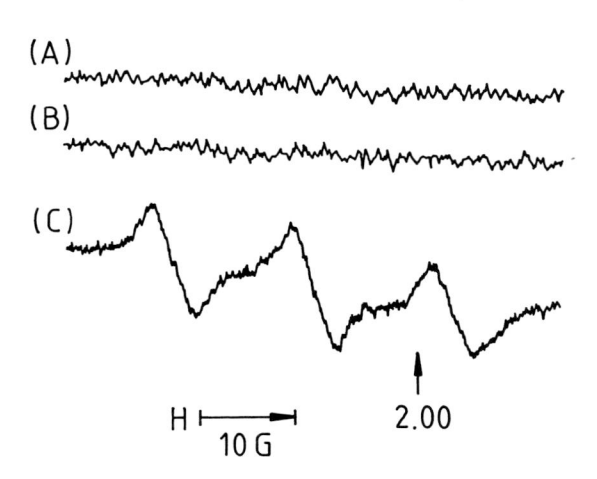

Fig. 193 Spin-trapped EPR spectra obtained from samples in the ultrasound-flow system: (A) flow solvent alone; (B) flow solvent and myocardium, no ultrasound; and (C) myocardium with ultrasound generation.

Since the ablation of tissue samples with pulsed laser radiation is often accompanied by visual and auditory evidence of acoustic activity at the tissue target site (15), we attempted to induce these same effects by direct ultrasonic disruption of cardiovascular tissue. A difficulty with both the laser and ultrasound experiments is in differentiating effects on the tissue target from those produced in the spin trap solution itself. This is particularly important in the case of spin trapping experiments, since the spin trap will intercept any radical formed, whether they originate in the direct reaction of the tissue targets, or

465

4. Laser Treatment

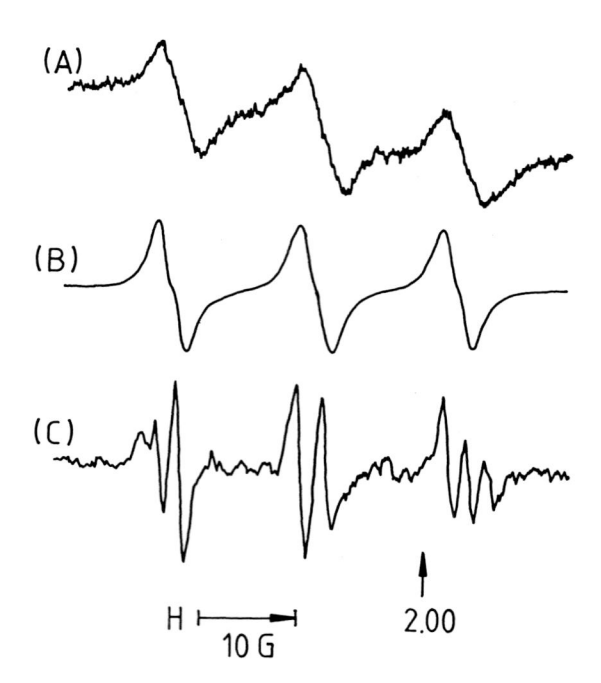

Fig. 194 Comparison of spin-trapped EPR spectra of myocardium produced by different irradiation sources: (A) ultrasound; (B) excimer laser (110 mJ/pulse at 308 nm), and (C) argon-ion laser (0.30 watts at 514 nm).

by the disruption of the spin trap or its accompanying solvent.

In the work described above the problem of isolating reactions of the laser light energy with the spin trap solution was eliminated by first examining the reactivity of the spin trap solution without any tissue sample present, and demonstrating that no laser-generated EPR signal was produced in the absence of the tissue sample in the light beam. In the case of the ultrasound experiments, however, the spin trap solvent alone did produce an EPR signal in the absence of tissue. Therefore, the flow apparatus was introduced to eliminate the background signal generated by the ultrasonic disruption of the spin trap itself.

A series of EPR spectra taken under cw argon laser, pulsed excimer laser, and under ultrasonic fragmentation of a myocardium sample is shown in Figure 194. The similarity of spectral features of the spin-trapped EPR from the excimer laser with those generated by ultrasound is obvious in the figure. Both cases produce strong EPR spectra with a dominant three line nitrogen hyperfine splitting and a barely resolvable secondary beta hydrogen hyperfine splitting built on each of the nitrogen peaks (19).

In contrast, the cw argon-ion laser produces a characteristic EPR spectrum from the spin trapped radical species generated by the thermal disruption of the tissue target that is distinctly different from that observed for either the excimer or ultrasonically generated radical. First, the EPR signals are weaker (by a factor of about 200) than the excimer or ultrasound cases. And, secondly, there is extensive hyperfine splitting of the nitrogen triplet in the EPR pattern with the cw laser.

Both the excimer laser and the ultrasonic probe produced tissue damage in our experiments that exhibited no gross evidence of thermal injury to the surrounding area. This observation for the excimer laser has been widely reported in its application to cardiovascular tissue (4,12,21). It is perhaps not unexpected in the case of tissue disruption by an ultrasonic source, as well, since sound waves are expected to break up a tissue sample mainly by ablative acoustic shock, with some accompanying heat generation. Although the exact identity of the radicals produced in the two experiments is not readily identifiable on the basis of the (limited) hyperfine structure observed in Figure 6, the observed EPR spectra are not inconsistent with the radicals being the same in both cases.

In contrast, the radicals produced under conditions of direct evidence for thermal damage to the tissue sample when the argon laser light energy is used are clearly not the same as produced under conditions of clean ablation by either the excimer laser or the ultrasonic probe. Again, the identity of the radical produced when the sample is charred by the argon laser is not readily identifiable on the basis of the spin- trapped hyperfine. But the fact that it is a different radical seems indisputable on the basis of the spectra displayed in Figure 6.

Even without a firm identification of the radical species generated in each of the spectra, we feel that the spectra provide important information about the mechanism of laser action in cardiovascular tissue. The observation of ablation of organic material, whether plastic polymer sheets or cardiovascular tissue samples, has been described as being accompanied by acoustic "popping" and high velocity expulsion of particulate debris (15,21,24). Such a process could well be effected by a photogenerated acoustic wave within the tissue, causing a shock wave of sufficient magnitude to disrupt the bonds holding together the protein chains that comprise the tissue or the polymer chains comprising the plastic. If this is the mechanism of clean cutting by the excimer laser, then the same behaviour would be expected of a purely acoustic source of energy released in these samples and capable of disrupting the same protein chains. The ultrasonic source provides just such an acoustic shock wave to the tissue and does seem to result in the same radical signature in its hyperfine pattern.

Of course, these experiments do not prove directly that the same acoustic disruption mechanism is active with the pulsed laser and the ultrasonication of the tissue sample. The results are only consistent with that mechanism. What is required are time resolved EPR experiments to identify directly the radicals produced in the pulsed, cw laser, and ultrasound experiments to provide a full picture of the events involved in the mechanism of ablation. These experiments should provide, for the first time, a direct view of the fragments produced in tissue disruption by laser light energy in the photoablation process.

Acknowledgement

This research was supported by the US National Heart, Lung and Blood Institute under Grants No HL36918-01 and HL32747-01.

4. Laser Treatment

References

1. NIH Workshop on laser and fiberoptic applications in cardiovascular research, sponsored by the NHLB, NIH, Washington DC, Sept 26-27, 1985.

2. (a) Clarke RH, Isner JM, Sarabia J, Aharon AS, Konstam MA, Cleveland RJ. Clinical Research 33, 742A, 1985.

   (b) Isner JM, Aharon AH, Donaldson RF, Deckelbaum LI, Clarke RH. Clinical Research 33, 742A, 1985.

3. Mueller D, Svrluga RS. Laser focus 21, 70, 1985.

4. Isner JM, Steg PG, Clarke RH. IEEE J Quantum Electronics QE-23, 1756, 1987.

5. Isner JM and Clarke RH. IEEE J Quantum Electronics, QE-20, 1406, 1984.

6. Isner JM, Clarke RH, Pandian NG, Donaldson RF, Salem DN, Konstam MA, Payne DD, Cleveland RJ. Am J Cardiol, 53, 1620, 1984; 55, 1192, 1985.

7. Isner JM, Clarke RH, Donaldson RF, Aharon AH. Am J Cardiol 55, 1192, 1985.

8. Deckelbaum LI, Isner JM, Donaldson RM, Clarke RH, Laliberte S, Aharon AH. Am J Cardiol 5, 488, 1983.

9. Anderson RR, Parrish JA. Science 220, 524, 1983.

10. Hayes JR, Wolbarscht ML. Aerospace Medicine 39, 474-480, 1968.

11. Welch AJ. IEEE J Quantum Electronics QE-20, 1471, 1984.

12. Srinivasan R, Mayne-Banton V. Appl Phys Lett 41, 576, 1982.

13. Grundfest W, Litvak F, Forrester J, Goldenber T, Swan HJC, Morgenstern L, McDermid S, Rider D, Pacala T, Laudenschlager J. J Am Cardiol 5, 929, 1985.

14. Clarke RH, Isner JM, Donaldson RF, Jones G. Circ Research 60, 429, 1987.

15. Isner JM, Steg PG, Clarke RH. IEEE J Quantum Electronics QE-23, 1756, 1987.

16. Clarke RH, Cerio FM, Isner JM. Chlorotetracycline-induced fluorescence from atherosclerotic plaque with UV laser excitation, J Luminescence, in press, 1988.

17. Clarke RH, Hanlon EB, Isner JM, Brody H. Appl Optics 26, 3175, 1987.

18. Swartz HM, Bolton JR, Borg DC. Biological applications of electron spin resonance, Wiley-Intersciences, New York, 1972.

19. Janzen EG. Accounts Chem Research 4, 31, 1971.

20. Janzen EG, Dehler UM, Haire DL, Kotake Y. J Am Chem Soc 108, 6858, 1986.

21. Srinivasan R. Science 234, 559, 1986.

22. Jelleneck HHG, Srinivasan R. J Phys Chem 88, 3048, 1984.

23. Keyes T, Clarke RH, Isner JM. J Phys Chem 89, 4194, 1985.

24. Koren G and Yeh JTC. Appl Phys 56, 2120, 1984.

4.9. Endoscopically Guided Laser Angioplasty - A New Laser Angioscope

D Richens, MR Rees, DA Watson

Cardiac Research Laboratories, Killingbeck Hospital, Leeds, England

Abstract

We have found a high incidence of complications of laser angioplasty in the coronary arteries when the end of the laser probe is in contact with the wall of the vessel. A method of angioplasty using non-contact laser surgery would have fewer complications but it would be necessary to have a system of direct viewing within the vessel. This would ensure that the tip of the laser catheter is not in contact with any tissue. It would also then be possible to aim the laser beam at the target, obstructive atheromatous plaques.

We have determined safe working limits for the use of laser energy fired from a bare fibre within the coronary tree. We also describe a method of performing coronary angioscopy using ultra thin angioscopes. We have used a technique of firing continuous wave Nd:YAG laser energy down a single optical fibre within a working channel of such an angioscope. An experimental model has been set up in intact postmortem human hearts.

Using this system, complications of laser coronary angioplasty are minimized. We have shown that it is possible to ablate atheromatous disease at energies lower than that required to perforate human coronary arteries. Once sufficient experience has been gained in the laboratory setting, this system could be used to treat ischaemic heart disease.

Introduction

It has been shown that laser energy can vaporize atheromatous plaques within human coronary arteries (1,2). There are differences between laser tissue interactions when the laser beam is fired in the contact as opposed to the non-contact mode (3). We have found that contact laser surgery leads to tissue adhesion and melting of the distal tip of the optical fibres carrying the light energy. In addition, the narrow end of these flexible optical fibres often caused intimal damage to the coronary arteries during passage down the coronary tree (4).

We think that the use of laser energy fired from bare optical fibres in the non-contact mode is a more controllable method of angioplasty, as the complications secondary to contact between tip and tissue do not occur. It is important, however, to have a method of direct viewing within the coronary tree to ensure that the tip of the fibre does not damage the coronary intima and is not in contact with the wall of the vessel during firing of the laser beam. Such a

4. Laser Treatment

method of direct visualisation would also enable the beam to be aimed at the target tissue (5,6).

Methods

Laser

A continuous wave Nd:YAG laser (Pilkingtons Fiberlase Mark 2) emitting laser light of 1064 nm wavelength was used. The laser beam was fired down to a 400 micron bare glass optical fibre.

Nd:YAG laser energy is invisible to the naked eye; in order to aim the laser beam, therefore, a second beam of light is constantly passed down the fibre from the laser. This aiming beam is red and is emitted from a helium-neon laser within the machine.

Angioscopes

Two different angioscopes were used.

1. Olympus PF18L Ultra thin Endoscope. This has an outer diameter of 1.8 mm with a working length of 800 mm. It has no working channel. The angle of view field is 75° with a depth of field of 3 mm to 30 mm. Still photography was performed down the scope using the Olympus SM-2S adaptor combined with an Olympus OM2 35 mm SLR camera. Exposure compensation for use with 150 watt light source was minus 3.
2. Trimedyne 2.5 mm Optiscope. This has a working length of 100 mm. It contains no integral light source fibres but, instead, has a channel for a removable light fibre. It has a further 0.2 mm channel for saline flushing. There was no adaptor for direct still 35 mm photography. It was possible to insert the 400 micron optical fibre connected to the Nd:YAG laser into the illumination channel of this scope. When this occurred the helium-neon aiming beam was used for illumination. The fibre can be extended from the tip of the scope under direct vision.

Both endoscopes are capable of sterilisation with ethylene oxide.

Video photography was used by coupling the endoscope to an ultra sensitive video camera (Sopro 33). This camera is capable of sterilisation in ethylene oxide. It is 7.5 cm by 6.5 cm by 3.5 cm in size and weighs 175 g. The video camera was attached to a video recorder and the image obtained was simultaneously shown on a colour TV monitor. The light source used in all experiments was a 150 watt Tungston Halogen projector lamp (Keylight MSA).

Tissue

In order to determine safe working limits for the use of the laser, cadaveric human coronary arteries were used. These were obtained within 24 hours of death. The arteries were dissected from the heart and opened longitudinally. They were then cut into 2 cm segments.

For angioscopy, intact post-mortem human hearts were used. These were obtained within 24 hours of death.

Measurements

Safe working limits for use of the laser were defined as the minimum time taken to perforate the coronary artery at each power setting of the laser. The power settings of the laser varied within the range of 3 watts to 100 watts. Using the bare fibre, the laser was fired at the dissected coronary arteries from 0 mm, 1 mm, 2 mm, and 3 mm away. The fibre was maintained at 90° to the tissue by means of two fully adjustable clamps. The laser fibre and tissue were immersed in normal saline at room temperature. The laser was fired at each power setting of the laser over the time range of 0.1 seconds to 99 seconds. The coronary artery was then placed in 10% neutral buffered formalin for subsequent histological examination. Minimum perforation time for each power setting was determined at each distance following histological examination.

Angioscopy

The angioscopes were passed into the coronary arteries in either an antigrade fashion through the aortic root and via the coronary ostia or in a retrograde fashion via distal ateriotomies. The coronary arteries were simultaneously flushed with saline solution which was infused into the aortic root with a cross clamp on the aorta.

Laser Angioplasty under Direct Vision

The 2.5 mm Optiscope was inserted into the coronary artery. Saline was infused via the flushing channel of the scope into the coronary vessel. The standard optical fibre connected to 150 watt light source was passed down the illumination channel of the scope until it reached the tip of the instrument (Figure 195). The scope was manoeuvered under direct vision until it was adjacent to a coronary stenosis. The illumination fibre was then removed and the 400 micron bare optical fibre attached to the laser was inserted into the illumination channel. Subsequent illumination was by means of the helium-neon aiming beam of the laser. The fibre was then extended from the end of the tip of the instrument under direct vision until it was touching the stenosis. The fibre was then withdrawn over a

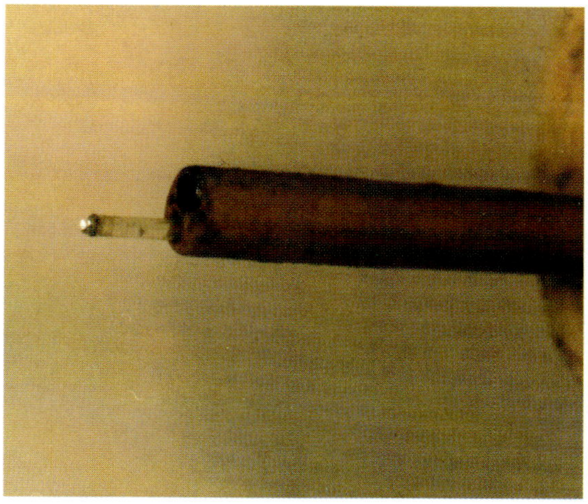

Fig. 195 Trimedyne 2.5 mm Optiscope. The optical fibre within the illumination channel has been extended from the end of the endoscope and emits a white light.

pre-set distance from the proximal part of the scope, such that the distance from the tip of the fibre to the stenosis was known. The most commonly used distance was 2 mm. Under direct vision laser energy was then fired at the stenosis.

Results

Safe Working Limits

A graph of the logarithm of the minimum perforation time for each power setting of the laser at each distance from the target tissue is shown in Figure 196.

Angioscopy

Very poor images were obtained with the angioscopes initially until simultaneous flushing of the coronary arteries was performed. This was due to collapse of the walls of the coronary arteries and resulted in impaction of the tip of the instrument on the wall of the vessel. Satisfactory images like those obtained in Figure 197 were obtained once the vessels were flushed with a clear solution. Better images were obtained with

4. Laser Treatment

MINIMUM PERFORATION TIME (S) BARE FIBRE SALINE

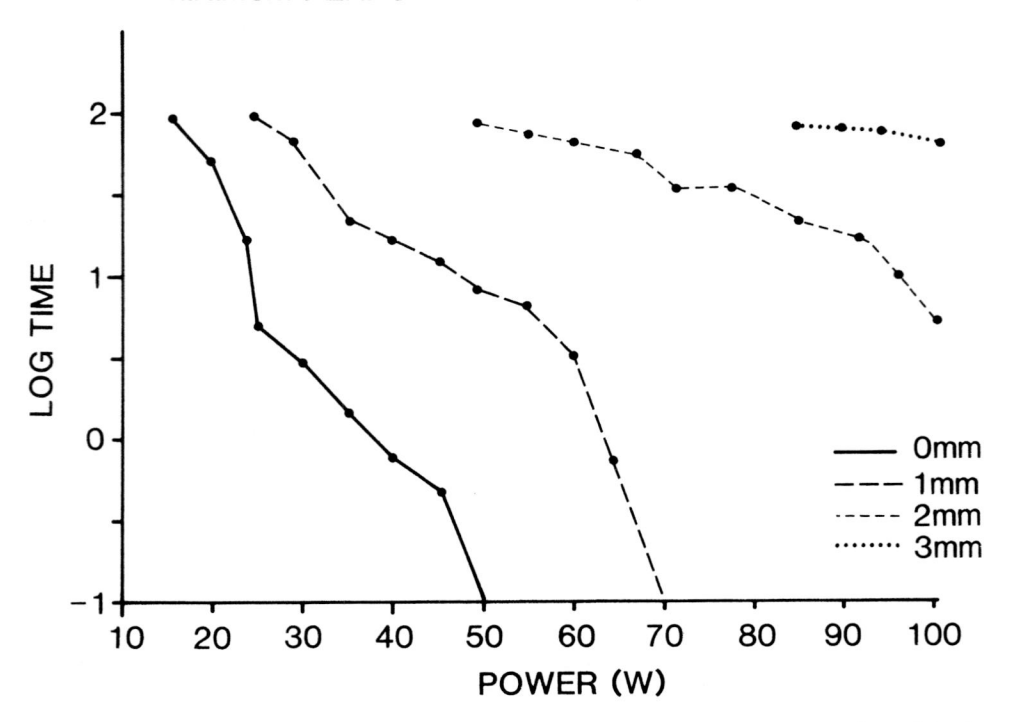

Legend: — 0mm, --- 1mm, ---- 2mm, ···· 3mm

Fig. 196 A graph of the minimum perforation time in seconds at each power setting of the laser. This is a linear log plot.

the Olympus instrument than with the 2.5 mm Optiscope. It was possible to assess 18 of the 27 coronary segments named by the National Heart Lung and Blood Institute Coronary Artery Surgery Study (7).

Laser Angioplasty under Direct Vision

The 2.5 mm angioscope could only be inserted into the proximal coronary tree of the majority of hearts studied. It was possible to fire the laser under direct vision without damaging the bare optical fibre or the endoscope, providing the fibre was not in contact with any tissue. Using saline flushing, it was possible to intubate the right coronary artery of the majority of human hearts without intimal damage secondary to passage of the instrument. This could be achieved up to the first acute marginal branch of the right coronary.

The laser was fired at each distance for times less than that required to perforate the coronary artery for that power setting of the laser. Using these lower energies, it was possible to ablate some atheromatous disease as seen in Figure 198.

Discussion

Safe Working Limits

It was possible to determine the minimum perforation times of fresh human coronary arteries. It can be seen from Figure 7 that, as the power setting of the laser increases, the time taken to perforate the coronary artery decreases. This is expected as power multiplied by time equals energy and higher energy beams vaporize greater volumes of tissue (8). It can also be seen that, as the distance from the tip of the fibre to the target tissue increases, so the minimum

4. Laser Treatment

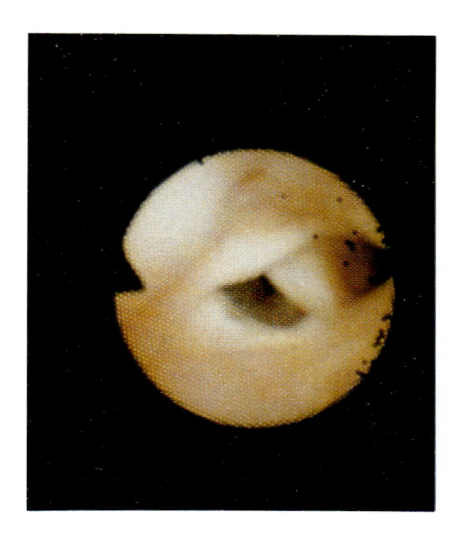

Fig. 197 The first diagonal branch of intact human coronary artery as seen down the Olympus PF18L Angioscope. There is a stenosis at the origin of this vessel due to atheromatous disease. The angioscope is within the left anterior descending coronary artery, the lumen of which continues in the 6 o'clock position of this figure.

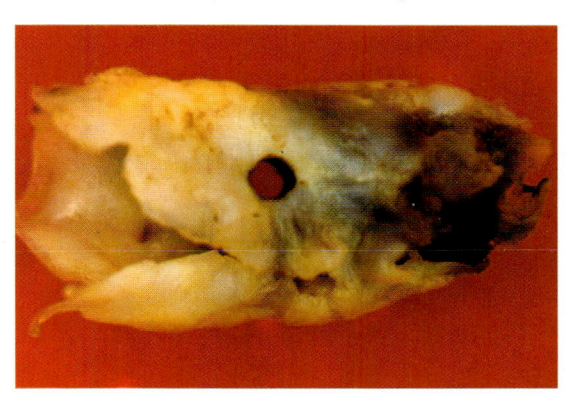

Fig. 198 Atheromatous plaque removed from the superficial femoral artery of a woman at femero-popliteal bypass. The plaque has been exposed to an Nd:YAG laser beam from a bare 400 micron optical fibre held 1 mm away from its surface at 90° to the target. Power of the beam was 55 watts and its duration was 4 seconds. This is within the minimum perforation time for this power setting of the laser at 1 mm.

perforation time increases. This is due to divergence of the laser beam as it is emitted from the bare fibre. This increases the diameter of the spot size on the target as the distance is increased. The greater the spot size, the lower the energy densities when the laser is fired (9).

It can be seen that the results have been plotted as a linear log curve. This is because the scale of time settings of the laser varies from 0.1 seconds to 99 seconds and the majority of times plotted on the Y axis are within the 0.1 second to 10 second range.

The range of power settings of the laser were 3 watts to 100 watts. At low power settings the perforation times greater than 99 seconds could not be recorded, and at high power settings perforation times of less than 0.1 of a second could not be determined.

These results provide safe working energy limits for the continuous wave Nd:YAG laser over the distances of 0 mm to 3 mm.

Coronary Angioscopy

The ultra thin angioscopes now available provide excellent definition of the anatomy of the coronary tree and other workers have demonstrated that they allow visualisation of disease not shown by conventional angiographic methods (10). The angioscope has both diagnostic and therapeutic capabilities.

Angioplasty under Direct Vision

Laser angioplasty under direct vision is now feasible in the human heart. The experimental set-up used is with a flaccid heart, with the coronary arteries full of saline. The authors feel that this technique should initially be used in the clinical setting with the patient on cardiopulsory bypass and the heart under cardioplegic arrest. There is obvious potential for development of a percutaneous system of angioplasty under direct vision.

Using laser energy within the limits previously described, it is possible to safely fire the laser inside a coronary artery. This laser beam can be aimed under direct vision. More work is required to look into ways of minimizing surrounding tissue damage by the laser energy, perhaps with the use of a pulsed laser system. As smaller angioscopes are developed, it will be possible to intubate the smaller branches of the coronary tree with a working endoscope. After experience has been accumulated in the laboratory setting, we feel that laser angioplasty using this technique could become a clinical reality.

Acknowledgements

The authors would wish to acknowledge Mrs Julie Brookes for the production of the manuscript, Mrs Helena Wright for technical assistance, and Miss Anne Schofield for production of the illustrations.

References

1. Geschwind HJ, Boussignac G, Teisseire, Benhaiem N, Bittoun R, Laurent D. Conditions for effective Nd:YAG laser angioplasty. Br Heart J 52, 484, 1984.

2. Abela GS, Normann S, Cohen D, Feldman R, Geiser E, Conti R. Effects of carbon dioxide, Nd:YAG and Argon laser radiation on coronary atheromatous plaques. Am J Cardiol 50, 119, 1982.

3. Ben-Shackea G, Spector ML, Morse DE. Hazardous by-products of laser irradiation - a qualitative and quantitative study. J Am Coll Cardiol 17, 46A, 1987.

4. Lee G, Seckinger D, Chan MC, Embi A, Stobbe D, Thomson R, Sanchez N, Ikeda R, Reis R, Mason D. Potential complications of coronary laser angioplasty. Am Heart J 108, 1577, 1984.

5. Lee G, Ikeda RM, Stobbe D, Ogata C, Theis J, Hussein M, Mason D. Laser irradiation of human atherosclerotic obstructive disease: simultaneous visualisation and vaporisation achieved by a dual Fiberoptic catheter. Am Heart J 105, 163, 1983.

6. Van Stiegmann G, Kahn D, Rose AG, Bornman PC, Terblanche J. Endoscopic laser endarterectomy. Surgery Gynecology and Obstetrics 158, 529, 1984.

7. Cass. The National Heart, Lung and Blood Institute Coronary Artery Surgery Study (CASS). Circulation 63-65, III-39, 1981.

8. Lee G, Ikeda RM, Stobbe D, Ogata C, Chan M, Seckinger D, Vazquez A, Theis J, Reis R, Mason D. Effects of laser irradiation on human thrombus: demonstration of a linear dissolution - dose relation between clot length and energy density. Am J Cardiol 52, 876, 1983.

9. Polyani TG. Physics in surgery with lasers. Clinics in Chest Medicine 16, 179, 1985.

10. Lee G, Garcia JM, Corso PJ. Correlation of coronary angioscopic findings in coronary artery disease. Am J Cardiol 57, 238, 1986.

4.10. Intraoperative Argon Laser Angioplasty in Coronary Arteries - First Clinical Results

FW Hehrlein, R Moosdorf

Department of Cardiovascular Surgery, Justus-Liebig-University, Giessen, FR Germany

Since the invention of LASER by SCHAWLOW and TOWNES (1) in 1958 several specialities of medicine showed an increasing interest in this new technology. It was Goldman (2) in 1962, who first used a Ruby-laser in dermatology and only one year later McGuff (3) performed the ablation of an atherosclerotic plaque from an arterial wall in an experimental setting. Different laser systems could soon be introduced into clinical use in dermatology, ophthalmology, otolaryngology, and in general surgery. However, further development of these first investigations in the cardiovascular system was limited by the lack of suitable laser systems and especially by the lack of flexible delivery systems for energy transfer within the small lumina of the vessels. Therefore it was only in 1983 that Choy (4) performed the first intraoperative laser angioplasty in a right coronary artery, during a coronary bypass operation, and Ginsburg (5) performed the first percutaneous recanalization of an occluded femoral artery in a patient. A major step to achieve clinical applicability was the availability of thin, flexible quartz fibres, which could be easily guided via different catheter systems, even within small coronary arteries.

Both of the above physicians used an Argon-laser system which, at that time, seemed to fulfil most of the conditions required for an optimal laser system for transluminal laser angioplasties:
- It should offer predictable tissue interactions with minimal thermal side-effects.
- It should to a certain extent be steerable.

Comparing the three commonly used laser systems in medicine, the CO_2-laser is the most precise cutting instrument with low tissue penetration and scattering, thus limiting the depth of thermal injury. In contrast, the Nd:YAG-laser shows a deeper penetration and even greater scattering in human tissue, distributing its heat in a greater volume and thus giving this laser a high coagulative potential. This system is thus preferable to arrest haemorrhage and for the ablation of vascular tumours. The characteristics of the Argon-laser show it to be localized in between the above, showing a deeper penetration than the CO_2-laser and a decreased scattering compared with the Nd:YAG-laser, therefore precise cuts or ablations can be performed with limited thermal injury. Moreover, this laser system fulfils a second condition

4. Laser Treatment

which is essential for use in the vascular system: its energy can be delivered by thin, flexible quartz fibres for intraluminal use. In addition, another distinct advantage is that the Argon-laser emits visible green light. In contrast the light of the CO_2-laser can only to date be transmitted by articulated mirror arms and therefore can only be applied to exposed surfaces or through straight tubes.

Because of these reasons we also chose an Argon-laser system for our first experimental work on laser angioplasty, which we started in 1984 (6). The continuous wave system was coupled to flexible quartz fibres of different sizes to transmit the energy.

In an initial series of investigations we exposed human atherosclerotic cadaver aortas to the beam of this Argon-laser system, varying time and intensity. Beginning with an energy of 5 Joule, we could demonstrate effective vaporization of atherosclerotic plaques. Increasing the energy, the laser crater showed a deeper penetration into the arterial wall. This uniformly produced the typical rim of carbonization at its surface, surrounded by a small zone of vacuolization and coagulation, indicative of thermal injury. Similar investigations performed under Ringer or cardioplegic solution (Bretschneider HTK)* showed no significant differences within this experimental setting.

Based on these first results, we then performed transluminal laser ablations in the coronary arteries of human cadaver hearts. Imitating intra-operative use, we introduced a flexible quartz fibre with a diameter of 0.6 mm, either through the coronary ostia or through a peripheral incision in the affected coronary artery. Power varied between 3 and 4 Watts using a pulsed mode with 3 second pulses. In 60% of a total of 15 cadaver hearts the Argon-laser proved to be effective in the direct ablation of atherosclerotic plaques or penetration of atherosclerotic occlusions. A high rate of perforations, however, was produced, an incidence of nearly 30%. Perforations especially occurred when the laser catheter was introduced via the coronary ostia, guided over a long distance or in cases of severely calcified excentric stenoses. These results are comparable with other groups (7), who also described high perforation rates using the unprotected open fibre. Reasons for this are the direct open beam, especially in curved segments or excentric lesions, as well as direct mechanical effects of the rigid and sharp fibre end. So the development of new probes which were totally metal-capped, promised a major improvement. On the one hand, they totally converted laser energy into thermal energy, removing the danger of the open beam, and on the other hand they caused less mechanical stress to the arterial wall because of their smoothly shaped metal heads (8,9). Using these probes in another series of investigations, we found them to be safe, and still retaining a good ablative potential with respect to atherosclerotic plaques. We therefore started our first clinical trial laser angioplasty with these probes in January 1987.

In this trial, laser angioplasty was not used as a single therapeutic procedure but as an additional adjunct to conventional coronary artery bypass surgery,

---

* Dr Franz Koehler Chemie, 6146 Alsbach-Hänlein, FRG

4. Laser Treatment

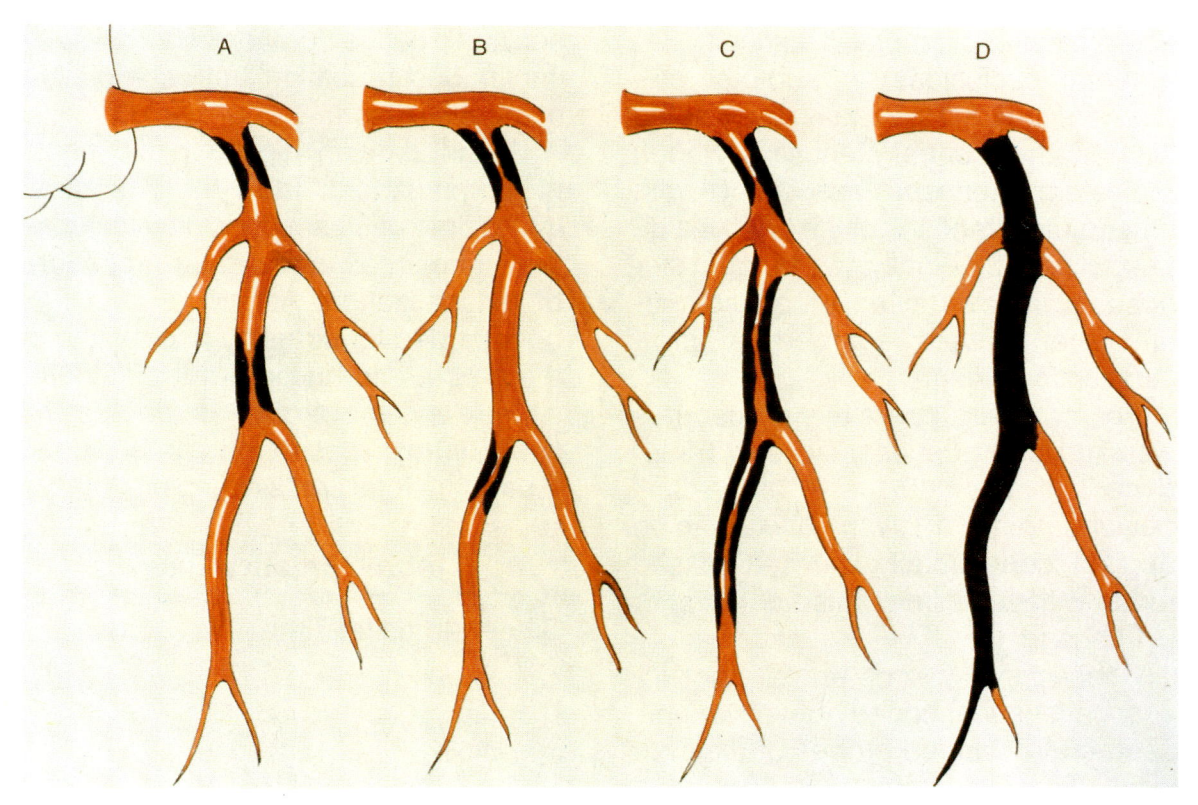

Fig. 199 Diagram of different types of atherosclerotic lesions in coronary arteries: a) tandem stenoses with entrapment of one or two major side-branches; b) "distal" tandem lesion entrapping all major side-branches; c) tandem lesion with a long diffuse stenosis; d) totally occluded vessel affecting major side-branches.

endarterectomy, and intra-operative balloon angioplasty. Specific indications for this modality were proximal tandem stenoses entrapping one or more major side branches (Figure 199a, b). Later on, longer subtotal stenoses or occlusions of the LAD, causing impaired flow from the bypass graft to one or more major branches, were also tackled (Figure 199c). Stenoses extending to the distal portion of the artery or total occlusions of the vessel over a long distance (Figure 199d) were excluded from laser angioplasty and conventionally treated by peripheral balloon angioplasty or endarterectomy. With diffusely diseased vessels, the highly calcified atheromatous core is extremely resistant to laser ablation and therefore offers a greater risk (Figure 199).

Between January and October 1987, 20 laser angioplasties were performed during coronary bypass procedures. Sixteen of these patients were male, 4 female, and the mean age was 57.8 years (49-67 years). The pre-operative clinical data of these 20 patients is summarized in Table 57.

Pre-Operative Data			
NYHA class	II (5)	III (11)	IV (4)
Cardiac index	3.95	(3.3-4.4)	
Ejection fraction	63.4%	(40%-83%)	
Myocardial infarction	10 (1x)	3 (2x)	

Table 57

Indications were tandem stenoses of the LAD in 9, typically entrapping major

4. Laser Treatment

diagonal and/or septal branches. Segmental occlusions or subtotal stenoses of the LAD in 7, again associated with another central stenosis. Two left mainstem stenoses associated with other major stenoses of the LAD or a diagonal branch. Finally, two tandem stenoses of the circumflex artery and marginal branch were regarded as an indication for lasing.

For our intra-operative procedures we used an Argon-laser system (Trimedyne Optilase 900)* with a maximal power output of 12 Watt. Power can be applied continuously or in a pulsed mode with a minimal pulse duration of 0.1 second.

Consequent to our preparatory investigations mentioned above, we only used metal-capped probes of different sizes. The first cases were performed with the typical hot tips* with different sized round or football-shaped metal heads. Later on we used the new Spectraprobe*, a so-called hybrid probe with a small sapphire window at the top of the metal cap. This emits a certain amount of direct laser energy (about 20%), while the major part of the laser energy still is converted into heat (about 80%). These probes were used in 7 patients, the conventional hot-tip in thirteen. Additional balloon angioplasties were performed in 3 cases in order to achieve sufficient luminal diameter, and in two cases this was followed by a final low power lasing to smooth the intraluminal surface. In contrast to laser angioplasty in peripheral vessels, we consider a reduced power of 5-7 Watt to be sufficient for the lasing in these small coronary vessels. It was applied in a pulsed mode with a pulse duration of 1 sec and a pause duration of 0.2 sec with continuous repetition until completion of recanalization.

Further data on this group of patients is summarized in Table 58. The mean lasing time of 30 seconds only includes the immediate intravascular procedure of recanalization. Additional time has been added for coupling and testing of the probe, introduction of the catheter sheath and the probe, as well as the final control. These times are included thus in the total cross clamping time.

Intra-Operative Data	
Cross Clamping Time	61 min (38-80 min)
Number of Anastomoses	2.8 (2-5)
Additional Endarterectomy	2
Mean Lasing Time	30 sec (15-20 sec)

Table 58

When performing intraluminal laser angioplasties, a sufficient amount of fluid irrigation is essential to minimize the risks. This prevents thermal damage to adjacent unaffected parts of the posterior wall as well as preventing sticking of the heated probe. In our coronary bypass procedures, cardiac arrest is achieved by perfusing cardioplegic solution (Bretschneider HTK)** through the aortic root. In some minor stenoses the continuous infusion of this solution is sufficient to cool and avoid sticking. In cases with severe stenoses or even occlusions, this technique is limited and we then prefer direct irriga-

---

* Trimedyne Incorporated, Santa Ana, California, USA
** Dr Franz Koehler Chemie, 6146 Alsbach-Hänlein, FRG

4. Laser Treatment

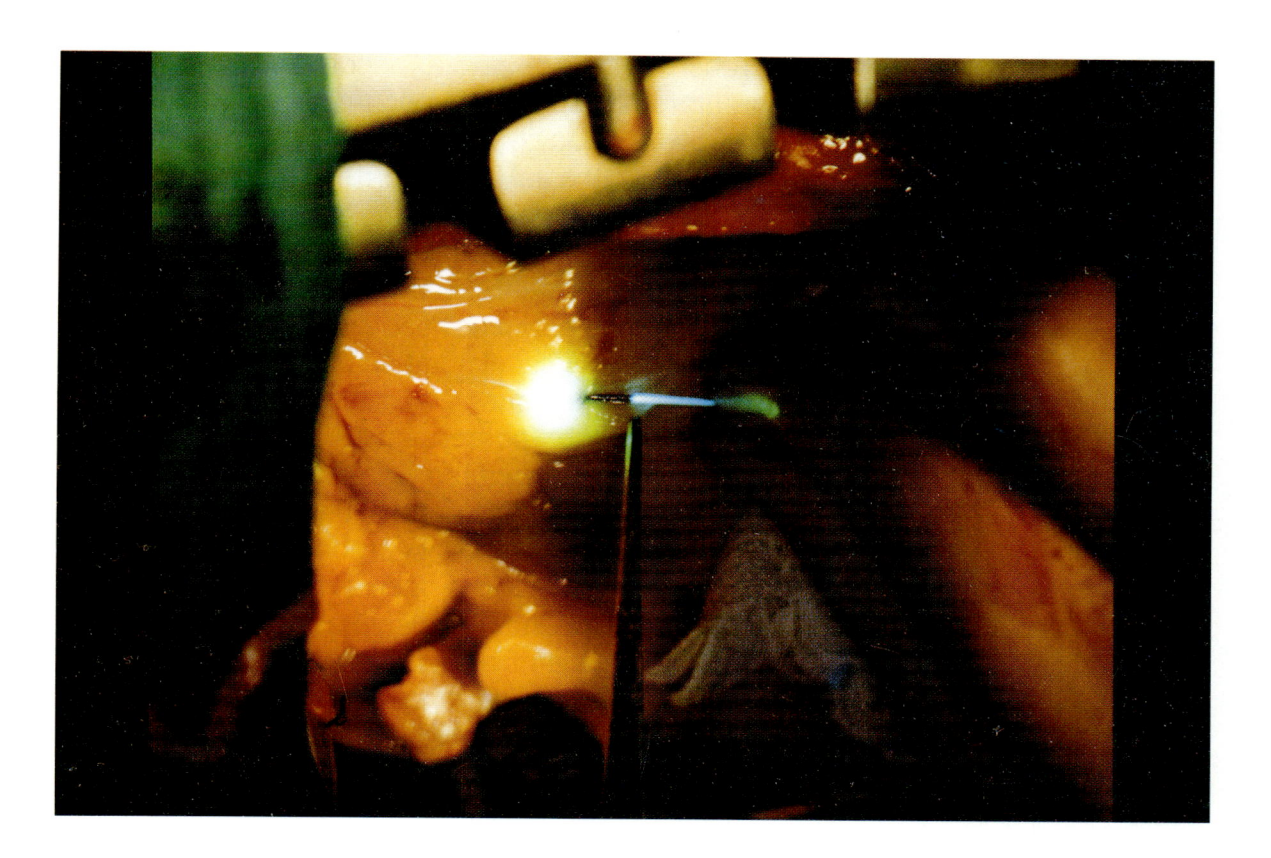

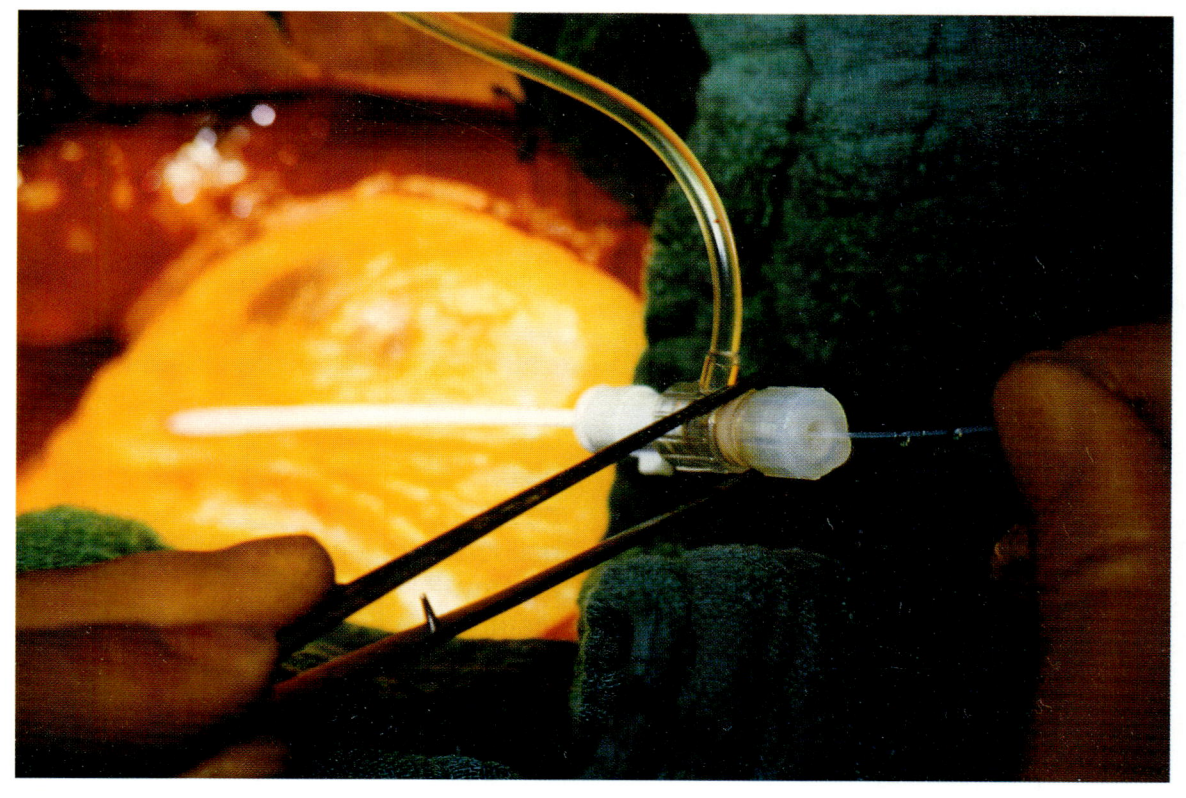

Fig. 200 a, b) Intra-operative view of a laser procedure of the LAD. Because of a total occlusion, a catheter sheath is introduced into the coronary artery, guiding the laser probe in its central lumen and enabling continuous fluid irrigation through a side port.

4. Laser Treatment

tion. We introduce a special 5 French catheter sheath with a sideport, through which cardioplegic solution is administered continuously while the laser probe is introduced through the central lumen for the lasing procedure (Figure 200). A new probe which has just entered first clinical trials, integrates these two characteristics in one system. The flushing medium can be administered and is emitted through small perforations in the heated metal head.

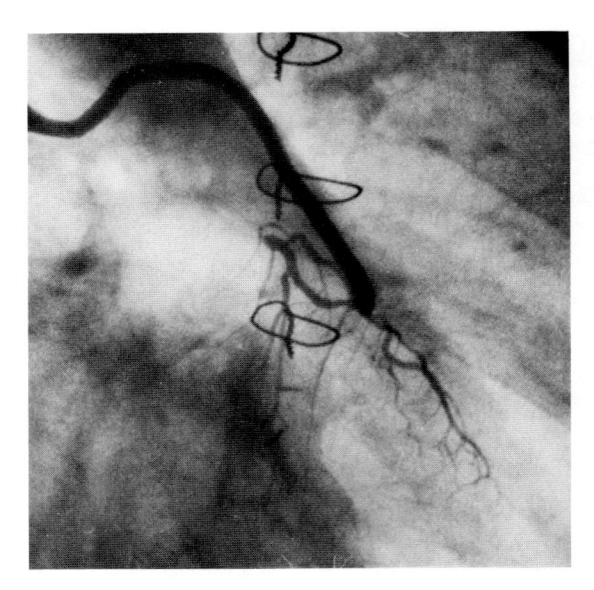

Fig. 201 Re-angiogram after laser angioplasty of a tandem stenosis of the LAD (RAO). The proximal occlusion has been left to avoid competitive flow. The second subtotal lesion is widely open, allowing an unimpaired retrograde flow to the large septal and diagonal branch.

In our 20 patients the laser angioplasty was successful in 17 cases. The laser probe could in these cases be passed through the distal portion of the aforementioned tandem stenoses or occlusions. The lumen, as well as effective reperfusion of the formerly interrupted branches could be demonstrated intra-operatively with calibrated probes, Cardiogreen-perfusion, angioscopy or fluoroscopy. In one patient a perforation occurred in relation to a heavily calcified excentric stenosis of the LAD, and in two other cases the lasing procedure had to be terminated because of similar findings that are at present unfeasible for laser angioplasty. In these three cases complete revascularization was achieved by conventional endarterectomy without further complications. Apart from these three cases, we saw no other intra-operative complications, no dissections, and no probe-related complications. Post-operatively all patients had an uneventful course and there were no deaths among this group of 20 patients. There were also no bleeding complications and only one patient showed signs of temporary myocardial ischaemia which later disappeared without any signs of a transmural infarction. Four patients had post-operative arrhythmias, two with ventricular extrasystolies, which in one case was present pre-operatively, and two with atrial fibrillation. These arrhythmias are quite common after bypass procedures and not specific or increased in this group. All patients could be treated successfully with medical therapy.

The first clinical trial demonstrated that intra-operative laser angioplasty can be successfully performed as an adjunct to conventional bypass surgery, besides the established methods of balloon angioplasty and endarterectomy. Its major advantage is that this method can be performed within a reasonable time. The immediate intra-operative success rate of 85% is comparable to the other two methods (10). The intra-operative as well as the post-operative complication rate is low and all of our patients had an uneventful post-operative course.

For further evaluation of this method, especially with respect to the long-term efficacy, prolonged follow-up and reangiography has to be awaited. Up till now we have performed two reangiograms between 4 and 6 months post-operatively, demonstrating a satisfactory result of laser angioplasty.

Further improvements can surely be expected with increasing experience with this method, as well as new developments of probes and laser systems. At present, laser angioplasty in coronary arteries is still not a routine procedure, but these initial results show some promising characteristics which, with further developments, may lead to an alternative, enabling the surgeon to achieve complete revascularization, even in cases with diffusely diseased coronary arteries (Figure 201).

References

1. Schawlow AL Townes CH. Infrared and optical Masers. Phys Rev 112, 1940, 1958.

2. Goldman L, Blaney E. Laser therapy of melanomas. Surg Gynecol Obstet 124, 49, 1967.

3. McGuff GE, Bushnell D, Soroff HS, Deterling RA. Studies of the surgical application of laser (light amplification by stimulated emission of radiation). Surg Forum 14, 143, 1936.

4. Choy DSJ, Stertzer SH, Myler RK, Marco J, Fournial G. Human coronary laser recanalization. Clin Cardiol 7, 377, 1984.

5. Ginsburg R, Kim DS, Guthaner D, Toth J, Mitchell RS. Salvage of an ischaemic limb by laser angioplasty: description of a new technique. Clin Cardiol 7, 54, 1984.

6. Moosdorf R, Glauber M, Scheld HH. Experimentelle Untersuchungen zur Frage der klinischen Anwendbarkeit des Argon-Lasers in der Herz- und Gefässchirurgie. Herz-Kreislauf 9, 427, 1987.

7. Abela GS, Normann SJ, Cohen DM, Franzini D, Feldman RL, Crea F, Fenech A, Pepine CH, Conti CR. Laser recanalization of occluded atherosclerotic arteries in vivo and in vitro. Circulation 71, 403, 1985.

8. Abela GS, Fenech A, Crea F, Conti CR. "Hot-tip": another method of laser vascular recanalization. Lasers in Surgery and Medicine 5, 327, 1985.

9. Sanborn TA, Faxon DP, Haudenschild C, Ryan TJ. Experimental angioplasty: circumferential distribution of laser thermal energy with a laser probe. J Am Coll Cardiol 5, 934, 1985.

10. Scheld HH, Görlach G, Kling D, Moosdorf R, Stertmann WA, Hehrlein FW. Technik der koronaren Endarteriektomie. Z f Herz-, Thorax- und Gefässchirurgie 1, 91, 1987.

Index

A

Allogenic endothelial cells	361
Alloreactivity	257
Alpha-1-antitrypsin	223
Angiogenesis	229
Angioscope	431
Angiotensin I	239
Angiotensin II	239
Antigen presenting cell (APC)	254, 364
Antilymphocytoglobulin in heart transplantation	79
Antithrombin III	219, 223 - 225, 283
Antithrombin III-deficiency	225
Argon and Krypton Lasers	403
Artificial heart	378
AT III	224
Atherogenic diets	417
Atherosclerotic-like plaque	417

B

B-lymphocytes	250
Basement membrane	275, 332, 337, 341 - 342
Bi-ventricular assist device (BVAD)	158
Biomaterials	380
Biomer	379, 382 - 383
Bioresorbable arterial prosthesis	274
Bradykinin	239, 243
Bridging for transplantation	175

C

CAM-1	260
Cape Town experience on transplantation	20
Carbon dioxide laser	401
CD4	251
CD8	251, 254
Class II histocompatibility antigens	257
Clinical endothelial seeding	285
Coagulation factor V	218
Collaborative Heart Transplant Study	51
Collagen	271, 289, 333 - 335, 342
Collagen IV	356
Collagen type I/III	335, 342
Collagenase	297, 313, 323, 327, 342, 372
Continuous wave Nd:YAG laser energy	452, 468
Cryopreserved endothelial cells	361
CTL	251, 255
Cyctotoxic granulocytes	366

Index

Cyto-Immunological monitoring 92, 98, 106, 142
Cytotoxic T-cells 261

D
Desoxyspergualine 138
Detection of acute rejection 92
Dispase . . . . 323, 325 - 327
Donor Selection 47
Donors 34
Double lung transplantation 34, 48

E
ELAM-1 260
Electromagnetically stimulated coronary artery 420
Emphysema 34
Endothelial cell 237, 316, 361
Endothelial cell growth factor (ECGF) 229
Endothelial cell seeding . . . . 282, 284, 288, 296, 303 - 304, 311, 341, 378
Endothelial derived relaxing faxtors (EDRF) 236
Endothelial leucocyte adhesion molecule 260
Epsilon-amino-capronic-acid 361
Excimer Laser 403, 424
Extracellular matrix . . . . 334 - 335, 374, 382 - 383

F
Factor VIII-related antigen 327
Fast-Fourier-Transformation 98
Fat microvessels 310
Fibrin . . . . 271, 332, 342, 363 - 365
Fibrin glue . . . . 342, 344 - 347, 361 - 362
Fibroblast growth factor (FGF) 229
Fibronectin . . . . 271, 332, 341 - 342, 344 - 347, 354 - 358, 373 - 374, 379 - 380, 382
Fluorescence spectral analysis 428
Free radical formation 461

G
Gamma interferon 253, 365
Gelatin 355
Glucosaminoglucanes 283
Glutaraldehyde-preserved . . . . 382 - 384
Glycoprotein laminin 344
Glycoproteins . . . . 332, 341 - 342

H
H^3-thymidine . . . . 379 - 380
HBGF-I . . . . 230 - 234
HBGF-II . . . . 230 - 234
Heart preservation 120
Heart transplantation to neonates 27, 92

Index

Heart transplantation 98, 120
Heart-lung or lung transplantation 33
Heparin-binding growth factors 232
Helper T-lymphocytes (TH) 251
Histopathology of acute rejections 138
HLA-antigens 253
Homologous endothelial cells . . . . 361 - 362
Hot metal caps 451
Hot tip probe 436
Hyperacute rejection 138

I
Immune interferon 253
In vitro endothelialization 361, 364, 366
Interleukin-1 (IL-1) 256
Interleukin-2 (IL-2) 253

L
Laminin . . . . 271, 289, 334, 337, 342 - 345
Laser anglioplasty 469, 478
Laser probes used in the contact mode 451
Laser basics 391
Latissimus dorsi muscle 182
Left and right ventricular (LVAD) 158
Leukocyte function antigen (LFA-1) 258
Leukotrienes 239
Luminescence spectroscopy 411
Lung-heart transplantation 49
Lymphokine-activated killer cell (LAK) 260

M
Major histocompatibility complex (MHC) 252, 364
Microvascular endothelial cells 378
Monoclonal antibodies 82, 88
Monocyte/macrophages 250
Multidonor 362

N
Nd:YAG Laser 402
Non-invasive rejection 98

O
OKT-3 prophylaxis against cardiac rejection 84
OKT-3 as treatment for advanced cardiacrejection 83
OKT-3 as treatment for advanced cardiac rejection 84
Oncogenes 232
Orthotopic heart transplantation 20

Index

P

PAF	244 - 246
PDGF	263, 276
Pellethane	379, 381 - 383
Percutaneous atherectomy	440
Preformed natural antibodies	128
Peyer's patches	259
Photoablation of tissue	460
Photons	394
Plasminogen activator inhibitor	218, 283
Platelet activating factor (PAF)	218, 240
Polypeptide mitogens	229
Postoperative Management	41
Prerequisites for laser anglioplasty	423
Procoagulant activity	222
Prostacyclin	365, 373
Protein C-system	219
Protein S	219, 222 - 223
Pseudo-neointima	378
Pulmonary Preservation	36
Pulsed mode laser	424

R

Recipient and donor selection	48
Rotating-tip (Kensey catheter)	432

S

Sapphire tipped probes	452
Seeded grafts	285
Seeding device	342, 362
Simpson atherectomy catheter	432, 440
Single lung transplantation	34, 47
Skeletal muscle conditioning	184
Skeletal muscle ventricle	182, 185
SMV construction	187

T

T-lymphocyte	364
Thrombogenicity index	287 - 288
Thrombomodulin	219
Thrombus-free surface	311, 314, 317
Tissue thromboplastin	218
Tissue-type plasminogen activator	218 - 219
Total artificial heart	158, 168, 175
Total lymphoid irradiation in clinical transplantation	106
Total lymphoid irradiation in experimental transplantation	64
Tumor necrosis factor	258
Two-dimensional echocardiography	98
Type I collagen	343

Index

Type I/III collagen . . . . 344 - 347
Type III collagen 343
Type IV collagen . . . . 337, 343 - 347, 357

U
Unilateral and bilateral lung transplantation 46
Use of anencephalic organs 28

V
Von Willebrand factor 218

X
Xenogeneic hyperacute rejection 127
Xenogeneic transplantation 127, 137
Xenografting the neonate 27